Manual of simulation in healthcare

Manual of simulation in healthcare

Edited by

Richard H Riley

Anaesthetist, Department of Anaesthesia and Pain Medicine,
Royal Perth Hospital and Clinical Associate Professor of Anaesthesia,
Department of Pharmacology, Medicine and Anaesthesia,
University of Western Australia

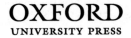

OXFORD
UNIVERSITY PRESS

OXFORD

UNIVERSITY PRESS

Great Clarendon Street, Oxford OX2 6DP

Oxford University Press is a department of the University of Oxford.
It furthers the University's objective of excellence in research, scholarship,
and education by publishing worldwide in

Oxford New York

Auckland   Cape Town Dar es Salaam   Hong Kong   Karachi
Kuala Lumpur Madrid Melbourne Mexico City Nairobi
New Delhi Shanghai Taipei Toronto
With offices in
Argentina Austria Brazil Chile Czech Republic France Greece
Guatemala Hungary Italy Japan South Korea Poland Portugal
Singapore Switzerland Thailand Turkey Ukraine Vietnam

Oxford is a registered trade mark of Oxford University Press
in the UK and in certain other countries

Published in the United States
by Oxford University Press Inc., New York

ISBN 978-0-19-920585-1

Printed in the United Kingdom by
Lightning Source UK Ltd., Milton Keynes

Whilst every effort has been made to ensure that the contents of this book
are as complete, accurate and up to date as possible at the date of writing,
Oxford University Press is not able to give any guarantee or assurance that
such is the case. Readers are urged to take appropriately qualified medical
advise in all cases. The information in this book is intended to be useful to
the general reader, but should not be used as a means of self-diagnosis or
for the prescription of medication.

Foreword

David H Wilks

There is a long history of using simple devices to simulate the real experience in healthcare education. A simple example would be teaching students to handle needles and sutures using a pig's foot or a piece of simulated skin. A more complex example is the use of the famous Resusci Anne™ to teach a partial task such as chest compressions associated with positive-pressure ventilation. The development of sophisticated, instrumented, mannequins coupled with computerized physiology and pharmacology programmes began a new era in healthcare simulation. These new mannequins had the ability to react to student interventions in a realistic and automatic manner not requiring instructor intervention. The mannequins were originally developed and popularized within the field of anaesthesiology. It was quickly realized that not only could these mannequins be used to simulate an anesthetist's interaction with a patient but that they can also be used for team building situations leading to the development of 'Crisis Resource Management'. In the short period of the past two decades, the use of mannequins to create simulated experiences has been adopted by diverse healthcare providers including nursing, various medical subspecialties and other allied health providers.

Healthcare educational institutions around the world are recognizing the need for providing their students with simulated experiences not only to enhance the educational experience but also to improve on patient safety. When embarking on the development of a simulation centre, some of the questions inevitably asked are:

- How large should the centre be?
- What types of rooms do I need in a simulation centre?
- How will I run the centre?
- What equipment should I buy?
- Who will the users be?

Dr Riley has chosen contributors for this book who have the experience necessary to answer these questions. Section one provides simulation centre logistics, section two discusses the various equipment available, and section four addresses the needs of the different subspecialties.

For me, the most important section of this book is section three – Education Components. A machine is simply a machine unless it is integrated into the learning environment using sound educational principles. The question concerning educational integration of the simulation modalities is often left off the initial list when planning a simulation programme. Dr Riley needs to be congratulated for devoting a large section of this book to education; education is the pivotal element in determining a centre's success.

2008
David H Wilks MD
Professor and Chair
Department of Anaesthesiology
West Virginia University
School of Medicine

Preface

The idea for this manual came to me during the inaugural Simulation and Skills Training Special Interest Group of the Australian and New Zealand College of Anaesthetists held in Perth, September 2000. At that time the chief references for those of us who had entered the world of medical simulation were David Gaba's book *Crisis Management in Anesthesiology* and his chapter in Miller's textbook of *Anesthesia*. Learning how to use the commercially available medical simulators was achieved through attendance at Dr Gaba's ACRM Instructor's Course at Stanford and old-fashioned on-the-job practice. Subsequent discussions with colleagues in this growing field made it apparent that many of us were struggling with common problems but that there were some very creative solutions. However, the process of mustering these collective talents and experiences was quickly subdued by the pressures of teaching and administration in a new simulation centre.

My association with local and international simulation meetings not only enriched my knowledge of simulation in healthcare but also brought me into contact with many leaders in simulation. I am deeply grateful that many of these simulation leaders have kindly shared their expertise with us. Thanks must also go to hospital and organizational administrators and Heads of Departments who have supported the simulation community. I thank those who have mentored and inspired me: David Wilks, Myroslav Klain, Peter Winter, and Peter Safar. I also would like to thank Sara Chare, Clare Caruana, Eloise Moir-Ford, Anna Winstanley, Catherine Barnes, Georgia Pinteau, Kelly Hewinson, Kate Wanwimolruk and the team from Oxford University Press who kept me on track. Finally, I wish to express thanks to my wife Vera who has been my support and strength through the simulation journey.

2008
Richard H Riley
Perth, Western Australia

Contents

Foreword *v*
David H Wilks
Preface *vii*
Contributors *xiii*

Part 1 **Simulation centre logistics**

1 Simulation and skill centre design *3*
Ross Horley

2 Simulation centre operations and administration *11*
Yue Ming Huang and Thomas Dongilli

3 Mobile simulation *25*
Frances C Forrest

Part 2 **Simulators, training aids, and equipment**

4 Lessons from aviation simulation *37*
Ray Page

5 Medium and high integration mannequin patient simulators *51*
Samsun (Sem) Lampotang

6 Airway training devices *65*
Harry Owen and Cindy Hein

7 Equipment *81*
Gary Hope and Chris Chin

8 Cardiopulmonary resuscitation and training devices *87*
Sheena Ferguson

Part 3 **Education components**

9 Teaching and learning through the simulated environment *99*
Iris Vardi

10 Developing your teaching role in a simulation centre *115*
Ronnie Glavin

11 Teaching in clinical settings *125*
Fiona Lake

12 Scenario design: theory to delivery *139*
Chris Holland, Chris Sadler, and Angie Nunn

13 Debriefing: theory and techniques *155*
Brendan Flanagan

14 Teaching a clinical skill *171*
Jeff Hamdorf and Robert Davies

15 Training and assessment with standardized patients *181*
John R Boulet and Anthony Errichetti

16 Team building and simulation *199*
Andrew Anderson

17 Problem-based learning for simulation in healthcare *213*
Russell W Jones

18 Research in simulation *227*
Alexander Garden

Part 4 **Applied simulation**

19 Simulation in nursing education and practice *241*
John M O'Donnell and Joseph S Goode Jr.

20 Crisis resource management in healthcare *277*
Geoffrey K Lighthall

21 Intern training: a national simulation-based training programme to
enhance readiness for medical practice *295*
Orit Rubin, Haim Berkenstadt, and Amitai Ziv

22 Non-technical skills: identifying, training, and assessing safe behaviours *303*
Rhona Flin and Nicola Maran

23 Simulation training programmes for rapid response or medical
emergency teams *321*
Elizabeth A Hunt, Nicolette C Mininni, and Michael A DeVita

24 Simulation in paediatrics *337*
Louis Patrick Halamek and Kimberly Allison Yaeger

25 Obstetric simulation *351*
Shad H Deering

26 Simulation in emergency medicine *375*
John A Vozenilek and Mary D Patterson

27 Cardiopulmonary bypass simulation *391*
Richard Morris and Andy Pybus

28 Simulation for military medical training *407*
Mark W Bowyer and E Matt Ritter

29 Incorporating simulation into the medical school curriculum *421*
Randolph Steadman and Rima Matevosian

30 Surgical simulation *435*
Roger Kneebone and Fernando Bello

31 Creating virtual reality medical simulations: a knowledge-based
design and assessment approach *449*
Dale C Alverson, Thomas P Caudell, and Timothy E Goldsmith

32 Respiratory medicine and respiratory therapy *465*
Brian Robinson

33 Role of cognitive simulations in healthcare *477*
Usha Satish and Satish Krishnamurthy

34 Effective management of anaesthetic crises: design, development, and evaluation of a simulation-based course *489*
Jennifer Weller

35 Simulation in high-stakes performance assessment *501*
Leonie Watterson

36 Simulation in sedation training for non-anaesthesiologists *519*
Mordechai Bermann, Bryan L Fischberg, and Malay Rao

37 Medical educational simulation: a European perspective *525*
Willem van Meurs, Doris Østergaard, and Stefan Mönk

38 Society for simulation in healthcare *529*
Daniel Raemer

Glossary of UK and US medical terms and abbreviations *533*

Index *541*

Contributors

Dale C Alverson
Professor of Pediatrics and Regents' Professor Medical Director, Center for Telehealth and Cybermedicine Research, University of New Mexico, Health Sciences Center, Albuquerque, USA

Andrew Anderson
Managing Director, Crawford Medical Limited, Banbury, UK

Fernando Bello
Senior Lecturer in Surgical Graphics and Computing, Department of Bio-surgery and Surgical Technology, Imperial College London, London, UK

Haim Berkenstadt
Deputy Director, The Israel Center for Medical Simulation (MSR), Director, Department of Day Care Surgery and Anesthesiology C. Sheba Medical Center, Tel Hashumer, Israel

Mordechai Bermann
Associate Professor of Anesthesiology, Director of Patient Simulation Center, Department of Anesthesiology, University of Medicine and Dentistry of New Jersey-Robert Wood Johnson Medical School, New Brunswick, USA

John R Boulet
Associate Vice President, Research and Data Resources, Foundation for Advancement of International Medical Education and Research (FAIMER), Philadelphia, USA

Mark W Bowyer
Professor of Surgery and Chief, Division of Trauma and Combat Surgery, The Norman M Rich Department of Surgery Director of Surgical Simulation, National Capital Area Medical Simulation Center, Uniformed Services University Bethesda, USA

Thomas P Caudell
Professor, Department of Electrical and Computer Engineering; Director, Center for High Performance Computing, University of New Mexico, Albuquerque, USA

Chris Chin
Associate Director of Barts and the London Simulation Centre, London, UK

Robert Davies
Urological Surgeon, Department of Urology, Sir Charles Gairdner Hospital, Perth, Australia

Shad H Deering
Staff Physician, Maternal-Fetal Medicine, Department of Obstetrics and Gynecology, Medical Director, Andersen Simulation Center, Madigan Army Medical Center, Tacoma, USA

Michael A DeVita
Professor Critical Care Medicine and Internal Medicine, University of Pittsburgh, Pittsburgh, Pennsylvania, USA

Thomas Dongilli
Director of Operations and Administration, Peter M Winter Institute for Simulation Education and Research; Administrator, Department of Anesthesiology, School of Medicine, University of Pittsburgh, Pittsburgh, Pennsylvania, USA

Tony Errichetti
Chief of Virtual Medicine, Director, Institute for Clinical Competence, New York College of Osteopathic Medicine, Old Westbury, USA

Sheena Ferguson
Director of Education, BATCAVE, University of Mexico, New Mexico, USA

Bryan Fischberg
EMS Educator, Robert Wood Johnson University Hospital, EMS & Trauma Education, New Jersey, USA

Brendan Flanagan
Associate Professor in Patient Safety
Education, Monash University, Faculty of
Medicine; Nursing and Health Sciences
Director, Southern Health Simulation Centre,
Monash Medical Centre, Moorabbin Campus,
Melbourne, Australia

Rhona Flin
Professor, Applied Psychology, University of
Aberdeen, Old Aberdeen, Scotland

Frances C Forrest
Medical Director, Bristol Medical Simulation
Centre, UK

Alexander Garden
Clinical Director Anaesthesia, Wellington
Hospital, Associate Professor and Clinical
Associate Director, Sleep Wake Research
Centre, Massey University, Wellington,
New Zealand

Ronnie Glavin
Scottish Clinical Simulation Centre,
Scotland

Timothy E Goldsmith
Professor of Psychology,
Department of Psychology, University of
New Mexico, Albuquerque, USA

Joseph S Goode Jr.
Instructor, University of Pittsburgh School of
Nursing, Nurse Anaesthesia Program, and
Staff Nurse Anesthetist, UPMC Presbyterian
Hospital Pittsburgh, PA, USA

Louis Patrick Halamek
Associate Professor, Division of Neonatal and
Developmental Medicine, Department of
Pediatrics, Stanford University; Director,
Center for Advanced Pediatric and Perinatal
Education (CAPE); Attending Neonatologist,
Packard Children's Hospital at Stanford,
Palo Alto, USA

Jeff Hamdorf
Surgeon; Professor of Medical Education,
The University of Western Australia, Perth,
Australia

Cindy Hein
Intensive Care Paramedic,
SA Ambulance Service,
Senior Lecturer, Department of Paramedic
Social Health Sciences, Flinders University,
South Australia, Australia

Chris Holland
Medical Education Fellow and Intensive Care
Medicine Specialist Registrar, Simulation
Centre, Barts and the London NHS Trust,
London, UK

Gary Hope
Operating Department Practitioner, Barts and
the London Simulation Centre, London, UK

Ross Horley
Founder and Managing Director of Medic
Vision Ltd., Melbourne, Australia

Yue Ming Huang
Assistant Professor, Department of
Anaethesiology, David Geffen School of
Medicine at UCLA, Director of Operations,
University of California Los Angeles
Simulation Centre, USA

Elizabeth A Hunt
Director, Johns Hopkins Medicine Simulation
Center, Baltimore, Maryland, USA

Russell W Jones
Director of Assessment, RACGP; Professor,
Centre for Medical and Health Sciences
Education and, Department of Anaesthesia
and Perioperative Medicine, Monash
University, Melbourne, Australia

Roger Kneebone
Senior Lecturer in Surgical Education,
Imperial College London, London, UK

Satish Krishnamurthy
Co-Director, Minimally Invasive Cranial
Neurosurgery Director, Pediatric Neurosurgery
Department of Neurosurgery Henry Ford
Health System, Detroit, Michigan, USA

Fiona Lake
Associate Professor in Respiratory Medicine
and Medical Education, Royal Perth Hospital
and University of Western Australia,
Perth, Australia

Samsun (Sem) Lampotang
Professor of Anesthesiology, Center for
Simulation, Advanced Learning and
Technology, and Department of
Anesthesiology, University of Florida,
Gainesville, Florida, USA

Geoffrey K Lighthall
Associate Professor of Anesthesia and Critical
Care Department of Anesthesia, Stanford
University School of Medicine, Stanford,
California, USA

Nicola Maran
Director, Scottish Clinical Simulation Centre,
Stirling Royal Infirmary, Scotland

Rima Matevosian
Associate Professor, Department of
Anaesthesiology, University of California,
Chair, Department of Anaesthesiology, Olive
View-UCLA Medical Center, USA

Nicolette C Mininni
Advanced Practice Nurse, Critical Care,
University of Pittsburgh Medical Center,
UPMC Shadyside, Pittsburgh, USA

Stefan Mönk
Simulation Centre for Anaesthesiology,
Johannes Gutenberg University, Mainz,
Germany

Richard Morris
Anaesthetist and Perfusionist, Department of
Anaesthesia, St. George Hospital, Sydney,
Australia

Angie Nunn
Centre Manager, Medical Simulation Centre,
Barts and The London NHS Trust, London,
UK

John M O'Donnell
Director, University of Pittsburgh School of
Nursing, Nurse Anesthesia Program, Associate
Director, Winter Institute for Simulation,
Education and Research (WISER) Pittsburgh,
USA

Doris Østergaard
Associate Professor, Danish Institute for
Medical Simulation, Herlev Hospital,
Copenhagen, Denmark

Harry Owen
Professor and Director, Clinical Skills and
Simulation and Skills Unit, Flinders
University, South Australia, Australia

Ray Page
Former Manager, Simulator Services,
QANTAS Airways; past Chair, IATA Flight
Simulator Technical Committee; Inaugral
Chair, Simulation Industry Association
Australia (SIAA)

Mary D Patterson
Medical Director Center for Simulation and
Research Pediatric Emergency Medicine,
Department of Pediatrics, Cincinnati
Children's Hospital Medical Center, USA

Andy Pybus
Anaesthetist, Department of Anaesthesia,
St. George Hospital, Sydney, Australia

Daniel Raemer
Director, Boston Simulation Centre, MA, USA

Malay Rao
Second year medical student, University of
Medicine and Dentistry of New Jersey,
Robert Wood Johnson Medical School,
Piscataway, New Jersey, USA

E Matt Ritter
Assistant Professor of Surgery, Assistant
Director of Surgical Simulation, National
Capital Area Medical Simulation Center, The
Norman M Rich Department of Surgery,
Uniformed Services University, Bethesda,
Maryland, USA

Brian Robinson
Director, National Patient Simulation Training
Centre, Wellington Hospital, Wellington,
New Zealand

Orit Rubin
MATAN–Attribute Focus Assessment Unit,
National Institute for Testing and Evaluation,
Director of Evaluation and Assessment, The
Israel Center for Medical Simulation (MSR),
Jerusalem, Israel

Chris Sadler
Anaesthetist and Director Medical Simulation
Centre, Department of Anaesthesia, Barts and
The London NHS Trust, London, UK

Usha Satish
Director, Simulation Laboratory, SUNY Upstate Medical University, New York, USA

Randolph Steadman
Professor and Vice Chair, Department of Anaesthesiology, Director, UCLA Simulation Center, University of California at Los Angeles, California, USA

Willem van Meurs
Associate Scientist, INEB – Instituto de Engenharia Biomédica, Porto, Portugal

Iris Vardi
Educational Consultant and Senior Project Officer, Curtin University of Technology, Perth, Australia

John A Vozenilek
Emergency Physician, Assistant Professor, Feinberg School of Medicine, Northwestern University, Division of Emergency Medicine, Evanston Northwestern Healthcare, Evanston, USA

Leonie Watterson
Director, Sydney Medical Simulation Centre, Royal North Shore Hospital, Sydney, Australia

Jennifer Weller
Associate Professor, Head of Centre of Medical and Health Sciences Education, Specialist Anaesthetist Faculty of Medical and Health Sciences, University of Auckland, Auckland, New Zealand

Kimberly Allison Yaeger
Director, Training and Research Center for Advanced Pediatric and Perinatal Education, Stanford University, Palo Alto, USA

Amitai Ziv
Director, Israel Center for Medical Simulation, MSR; Deputy Director, Sheba Medical Center; Director, Risk Management and Quality Assurance; Sheba Medical Center, Tel Hashomer, Israel

About the editor

Dr Richard Riley is a practising anaesthetist at Royal Perth Hospital, having trained in anaesthesia in both Australia and the USA. His interest in medical simulation began in 1997. He became Clinical Director of the Centre for Anaesthesia Skills and Medical Simulation at the University of Western Australia in 2002. In 2006 he was the meeting Chair for the International Meeting on Medical Simulation. He also has interests in difficult airway management and obesity. He is also the Chief Editor of the *Australasian Anaesthesia Journal*.

Part 1

Simulation centre logistics

Chapter 1

Simulation and skill centre design

Ross Horley

Overview

- Key elements in the design of a skills training facility are building form, room usage (function) and technology.
- Important design criteria are space planning for traffic flow, adequate breakout spaces, storage, entrance and exit design.
- Room usage includes mock operating theatre, control room, procedure room, debriefing rooms, communications room, lecture theatres, e-learning pods, external areas, breakout spaces and cafeteria.
- Technical aspects include a high level of lighting and flexible control, air handling system with fresh air cycle, access control security system connected to a CCTV system, high level of sound insulation and master audiovisual system permeating all training areas.
- The skills training facility needs to connect to broadband and telecommunications networks to facilitate telemedicine and videoconference applications.

1.1 Introduction

Simulation and skills centre design can be broken into a number of key components, which include building form, room usage (function) and technology.

Building form references how the building or space appears. Room usage is the actual function of the room or space referencing the types of training or the types of activity that will be carried out in those rooms. The technology component focuses on using technology to best enhance the educational process. A simulation and skills centre is an educational facility in a clinical setting; the technology, the location and relationships of the rooms should all be taken into account during the design process to facilitate augmenting the educational process.

1.2 Building form

The building form or visual architecture of a skills centre, while often varied, needs to be complementary to the clinical and educational process. The facility should be designed to enhance the transfer and acquisition of medical, surgical and communication skills.

Elements such as colour, brightness, energy efficiency, and building finishes are all important to create the clinical and educational ambience. However, a simulation and skills training centre is not a hospital. It doesn't need to represent the total clinical aspects of a hospital, but it does need to emulate a medical facility and remain a learning centre.

1.2.1 Space planning

One of the areas that is critical in the planning of the space is traffic flow, efficiently catering for the diverse activities that are carried out in the skills training centre. Many skills training centres are single service (catering for a single clinical discipline). However, a more sustainable and increasingly used model is for a multidisciplinary skills training centre, which can deliver a diverse number of training activities to medical practitioners and health workers. As the target market for a multifunctional skills training centre includes surgeons, nurses, anaesthetists, paediatricians, allied health workers, and paramedics, among others, traffic flow and very efficient space planning become important elements in the management of the training activities of these different groups. Breakout spaces, circulation, storage, and access to the building, are design elements that need a high priority in the development of a skills training centre.

1.2.1.1 Breakout spaces

In the design of skills training facilities there needs to be significant emphasis placed on the management of traffic flow during breaks in training events and to direct traffic to nominated breakout areas without disruption to the other users of the centre.

The following situation could easily occur: surgical training is taking place in one section of the skills centre, anaesthesia training in another and nurse training in a third area, but all 'breaking' at the same time. There needs to be logical areas for these groups to congregate separately without interfering with the other groups. The process of casual discussion relating to the course experience can be very important when it comes to the learning process.

A number of breakout areas within the centre may be required. Each breakout area should be fairly insular in regard to other breakout spaces. Mixing the different disciplines at this point, between participants who have just finished one course with participants who have just finished a separate course, could hinder the flow of communication, discussion, and reflection.

A further issue is the confidentiality of those who attend courses and how well they performed in the course. Thus, breakout spaces need to be well designed in the skills training facility, so that there is sufficient number of them that when a course breaks, the participants can go to their own breakout space. Ideally, the breakout spaces are separate or the spaces are large enough to accommodate pockets of groups. A centralized cafeteria can be a solution with obvious benefits. Effective breakout spaces are very important, and many times in the planning phase their significance is underestimated.

1.2.1.2 Technical traffic flow

The flow of traffic for technical staff and the visitors to the centre is quite critical and has a significant impact on the efficiency of the skills training centre. The best situation is to have dedicated technical circulation space separate from space for the users of the building. This is not dissimilar to what happens in a hotel, for example, where the back of house area is where most maintenance and general staff transfer and avoid the public space. This is sometimes very difficult to achieve in skills centres, because of space limitations. Problems may develop when there is a number of concurrent training courses, all of different durations, and the setting up of one course interferes with the running of another. The technical corridors or technical space is a solution for this. The desired plan is that training rooms can be set up and cleared away without ingress into the normal circulation space that the public would tend to be in. Effective technical traffic flow will considerably add to the efficient running of the skills training centre.

1.2.1.3 Storage

Storage is one of those elements within a skills training centre that is never adequately considered. Although electronic education, such as e-learning and computer-based simulation, is replacing paper-based educational material, there are still large pieces of equipment used in the training process. In a multifunctioning skills training centre, the skills training rooms are generally generic and the equipment that is used for one course will need to be removed from that room and stored because different types of equipment may be used for the next course. A minimum of 20% of the entire floor area should be allocated for storage. Storage should always be in close proximity to the training space and where possible it should be expandable. Offsite storage can be advantageous for equipment that is used infrequently.

1.2.1.4 Building entrances and exits

First impressions of a skills training centre are important. There needs to be a designated point of entry and exit for the users, equipment, and staff, and a point for participant registration. Even when skills training centres are located within a teaching hospital there is still a need for a controlled point of entry and exit. Furthermore, a controlled point of reception is desirable. Such a reception has two critical roles:

- To meet and greet course participants to guide them to the appropriate area, answer questions, facilitate storage of personal items (coats, laptops, and other equipment that people bring).
- Create a point of security, because theft is a considerable problem in many skills centres.

  The design of the skills centre needs to accommodate efficient and effective entry and exit, and the marshalling of people into appropriate areas while maintaining a high level of security.

1.2.2 Room usage

Depending on the focus of the specific simulation and skills training facility, the layout of the rooms and the number or type of those rooms will vary. However, the following rooms are identified as common in a multifunction skills training facility:

- mock operating theatre
- associated control room
- procedure room
- debriefing rooms
- communication rooms
- lecture theatres
- e-learning pods
- external areas for external training activities
- breakout spaces
- cafeteria or coffee and tea making facilities.

1.2.2.1 Mock operating theatre

Many skills training facilities have been established around a mock operating theatre concept. This type of skills training facility is generally associated with mannequin-based training and not necessarily surgical training. In a multifunctional skills training facility the mock operating theatre is a mandatory inclusion, even where a skills training centre is focused more on surgical skills training.

The mock operating theatre needs to be a similar size to an actual operating theatre, approximately 50 m². The size can be reduced to around 40 m² if necessary. The theatre does not always need medical gases, a specialized air handling system, equipotential earthing system, or any of the specific hospital based services that exists in an actual operating theatre. However, some anaesthesia and respiratory medicine equipment may require the use of medical-grade gases to avoid loss of warranty. A mock theatre recreates the environment where training activities are centred around a simulated patient. This room is aimed at replicating the experience of the operating suite, therefore the room construction can be more conventional rather than medical-grade. For example, the ceiling system can consist of lay-in tiles rather than flush plaster. The light in the centre of the operating theatre is just there as a prop. It does need to work, but it does not need to be anything greater than a light that represents an operating theatre light. The same applies when it comes to surgical and anaesthetic pendants.

One important exception is when the simulated operating theatre has a high fidelity mannequin that fulfils the role of the patient. High fidelity mannequins do require gas such as nitrogen, oxygen, carbon dioxide, nitrous oxide, and compressed air. These gases are required at the mannequin location. In many cases the gases are installed in the mock anaesthetic pendant but in other cases these services are brought through channels in the floor.

In the design of the operating theatre, it is also important that there is sufficient piping and cable capacity to allow for future pipes and services. Floor trenches are better and more cost effective than raised floors; however, services can also be installed down the surgical and anaesthetic pendants. In a mock operating theatre, space needs to be relatively flexible. If floor duct is possible, the floor ducts are preferably installed in a cross configuration (north/south/east/west) through the centre points of the room.

1.2.2.2 Control room

A control room is required immediately adjacent to the mock operating theatre fitted with one-way glass, so that the people in the control room can view the operating theatre but the participants in the operating theatre cannot view into the control room. It is preferable that the glass is angled slightly and the lighting system in the control room is equipped with low brightness luminaires and is dimmed.

The audiovisual and technical requirements of the control room will be covered later in this chapter. The control room is a logical space to locate communication racks and audiovisual equipment, and needs to be relatively soundproofed, as does the operating theatre. The requirement for soundproofing the control room is to eliminate sound transfer into the training areas from the control room. Audible activity within the operating theatre can become quite loud, because of the severity of the trauma that is being simulated.

Many skills training facilities have simulated procedures rooms that are similarly set up like the operating theatre, albeit to a lesser technical specification. These too require a control room to view into the training space. This usually means that there are two control rooms: one for the procedure room and one for the operating theatre. Common control rooms are not efficient when there are concurrent training activities.

1.2.2.3 Debriefing rooms

A simulation and skills centre requires a number of debriefing/discussion rooms. The debriefing rooms should generally be able to accommodate about 10 people, but there needs to be the ability to accommodate larger crowds when necessary.

The debriefing rooms serve a number of functions. One is for the debriefing of activities that have concluded in a mock simulation. The participants return to the debriefing room where the facilitator can walk them through the appropriateness, or otherwise, of their actions; and review what they did well and what they might do differently next time.

Debriefing rooms can also be used as small meeting rooms or locations for video conferencing. Debriefing rooms can fulfil the role of an observation room so that people who are associated with the skills training course, but are not actually located within the mock operating theatre, can view what is happening. It is desirable that multiple video links are provided into a debriefing room; at least three or four cameras need to be viewed simultaneously. This concept is an alternative to providing observation windows into the operating theatre, which just gives a single dimensional view. Debriefing rooms should also be in close proximity to the operating theatre or procedure room training areas.

1.2.2.4 Communication/human factors rooms

An emerging activity used in skills centres is communication training and human factor analysis. Training focuses on the communication within teams, or communicating adequately to patients. Effective communication is a very important skill but has not previously been addressed adequately in health education. Significant emphasis is now placed on improving communication skills to enhance patient care and communication skills among healthcare teams.

The skills training centre will need space designed to support communication training. The space includes small surgical communication suites centred around a control room to view and record the communication activities. The suites can be set up as a doctor's office, a day surgery facility, a consultation room, or any variation on this theme. Actors play the part of patients or as part of a team, and the trainee or participant is immersed into the scenario and their actions are video recorded for analysis and assessment.

A good layout for a series of communication rooms is a hub and spoke arrangement: the control centre is at the hub and the communication rooms are the spokes. There have been numerous other configurations, such as a corridor design, where the control room is a service corridor behind the communication rooms. The participants enter the communication rooms through the opposite side to the technical corridor. The layout is very much dependent on how much space can be allocated within the skills training facility.

1.2.2.5 Lecture theatre

It is important that at least one lecture theatre is provided within the skills centre that can cater for a significant number of people, preferably greater than 50. The lecture theatre can be level or tiered. It is preferable to have lectures theatres flat because this style enables reconfiguration and it can be part of a multifunctional concept. If the lecture theatre is tiered, it means that it is limited to a lecture function. If the lecture room is not tiered the ability to view adequately is diminished. The style of lecture theatre needs to be assessed at the time of design. It should be equipped with appropriate audiovisual and communication equipment to not only view multimedia content but also to participate in video conferencing, and to record activities that are happening within that lecture theatre.

1.2.2.6 E-learning pods

There is a transition to electronic forms of learning (e-learning). The skills training facility needs to accommodate e-learning activities and therefore e-learning pods or carrels are recommended. Whether the e-learning activities relate to role-play, real-time gaming, static learning or interactive individual learning, such as reviewing educational materials, there needs to be a space within the skills training centre for this type of activity. The traditional carol type layout may be appropriate. Depending on the size and needs of the skills training centre the number of bays and carrels will vary.

1.2.2.7 External training areas

Where possible, it is beneficial to incorporate an external training area as a component of the skills training facility. External training areas may be fitted out with props, such as wrecked motor vehicles, building rubble or ambulance facility, that aim to provide a realistic training environment in an external space. Audiovisual devices can link this external space back into the skills training centre so that the activities are captured on video and audio and then used within the debriefing rooms.

1.2.2.8 Breakout spaces

Break out spaces need to be designed as a relaxing environment to facilitate freedom of communication and encourage discussion by participants. There may need to be some e-learning facility in close proximity to the breakout space so that further information can be accessed during this time.

In close proximity to these breakout spaces there should be beverage facilities.

Many skills training courses will be longer than a half day, so catering needs consideration. Whether food is brought in or catered onsite, refreshments need to be provided. It is better for continuity if the participants do not leave the skills centre to purchase lunch or for any tea breaks.

1.3 Technical aspects of a simulation and skills centre

1.3.1 Lighting

Lighting is very important to generate the appropriate ambience and to create the feel of the environment. Lighting needs to be variable, low glare and cost effective. Lighting levels need to be at least 1000 lux within the surgical training areas, greater than 800 lux within the mock training centres and similar lux levels to match the teaching and learning areas within the rest of the building. The lighting should be controllable, and the ability to vary the intensity of the light is important. Task lighting should be used where appropriate and, in surgical training laboratories, colour rendering is important.

1.3.2 Air handling systems

Air handling systems should be designed for the maximum occupancy of the building. The system should be based on fresh air to suit local building bylaws and requirements. Air handling systems in surgical training areas need to be fully compliant with environmental laws pertaining to the activities being carried out within those spaces, especially if there is cadaveric or animal material or any other preserved material that emits gases. Specific air handling for mock operating theatres is not required, as generally the type of activities within those spaces has no requirement for any further air treatment apart from what is expected in an educational facility.

1.3.3 Security

An access control system should be provided within the skills training facility. If the skills training facility is a part of a hospital, it would be expected that the access control system would be extended from the hospital system. If the skills centre is stand alone, it would require a stand alone security system. The importance of the access control system is to monitor movement in and out of the building. Access control systems serve a number of purposes: to secure the space and to enable authorized after-hours access to simulators. A skills training centre, therefore, needs to be as accessible as possible; however, it also needs to be as controlled as possible, because of the risk of theft or damage to equipment. Access control systems can adequately monitor or give access to approved personnel for training; they monitor the time personnel log in and the time they log out, and provides them with access to specific areas. Access control systems connected to a CCTV video and audio system can record after-hours activities, and provide an enhanced level of security.

1.3.4 Acoustic treatments and sound transmission

In the case of a multifunctional skills training centre, each of the training spaces should be acoustically isolated from each other so that the transmission of sound from one training environment to another is minimized. Even when operable walls (partitions) are provided to greater flexibility of the space, sound transmission should be minimized. There is a considerable reduction in the effectiveness of a training session when there are activities that can be heard in an adjoining room. A further important element is confidentiality and respect for the people that are undergoing the training in adjacent areas. Sound insulation should be provided within the walls and the room layout designed to minimize sound transfer from training spaces.

1.3.5 Audiovisual system

The audiovisual system within a skills training centre is a critical component, as much of the activity that occurs within the centre is videotaped and replayed during debriefing or for subsequent analysis or assessment. Therefore, good video imagery and audio clarity is important. The ability to record multiple feeds, to take multiple camera shots from each of the training spaces, to route that video and audio signal to a remote destination, and to receive multiple inputs from external spaces, such as operating theatres or other skills training centres, and then display those feeds in a lecture environment within the skills centre is essential. The audiovisual system should permeate all training areas and as such should be designed as one master system, or at least the concept of the design of the audiovisual system needs to be one that works as a common master audiovisual control system. Individual devices, however, should be controllable from within those spaces. Current systems using touch-screen technology (such as AMX or Crestron) or other types of systems, may adequately provide this feature. It is recommended that audiovisual systems be designed as a digital system to record audiovisual content directly to computer hard drive systems (file servers). There are commercial video file management programs that allow facilitators to annotate and save video segments for easy retrieval during or after the scenario.

Management of these file servers, and an archiving policy need consideration. Access to content from multiple locations is a base level of functionality so that the trainer can present the appropriate content in the specific training area, lecture theatres or other group learning area. The system shall also limit access for unauthorized people to view the content. The file recording system, the archiving of the system, and the management of the system needs to be well defined.

The audiovisual system should be connected to significant broadband connections to enable video conferencing and tele-education to external locations. The inter-connectivity to external networks and therefore other skills training facilities can enhance the activities of the skills centre, including linking into actual operating theatres at remote hospitals or to educational facilities. The function encourages collaboration, to participate in remote training activities but also be a point of destination for educational curriculum.

1.4 Conclusion

The key elements in the design of a skills training centre relate to building form, room usage (function) and technology. The building should be designed to cater for healthcare training and achieved in a simulated clinical setting. To achieve a good design there are numerous factors to consider, such as storage, traffic flow, interrelationships of the rooms, the ambience, and the technical components. Understanding these concepts will assist greatly in the design of an efficient and effective skills training centre. Above all, the training space needs to be flexible to cater for a multitude of training activities and future training technologies. Consideration for flexibility and the seamless incorporation of new technologies is fundamental to good design process. The success of a skills centre starts with a clear understanding of the issues associated with the training activities at the design stage, and the ability to provide design solutions to overcome these issues.

Chapter 2

Simulation centre operations and administration

Yue Ming Huang and Thomas Dongilli

Overview

- This chapter presents a practical approach to simulation centre operations, with ideas from two simulation centres that have both been in operation for over 12–14 years, and a combined 20-year personal experience working in simulation.
- Begin with defined roles and responsibilities for the simulation centre personnel team.
- Establish an organizational system for labeling, filing, and record keeping. Follow it diligently. Meticulous documentation is critical – create logs to document everything, from simulation utilization to evaluations.
- Use checklists to ensure thoroughness of simulation set up, and consistent and comprehensive facilitation of course objectives.
- Schedule simulation sessions, rooms, equipment and personnel realistically and balance daily operations with routine simulator maintenance, scenario programming and testing, troubleshooting, administrative work, and program development. Block off time for planning and preparation on the simulation calendar.
- Develop and program scenarios using a systematic process, beginning with learning objectives that are integrated with existing curriculum, and continuing with routine reviews to ensure timely incorporation of feedback from sessions.
- Train staff and faculty to allow succession of skills and to assess the quality of the established organizational infrastructure.
- Create a simulator website to serve multiple functions, including marketing and publicity, online scheduling, course management, and a common communication forum for internal users.
- Be prepared for real emergencies in your simulation centre.

2.1 Introduction

It is 7:45 on a Monday morning after a long weekend and you are experiencing a crisis in the simulation centre. No, this is not a simulated critical incident scenario, but a real logistical nightmare. You have an 8:00 team training session with a community physician, two anaesthesia residents, one surgery resident, one operating room nurse and three faculty instructors. Additionally, you have three visitors from out of town who are interested in seeing how you run your sessions, and one of them has potential funding opportunities for simulation research. You have run many simulation sessions before but today, the stakes are higher with a paying participant, a multidisciplinary team training approach and a number of observers evaluating your work. Unfortunately, everything that can go wrong is going wrong today. The simulator has malfunctioned and you cannot mask ventilate as usual. The main overhead camera has a poor image coming through. Two of your visitors are here and looking to you for direction. The other visitor has called and asked if you could meet him outside because he is lost. Your participants are slowly arriving and accumulating in the conference room. The extra copies of the handouts you made 2 days ago are nowhere to be found. The copying machine nearby is broken so you have your assistant running upstairs to use a different copier. Meanwhile, you get paged that one of the residents is caught in traffic and will be running late. The phone is ringing with someone inquiring about scheduling for a tour of the simulation centre. Your instructors have questions about the course materials. The simulator is not ready and the clock is ticking fast . . .

While this may be a worst-case hypothetical scenario, all of us working in simulation have experienced a number of real-life operational problems while running a simulation centre. Those new to simulation will inevitably experience these 'growing pains'. Most of us improvise when faced with logistical or technical difficulties. Sometimes, the problem is a quick fix that reminds us of the limitations of simulation and the holes in our system. Other times, they require extensive troubleshooting that forces us to use contingency plans in place of actual simulation sessions. This is when we can truly appreciate the administrative and organizational efforts of the simulation team, which help anticipate and minimize such disasters. In this chapter, we share our experience and ideas on how to establish and maintain an operational infrastructure that not only looks out for the present operations but also ahead to the future in the development of a simulation centre.

2.2 **Administration**

A successful simulation centre will inevitably have a staff to support the administration and operation of the centre. Regardless of whether there is a single specified person in charge of administration or the work is shared among directors and multiple coordinators of a simulation centre, there are defined responsibilities and roles to operating a simulation centre. Here, we break the administrative tasks into three timeframes: preparations, performance, and post-simulation administration.

2.2.1 **Preparations before the simulation**

Never underestimate the amount of time you will need for designing and setting up a simulation course. Planning activities must occur long before the actual training sessions. The list below illustrates the extent of work required prior to the participants' arrival.

Create a budget to assess whether you have the financial and personnel resources to carry out your simulation course.

Establish the simulation course per institutional or organizational policies. This could take a while depending on institutional practices regarding course establishment and accreditation. A needs assessment and a course syllabus describing learning objectives and evaluation methods are necessary to begin the process. For courses offering credit (official student clerkships and electives or continuing education courses), follow the required guidelines.

Make course-specific checklists to include:

- Instructional material such as journal articles, X-rays, MRIs, CTs, TEEs, photo images, and props to enhance the realism of the scenario.

- Equipment and personnel needed for the course, including simulator, room requirements, audiovisual capabilities, props and instructors.
- Logistics, including traffic flow, room set-up instructions (best illustrated with photos and diagrams), scenario scripts, and simulator software programming codes.
- Prepare two folders, a paper-based version and an electronic format, of everything related to the course, including the checklists and course syllabus, descriptions, handouts, simulator instructions and scripts, programming codes, and any other educational references for evidence-based debriefings. Pictures are extremely helpful.
- Make copies of handouts, consents, confidentiality and disclaimer forms for participants and scripts for instructors, evaluations, and surveys for participants etc. – it is best to have enough for several sessions in order to avoid rushing around to make last-minute copies.
- Advertise course and schedule groups.
- Arrange directions, parking and accommodations for participants if necessary.
- Order food if appropriate.
- Check supplies, conduct inventory with checklists and order missing items.
- Inform participants and instructors of pre-course reading/assignments – these can be posted online.
- Send reminder emails to participants and instructors a couple of days before session.
- Prepare name labels and sign-in sheets.
- Test equipment and prepare rooms.
- Place everything in a common place that the faculty and staff can access – all simulation personnel should know where the files and equipment are in the simulation centre and on the common computer server.

2.2.2 Performance on the simulation day

On the day of the simulation course, checklists should be used to ensure that last-minute troubleshooting and preparations are accounted for. Ideally, everything should have been checked the day before, but if time constraints do not permit advance preparations, allow a minimum of 1 hour for set-up.

Set up food if applicable Make sure the food arrives on time with utensils. Coffee-break room should also be well stocked for staff and visitor use.

Conference or classroom set-up Turn on television or viewing screen; test LCD projector and laptop synchronization to avoid technical problems with projections during debriefing; have presentations and handouts ready. For example, if participants are first gathering in conference room for orientation, display instructions and give participants necessary handouts (confidentiality agreements etc.) to read.

Simulator control room set up test audiovisual equipment, recording devices and supplies (hard drive space, DVD disks), computer connections, intercom systems, wireless communication systems and display monitors.

Simulator room set-up Test equipment such as anaesthesia machines, defibrillators, laryngoscope blades, test audio and video functions, prepare props, etc.

Simulator set-up Power on and run through the simulator features from head to toe for functionality; have orientation case or first case set up and ready for demonstration.

Participant arrival Greet and welcome participants as they arrive, direct them to appropriate rooms (use signs or have designated staff ushers), show them where to place their belongings (if lockers are provided), where the restrooms are, and provide proper clothing if they did not arrive in proper attire (white coat, scrubs, gowns, masks, caps as required for specific course). Provide nametags, ask them to sign in, sign confidentiality forms, consent forms for research, media release forms for videotaping, etc.

Orientation A simulation team member should explain session format and expectations, answer questions, and provide a hands-on orientation to the simulator equipment (capabilities and limitations). This is where you can decrease performance anxiety and set the tone for a safe learning environment for your participants.

Simulation experience Simulation staff may play multiple roles during a scenario, as facilitator, operator and confederate in the case.

Debriefing As the learning occurs in the post-simulation discussion, make sure that supporting documents, handouts, and video playback system are ready.

Participant feedback and programme evaluation Appropriate forms should be distributed at the end of the session.

Certifications Make sure participants complete forms for CME credit; issue certificate/letter of attendance if needed.

Data collection Designate someone to collect or a place for completed forms before participants leave.

2.2.3 Post-simulation administration

It is often tempting to leave after a long day of simulation, particularly since emails and other responsibilities await us. However, reflection and feedback from the sessions are just as important as the preparation and operation of the sessions themselves. After each teaching session, the following are recommended.

2.2.3.1 For internal purposes

Debrief instructors Build in at least 10 minutes at the end of a course to sit down with the instructors and discuss the sessions with them, how they feel, what are the good points, what could be improved, new ideas, etc. If time does not permit a formal discussion, a follow-up email may solicit feedback from the instructors.

Debrief staff This may occur with the instructors or separately and is meant to obtain feedback regarding programmatic issues and troubleshooting strategies; create a list of action items to incorporate for the next session or make the changes as soon as possible.

Collate documents There will be paperwork strewn all over the place or lost if they are not systematically collected. Designate someone to collate important papers into a specified folder for better organization.

Enter data Make sure you record all course information on your simulation usage log (include names of instructors, staff, participants, level of training, date, time, room, number of simulator hours, type of simulator used, title of session, simulator problems, etc.). To improve on cases for the next session, it is important to enter and review data as soon as possible. Research projects may call for specific timelines for data entry and analysis.

Update simulation logs

Evaluate simulator scenario, course and overall programme Review evaluation forms to gauge progress and set goals for improvement; review resources for budget re-analysis.

Generate reports based on collected data: this could be useful to update the simulation centre team during regular meetings or for reporting to funding sources or other authorities.

2.2.3.2 For external purposes

If appropriate, send follow-up or thank you email Include survey if conducting research and participants have signed consent forms. Notify students of examination scores or individual written feedback.

Send link to online evaluation If paper copy was not distributed and collected on site.

Send CME forms to appropriate office.

Compile required documentation and reports as necessary.

2.3 Simulator maintenance

Simulation training relies heavily on the fidelity and functionality of the available equipment. For simulation instructors and staff, nothing is more frustrating than planning a course, showing up for the session and having the equipment malfunction. What is worse, and more embarrassing, is the realization that the problem was something that should have been dealt with before the start of the course. Since most multidisciplinary centres offer a broad range of courses, it is anticipated that the sheer number of users and the specific types of courses would cause trauma and wear-and-tear to the simulators. Understanding the specific nature and use of the simulator for a particular course will allow the operational staff to identify these problems after the course, as well as to ensure that those specific functions are checked before the simulation sessions.

2.3.1 Routine maintenance

Almost every piece of equipment requires some form of routine maintenance. Recommendations from the manufacturer are usually provided via an operations manual. We suggest contacting the manufacturers' service support for all equipment related questions. Along with an inventory list, we suggest creating a routine maintenance checklist for each piece of equipment in your centre. Simulator equipment should be treated like regular patient care equipment that requires scheduled inspections. A regularly scheduled routine maintenance day should be placed on your simulation calendar and recorded in the routine maintenance log. Custodial work such as dusting electrical devices and cleaning the simulator with alcohol and recommended solvents should be included in the routine maintenance.

2.3.2 Course-specific simulator maintenance

An equipment checklist is mandatory for course-specific simulator maintenance. Prior to each course, the equipment in the room must be tested and ready for use. The tests apply to the audio and video equipment, the functionality of the simulator(s), and any other equipment that may be used. A log of the testing procedure should be recorded for each piece of equipment, as this information will be useful for future reference and repair tracking. Similarly, after each course, the same checklist should be re-evaluated so that the equipment will be ready for the next user.

2.4 **Data organization**

A systematic way of organizing the copious amounts of paperwork and data generated from operating a simulation centre is invaluable to a centre's success. Every simulation centre will at some point be asked to review and report their records, whether for budget and quality assurance reasons, or for national conferences and research purposes. Whether your centre is driven by teaching and assessment or by research, all institutions are potential prey to data excess and chaos as they grow and expand. Therefore, starting with a clear idea of the organizational structure of your centre will help minimize growing pains and enable quicker expansion. Below are some tips on establishing a system of organization within your centre.

- Have dedicated storage space for simulation material (secure, physical space for equipment and computer/server hard drive space with back-up system for electronic files).
- Create logs to track simulation usage, instructional hours, troubleshooting and repairs, routine maintenance, inventory checks, ideas, budget and expenses, anything that you might want to generate data with later.
- Create hard copies of everything and organize in tabbed folders for each course.
- Establish a clear filing and document labeling system. Save electronic files using same format, (i.e. each document should have file name/path and revision date as a footnote to help users access file on server).
- Colour-label your equipment and clearly indicate cable connections.
- Photograph and/or diagram room set-up, equipment connections and patient profiles include these in course folders.
- If possible, use online evaluations and examinations that can be accessed through secure internet or networked system and are downloadable to a database for report generation.
- Research data should be maintained in separate folders for each study/project with intermittent analyses to gauge progress of study.

2.5 **Scenario development and programming**

Let's face it – designing curricular material takes an enormous amount of time and effort. Thus, case contribution by your instructors is critical to the development of a simulation curriculum. Increasing the repertoire of cases in your simulation library not only allows flexibility in choice of scenarios to use for students who come back for more than one simulator session, but also provides new instructors with examples of solid instructional material to use. However, scenario development is not as simple as making up a case stem and running the simulator 'on the fly'. The operational and administrative team should enforce systematic standards for scenario development.

To aid instructors in scenario design and to make the programming process easier, a template is recommended. Gleaning from the *Journal of Simulation in Healthcare* template for case submissions and other open-source templates, the following components are recommended for inclusion on the scenario template:

- Name of person writing the case (author)
- Date
- Simulation hardware and software
- Case title

- Case diagnosis and prognosis – if using a real case, make sure that links to patient information are coded to protect patient privacy
- Target audience discipline and level of training
- Educational rationale – why is this scenario important?
- Learning objectives or teaching points
- Course prerequisites and/or guided study questions for participants
- Assessment instruments (such as checklists or pre-simulation and post-simulation questions)
- Equipment list
- Scenario events – how the case unfolds
- Simulator set-up information
- Simulator script for operator – vital signs at each state, prompts for programming purposes
- Instructor script – include lines for any supporting role that the instructor or other member might play in the scenario
- Case stem – patient information for students
- Supporting materials (CXR, ECG, TEE, etc.)
- Debriefing questions for facilitator to use
- References and web links

Regardless of the brand of simulator you use at your facility, there are some general core procedures that should be followed when developing and programming scenarios to be included in your scenario library. A meeting with the case contributor to establish a clear set of goals and objectives is the first step. One can easily spend hours programming complicated software and covering broad areas of education without a structured approach only to discover that the learning objectives could not be met by the particular simulator or in the programmed fashion. The programmer should ideally work with the case developer/content expert throughout the scenario development. A common misconception of many first-time simulation users is to integrate everything into one scenario. Most of the time, this is not possible because of logistics or the amount of time it would take to program every single possible path. Below are our recommended steps:

- Meet with a simulation team member to discuss feasibility of scenario re-enactment with the current simulators.
- Create specific goals and objectives for the training session. Depending on the participants' level of experience, you may want to keep this simple.
  - Example: anaphylaxis can be quite complicated and may advance in different directions. In a single scenario, you may want the trainee to recognize anaphylaxis and start the first round of treatment.
- Specify evaluation points based on your goals and objectives.
  - Example: assess if the student:
    - i. recognized anaphylaxis
    - ii. discontinued antibiotic
    - iii. called for help
    - iv. started an intravenous drip
    - v. administered epinephrine.

While there are many other points to assess, these may be the learning objectives and outcomes most appropriate for this audience.

- Identify and plan the logistics (order of events, timing) of the scenario.
  - Example: You have 5 minutes to run the entire scenario.
  - Students should recognize anaphylaxis within the first 3 minutes.
  - Students should discontinue the triggering agent, then give epinephrine.
- Write out the entire script from start to finish. Make sure it makes sense to someone else and that the scenario can be completed in the allotted time.
- Program the scenario, keeping in mind simulator capabilities. Using a head to toe review method to change necessary parameters for intended outcomes.
- Test the scenario prior to implementation. Pilot it with the target audience.
  Look for specific things such as:
  i. Does it run the way I programmed it?
  ii. Medically – does it make sense clinically?
  iii. Logistically – are the order and equipment set-up feasible?
  iv. Check for timing. If events are supposed to occur over a certain time, make sure they are standardized and consistent. Also make sure that your scenario does not go over the specified time allocation, to allow for enough time for debriefing.
- Maintain a log of changes to the scenario and clearly label a printout of the latest version of the programming code or scenario frames.
- Create checklists for each course (list equipment and educational material needed as well as steps for setting up the simulation, instructor notes and simulation programming codes).
- Create a summary page for each case, listing all related files and locations.
- Store everything electronically and physically in a common location.
- Hold regular instructor meetings to review existing scenarios and develop new ones.

2.6 Calendar and booking system

As your centre grows, so will the request to use it. With that understanding, it is crucial for a simulation centre to develop procedures that can ensure accuracy and ease of use. The operational schedule of a simulation centre can be a logistical monster if not systematically controlled. Consider a scheduling problem such as overbooking a room. This has bigger implications than what meets the eye. Taking into account the amount of time, resource and efforts needed for a single simulation session, one can appreciate the frustrations of the two parties standing there to use the same simulator equipment. Sometimes, it seems as if the stars must be aligned for certain groups to attend the simulation training sessions. Instructors and students may have been pulled from clinical duties to teach or train, and each person may have had to travel quite a distance to the simulation centre. Clinical departments that are contributing to the operational finances of the simulation centre will not pay for such services for very long if space and time conflicts occur frequently.

Since scheduling is a key component to the operational infrastructure of a simulation centre, we need to balance maximal accommodation of users while maintaining control of the logistics. There are many aspects to scheduling or booking that need be considered, from room assignments to coordinating instructor training, to making time for equipment repair and scenario programming. What follows are various considerations and scheduling systems used at many simulation centres.

2.6.1 **The reservation process**

The operational infrastructure of a simulation centre depends on an established process for scheduling training sessions, reserving rooms and equipment. One or two key individuals should manage this process. Too many people would lead to confusion, yet a single person bottleneck situation is not ideal either. Generally, it is not wise to have an open calendar for anyone to reserve times individually, as most people do not have the bigger picture of the simulation centre operations in mind. The optimal scheduling system would have a feedback mechanism to the requestor as well as an internal checking system for the scheduler. This could be accomplished manually or automatically and electronically.

2.6.2 **The manual calendar**

The manual process for reserving rooms is used at many simulation centres. This is often a paper system, which is inexpensive, but also has more room for errors compared with other formats. However, a meticulous coordinator could make this an efficient and reliable system. A schedule request form can be created and a master calendar would be maintained. Instructor name, course name, number of rooms, dates, number of people attending and equipment needed are examples of the type of information needed on the form. These request forms could be mailed, faxed, or even scanned and emailed. The person responsible for maintaining the master simulation centre calendar must ensure up-to-date accurate records of requested and confirmed dates, as well as cancellations and other pertinent information relating to each scheduled session. This information may be critical to funding or staff performance reviews. By maintaining accurate records, you can also show increase in utilization by certain groups, or number of courses taught by certain instructors. One major complaint with such a manual scheduling system is the inability to view the calendar by those requesting dates. The turn around time for this process can also be painfully long as it often depends on the availability of the scheduler as well as waiting on others to finalize the calendar. However, on the whole, this system works well at most sites.

2.6.3 **The blocked time concept**

Blocked time for instructional sessions address problems related to workforce or instructor availability, such as "I can only get my anaesthesia residents out of the operating rooms on Tuesday afternoons" or "I can only teach on Wednesday mornings." These are common issues that hospital-based simulation centres face every day, struggling to balance real patient care with simulated lessons. The blocked time concept simply means that based on the end users' needs, a common time and day would be identified and reserved on the simulation centre calendar on a recurring basis. This works particularly well for smaller centres and for regularly scheduled courses. A specific time and day would then be reserved each week for these users, for example, every Tuesdays from 1:00–5:00 for anaesthesia resident simulation training. If the regular users feel that they may not be there every week, then allow them first right of refusal for others requesting the same time and date.

2.6.4 **Electronic or web-based scheduling**

Using an internet based request system for scheduling teaching sessions is ideal for simulation centres. A room request form should be accessible on your website. It should be kept simple by providing multiple choices with drop-down boxes, which would make completing the form quick and easy. Submission of this form should automatically generate an email to the master scheduler to check the calendar for conflicts and approve or deny the request. There should be only one accountable person with a trained back-up person. Revisions to the calendar should also be submitted electronically. This process helps decrease human error and minimize the time spent on correspondence with all the requests that come in or get changed.

There are many benefits to using a web-based calendar. Multiple users, including the course director, the course instructor, and the participant could access the calendar for information relating to courses, including time and location of simulator sessions. Schedule changes can be done quickly and updates would be available immediately online. This also allows the requester the opportunity to plan ahead before submitting the request. To facilitate such correspondences, a web-based schedule should include the course date, name of course, location of course, and names of the instructors. The schedule should also include use of the conference rooms or any other training rooms. Linking equipment with room use would also prevent conflicts in scheduling. For example, one would not be able to schedule the use of a particular simulator that requires gas use without also scheduling for a room with gas outlets.

2.7 Scheduling tips

2.7.1 Schedule down time

A common oversight to avoid is not scheduling 'down time' for maintenance and repairs. While we would like to tell others that we use our simulators every hour of the day, it is not possible logistically. Whether you have a small or large simulation centre, it is critical to your operations to maintain and repair simulator equipment in a timely fashion. Therefore, placing dedicated time on the calendar for operational reviews is as important as scheduling actual student sessions. Take advantage of this down time to also check inventories, order supplies, and accomplish other related duties. Operations staff should allow 1–2 hours per week per room for these activities.

2.7.2 Instructor and staff training

As your centre expands, so will the need to increase instructional and operational staff. Instructor and staff training time will become a regularly scheduled course. This training will range from teaching instructors how to run the simulator, to course design, to programming the simulator software. Regardless of whether you have formal courses or if you conduct faculty and staff training informally, learning at the simulator is an important aspect of the training. Keep in mind that a fair amount of time will be needed for individuals who are novices in healthcare simulation. Set a standard time aside each week for this training, as well as for staff development and meetings to improve the simulation programs.

2.7.3 Back-to-back courses

When running courses back-to-back, allow time for room turn over, equipment set-up, and instructor and participant orientation. Simulator preparation inevitably takes time, particularly if the sessions require an elaborate set-up. Consider that trainees will need to leave, equipment will need to be moved and cleaned, and new equipment will need to be set-up and tested. You should allow at least 15 minutes between courses, although most have a standard 30-minute turn over. Even without any need for a room turn over, the simulation centre staff would appreciate a restroom or coffee break.

2.7.4 Running multiple rooms simultaneously

For facilities that have multiple simulation rooms, there are some basic considerations that can make the operational flow of the centre smoother. If a course will be using more than one room, schedule those courses next to each other if logistics allow. This will permit a central location of equipment, instructors and students, and course support will be easier. Ideally, control rooms should be designed to facilitate operation of a simulator from any room. This would allow multiple, highly scripted scenarios to run from a single control room. However, more than one simulator operator will be needed to run simultaneous sessions, and soundproofing may be a concern if both are in the same room.

2.8 Publicity

Whether it is the grand opening for your simulation centre or a special event to mark a milestone, you will want to have a venue for advertising your simulation centre activities. Some degree of publicity is needed to promote your programme and increase interest in simulation training, particularly for a developing centre that would like to reach out to potential donors from the community. The amount of publicity that you would like for your simulation centre depends on your goals. If the centre mission is to serve the institution only, an institutional announcement may suffice. However, if you wish for your simulation centre to be known outside of your institution, media relations may need to play a larger role. Marketing your centre can be accomplished through the use of newspaper advertisements, flyers, brochures, list serves, internet websites, or through word-of-mouth. Simulation centres should be prepared to deal with public inquiries once the word is out that you have an innovative training centre with high-tech simulators.

Public inquiries may come in two forms: from the media, such as the local TV station or newspaper, or from outside users and interested parties. The first, public media, are often handled through your institutional policies on dealing with media relations. If available, knowing who your media relations person is helpful. This person could confirm whether or not a specific news event warrants publicity in the community or national coverage, and if so, puts the centre in touch with the appropriate liaison from the respective news centre. The media relations person could also ensure that media requests align with the institutional policies, such as compliance to privacy and confidentiality regulations. The local media is a good way to showcase your simulation centre to the lay public, as well as to promote simulation news between departments and schools within a university. However, as with any media, keep in mind that despite the large amount of time spent on responding to the public media, much of it may end up in the cutting room and not in the news.

The second group of public request comes from outside users and interested parties who contact the simulation centre for various reasons, such as for course information, tours and demonstrations, or meetings to discuss potential training contracts. Some may even show up at your door unannounced. Many of these individuals are looking for information on your centre's operational infrastructure or how you run simulation sessions, because they are in the process of building their own simulation centres. Others may want to tour your site or ask for assistance with case scenario development. For these requests, it is important to develop policies for your centre, such as procedures for visitors, standards for sharing cases, dealing with requests for onsite observations, signing media release forms and responding to visitors. These policies could be as simple as form letters to reply to email solicitations, or more elaborate procedures on how visitors must obtain permission to observe teaching sessions.

Outside solicitations can consume a lot of your time. One phone call may lead to another and soon your day is filled with phone consultations and requests for follow-up visits. While many of these solicitations are often opportunities for sharing and collaboration, they nonetheless distract from the daily work. Rather than becoming overwhelmed with the entourage of solicitations, it is better to view them as marketing opportunities to engage interested parties, expand the scope of simulation, distribute work, and disseminate information to a larger audience. Having established centre policies will provide an organized approach, with consistency and fairness in dealing with both internal and external requests.

2.9 The simulation centre website

A dedicated website for your simulation centre is not only a useful tool for your users, but could also be a valuable resource for your staff and a showcase of your facility. The website could be a central access point that links the centre staff, instructors, students and learning material. If organized in a systematic, user-friendly way, the website could be the online source for all simulation-related activities. The problem is that most centres do not have a dedicated simulation centre computer support personnel or a webmaster to do the cumbersome, time-consuming task of maintaining and updating the web pages. Thus, before embarking on the development of an elaborate website, consider the following questions:

◆ Do you have the institutional information technology support to design, program and maintain your website? Who will be Webmaster?

◆ What are the server requirements for what you want? Consider what you want on the website; fancier web pages with flash media and video clips will require more computing (and personnel) power.

◆ Are there any security issues? Do you have any intranet sites requiring password entries?

After you have decided to host a website for your simulation centre and have acquired the resources to do so, the next step is to consider the content of your website. The following is a list of sections that you may want to include on your website:

Homepage with mission statement What does your simulation centre provide to the school, to the potential users and to the community?

Facility description You may want to include floorplans, size and types of rooms, simulator equipment and task trainer descriptions, history of simulation centre.

Faculty and staff information Your operational and instructional team – your instructors, their title/position and contact information; photos would be helpful.

Directions and map to facility Driving and parking directions, diagrams and maps will help outside users locate your facility; include a section on accommodations near your centre for out-of-town visitors.

Contact information List your centre address, telephone and facsimile numbers, and email address of webmaster.

Course catalogue with description and syllabus Include course title, location, available dates/times, instructors, learning objectives, prerequisites, target audience, registration information/form, cost and whether credit is provided.

Calendar and/or scheduling system Calendar view of centre activities; instructions on how to sign up for a course; automatic generation of reminders.

Educational resources for faculty and students Links to course prerequisite reading material and additional web-based simulation sites; orientation material and confidentiality policies may be posted here.

Virtual tour and photo gallery Show off your centre activities and facility with pictures and/or video clips.

News and events Announcements and news related to the simulation centre; advertisements for course/meeting registration; highlights and special recognition of awards and activities.

Simulation reference library Develop an online repository of articles on simulation and links to simulation centres and simulator manufacturers.

Research information Focus on publications and research projects conducted by your centre, include information on opportunities for collaboration.

Giving opportunities Recognize those who have given to the centre and attract additional donors for funding and support.

User portfolio accounts An option for users to register and create an individual account in order to manage their coursework and track their learning.

Search engine function Ability to search within your web pages as well as links to other simulation centres.

Intranet Password-protected site for confidential files, instructor materials such as scenario templates and complete case information.

2.10 **When things really go bad: real-life emergencies**

You are in your simulation centre and someone yells for help. The call is ignored because there are courses going and that is a usual request that you hear. The problem, however, is that this time it is a real call for help. We practice emergencies all the time in simulation, but are we prepared for the real ones that take place in our centre? What can we do when a real emergency occurs during a simulation session, particularly for simulation centres that are not located within a hospital system? The following are recommendations for making sure your centre is prepared for real life crises.

- Establish a protocol for emergencies:

   Who will activate the emergency medical services?

   Or who to call in house if you are located in a hospital (designated number for in-hospital paging system).

- Establish a phrase that will trigger a real response (e.g. Code Blue).

- Establish an area in your centre where real resuscitation equipment will be housed. Make sure you label that equipment 'Not for Simulation'!

- Your emergency kit or crash cart should contain everything that a real crash cart would contain, including but not limited to:

   Smelling salts

   AED/defibrillator

   Bag-valve mask

   Nasal cannula

   Non-rebreather face mask

   Ice pack

   Oxygen tank with regulator

   Flashlight

   Intravenous start kit

   ACLS algorithms and medications such as epinephrine

- Use local recommendations to prepare emergency kits for natural disasters such as earthquakes.
- Clearly illustrate your fire and disaster escape routes (simulation centre staff should know them without need to refer to a diagram).
- Make sure all of your emergency kits are located in a central location clearly marked and always stocked.
- Know where your fire extinguishers are located and how to use them.
- Run routine simulation drills to practice real-life emergencies.

2.11 **Concluding remarks**

Just as we teach our students through simulation to anticipate the worst and prepare for all types of crises in the real world, the simulation centre operations team should also be primed to deal with real-life crises, whether they are life threatening or logistical nightmares. We hope that by sharing our experiences and ideas to create systematic procedures and standards, you will be able to apply some of these tips to successfully manage your simulation centre operations. The themes throughout this chapter have been to document best practices, consistently follow procedures, and routinely check the established system for ways to improve and renew. As with any organization, a simulation centre is as good as the people working in it. Learning does not occur without good teachers and a functional infrastructure to support the instruction. Teamwork and a strong foundation are crucial to smooth operations. We wish you and your team all the best in developing and maintaining your simulation centre.

Chapter 3

Mobile simulation

Frances C Forrest

Overview

- Dependant on the portability of the simulator, a user may be able to move a simulator from one teaching location to another or to teach a scenario on the move. Both aspects of mobility are useful in extending the scope of simulation to a wider audience or repertoire of scenarios.

- Good organization and preparation are vital to the success of moving a simulator to a temporary location. The process is more complex when the dedicated simulation environment is left.

- Transportation of simulators requires care and technical support. Investing in a specific vehicle for moving simulators can be useful. Some centres have purchased vehicles such as ambulances to support clinical scenarios in the field.

- Choice and design of scenario is crucial to success of any mobile programme.

3.1 Introduction

This chapter is based on experiences at Bristol Medical Simulation Centre (BMSC). The content refers to mannequin simulators that are hardware based and either script or model controlled[1]. Running a scenario where the simulator has to move location (for example, transferring a head injured patient from one site to another) is the ultimate challenge for teachers. Most simulators are not up to this task because they are not completely wireless controlled or battery driven. Thus there are restrictions imposed by computer control, power or gas supply. This chapter will review our experience with a mobile simulation capability.

3.2 Reasons to move simulators

In 2002 BMSC moved to a new purpose built simulation centre. Moving simulators onsite and offsite was a key necessity in the new BMSC business plan.

The new centre was designed with multiple rooms capable of running different fidelity simulators. Each room could be used to recreate a different clinical area. However, finances were insufficient to purchase a simulator for each area and therefore simulators needed to be moved from area to area depending on the teaching need. This had to be done without damage to the simulators or the environment.

At the time BMSC relocated, it also became clear that there was a market for offsite simulation. There were a number of groups who wanted simulation brought to them, rather than for the student group to travel to the centre. Each group presented an opportunity for new business.

It appeared there were two reasons for this. Firstly, groups believed that it was more cost and time effective to take simulation out to them, and secondly it was difficult to free up a team of healthcare workers to attend and train at a distant centre together.

Another reason for moving simulators has now arisen. The development and subsequent marketing of two new baby simulators, SimBaby® [2] and BabySim®[3], requires creation of complex paediatric environments such as the operating theatre and Paediatric Intensive Care Unit by the user community for teaching. This is expensive (purchase of appropriate props and equipment) and requires additional space and storage not necessarily planned for by existing centres. Consequently, and perhaps particularly relevant when the simulators are physically smaller and lighter, taking paediatric simulation to the real clinical environment is an appropriate and cheaper alternative.

In all cases the luxury of taking a simulator out to a peripheral site, be it a walk-in centre, GP practice or specialized hospital unit, allows people to train together in the teams they work in and in the real workplace. This is the most important reason for teachers to consider developing a mobile programme.

3.2.1 First experiences

In 1998, on secondment to the Harvard Simulation Centre in Boston, the author worked with Dan Raemer, Director of the Harvard Simulation Center. During this secondment an experiment was undertaken to run 'mock codes' (cardiac arrest drills) in a local hospital. The simulator in use was an Eagle simulator, now no longer manufactured[4], and included a full sized adult mannequin, control computer and stack system. The reason for running this experiment was to show a variety of healthcare workers the value of simulation as a tool for learning; at that time there was hesitancy from staff in the different Boston Hospitals to attend the offsite simulation centre.

The logistics of this operation were complex and costly in terms of time and staff. Particular issues that needed to be addressed (and apply to any attempt to move offsite) included:

♦ Communication and planning with the local site team.

♦ Identification of an appropriate place and time for training.

♦ Pack up, transport and set up the simulator (and props).

♦ Design of a suitable scenario.

♦ Running the scenario in a 'foreign' environment (i.e. without the usual technical support).

♦ Returning to base.

This experience highlighted some of the real difficulties in transporting and setting up a high fidelity simulator for a short time. With newer less complex simulators some of these aspects of mobility have been made easier.

The results of this experiment were presented at the Society for Technology in Anesthesia Meeting in Tuscon, Arizona, 1998[5].

3.3 The mobility of simulators

There are now a considerable variety of simulators on the commercial market[1]. Screen-based simulators are usually compact and easy to transport – either software on a CD or a laptop computer with the software installed. Some hardware-based simulators, such as Laerdal's SimMan [2] and Medical Education Technologies Inc. Emergency Care Simulator (METI-ECS®)[3], were designed to be portable, enabling trainers to take mannequin-based simulation out to the workplace. These models post-dated the higher fidelity systems, such as the Eagle simulator[4] or METI's Human Patient Simulator (METI-HPS®)[3], which were designed to remain in one place or be moved only rarely. The development of more portable, and often cheaper, systems reflected the need of the user community. Those wishing to develop simulation programmes were often without the luxury of adequate budgets or dedicated simulation centres. Cheaper systems, that could easily be unpacked and used in the workplace, and put away and stored later, seemed an ideal solution. Furthermore, healthcare workers based in the field (paramedics, firecrew and the military) were as interested in simulation and its potential for training as those based in a hospital setting. For these groups, a portable system was essential if scenarios were to recreate working situations.

Portability has previously been associated with loss of simulator sophistication. For example a simulator such as the Anaesthesia Computer Controlled Emergency Situation Simulator (ACCESS®)[6], is easy to pack and move and take to any classroom or clinical situation. It is a hardware-based, script driven simulator and consists of a Laerdal airway mannequin, with some airway modifications, and a separate computer and screen. There are no cables linking the scripted computer to the mannequin and no driving gases – hence its simplicity. While it can be defined as a simulator capable of teaching psychomotor and cognitive skills[1], the manner in which it can be used for such purpose is only as good as the teacher's ability to manage the scenario, the student's ability to suspend disbelief and the environment in which it is used.

At the other extreme, the hardware-based model driven simulator HPS, enables the teacher to design scenarios that are far more realistic and demanding of the student. The mannequin, driving computer and stack system are heavy and cumbersome and include hundreds of cables and connections between the stack, computer and mannequin. The system is simply not designed to be portable. The system is designed to look like a human and reproduce sophisticated physiological responses to drugs and interventions and thus enable development of realistic clinical scenarios. To achieve this aim, early simulators were completely static and took up considerable space. Later systems are more compact but still bulky, and moving these systems can be fraught with problems.

The development of SimMan® and METI-ECS® brought both portability and some degree of sophistication. Both systems can be packed up and transported to a new site for a teaching session with relative ease. As such, both systems can be considered mobile. Thus it is easy to take SimMan® to a Recovery Ward or METI-ECS® into a real operating theatre for a teaching session. The scenarios used should take into consideration the limitations of each model. They are not necessarily translatable. In other words what works well on one simulator, can be a disaster on another! For example, SimMan® has no pharmacological modelling so using this for a complex cardiovascular scenario is not easy (but not impossible), whereas METI-ECS® does have cardiovascular modelling, making it ideal for complex ACLS scenarios. SimMan® has a straightforward airway for bag and mask ventilation and affords a Grade 1 intubation in normal working mode. METI-ECS® is harder to bag mask ventilate and the intubation is graded 'difficult' depending on the experience of the user. Thus it is more sensible to use SimMan® rather than METI-ECS® for scenarios that focus around airway issues.

Not all simulator users have access to multiple simulators, and choosing a simulator to best suit the teaching requirements needs to be well planned and considered before money is spent. Newer portable systems are now coming on to the market that may offer good value for money.

HAL®[7,8] is a mannequin-based, script-driven simulator. Outwardly similar to SimMan®, its launch onto the market was met with enthusiasm by user community as it offered similar teaching potential to SimMan but with improved portability; the compressor was built into the leg of the simulator and a wireless control laptop meant the simulator could be controlled up to 300 metres away. Sadly, at BMSC geographically located in the south of England the technical support we required from the host company located in Florida, USA, was unsatisfactory for our needs as a UK user. This is a salutary lesson to all simulator users, new or experienced, that ongoing technical support and guidance is essential before purchasing any new piece of equipment (the author takes all responsibility for the decision making in this example!).

New to the market in February 2007 is iStan® launched by METI. This simulator may address many of the shortcomings of other portable simulators linking model driven simulation with wireless control. (The author has no experience of this system.)

As a rule of thumb it is always easier to work within a dedicated centre designed to run simulator equipment. The reasons are logical. Such an area can be designed and maintained for the purpose of simulation training with dedicated staff to run it. Back-up simulators or teaching aids are readily available to staff should they be required at short notice. Maintenance equipment is on hand. Running simulations is never entirely straightforward, and good preparation and anticipation of the unexpected is always essential. This is even more important when attempting to work offsite.

3.3.1 Moving equipment onsite

If a centre is designed to run simulators in different rooms it should be possible to minimize the problems of moving equipment from one room to another. At BMSC three locations were designed to run the METI-HPS®. This equipment, like any of the larger lifelike simulators, is heavy and cumbersome, and staff needed to be trained in manual handling. Damage can easily happen in transfers. Common problems are cable disconnections, evulsion of tubing or wires and reconnection mistakes. Problems usually occur because staff forget or fail to use checklists to test the simulator after movement. It is advisable to power up any simulator after it has been moved and dummy run a scenario.

3.3.2 Moving equipment offsite

Whatever the simulator, such endeavours need to be run like a military operation if they are to be successful. Over the years BMSC has taken low fidelity and mid fidelity simulators to hospitals, walk-in centres, cottage hospitals, church halls, A&E departments, exhibition halls and hotels, as well as setting scenarios in the back of an ambulance. The most difficult environments to work in are exhibition halls or hotels because they are so unclinical. If you are asked to run scenarios in such areas it is advisable to ask the simulator manufacturer to set up the equipment, bring props and run the scenarios, because they are expert at it

Here is a checklist of considerations before simulating offsite; remember to start planning weeks or months ahead.

- Identify the team. Make sure that there is a leader and enough staff with the skills to move, set-up, run and teach a simulation.
- Ensure the team members can communicate with each other on the move and at the destination (use either radio headsets or mobile phones). Make sure that there are contact numbers and names for the destination.
- Take money or credit cards for food petrol and unexpected events.
- Label all the equipment so that it is owner-identified for return.
- Use a list to check equipment in and out. Design this in sections:
  - mannequin
  - driving equipment (e.g. gas cylinders, compressors, lap tops, extension cables)

- props
- paperwork
- teaching aids

◆ Ideally visit the area first. Plan where to park, how to offload and whether there are appropriate ramps or lift access.

◆ Charge all battery operated (or backed up) equipment from the night before transfer. Electrical connections, lack of extension cables and sockets are the biggest problem. Remember to check if the simulator has USA configuration, in which case you will need a transformer.

◆ If planning to leave equipment overnight, make sure there is appropriate security.

◆ Check insurance details – of yourselves and of the equipment for damage.

◆ Consider the vehicle for transfer. An ambulance is ideal; small lorries may require special driving licences and may be difficult to lift gear in and out.

3.4 Transporting equipment

Small simulators or larger ones that can be broken down into small lightweight parts can be transferred in any vehicle large enough to accommodate all the pieces. However, this means time is required to disassemble and reassemble the kit and there is more likelihood of technical problems because of this. Larger simulators can be professionally packaged and sent by carrier, but this brings the inconvenience of relying on other companies.

An ambulance makes the perfect vehicle for transferring simulators. Simulators can be loaded onto purpose built emergency vehicle trolleys. These are specifically designed to go up or down to the appropriate height for entrance or exit of the vehicle. Lifting equipment on an ordinary patient trolley is very heavy and would require a vehicle with a tailgate mechanism.

3.4.1 An ambulance as a vehicle for simulator transport

In 2003 BMSC purchased a decommissioned square bodied, Chevrolet ambulance for £2000 sterling. This came with an intact interior, an ambulance trolley, and working sound and lights. All labelling (determining it as a working ambulance) had been removed.

There is a good secondhand market for ambulances in the UK. The local ambulance Trust may have vehicles that they wish to sell. These are available through private sale or through car/vehicle auction. Once acquired the vehicle requires regular maintenance (Ministry of Transport inspection, and servicing), taxing and insurance.

BMSC developed a business plan for the purchase of the ambulance that included use of the vehicle for transporting simulators offsite and specific ambulance scenarios. Before embarking on such a purchase the following considerations should be made:

◆ Establish how the vehicle will be insured: no regular insurance company in the UK will undertake vehicle insurance for transfer of medical equipment and training. (The local hospital to which BMSC is affiliated undertook this role for us.)

◆ Establish that there are staff members whose driving licence allows them to drive an ambulance. Newer British licenses do not allow for this. Staff would then have to undertake an HGV license course, which is expensive. (All staff driving the vehicle were named to the Trust for insurance purposes.)

◆ Establish that there is a local garage that will maintain the vehicle. (A Chevrolet ambulance is American in origin and some garages would not undertake this work.)

- Establish links with the local paramedics to help with general maintenance and input to design of scenarios.
- Work out a business plan to cover running costs each year.

3.5 Mobile scenarios

Scenarios that work well onsite may be a disaster offsite. Working in a nonclinical hostile environment is a real challenge. The pressures associated with this are only heightened when customers want value for money. In choosing or designing a scenario the following steps should be considered:

1 Establish the teaching aims for the session.

2 Design a scenario.

3 Evaluate which simulator is best to provide this; you must know the strengths and limitations of each simulator. Scenarios are not translatable between simulators.

4 Consider if the simulator can be moved to the planned environment (if not reconsider 1, 2 and 3).

5 Review the additional props required. If needed, assess whether these can be run offsite.

6 Plan emergency action (if equipment fails).

Keep the scenarios simple. A bad demonstration will lose you credibility and potentially upset the delegates. Without a simulation suite it is extremely difficult to run a simulator discreetly. Full operating theatre scenarios fail by being too ambitious and are a route to failure. It is often best to adopt the tutorial format or undertake a 'static' scenario where the status of the patient does not change much during the course of the scenario. An example of a static scenario would be a patient with abnormal physiology (tachycardia, hypotension, tachypnoea) requiring assessment and stabilization before an operation. The trainee would be expected to assess through communication and examination the status of the patient and instigate basic treatment and investigations.

Ultimate mobility consists of designing and running scenarios on the move (e.g. transferring a patient between hospitals). None of the simulators on the market have been capable of *easily* sustaining a sophisticated simulation while being actively moved in and out of rooms or vehicles (at the time of writing iStan® has not been evaluated by the author). Limitations resulting from the weight and size of kit, or electrical or gas supplies, are the cause of such restrictions. HAL® [7] is marketed with wireless control, in theory allowing the trainer to control the simulator from as far away as 300 metres. Despite considerable effort BMSC was unable to make this function work reliably. Such an ability would be extremely useful, enabling users to develop scenarios where the simulator can be freed of all cables and moved while the scenario continues to function and the monitors continue to show physiological parameters. This would open up a whole host of new training opportunities for medical staff involved in the repatriation or transfer of patients.

Currently at BMSC trainers design scenarios that cover aspects of patient transfer up to the point of moving a patient. If the trainer wishes to take the scenario further they have to consider the limitations of the specific simulator they are using.

For example, Table 3.1 refers to the staging and teaching aims of a SimMan® scenario. This scenario is used for teaching inexperienced anaesthetists how to stabilize and package a patient with an acute head injury for transfer to another hospital. The scenario is designed to be run on SimMan® rather than METI-ECS® because the simulator has an easier airway (the scenario requires the patient to be intubated by the student) and is smaller and lighter to move on a trolley.

Table 3.1 Example of an acute head injury scenario using SimMan®

Simulation	Head injury
Type of simulator	◆ SimMan® in ward area ◆ Run off compressor ◆ On movable trolley
Faculty required	◆ SimMan® controller ◆ Observer/debriefer
Scenario information	◆ 20-year-old male ◆ Assaulted in the early hours of the morning ◆ Paramedics called by friends because patient started to talk 'funny' ◆ Closed head injury with variable consciousness
	At scene: ◆ Treated by paramedics: collar, oxygen IV access ◆ Brought to A&E
	In A&E: ◆ Vitals reviewed (same). N/Saline started. C-spine/neck and pelvis clear. Bloods sent. ◆ D/W neuro unit between A&E consultant and Unit – need for anaesthetist to come and take patient for urgent scan and admit for Obs in unit
Staging	◆ On trolley, neck collar, oxygen through HM blood on head (i.e. look like head injury) ◆ IV access and drip attached (N/Saline), ◆ Anaesthetic trolley, whiteboard and pens ◆ A&E chart filled in, anaesthetic chart available (oxylog ventilator and O_2 cylinder available) ◆ Compressor for SimMan® ◆ Movable trolley
Learning outcomes	◆ By the end of the scenario the participants will have stabilized the patient, packaged and moved him out of the building and down the street and back

Simulation settings – settings altered 'on the fly' in response to trainee interventions

	RR	O₂ Sat	CO₂	HR	ABP/ NIBP	GCS	Temp	Sounds	Other
Start	9	94		90	160/85	8–9 eyes open to pain = 2 sounds only = 2 or nothing = 1 localizes to pain	37.0	Bilateral vesicular	

Debrief

◆ Remember A,B,C,D,E assessment
◆ GCS assessment, decision to intubate
◆ Stabilize: GA with RSI
◆ Package
◆ Did they have any problems on transfer?

Part of the scenario is designed to show the problems of moving patients up and down corridors or into a lift. When using SimMan® all monitoring is lost once the electricity supply is disconnected. The air compressor requires electricity, and chest movement and pulses are lost to the mannequin unless it can be replaced. This requires a portable air cylinder with appropriate cabling and fittings, and should be easy to remedy.

To address the loss of monitoring, the teacher has two different options.

Option one An extension cable would provide electricity supply for movement along the horizontal for both the monitor and compressor. However, the distance that can be moved is limited to the length of the extension cable and does not allow movement into a lift.

Option two The teacher can do away with the monitor, control computer, chest movement and pulses, and continue to tell the students the physiological parameters, but fidelity is lost.

These issues will continue to plague the fidelity of scenarios. By advanced consideration and careful scenario design the teaching aims can be achieved despite these drawbacks. Here is a summary of BMSC recommendations for mobile scenarios.

- ◆ What works:
  - Practical demonstrations (e.g. new equipment such as airway devices)
  - Drug demonstrations, especially if they can be linked to complimentary screen based simulations (e.g. gas inhalation and uptake display GasMan® [8])
  - Basic scenarios based on non-changing physiology (e.g. communication or physiological assessment)
  - Basic or intermediate life support type scenarios
  - Tutorials on running or maintaining simulators
  - Scenario design
- ◆ What doesn't work:
  - Full theatre or anaesthetic scenarios requiring anaesthetic machines (unless in a clinical environment)
  - Complex scenarios with rapidly changing physiology
  - Scenarios on the move

3.6 **Conclusions**

The staff at BMSC gained experience in moving simulators the hard way through trial and error. At times this was damaging to our business when scenarios failed or when delegates were unimpressed. Moving simulators onsite is not without problem, and taking simulators out to new audiences is a challenge and can be both good fun and rewarding. It is hoped that this chapter is of practical help.

The ultimate in mobility comes from groups who have conquered using simulators in unusual situations. The military have used them in the field teaching and preparing primary and ancillary medical staff to prepare for triage, resuscitation, and management of injured patients in war zones. Other groups have taken them in the air in helicopters or fixed wing planes. Perhaps the most testing and dramatic experience has been the use of simulation to teach astronauts how to deal with medical emergencies in the weightless environment of simulated space[9].

References

1. Cumin and Merry (2007). Simulators for use in anaesthesia. *Anaesthesia* **62**: 151–62.
2. Laerdal: http://www.laerdal.com

3. METI: http://www.meti.com

4. Cooper JB, Taqueti VR (2004). A brief history of the development of mannequin simulators for clinical education and training. *Quality and Safety in Health Care* **13**: 11–18.

5. Raemer DB, Maviglia S, Van Horne C, Stone P (1998). Mock codes: using realistic simulation to teach team resuscitation management. Presented at *The Society of Technology in Anesthesia Conference*, Tuscon, Arizona.

6. Byrne AJ, Hilton PJ, Lunn JN (1994). Basic simulations for anaesthetists. A pilot study of the ACCESS system. *Anaesthesia* **49**: 376–81.

7. Gaumard: http://www.gaumard.com

8. GasMan: http://www.gasmanweb.com

9. Doerr H, Murray B, Cuttino M, Borderick TJ (2006) Training astronauts to manage trauma (emergencies): Integrating Human Patient Simulations into medical operations for national aeronautics and space administration (NASA) ITACCS **16**(1): 26–30.

Part 2

Simulators, training aids, and equipment

Chapter 4

Lessons from aviation simulation

Ray Page

Overview

- Flight simulation is now an integral part of all airline operations providing training that can no longer be carried out effectively or safely in the actual aircraft.
- Aviation experience with the development and use of simulation now dates back almost one hundred years and has resulted in the credibility and acceptance of simulation for training and testing.
- The success of flight simulation has resulted from the establishment of standards for data, design, modelling, performance, and testing, with international agreement for accreditation at defined levels of fidelity.
- Training analysis is an essential element in the decision of the fidelity level of any simulation device, along with a training programme for its use.
- Transfer of knowledge from the simulator must apply to the real aircraft without any modification or excuse.
- Simulation is a science in its own right with recognized problem areas, which must be addressed and tested in any simulator design or application.
- Accreditation testing to a specified standard or level is essential in guaranteeing that standards are achieved and then maintained through a scheduled retesting programme.
- In the aviation industry, enforcement of simulation standards has come through regulation; however, the actual standards were developed by the industry and not through regulation.

4.1 Introduction

Simulation is now a multi-million dollar industry with applications spread over a vast number of training and analytical areas. While those involved with simulation readily identify its origins from the flight simulator, there is little concept of the efforts made by the world airlines to introduce standards and testing criteria, which provided the credibility and acceptance for the use of simulation as a training tool.

The technology now available for the simulation task is unbelievable by comparison to that of the past. Many of the early problems such as data, modelling and standards, which plagued the flight simulator from its inception, are now evident in other domains using simulation for training. Also, the science of simulation has evolved and many lessons were learned along the way. In order to produce quality simulation for training and testing it is essential that new simulation design engineers have an understanding of this science and not just the academic knowledge of what is being simulated.

Those who wish to use simulation as a source of training, testing or regulation would therefore be well advised to have some understanding of the lessons learned by the aviation industry in order to establish their own standards and specifications. Also, the design, construction and level of fidelity requirements for the task of simulation training, and especially for the need of testing and accrediting such devices, should be appreciated.

4.2 **History of flight training devices**

The history of flight training devices is an enormous subject and therefore it is only possible to skim briefly through some of the better known devices to illustrate the development from manual assisted trainers to automation with man-in-the-loop-training. Advances in technology, from levers and springs to analogue and digital computation, the addition of features such as motion and visual systems, have led to the modern flight simulator (Fig. 4.1).

Each of these developments advanced the training ability of the flight simulator though in turn often producing new sets of problems, which had to be addressed and overcome. The end result is that the aviation industry was provided with a unique comprehensive training in the developing science of simulation. It was from this experience that the world's airlines united to establish standards and testing criteria, which have an application to all simulator-training devices.

Many of the very early devices attempted to achieve simulation for testing new aircraft prototypes by using actual aircraft supported by balloons, overhead gantries or railway bogies. Related to these ideas were the first proposals for truly ground based trainers, which in effect were aircraft tethered to the ground but capable of responding to some aerodynamic forces.

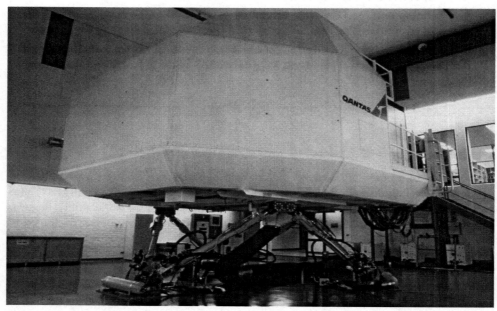

Fig. 4.1 A modern flight simulator. Estimated value is $US 25 million.

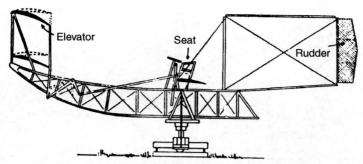

Fig. 4.2 The Sanders Teacher. (Presented at the *50 Years of Simulation* conference, Royal Aero Society, London, 1979).

4.2.1 **The Sanders teacher**

One such device was the Sanders Teacher [1], which the 1910 December issue of *Flight* stated: 'The invention therefore of a device which will enable the novice to obtain a clear conception of the workings of an aeroplane and conditions existent in the air without any risk personally or otherwise is to be welcomed without doubt. Several have already been tested and the Sander's Teacher is the latest to enter the field.'

The Sander's Teacher (Fig. 4.2) was constructed from actual aircraft components and in reality became an aircraft mounted on a universal joint and installed in an exposed position facing into the prevailing wind. While this type of trainer did not require any manual assistance, it did rely on the prevailing wind for simulation. Unfortunately many of these devices were not successful because of the unreliable and irregular nature of the wind. It is interesting that these properties of the wind drove the requirements for increased fidelity some 60 years later so that complete crosswind training could be carried out successfully in the modern flight simulator. One example of an application of the principle of the Sanders Teacher was that of the Eardley Billing type trainer as shown in Fig. 4.3.

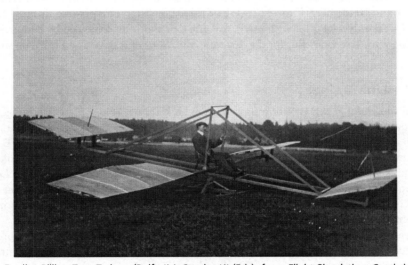

Fig. 4.3 Eardley Billing Type Trainer. (Rolfe JM, Staples KJ (Eds), from *Flight Simulation*, Cambridge Press, 1988. Reproduced with permission of Flight International.)

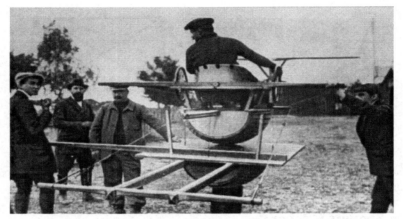

Fig. 4.4 The Antoinette Trainer. (Rolfe JM, Staples KJ (Eds), from *Flight Simulation*, Cambridge Press, 1988. Reproduced with permission of Flight International.)

4.2.2 **The Antoinette trainer**

Also in this period was the first truly synthetic flight training device, which was advertised in a 1910 Antoinette Catalogue (Fig. 4.4). This consisted of two half sections of a barrel mounted and moved manually by training assistants so as to represent the pitch and roll of the aircraft. The prospective pilot sat in the top half section and was required to control the device in order to line up a reference-bar with the horizon.

The next step in the evolution of the flight trainer was the replacement of the human assistants with mechanical or electrical actuators linked to the trainer's controls. The aim of these now automatic devices was to rotate the trainee pilot's fuselage into an attitude corresponding to that of the real aircraft in response to the trainee's inputs. Provision was usually made for an instructor to introduce disturbances in attitude to simulate the effects of rough air and to introduce control problems to the student. One example of this technique was a family of devices described by Lender and Heidelberg[2] in 1917. One of these consisted of a pivoted dummy fuselage mounted on a universal joint with pitch, roll and yaw motions produced by compressed air motors and introduced, possibly for the first time, variations of response and feel with simulated speed.

4.2.3 **The Link Trainer**

The most successful of this type of trainer was the Link Trainer (Fig. 4.5), which is regarded as the foundation of flight simulation. Edwin Link gained his early engineering experience with his father's firm 'The Link Piano and Organ Company of Binghamton New York'. In fact, Ed Link's first patent was granted for an improvement in the mechanism for player pianos. Ed Link was an intrepid pilot and his trainer was developed in the period 1927–9 in the basement of the Link factory using some of the pneumatic mechanisms from player pianos. The first Link Trainer[3] was patented in 1930 and advertised as 'An efficient aeronautical training aid and a novel, profitable amusement device.' An electrical driven suction pump mounted in the fixed base fed the various control valves operated by the stick and rudder, while another motor driven device produced a sequence of attitude disturbances. This trainer turned through 360° and was the first fully automatic device though in common with all trainers of the day was adjusted by trial and error until the 'correct feel' was obtained.

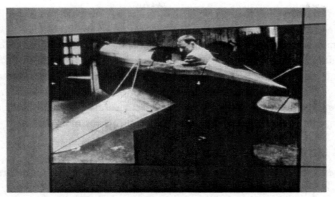

Fig. 4.5 The Link Trainer. (Rolfe JM, Staples KJ (Eds), from *Flight Simulation*, Cambridge Press, 1988. Reproduced with permission of Flight International.)

However, despite 20 years of inventiveness, synthetic trainers had not caught on and simulation was not seen as a realistic substitute for actual flight training, and acceptance of simulated flight had to wait for further developments in the science of simulation. What is significant, however, is that Ed Link[4] became known as 'the father of flight simulation' and went on to establish the Link Company which, over the next 60 years became the world's largest simulator manufacturer. It was a pioneer in most forms of simulation development, both commercial and military (including the development of an anaesthesia simulation device), as well as all of the simulators used in the NASA space programme. Unfortunately the Singer-Link company was the victim of a massive corporate raid in the 1990s, broken up and sold off piece by piece.

4.2.4 Simulated instrument training

In the late 1920s a new stream of development began as the need became recognized for effective training of pilots in the skills of blind-flying or instrument flying, and existing trainers were fitted with simulated navigation instruments. Blind-flying training was started by Link in the early 1930s and when the importance of this type of training was recognized by the US Army Corps, a contract was awarded to carry the US mail. This was the start of recognition of simulation for pilot training. The 1930s were indeed the years of the Link Trainer and this device was produced in many versions and sold to countries such as Australia, England, Japan, France, Germany and the USSR.

4.2.5 World war II

In the early stages of World War II the need arose for the training of a very large number of pilots involved in the operation of a variety of military aircraft with all basic pilot training being performed in part on Link Trainers. Developments in aircraft design such as variable pitch propellers, retractable undercarriages and higher speeds made training in cockpit drill essential and complete fuselage mock-ups were introduced.

4.2.6 Analogue simulation

The major advances in electronics during World War II and the development of the analogue computer now made the technology available to solve the flight equations of the aircraft allowing the simulation of the response to aerodynamic forces rather than empirical duplication of their effects. In the period following the war the first generation of analogue devices were developed, though many contained both forms of simulation. Some trainers were indeed true analogues and these were certainly the direct ancestors of the modern flight simulator. One of the major limitations to this time had been the lack of accurate flight and engine performance data, and manufacturers were committed to *ad hoc* methods to obtain desired performance. This began to change with the large post-war subsonic jet transport aircraft, where airframe manufacturers began producing more complete data and improved flight performance testing.

4.2.7 **Digital simulation**

Despite improved hardware design, the reliability of the large analogue simulators failed to meet training demands. These computers were also difficult to maintain and extremely costly to modify, reducing the potential for increased fidelity for flight simulation. In the early 1960s there were now a number of manufacturers attempting to develop digital simulation and many hybrid devices were introduced that also proved unreliable. During this period Link, now Singer-Link, developed the Mark 1, which used three parallel processors for arithmetic, function generation and navigation and radiostation selection. This was a major breakthrough, and simulators using this system were purchased by most of the major world airlines and a very large quantity for the US Military. These early digital computing devices went through a number of development stages though speed of computation and storage capacity were major limiting factors in the fidelity of simulation able to be provided.

By the 1970s general purpose computers had improved to the extent that some could now be considered for flight simulation, and from this time onwards computer selection became a major issue for each simulator manufacturer. Not all these decisions resulted in good simulation and many lessons were learned in terms of resolution, speed, and capacity requirements.

4.2.8 **Motion systems**

Apart from the very rudimentary motion system of the early Link trainers, flight simulators up to the mid 1950s had no fuselage motion systems. This was often justified by statements that pilots no longer flew 'by the seat of their pants'; however, the fact remained that the simulators did not feel completely like the aircraft they simulated. It was found that some improvements could be introduced by empirical adjustment of the simulator control-loading and aircraft dynamics, which gave some compensation for the lack of motion.

In 1958 simulator manufacturer Redifon produced a single axis pitch motion system under contract for a BOAC (British Overseas Aircraft Corporation, now British Airways) Comet IV simulator. More complex motion systems followed with two, three, four, five and finally six axes, which was by then considered essential to provide the lateral acceleration required for aircraft such as the Boeing B747. A great deal of research on motion systems has been carried out by NASA, and the landing of the Lunar Landing Module, for example, presented an unusual challenge that required extensive simulation training.

4.2.9 **Visual systems**

Visual Systems, providing out-of-the-window visual scenery had been proposed and constructed since the inception of the flight trainer. Some of the early Link trainers were mounted inside a panoramic display to give the illusion of flying high. It is well beyond the scope of this chapter to even attempt to discuss the numerous concepts for visual systems that have been tried over the history of the flight simulator, and therefore only a few of the more successfulwill be discussed here.

The light-point source projection or shadowgraph method enjoyed some popularity in the 1950s. However, shortcomings of the shadowgraph seem to have limited the success of this system. During this period another method of visual presentation was developed using film and an anamorphic optical system known as visual anamorphic optical system (VAMP), which produced a good quality picture but was limited by the inability to fly outside the area of interest contained on the filmstrip.

Closed-circuit television (CCTV) systems followed, where the scene was constructed on a moving belt and viewed by a camera through an optical probe, which allowed for pitch, roll and rotation then to be projected onto a flat screen mounted in front of the flight simulator cockpit. Large rigid models subsequently replaced the belt, where the camera moved over a terrain, which was now capable of containing models of actual towns and country with lighting for night-time simulation. These systems usually operated with a scale factor of 2000:1 and remained in service well into the 1970s.

The first computer-generated image (CGI) systems for simulation were produced by General Electric (USA) for the space programme. Progress in this field was rapid and closely linked to developments in digital computer hardware, with a parallel development taking place using calligraphic or stroke writing rather than raster scan, which enabled a superior reproduction of light points for runway lighting. All of these systems were displayed on a picture tube and viewed through a beam splitter from a mirror mounted in front of the display. While the quality of the displays was quite acceptable there were limits to the size of the scene able to be produced, and displays were mounted in juxtaposed locations in an attempt to improve the field of view.

The final development, which is still in operation on modern flight simulators, moved to a projected picture produced on a curved screen to allow continuous viewing in excess of 180°, thereby allowing training for a circling approach. In addition, the quality and content of the displayed picture improved, as well as modelling techniques that provided photo texture, allowing actual route familiarization to be accomplished in the flight simulator.

4.3 Flight simulator standards

From the evolution of the flight simulator it can be seen that at every stage of development technology was both a driving force and a limiting factor. However, these successes, as well as the failures, led to an understanding of a new science of simulation along with its philosophy for training.

In the beginning there were no standards and each simulator manufacturer produced what they believed was desirable for the airlines training needs and it would be no exaggeration to state that no two flight simulators from the same manufacturer, representing the same aircraft, performed or felt the same. This resulted from the complete lack of standards for data and performance as well as lack of objective acceptance testing criteria, leaving each simulator to be 'tuned' subjectively to please the pilots accepting the flight simulator.

Airlines bought flight simulators in good faith and then found they had great difficulty maintaining some standard that had never been defined. Their acceptance was based only on subjective pilot assessment. This situation also did little for pilot confidence in flight simulation or provided any incentive for the regulating authorities to grant training credits for the use of the flight simulator instead of the aircraft.

4.3.1 International Airline Flight Simulator Technical Association

In the early 1970s the simulator engineering organizations of a small number of the world's airlines joined together to form an association to be known as International Airline Flight Simulator Technical Association (IAFSTA), and several meetings were held to which the simulator manufacturers of the day were also invited. These meetings were an open forum discussion on problems experienced with both flight simulators and their respective manufacturers. Several of the simulator manufacturers at that time did not react kindly to public criticism and there were suggestions of legal challenges. IAFSTA had no legal protection for its members and the airlines looked to International Air Transport Association (IATA) to form a flight simulator technical committee under the umbrella of this organization. In October 1973 the first meeting of the IATA Flight Simulator Technical Committee (FSTC) was held in Denver, USA.

4.3.2 IATA FSTC

This organization now set about the task of forming working groups to examine what was needed to establish standards for constructing, testing and accrediting flight simulators. These working groups invited participation from simulator, airframe and avionics manufacturers and a new wave of cooperation was established to develop standards for data and performance requirements to be used in the construction and testing of flight simulators. This resulted in the publication of an official IATA document *Flight Simulator Design and Performance Data Requirements*, which then formed a contractual part of all airlines specification of requirement in the construction and acceptance of their flight simulators. This process was achieved with considerable effort by a small dedicated group from the airline industry with many traumas and confrontations, resulting in numerous closed sessions along the way.

What was extremely difficult for the airframe manufacturers to appreciate was that the data requirements for high fidelity simulation required flight data collection at a level of accuracy and content far greater than that required for the certification of the actual aircraft. In this regard Boeing must be credited for their foresight and cooperation in providing data packages for their aircraft. A QANTAS Airways simulator engineer who actually controlled the aircraft flight tests was nominated by the FSTC to collect these data for the Boeing B747–400.

4.4 Regulation

The whole of the aviation industry is highly regulated and as a basic element of flight safety, aircrew training and the use of simulation is included in these regulations. Once standards had been established, the regulatory authority in the USA, known as the Federal Aviation Authority (FAA), gave approval for credits from the flight simulator to replace aircraft training, following a proposal by the FSTC. The FAA agreed to an incentive programme with the landing credit being the initial goal. This was the start of a long process of driving technology and testing to achieve 'zero flight time', which is the ability to use the flight simulator as a total replacement for pilot training and testing.

In 1992 agreement was reached to produce the International Civil Aviation Organisation (ICAO) *Manual of Criteria for the Qualification of Flight Simulators*, which now forms the basis of most nations' regulations. These regulations cover the testing for the level of use and dictate ongoing maintenance and support requirements, including approvals for all modifications as well as retesting. This guarantees the ongoing fidelity of any approved flight simulator.

4.5 Fidelity

Flight simulation is the process of reproducing the task of flying in the real world to one in a safe, ground-based environment. The degree to which the real world is reproduced or simulated is known as the fidelity of simulation.

The flight simulator is a pilot-in-the-loop device, which relies on a number of components to produce a complexity of stimuli to which the pilot must react and learn to respond. Learning takes place through regular practice. Practice is the process of performing specific cognitive or psychomotor activities in response to stimuli indicating the need for such actions.

The level of fidelity can be described where all relevant stimuli are made available for recognition and practice and where such stimuli change realistically with variations in the inputs and responses to and from the pilot.

Also, recognition of those stimuli, which are not relevant to the task, is an equally important aspect of the learning process.

Specification of these components and the tolerances required for their performance have been established by standards defining the levels for which accreditation and approvals are available from regulatory authorities. These levels in turn relate to the training permitted to be carried out in the referenced flight simulator device based on the fidelity of simulation available.

Hence, the fidelity of any simulation device is limited by the weakest component producing stimuli. This may be the flight data or it's implementation, flight controls, motion, visual systems or even the sound system where pilot reaction may be alerted through subcognitive recognition. When we discuss how much fidelity is enough or cost trade-offs, we must be mindful of the consequences of not properly accomplishing the mission. Transfer of training is the major issue and the same knowledge learned in the flight simulator must apply to the real aircraft without modification or excuse.

While the use of flight simulation has provided huge cost savings to airline operations, the use of high technology solutions to provide the high fidelity simulation has in turn resulted in higher costs in procurement and ongoing support. In our current, cost-conscious environment this has raised questions regarding levels of fidelity currently demanded and considerable pressure to get more credits for reduced fidelity. As a classic example to produce cost savings, the necessity for motion systems was challenged in the early 1990s, and references made to studies carried out in the 1980s that suggested that no incremental training benefit was produced by the use of motion.

Unfortunatel,y these studies involved the use of earlier generation hardware and software that was not only limited in performance but also possibly even producing negative training cues, which was an unfortunate aspect of some early motion systems. The Rand Report commissioned by the US Air Force likewise dismissed these studies as well as the Gilliom Report commissioned by the FAA, both fully supporting the use of motion systems for flight simulation. In the late 1990s this subject was again raised in respect of the high cost for Regional Carriers to have to use motion based flight simulators for training. This resulted in a further study and a report published in the *International Journal of Aviation Psychology*[5], which concluded that no definitive conclusion could be drawn to warrant any modification to the current regulations that required the use of motion based flight simulators.

4.6 **Motion systems**

Virtually all cueing in flight simulators relates directly or indirectly to representing the motion of the aircraft, and just as when walking, riding or driving, we maintain our inertial orientation through a number of sensory systems. Each system is tuned to a different facet of the motion environment and makes its own contribution to the orientation process.

The eyes are without doubt the most important motion sensing system. They do not operate in isolation from the other sensors and while they provide the most accurate information, they operate at a slower rate than the other sensors. This was highlighted in a study by De Berg *et al.*[6] on engine failures with Boeing KC-135 aircraft. When an outboard engine fails with this aircraft on takeoff, it yaws. This produces obvious cues on the flight deck instrumentation, as well as with the visual scene. However, the time lapse for detecting and interpreting these cues in isolation without motion does not allow for correction of the yaw before the aircraft leaves the runway.

In some situations the visual cues are so strong and important that experienced pilots may be able to ignore all other information. For example, when a pilot is exposed to unusual circumstances, such as wind shears and system failures, in the absence of prior aircraft exposure or experience, the entire spectrum of cues is vital for maintaining control and for training in the unique characteristics of the situation or the aircraft being simulated.

While the visual receptors can provide highly accurate motion information, they require more time to generate useful control information than the other sensors.

In essence the visual system senses rates of motion by accumulating information from a number of scans. When response time is not critical and good visual information is available, flight control by visual reference only can be timely and accurate. However, when response time requirements are more demanding than the visual scanning capability, other more rapidly processed motion information is required.

The relationship between visual and motion sensory systems is illustrated in the findings of Young[7] who determined that tracking with only visual inputs was quite accurate at display frequencies below 1 Hz. When motion stimuli were provided to the vestibular and neck muscle sensors though, the tracking capability of the eye was raised to 2.5 Hz.

4.6.1 Skin and muscle sensors

In 1972 Gum[8] modelled the skin and muscle receptors and concluded that information from these receptors provided motion information to the central nervous system more rapidly than the vestibular receptors, as well as providing signals to the eyes to stabilize them in space. In evaluations[9] of the US Air Force Simulator Air-to-Air Combat Simulator (SAAC) it was found that using a compartmented, dynamic g-sensitive seat, which simulated the skin pressures associated with motion, the F-4 pilot's ability to perform overhead manoeuvres and tracking target aircraft was so greatly improved that it was almost as accurate as with the actual aircraft. The conclusion was that the simulation of skin pressure greatly simplified the use of the visual cues in this high performance situation.

4.6.3 Vestibular system

The non-auditory sensors in the inner ear do not respond to motion but to the accelerations associated with angular and linear motion. They are extremely sensitive and respond significantly faster than the visual sensors, as they do not require any interpretation of sequential events or information scans.

Meiry[10] modelled the visual, vestibular and neck muscle sensory systems and concluded that a major function of the non-visual motion sensors is to maintain the eyes stationary with reference to the visual object being tracked. Dichgans and Brandt [11] investigated a relationship between the vestibular and visual sensory systems where a sense of motion is perceived in a fixed base simulator by moving visual stimuli, which explains commonly experienced vertigo in this type of training situation.

4.6.3 Vertigo

Spatial disorientation and motion sickness like symptoms experienced in some simulators are now understood to result from pilot perception of discrepancies in the timing of patterns of information presented to those experienced in the aircraft under corresponding circumstances. While pilots are able to adapt to many discrepancies, complex neural interactions between visual and other sensory systems make the absence or delay of non-visual stimuli (motion) in the presence of strong visual cueing difficult to reconcile.

4.6.4 Latency

Latency, or throughput delay, are terms used to define any perceived time delay in aircraft response to pilot movement of flight controls. Without doubt any abnormal delay from pilot input to response from motion, visual scene, controls or instrumentation, has been a major cause of problems resulting in pilot-induced oscillation, where overreaction and control result from trying to anticipate the required response times. This was a major problem in the earlier digital simulators caused by inadequate computer processing speed and often inappropriate arrangement of computer programs. In addition, poor response times of the digital controls systems providing the actual feel to the pilots often resulted in delays, minute pulsing or shudder, which led to more rigid testing of flight simulators before any device can be certified for training.

4.7 Data

The most commonly accepted area for discussion relating to fidelity without doubt is data and the mathematical models used to provide accurate performance and characteristics of the aircraft being simulated. While in the past, data quality has been a problem, standards are now fully established that demand that these data be generated from actual aircraft flight tests with the scope and tolerances defined through the IATA document *Flight Simulator Design and Performance Requirements*.

4.8 Acceptance testing

The proof of simulator performance depends on a rigorous testing programme carried out before acceptance, where performance of both flight and systems are tested to the tolerances agreed in the Acceptance Test Guides. This usually commences with testing of all physical elements such as instrument and controls calibration and operation. An aircraft such as a Boeing B747 can usually be accepted by a flight crew in 2 days, whereas a flight simulator for this aircraft can take up to 10 weeks using both simulator engineers and pilots. Simulator performance and fidelity also relies on an operation free from any interruptions, such as computer 'glitches' or any problem that interferes with the reality of the training task being undertaken. This is usually verified following formal acceptance, where the simulator must then demonstrate continued reliability over a 90-day period in full training.

4.9 Training and skill learning

The long history of flight simulation has led to greater understanding of the learning process and its application to the training task. When considering the requirements of the fixation and automation stages of learning, it is easy to rationalize on the benefits of using the flight simulator *versus* the aircraft both in terms of safety and cost. It is also interesting to note that when the integration of these skills and responses within the whole task context is near completion, training may well be accomplished in a simulator incorporating only fragmentary cues needed to trigger the response to be integrated.

4.9.1 Transfer of training

The effectiveness of simulation is most graphically expressed in the terms of 'Transfer of Training', which is the degree to which practice in the simulator results in proficiency in the actual flight environment. This can be assessed readily where direct comparisons can be made for normal flight tasks. However, many of the flight situations in which simulation is of major benefit cannot be practised safely in actual flight, providing great difficulty in assessing transfer effectiveness through actual in-flight performance measurement.

4.9.2 Training analysis

Without doubt there has been some confusion in regard to the specification of flight simulation to meet training requirements. However, the need to carry out a training analysis is now well understood and has resulted in training programmes that use high fidelity flight simulators, lower level devices and even part task trainers, to provide the required training sequences and results.

The level to which a flight simulator is accredited is totally related to the complexity of the stimuli to which the pilot must learn to respond at a specific step or level in the training process. Lower level devices and part task trainers are economical and efficient in the development of skills, which may then be integrated in more advanced or complex trainers or simulators. Determination of the required stimuli, skill level/device relationship are crucial processes that require a complete understanding of the operational requirements as well as the optimum method of developing that skill through the discrete levels and their related value at each level.

4.10 Aircraft management

Beyond the skill learning process there exists the need to train pilots how to operate efficiently as a crew, how to assess and manage unusual and emergency situations, as well as the maximization of the resources available to them for decision-making under such circumstances. This crew training is carried out on commercial airlines by a procedure known as Line Oriented Flight Training (LOFT) and the management skills derived from the emergency training aspects are referred to as Cockpit Resource Management (CRM) and, more recently, as Crew Resource Management.

4.11 Conclusion

Flight simulation is now an integral part of all airline operations, providing training that can no longer be effectively or safely carried out in the actual aircraft. With experience gained from the aviation industry, simulation is now recognized as a science and is used in a broad spectrum of training applications.

This brief history of the development of flight simulation is intended to show how each step has harnessed the latest technology available, often producing its own unique set of problems, which in turn has provided an exceptional understanding of simulation for man-in-the-loop training. For those now involved in the task of simulation there should be an understanding of the problem areas identified, as these are not unique to aircraft simulation.

Without doubt the success of simulation in the aviation industry hasresulted from the establishment of standards for data, design, modelling, performance and testing with international agreement on standards for accreditation.

In conclusion, it must be understood that enforcement of these standards has come about through regulation. However, the actual standards were developed and established by the industry and not through regulatory agencies.

References

1. Haward DM (1910). The Sanders Teacher. *Flight* 2, **50**: 1006–7.
2. Lender M, Heidelberg P. British Patent 127,820 First Filed 1917; British Patent 158,522 First Filed 1917.

3. Link EA Jnr. US Patent 1,825,462 Filed 1930.

4. Kelly LL (1970). *The Pilot Maker*. Grosser & Dunlap, New York.

5. Burki-Cohen J, Soja NN, Longridge T. (1998). Simulator platform motion – The need revisited. *International Journal of Aviation Psychology* **8:** 293–317.

6. De Berg OH, McFarland BP, Showalter TW (1976). The effect of simulator fidelity on engine failure training in the KC-135 aircraft. Paper presented at the AIAA Visual and Motion Simulation Conference, Dayton, Ohio April 1976.

7. Young LR (1962). A sample data model for eye training movements. Doctoral Thesis Massachusetts Institute of Technology.

8. Gum DR (1972). Modelling of the human force and motion sensing mechanisms. Master's Thesis, The Ohio State University.

9. Stark EA (1976). Motion perception and terrain visual cues in air combat simulation. AIAA Visual and Motion Simulation Conference, Dayton Ohio, April 1976.

10. Meiry JL (1968). The vestibular system and human dynamic space orientation. NASA CR-628 1968.

11. Dichgans J, Brandt T (1972). Visual-vestibular interaction and motion perception. *Bibl Ophthalmol* **82:** 327–38.

Chapter 5

Medium and high integration mannequin patient simulators

Samsun (Sem) Lampotang

Overview

- Researchers in anaesthesia helped create the first generation (ca. 1969) and the second generation (ca. 1987, with support from the US Anesthesia Patient Safety Foundation) of mannequin patient simulators as well as the first screen-based patient simulators.

- As an emerging and rapidly growing field, simulation in healthcare has not yet standardized its terminology. As early as possible, standard terminology should be established and uniformly adopted, facilitating communication and collaboration between personnel from widely different backgrounds.

- The term 'mannequin patient simulator' is suggested to distinguish simulators based on mannequins from display-based (screen-based) patient simulators.

- Fidelity is in the eye of the application (subjective to the end-use and learning objectives). Instead of 'fidelity', mannequin patient simulators should be classified according to objective measures such as the level of integration between models, simulator input (user interventions) and simulator output, and model accuracy and scope (number of fundamental parameters modeled).

- To the extent possible, instructors should not be required to function as sensors of user interventions and/or to improvise simulator response but should be allowed to focus on teaching. Conversely, mannequin patient simulators should not teach, that is, they should not be used by trainees without instructor supervision.

- Assuming that the requisite sensors, actuators and models are integrated, automaticity of simulator response can be accomplished via scenarios that orchestrate changes in model parameters based on trigger events (time, concentrations, thresholds, etc.). Scenario editors provide the ability to create custom scenarios or edit those provided by manufacturers and other users.

- We cannot simulate what we do not know. Our knowledge about patients is incomplete, imperfect and inconsistent. Arguably, there is more that we do not know about the human body than we do know. This must be a fundamental consideration when comparing patient simulation (mannequin or display-based) to simulation of finite, man-made systems like aircraft.

- In 'inside looking out' simulators for aircraft, submarines, tanks, ship bridges, nuclear reactors, users are inside the simulator and exterior appearance and size need not be like

Overview *(continued)*

the system being simulated, unlike mannequin patient simulators where users are outside the simulator. In tetherless designs, the finite volume of a mannequin cavity effectively limits how much hardware can be imbedded inside.

◆ Mannequin patient simulators are not encyclopaedic. Desired features may be unavailable from commercial off-the-shelf mannequin patient simulators. Some simulator designs support an application programing interface that allows simulator personnel with the requisite knowledge and skills to add desired features, in consultation with the manufacturer.

◆ The real value of simulation may lie in its ability to focus on the essential characteristics of a system and de-emphasize or eliminate distracting, irrelevant details that some might construe as a reduction in fidelity. Demanding higher fidelity simply for the sake of fidelity may needlessly throttle the continued enhancement, adoption and benefits derived from mannequin patient simulators.

5.1 Introduction

This chapter is about mannequin patient simulators such as the Medical Education Technologies Inc. Human Patient Simulator (METI-HPS®), SimMan® and NOELLE® implemented *via* life-size, computer-controlled mannequins (sometimes spelled as manikins) that, independently of the instructor or simulator technician, can simulate a range of physiological, pharmacological and clinical parameters, processes and conditions, commensurate with their level of integration and mathematical modeling. The chapter is written from the perspective of a developer and user for users and developers of mannequin patient simulators. It will devote a large part to terminology and concepts relevant to mannequin patient simulators rather than attempting to provide an exhaustive list of currently available simulators and their features, perishable information readily available from vendors. While such a feature-based simulator list will eventually become obsolete, there will always be a need for users and developers of mannequin patient simulators to share a common terminology so that communication is clear and effective and expectations remain manageable. Proper use of terminology can help mannequin patient simulators deliver on their potential as smoothly and quickly as possible in areas such as healthcare personnel training, clinical, patient safety and research applications, the science of learning and training with simulation and simulation technology. Scenario editors and applications of mannequin patient simulators are not discussed in depth because they are covered elsewhere in this manual.

5.2 Terminology

As a discipline evolves, terminology can become a problem. Most will agree that the nascent field of simulation in healthcare has evolved very rapidly at the beginning of this new millennium, if one is to judge from attendance and the number of abstracts presented at, for example, the Annual International Meeting on Simulation in Healthcare. Such a fast evolution exacerbates the problem, with terminology struggling to keep pace and a proliferation of different terms that describe essentially the same thing. As an example mannequin patient simulators, the topic of this chapter, have been described by a multitude of names that can be quite confusing to novices (more upon that later).

More established simulation fields like aviation and the military have been of tremendous value and guidance to simulation in healthcare. For example, the anaesthesia crisis resource management (ACRM) simulation programme originating from Stanford[1,2] was inspired by aviation's crew resource management (or cockpit resource management). Similarly, we can also look to flight and military simulation for insight about terminology and to illuminate discussions about fidelity[3].

The patent for the Link Trainer (considered as the first true flight simulator) was issued in 1931[4]. Yet, a 1999 Fidelity Implementation Study Group report[3] whose authors included flight and military simulation experts observed that 'fidelity' is one of the most inconsistently used terms in the modeling and simulation community while paradoxically being one of the most commonly used terms in simulation descriptions. This striking observation, almost 70 years after the Link patent was issued, should caution the simulation in healthcare community about the importance of terminology and the wisdom and enormous benefits of standardizing terminology as early as possible.

The multitude of names to describe mannequin patient simulators may be partly due to the perception that all are partially correct and none provides a fully accurate description like the proverbial tale of six blind men (including this author!) each touching different parts of an elephant and providing an only partially accurate description[5]. The terms 'whole body simulator'[6] or 'full body simulator'[7] have been used to describe mannequin patient simulators, but the descriptors apply more to the inanimate plastic mannequin than what is being dynamically modeled (mathematically, physiologically or pharmacologically). The terms whole-body or full-body simulator do not mean that the entire body and all the organs, subsystems and processes within it are simulated or modeled. For example, simulation and modeling of electrical activity of the brain is currently not a standard feature in commercially available mannequin patient simulators. Harking back to the early days of mannequin patient simulators when most of the development and applications were primarily in anaesthesia, they have also been called 'anesthesia simulators'[8,9] or 'anaesthesia simulators'[10,11], terms that in hindsight were self-limiting and not inclusive of other healthcare disciplines.

Mannequin patient simulators have previously been described as full-scale simulators[12,13], full-scale computer simulators[14], mannequin-based simulators[15], mannequin simulators[16], physical simulators, macrosimulators[17], integrated simulators[18], model-driven simulators[18], model-driven full human simulator[19], instructor driven simulators[18], intermediate fidelity simulators[18], and high fidelity simulators[20].

Other terms are based on the training purpose of the simulator: whole task simulators or trainers[21] and full mission simulators[22,23]. A part-task trainer focuses on a particular training task (such as applying cricoid pressure during intubation) and simulates only the part of the patient or task that is of interest[24]. In contrast, Schaefer defines a whole task trainer or simulator as replicating all relevant aspects of a task such as tactile, visual, and auditory feedback similar to performing a fibreoptic bronchoscope intubation on a patient. A full mission simulator reproduces all the features necessary to realistically simulate an entire mission. For example, in the case of general anaesthesia, a full-mission simulator must be able to respond realistically during the entire anaesthesia mission: induction, maintenance and emergence. Such a full mission mannequin patient simulator designed for anaesthesia would thus need to be able to physically absorb volatile anaesthetic vapour during induction and excrete it during emergence. A full-system simulator recreates the entire system such as the healthcare environment, personnel, equipment, supplies and the patient[25].

Some of these previous definitions are based on what mannequin patient simulators are the opposite of, that is, what they are not (e.g. whole-task *versus* part-task; full-scale *versus* reduced or magnified scale; macrosimulators *versus* microsimulators where the patient is instantiated on a computer screen instead of a mannequin). Other definitions are based on how they are driven (model or instructor driven) and disputably mapping the driving mode to high or intermediate fidelity, respectively.

The Merriam-Webster Online Dictionary[26] defines full-scale as:

- identical to an original in proportion and size
- involving full use of available resources.

Some simulations are for practical reasons at a reduced scale like an airplane model in a wind tunnel. All mannequins used in patient simulators are at full scale (actual size) enabling use of regular endotracheal tubes and medical instruments, devices and supplies with them. Thus the term full-scale simulator (referring to physical proportion and size) appears to describe more the mannequin than what is being actively simulated and modeled. If full scale is interpreted as in a scale of musical notes, the term still falls short when applied to a simulator because the full spectrum of processes in a human body is not simulated.

In this chapter, we will use the term simulator to mean only the mannequin patient simulator whereas the term simulation refers to an exercise that includes a mannequin patient simulator. The previous terms included simulator as one of the words while the following terms are used with simulation (the simulator and everything that is used together with the simulator): full-scale simulation[27], high fidelity simulation[28], and full-system simulation[25]. In full-scale simulation or full-system simulation, the entire environment or system is reproduced and a mannequin patient simulator, that is only a part of the simulation, is used with actual medical personnel and equipment (full use of available resources). Depending on the scope of a full scale simulation exercise, the simulation theater could be for example a single operating room (OR), a suite of ORs, a hospital ward, an entire hospital or a regional or national healthcare system.

5.2.1 The case for mannequin patient simulator

If screen-based patient simulators[29,30] that do not use mannequins did not already exist, the most concise term would be patient simulator (similar to aircraft or flight simulator). Thus to distinguish patient simulators implemented via mannequins against screen-based patient simulators, the term 'mannequin patient simulator' is proposed. The proposed term describes what is being simulated (a patient) and how it is being simulated (via a mannequin) distinguishing it from other forms of patient simulation like display-based patient simulators or standardized patients.

5.2.2 The case for using integration, instead of fidelity, for classifying mannequin patient simulators

A mannequin patient simulator can be considered from an engineering perspective as an input/output system implemented via a set of interlinked data acquisition and control systems (DAC) distributed over the entire mannequin and its ancillary equipment (such as a drug syringe label bar code reader). Fidelity is ultimately dependent on the application, the desired learning objectives and the individual threshold for achieving suspension of disbelief. In that sense, fidelity is subjective relative to the application and the eye of the beholder and useless or at best inconsistent in describing a mannequin patient simulator. For example, the METI-HPS®, which most would describe as a high fidelity mannequin patient simulator is high fidelity when used to learn about cardiovascular learning objectives but may be considered as low or no fidelity if electroencephalography is the learning objective. Fidelity is not necessarily uniform in any given mannequin patient simulator design.

Integration is a more objective descriptor, compared with fidelity, of the realism and level of automation and consistency of:

◆ detection and quantification of trainee interventions or resulting effects

◆ the response of the simulator to trainee interventions or lack thereof.

Integration as a descriptor is quantifiable and objective and is a measure that can be adjusted upwards as technological advances facilitate enhancements in the level of integration and modeling.

In the early days of mannequin patient simulators, naïve prospective users who were contemplating acquisition of such units would query how many scenarios were available with a given mannequin patient simulator design. Using the number of scenarios as an indication of the capabilities of a mannequin patient simulator may open the door to creative accounting of scenarios whereby multiple small variations upon a core scenario are counted as 'separate' scenarios. An appropriate analogy is that scenarios (such as malignant hyperthermia) are recipes and simulated basic parameters (such as oxygen consumption, pulmonary shunt or respiratory quotient) are culinary ingredients. The more ingredients (basic parameters) that are available, the more recipes (scenarios) that can be implemented, giving free rein to the imagination of instructors in customizing scenarios that facilitate acquisition of specific learning objectives.

5.2.3 Output

Thus, an objective measure of the capabilities of a mannequin patient simulator is the number of basic parameters that can be controlled and altered via a scenario editor or manually so that the resulting perceptible changes provide trainees an external representation of patient status. In turn, the number of physiological, pharmacological and clinical parameters that can be simulated is determined by the hardware necessary to output the external perceptible manifestations of changes in that parameter (e.g. a servomotor that moves a thumb to simulate twitch response to ulnar nerve stimulation as an indicator of neuromuscular blockade). Perceptible outputs from a mannequin patient simulator are comprised of clinical signs and data monitored via instruments such as multi-parameter physiological monitors. Clinical signs include movement (e.g. unilateral or bilateral chest movement, thumb twitch), palpable outputs (radial, carotid, femoral, pedal pulses), audible outputs (normal and abnormal breath, lung and bowel sounds), eye signs (normal and blown pupil response) and haptic outputs (when evaluating thumb twitch response by placing the palm against the thumb to prevent thumb motion, a stronger force is generated when a thumb excursion of larger amplitude is prevented[31]).

Outputs that are generated via monitors include numerical data such as arterial oxygen saturation determined by pulse oximetry and systolic and diastolic blood pressures and graphical data such as waveform data that includes electrocardiograms (normal and abnormal with various arrhythmias), capnograms and invasive blood pressure traces. In general, stimulation is used for displaying monitored data, that is, actual monitoring equipment such as multiparameter physiological monitors, including capnographs, pulse oximeters and electrocardiographs are interfaced to the mannequin patient simulator. The monitoring equipment is supplied (stimulated) by the mannequin patient simulator with the appropriate modulated gas concentration, current, voltage and pressure input to provide a realistic simulation output. Use of actual monitoring equipment with the mannequin patient simulator is an example of 'full-scale' simulation and provides trainees the opportunity to explore the 'buttonology' of the actual monitoring equipment in a realistic yet safe (to the patient) environment.

5.2.4 **Input**

A simulation exercise is characterized by its interactive nature whereby trainees can not only attempt to infer the status of the patient from the output of the simulation but also have to make decisions or diagnoses and intervene accordingly in real time. Thus, a high-integration simulator must be able to automatically sense user interventions without the need for simulation instructors or technicians to act as human sensors, a chore that may distract them from the instructional mission. From an engineering perspective, the input function in a mannequin patient simulator relates to the data acquisition part of the DAC system. Examples of sensors are fast gas analysers used to sample gas concentrations in bellows representing the alveolar space and bar code readers that read bar code labels affixed to syringes that encode the name and concentration of the drug in the syringe. In a medium-integration simulator, the instructor or simulation technician may have to observe and enter the identity and concentration of drug administered or the flow rates of oxygen and nitrous oxide. If the instructor or technician is distracted or overburdened, trainee interventions may be missed altogether or entered incorrectly creating risks of inconsistent and negative teaching or incorrect assessments in high stakes simulation.

5.2.5 **Models and scripts**

In the same way that instructors or simulation technicians acting as sensors can be fallible, they may also be inconsistent or not possess the requisite knowledge or be unable to improvise appropriately and in real time when called upon to drive the output of a simulator (e.g. to determine the time to recovery from neuromuscular blockade as determined by spontaneous breathing and thumb twitch response from a dose of rocuronium in the presence of potentiating volatile anaesthetics).

Models and scripts provide a consistent means to drive a simulator and allow instructors to concentrate on teaching, their core mission. A script is a preordained series of events based on time and the occurrence of specific events. Scripts are quicker to implement but less flexible than mathematical models. To work well, a script must anticipate ahead of time all possible user interventions or developments that have an impact on the scenario that the script controls and the mannequin patient simulator must have the requisite sensors that are able to detect (and in some instances quantify) all relevant user interventions or their effects. For example, a simple script may call for arterial oxygen saturation determined by pulse oximetry (S_pO_2) to fall (oxygen desaturation) two minutes after apnoea has been triggered. But, if the patient's lungs had previously been pre-oxygenated such that the oxygen concentration in the lungs at the beginning of apnoea was 80% and if there is no gas analyser to measure the actual 'alveolar' oxygen concentration, the above simple script would not provide a realistic simulation because desaturation occurs too quickly at 2 minutes after the start of apnoea.

A model is more flexible than a script because in a high-integration simulator, it can handle events that were not explicitly anticipated during development. A model is not based on a preordained series of events but instead relies on broad principles typically expressed in the form of mathematical equations. A model is more time-consuming to develop and validate than a script. Data from the literature is used to create a first iteration of the model. If data are not available in the literature, then experiments may need to be performed to acquire the needed data. Once a model has been developed, the model needs to be validated against the literature and with subject matter experts, a time consuming iterative task. A model provides 'liveliness' in a simulation and, when well integrated into a mannequin patient simulator, may even surprise the simulation developers.

As an example, assume that a model takes into account partial pressure of oxygen to generate the spontaneous breathing rate and the gas analyser sampling gas in the bellows representing the alveolar space has a barometric pressure sensor. If all the data is properly integrated in the simulator, then at high altitude without explicit input from the simulation developer or instructor, the model will cause the simulator to hyperventilate because of the reduced partial pressure of oxygen due to the lower atmospheric pressure. This is exactly what happened with an early version of the human patient simulator (HPS) that was exhibited at a meeting in Colorado and surprised the developers when first used at high altitude. While models are more powerful and flexible than scripts, the latter also find use in simulators equipped with scenario editors because certain scenarios require a script to trigger the start of an incident such as malignant hyperthermia, for example, 1 minute into a scenario. Thus, the HPS, a high-integration mannequin patient simulator is described as script-controlled and model-driven[13].

A scenario editor is used by instructors and simulation technicians to program scenarios *via* the user-adjustable parameters that can be controlled via the scenario editor. The scenario editor generates a script that can be considered as a finite state machine consisting of discrete states. The transition from one state to another can be triggered by time or the value of certain parameters (blood concentrations, alveolar O_2 or CO_2, S_pO_2, etc.) reaching given thresholds.

From the previous descriptions and examples, a high-integration simulator does not make use of instructors or technicians as sensors or to improvise the output of a simulator. It relies instead on models and scripts to drive the simulator output, on actuators such as a servomotor generating a physical thumb twitch to externalize the model's output and on sensors such as gas analysers to detect and quantify the effects of user interventions in real time. A high level of integration between input (sensors), models and scripts, and output (actuators) provides for a more realistic simulation experience. Hence, the recommendation to classify mannequin patient simulators according to the level of integration instead of fidelity. A high level of integration is also expensive because of the additional sensors and actuators required and the cost of model development and validation.

Various valid arguments have been made against unsupervised use of mannequin patient simulators. An additional consideration is that mannequin patient simulators cannot teach, in most cases. Just like instructors should not be performing the simulator's functions by acting as sensors and improvising simulator response, simulators cannot accomplish an instructor's functions, in the same way that a blackboard cannot provide instruction by itself. A mannequin patient simulator can be considered as an expensive blackboard that vastly enhances the capabilities of an instructor for teaching, training and assessment.

5.3 The fidelity trap

Fidelity in simulation at first appears to be a simple concept that is, in fact, a complex and multifaceted issue. Fidelity, as a lay word in common parlance, has many desirable connotations that may explain the knee jerk response that a higher 'fidelity' mannequin patient simulator must be a better simulator which:

◆ is not always true
◆ begs the question of defining what 'fidelity' and 'better' mean.

Fidelity is described at the Merriam-Webster Online Dictionary[26] as: "accuracy in details: exactness" or "the degree to which an electronic device (as a record player, radio, or television) accurately reproduces its effect (as sound or picture)". Generally, fidelity at its most abstract level implies a truthful connection to a source, for example, how accurate a reproduction is to its original. While a hi-fi (high fidelity) audio device may be what most have experience with, and therefore in mind, as an analogy to fidelity in mannequin patient simulators, it is inappropriate for many reasons. The use of fidelity in connection with simulators has many more dimensions compared to audio playback fidelity. Currently, simulation in healthcare researchers are grappling with many different kinds of fidelity such as educational, procedural, visual, operational, physical and functional fidelity.

In the case of fidelity as it refers to playback of recorded music, the source is complete (everything that is to be known about the source is known and captured in the storage medium), perfect and consistent and the domain to be reproduced is finite and bounded. Such is not the case with a human patient as will be discussed later. Also, in the human body one can zoom in deeper and deeper from representing a body by a central and peripheral compartment to finer details down to simulating the body or its subsystems by reproducing interactions at the cellular level or even lower. Also, when playing back recorded music, sounding as close to the source is the goal. With mannequin patient simulators, the ultimate goal is not necessarily behaving as closely to a human patient as possible but is usually determined by the many different applications where they are used.

To discuss simulator fidelity, the terms 'simuland' and 'referent' are helpful in conveying key concepts. A simuland is defined as "the system being simulated by a simulation"[3]. In mannequin patient simulators, the simuland is a human patient. In an anaesthesia crisis resource management simulation, the simuland includes the anaesthesia and surgical care teams, the OR environment and equipment as well as the mannequin patient simulator.

A referent is defined as "A codified body of *knowledge* about a thing being simulated"[3]. A referent in the case of a mannequin patient simulator could be pharmacology or physiology with the 'thing' being a human patient. At first encounter, simuland and referent appear to describe the same concept. Upon closer analysis, the term referent implicitly acknowledges that our knowledge about the simuland, a human patient, is incomplete, imperfect and inconsistent. For example, researchers are still trying to identify and understand the actual mechanism of general anaesthesia[32] or how certain types of diseases like cancer and multiple sclerosis are triggered. Much information about human patients is unknown and may actually not be knowable.

Thus a developer or user can at best attempt to simulate all that is *known* about a human patient but not the human patient itself *in toto*. We cannot simulate what we do not know. This brings to mind a drug company executive who inquired, during the early days of HPS development, whether it could be used instead of patients for clinical trials of a new drug! In general, we cannot use simulators to learn what we do not know. Incomplete knowledge about a human patient argues against the appropriateness of such absolute and extreme descriptors as full-scale, full-body, whole body and high fidelity simulators.

Furthermore, most simulation developers can recall instances where in spite of faithfully following pharmacological and physiological equations and data from peer-reviewed publications and reference textbooks in a mathematical model driving a simulator, the model needed additional tuning before the output matched the expectations of subject matter experts and clinicians (imperfect knowledge). In addition, knowledge may not be consistent. As an example, there are many pharmacokinetic models for the anaesthetic drug propofol and the output from these different models can vary significantly, even from a clinical perspective[33].

Another hypothetical situation to ponder is that should perfect fidelity be attained and mannequin patient simulators become indistinguishable from humans, then one might argue that the enormous effort and cost to achieve perfect patient simulators could have been avoided by simply using humans in the first place, in those instances where it is ethically acceptable, such as standardized patients, actors simulating specific ailments.

Higher fidelity may require more complex and sophisticated models that overload learners with overwhelming information and details that may actually detract from the effectiveness of a simulator by overshadowing the real learning objectives, a phenomenon that has been described as the 'seductive details' hypothesis[34]. Some would argue that the real value of simulation is its ability to focus on the essence of a system and de-emphasize or eliminate distracting, irrelevant details which others might construe as a reduction in 'fidelity'. In a recently completed study, a transparent reality simulation with lower visual fidelity provided more effective learning about the anaesthesia machine compared with a photorealistic simulation[35]. In yet another study, a surprising finding was that motion in some flight simulators did not result in a more effective simulator for certain tasks. "The results of the study indicate that the motion provided by the test simulator did not, in an operationally significant way for the tasks tested, affect either evaluation, training progress, or transfer of training, acquired in the simulator with or without motion, to the simulator with motion."[36]

To summarize, if simulation was an end onto itself, then admittedly higher fidelity in the sense of the simulator being as realistic as possible would be the ultimate goal. But in practice, a simulator is a means to an end that could be education, training and research and fidelity has to be viewed in the context of the desired application. Thus, when selecting a mannequin patient simulator, one should not fall into the fidelity trap but instead consider effectiveness and affordability for the intended applications (present and future). While there remains considerable room for improvement in mannequin patient simulators, users should appreciate the challenges facing developers and manufacturers. For most applications, current mannequin patient simulators are good enough. Users should do what they can with what currently meets their needs rather than fall into the fidelity trap and wait endlessly for the mirage of perfect 'fidelity'.

5.4 History and development of mannequin patient simulators

In the 1960s, an engineer and a physician (Abrahamson and Denson) were the first to create a computer-controlled mannequin patient simulator, SimOne®[37], that was ahead of its time. Reportedly, the computer that ran SimOne® occupied an entire wall of a room (personal communication, JS Gravenstein). In the mid-1980s, teams at Stanford and the University of Florida, independently and unaware of the other team's research, started working on the next generation of mannequin patient simulators. The history and development of the Stanford CASE® (Comprehensive Anaesthesia Simulation Environment) system developed by Dr David Gaba, an anaesthesiologist and his colleagues has been previously documented[16,38]. CASE® was licensed to CAE-Link and went on to become the first commercially available mannequin patient simulator (SimOne® was never commercialized). Among its many accomplishments and applications, CASE® was used to develop ACRM. The Stanford design was subsequently licensed to different companies. The last CASE® licensee, Medsim, discontinued production of mannequin patient simulators.

The initial implementation of the Florida simulator was built in the summer of 1987 during this author's industrial externship with Tom Clemens at Ohmeda Anaesthesia Systems (now GE Healthcare) in Madison, Wisconsin. It was a discarded anaesthesia machine rigged with computer controlled faults. The 'patient' was essentially a donated mechanical lung model modified to produce carbon dioxide[39] also used in industry as a platform for developing and testing capnographs (personal communication, Eben Kermit, Nellcor). The original computer that controlled triggering of the mechanical faults was one of the first 1000 original IBM PCs (discarded by the Ohmeda accounting department but much more portable than the SimOne® computer!). It is fair to say that the advent of inexpensive personal computers, coupled with increasing realization of the need to conduct research in patient safety, facilitated the rebirth and successful commercialization of mannequin patient simulators. Unmodified monitoring equipment (e.g. gas analyser, capnograph, ECG, blood pressure and heart rate monitors, pulse oximeter) were stimulated so that they could be used to detect and identify anaesthesia machine faults. The mannequin consisted of only a torso and an intubation head whose trachea was connected to the modified mechanical lung model. No clinical signs were simulated and diagnosis was done mainly via monitoring equipment. Subsequently, the Anaesthesia Patient Safety Foundation not only provided crucial funding to both Florida and Stanford but also encouraged the simulation of clinical signs such as palpable pulses, chest movement and breath and heart sounds. In hindsight, this heralded the shift in emphasis from anaesthesia simulation to patient simulation because many of these clinical signs had applications beyond anaesthesia. The Florida simulator was initially named the Gainesville Anesthesia Simulator (GAS), after the city where the University of Florida campus is located.

A distinguishing feature in the Florida core research and development team was the contribution of academic engineers who, as full time faculty members of the anaesthesiology department, also used the HPS to teach courses[40]. This first-hand experience as simulator instructors helped the engineers, R Carovano Jr, S Lampotang, and W van Meurs working with ML Good and JS Gravenstein, and other clinicians, to obtain a deeper appreciation of the need for automation of data capture and patient response so that instructors could focus on teaching rather than on running the simulator and improvising patient responses. This emphasis on automation led to patented innovative designs[41–51] and mathematical models[52] and was considered the main differentiating factor between the early Stanford and Florida designs[16]. Tellingly, both the Stanford (CASE®) and Florida (GAS®) simulator names initially included anaesthesia in the acronym. As the realization dawned that the scope of applications was much wider than anaesthesia, the name GAS® was changed to Human Patient Simulator® (HPS®). The HPS® technology was licensed by the University of Florida to Loral Corporation. When Loral was acquired by Lockheed Martin, a group of Loral employees led by Lou Oberndorf formed Medical Education Technologies Inc. (METI), headquartered in Sarasota, Florida in 1996.

5.5 Design considerations of mannequin patient simulators

As previously discussed, integration adds cost to a simulator but may be necessary for certain applications. Mannequin patient simulators are not inexpensive and discussions about cost-effectiveness and how to obtain funds to purchase them have always been present since their commercialization. Placing as many features as possible in a given design so that it can be used by as wide an audience as possible from multiple disciplines allows different departments with varied learning objectives to pool their resources together to acquire a simulator. If a simulator is designed to be modular in addition to providing an extensive list of features, it allows users to configure their simulator by selecting only those modules or features that they will actually use. For example, the Twitcher[31] module of the METI-HPS® can be removed when used with trainees who do not use neuromuscular blockade (NMB) agents and NMB monitoring and do not need to learn about it.

Mannequin patient simulators cannot be encyclopaedic and simulate all the known processes in a human body because, among other reasons, the space available inside a mannequin to house different actuators and sensors is limited. Thus, there might be features that are not provided by commercial off-the-shelf (COTS) simulators that an instructor may need to teach certain learning objectives. In that instance, an open architecture such as that available in the METI-HPS®, Emergency Care Simulator (METI-ECS®), PediaSim®, BabySim® and iStan® allows users to create and integrate add-on modules to the COTS simulator to support unmet learning objectives. In the case of the METI-HPS®, the HPS Internal Data Exchange Protocol (HIDEP) is used to send and receive data in real-time between the add-on module and the simulator using different protocols (RS-232, TCP/IP). A concrete example of a HIDEP application is a locally developed module for intracranial pressure[53].

Much has been written about the similarities between aircraft and patient simulators. A significant difference is that for an aircraft simulator that includes motion, trainees are inside looking out and do not see, for example, the hydraulic rods that are pitching and rolling the simulator. In other words, there is no size or visual constraint about the external appearance of an aircraft simulator. Trainees are looking at the 'outside world' via cockpit windows where the appropriate view can be projected at the right time, a form of screen-based simulation. The actual controls in a real cockpit are used in the flight simulator such that there is no tactile difference between the two. In contrast, one of the main user complaints about mannequin patient simulators from the start has been the unrealistic feel of the skin.

In mannequin patient simulators, trainees are outside of the simulator looking and touching the outside appearance and feel of a mannequin. In addition to tactile realism relating to the feel of the skin, this places visual realism (actuators cannot be protruding from the mannequin) and size constraints because only so many electromechanical components can be crammed into the hollow space in a life-size mannequin, especially for a tetherless mannequin patient simulator. In earlier designs, the mannequin proper was permanently mounted on top of a cart where much of the hardware was placed and hidden behind medical drapes (Fig. 5.1).

There are many mannequin patient simulators of varying levels of integration that have been developed over the years (CASE®, METI-HPS® and its derivatives, SimMan®, NOELLE®, Leiden, Sophus®, Access®). It is not the intent of this chapter to be encyclopaedic. We will briefly describe commercially available mannequin patient simulators only. Mannequin patient simulators are not limited to adult humans but also include paediatric and neonatal patients represented by life-size mannequins with dimensions appropriate for the age of the simulated patients. Available mannequin patient simulators simulate different patients: adult (METI-HPS®, SimMan®, and the

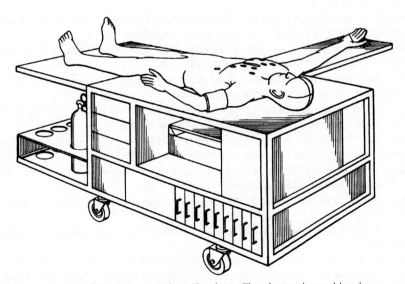

Fig. 5.1 An early version of the Human Patient Simulator. The electronics and hardware were housed in a cart on which the mannequin was fixed.

tetherless iStan®), obstetric (NOELLE®), paediatric (PediaSim®) and infant (BabySim®, SimBaby®). Just as the simulation designer has to let the learning objectives drive the features present in the simulator, the educator has to select which simulator to acquire based on current and future learning objectives.

Mannequin patient simulators have the potential to enhance patient safety by providing a means for healthcare personnel to learn by doing, individually and in teams, without risk to patients and to experience rare and dangerous events. As they become even more widespread, the applications of mannequin patient simulators will continue to increase. The challenges facing mannequin patient simulator developers and users are significant. Adoption of common and standardized terminology and an appreciation of the fundamental limitations facing mannequin patient simulation engineers can facilitate the dialogue, expectations and interaction between users, instructors, developers and manufacturers from diverse backgrounds.

References

1. Gaba D, Howard S, Fish K, Yang G, Sarnquist F (1991). Anaesthesia crisis resource management training (abstract). *Anesthesiology* **75**: A1062.

2. Gaba D, Fish K, Howard S (1994). *Crisis Management in Anesthesiology*. New York: Churchill-Livingstone.

3. Gross DC, Redactor (1999). Report from the Fidelity Definition and Metrics Implementation Study Group (FDM-ISG), 99S-SIW-167, 1999 Spring Simulation Interoperability Workshop (SIW), Simulation Interoperability Standards Organization (SISO), Orlando, FL, March 1999. [RPG Reference Document, *SIW Fidelity Report*.]

4. Link EA, inventor (1931). Combination training device for student aviators and entertainment apparatus. United States patent 1,825,462. 1931 Sep 29.

5. Retrieved on July 15, 2007 at Wikipedia web site http://www.wikipedia.org/wiki/Blind_Men_and_an_Elephant

6. Forrest F, Tooley M, Glavin R, Maran N (2001). Setting up and running a whole body Simulator Centre. *R Coll Anaesthetists Bull*; 5.

7. Goodwin JA, van Meurs WL, Sa Couto CD, Beneken JE, Graves SA (2004). A model for educational simulation of infant cardiovascular physiology. *Anesth Analg* **99**: 1655–64.

8. Gaba DM, DeAnda A (1988). A comprehensive anaesthesia simulation environment: re-creating the operating room for research and training. *Anesthesiology* **69**: 387–94.

9. van Meurs WL, Beneken JEW, Good ML, Lampotang S, Carovano RG Jr, Gravenstein JS (1993). Physiologic model for an anaesthesia simulator, abstracted. *Anesthesiology* **79**: A1114.

10. Chopra V, Gesink BJ, de Jong J, Bovill JG, Spierdijk J, Brand R (1994). Does training on an anaesthesia simulator lead to improvement in performance? *Br J Anaesth* **73**: 293–7.

11. Riley RH, Wilks DH, Freeman JA (1997). Anaesthetists' attitudes towards an anaesthesia simulator. A comparative survey: USA and Australia. *Anaesth Intensive Care* **25**: 514–9.

12. Hesselfeldt R, Kristensen MS, Rasmussen LS (2005). Evaluation of the airway of the SimMan™ full-scale patient simulator. *Acta Anaesthesiol Scand* **49**: 1339–45.

13. van Meurs WL, Good ML, Lampotang S (1997). Functional anatomy of full-scale patient simulators. *J Clin Monit* **13**: 317–24.

14. Wong AK (2004). Full scale computer simulators in anaesthesia training and evaluation. *Can J Anesth* **51**: 5; 455–64.

15. Nyssen AS, Larbuisson R, Janssens M, Pendeville P, Mayne A (2002). A Comparison of the Training Value of Two Types of Anaesthesia Simulators: Computer Screen-Based and Mannequin-Based Simulators. *Anesth Analg* **94**: 1560–5.

16. Cooper JB, Taqueti VR (2004). A brief history of the development of mannequin simulators for clinical education and training. *Qual Saf Health Care* **13**: 11–18.

17. Christensen UJ, Heffernan D, Barach P (2001). Microsimulators in medical simulation: An overview. *Simulation & Gaming* **32**: 250–62.

18. Maran NJ, Glavin RJ (2003). Low- to high-fidelity simulation – a continuum of medical education? *Medical Education* **37**(Suppl. 1): 22–8.

19. Murray WB, Good ML, Gravenstein JS, van Oostrom JH, Brasfield WG (2002). Learning about new anesthetics using a model driven, full human simulator. *J Clin Monit Comput* **17**(5): 293–300.

20. McFetrich J (2006). A structured literature review on the use of high fidelity patient simulators for teaching in emergency medicine. *Emerg Med J* **23**: 509–11.

21. Schaefer JJ (2004). Simulators and difficult airway management skills. *Pediatric Anaesthesia* **14**: 28–37.

22. Owen H, Mugford B, Follows V, Plummer JL (2006). Comparison of three simulation-based training methods for management of medical emergencies. *Resuscitation* **71**, 204–11.

23. Beaubien JM, Baker DP (2004). The use of simulation for training teamwork skills in healthcare: how low can you go? *Quality & Safety in Health Care* **13**(Suppl 1): i51-i56.

24. Owen H, Follows V, Reynolds KJ, Burgess G, Plummer J (2002). Learning to apply effective cricoid pressure using a part task trainer. *Anaesthesia* **57**: 1098–101.

25. Retrieved July 15, 2007 from Federal Aviation Authority web site http://www.hf.faa.gov/Webtraining/Training/Training019.htm

26. Retrieved July 15, 2007 from Merriam-Webster Online web site http://www.m-w.com

27. Seropian MA (2003). General concepts in full scale simulation: Getting started. *Anaesthesia & Analgesia* **97**: 1695–1705.

28. Issenberg SB, McGaghie WC, Petrusa ER, Gordon DL, Scalese RJ (2005). Features and uses of high-fidelity medical simulations that lead to effective learning: a BEME systematic review. *Medical Teacher* **27**(1): 10–28.

29. Smith NT, Starko KR (2005): The physiology and pharmacology of growing old, as shown in Body simulation. *Stud Health Techno Inform* **111**: 488–91.

30. Schwid HA, O'Donnell D (1993). The Anaesthesia Simulator Consultant: simulation plus expert system. *Anesthesiol Rev* **20**(5): 185–9.

31. Lampotang S, Good ML, Heijnen PMAM, Carovano R, Gravenstein JS (1998). TWITCHER: A device to simulate thumb twitch response to ulnar nerve stimulation. *J Clin Monit Comput* **14**: 135–140.

32. Orser BA (2007). Lifting the fog around anaesthesia. *Scientific American* June issue: 54–61.

33. Retrieved July 15, 2007 from Virtual Anaesthesia Machine web site http://vam.anest.ufl.edu/simulations/propofolpharmacokinetics.php

34. Carey S (2000). Science education as conceptual change. *J Appl Dev Psychol* **21**: 13–19.

35. Fischler I, Kaschub CE, Lizdas DE, Lampotang S (2008). Understanding of anaesthesia machine function is enhanced with a transparent reality simulation. *Simulation in Healthcare* **3**:26–32.

36. Longridge T, Bürki-Cohen J, Go TH, Kendra AJ (2001). Simulator fidelity considerations for training and evaluation of today's airline pilots. Proceedings of the 11th International Symposium on Aviation Psychology, Columbus, Ohio, USA.

37. Denson JS, Abrahamson S (1969). A computer-controlled patient simulator. *JAMA* **208**(3): 504–8.

38. Smith BE, Gaba DM (2001). Simulators. In: Lake C, Blitt C, Hines R, Eds. *Clinical Monitoring: Practical Application*. WB Saunders Company, New York: 26–44.

39. Lampotang S, Gravenstein N, Banner MJ, Jaeger MJ, Schultetus RR (1986). A lung model of carbon dioxide concentrations with mechanical or spontaneous ventilation. *Crit Care Med* **14**: 1055–7.

40. Lampotang S, Öhrn M, van Meurs WL (1996). A simulator-based respiratory physiology workshop. *Acad Med* **71**: 526–7.

41. Lampotang S, Good ML, Gravenstein JS, Carovano RG, inventors; University of Florida Research Foundation, assignee. Method and apparatus for simulating neuromuscular stimulation during medical surgery. United States patent 5,391,081. 1995 Feb 21.

42. Lampotang S, van Meurs WL, Good ML, Gravenstein JS, Carovano RG, inventors; University of Florida Research Foundation, assignee. Self regulating lung for simulated medical procedures. United States patent 5,584,701. 1996 Dec 17.

43. Lampotang S, van Meurs WL, Good ML, Gravenstein JS, Carovano RG, inventors; University of Florida Research Foundation, assignee. Apparatus for and method of synchronizing cardiac rhythm related events. United States patent 5,769,641. 1998 Jun 23.

44. Lampotang S, van Meurs WL, Good ML, Gravenstein JS, Carovano RG, inventors; University of Florida Research Foundation, assignee. An apparatus for and method of simulating bronchial resistance or dilation. United States patent 5,772,442. 1998 Jun 30.

45. Lampotang S, van Meurs WL, Good ML, Gravenstein JS, Carovano RG, inventors; University of Florida Research Foundation, assignee. An apparatus and method of detecting and identifying a drug. United States patent 5,772,443. 1998 Jun 30.

46. Lampotang S, van Meurs WL, Good ML, Gravenstein JS, Carovano RG, inventors; University of Florida Research Foundation, assignee. Apparatus and method of simulating breathing sounds. United States patent 5,779,484. 1998 Jul 14.

47. Lampotang S, van Meurs WL, Good ML, Gravenstein JS, Carovano RG, inventors; University of Florida Research Foundation, assignee. Apparatus and method for simulating lung sounds in a patient simulator. United States patent 5,868,579. 1999 Feb 9.

48. Lampotang S, van Meurs WL, Good ML, Gravenstein JS, Carovano RG, inventors; University of Florida Research Foundation, assignee. An apparatus and method for quantifying fluid delivered to a patient simulator. United States patent 5,882,207. 1999 Mar 16.

49. Lampotang S, van Meurs WL, Good ML, Gravenstein JS, Carovano RG, inventors; University of Florida Research Foundation, assignee. Apparatus for and method of simulating the injection and volatilizing of a volatile drug. United States patent 5,890,908. 1999 Apr 6.

50. Lampotang S, van Meurs WL, Good ML, Gravenstein JS, Carovano RG, inventors; University of Florida Research Foundation, assignee. Apparatus and method of simulating the determination of continuous blood gases in a patient simulator. United States patent 5,941,710. 1999 Aug 24.

51. van Meurs WL, Lampotang S, Good ML, Euliano TY, *et al.*, inventors; University of Florida Research Foundation, assignee. Life support simulation system simulating human physiological parameters. United States patent 6,273,728. 2001 Aug 14.

52. van Meurs WL, Nikkelen E, Good ML (1998). Pharmacokinetic-pharmacodynamic model for educational simulations. *IEEE Trans Biomed Eng* **45**: 582–90.

53. Thoman WJ, Gravenstein D, van der Aa JJ, Lampotang S (1999). Autoregulation in a simulator-based educational model of intracranial physiology. *J Clin Monit Comput* **15**(7–8): 481–91.

Disclosure: As coinventor of the Human Patient Simulator,® Samsun (Sem) Lampotang receives a fraction of the royalties that the University of Florida obtains from Medical Education Technologies, Inc. He is also a creator of the Virtual Anaesthesia Machine website and its web-enabled, display-based simulations at http://vam.anest.ufl.edu/wip.html.

Chapter 6

Airway training devices

Harry Owen and Cindy Hein

Overview

◆ There are many devices for assisting education and training in airway management. Choice of aids needs to be based on learning objectives and the level of achievement of students or trainees.

◆ Airway training using simulators can be structured to provide the most efficient training but this training must be integrated with clinical training for it to be most effective. Motivation is required to achieve superior performance.

◆ Airway training models do not always replicate normal anatomy or may not allow practice guidelines to be followed. This can interfere with learning by students and trainees and adversely impact on clinical care.

◆ Perceptual focusing is common during crises so endotracheal intubation training must stress when to abandon attempts and also emphasise rescue techniques for when intubation cannot be achieved promptly.

◆ Expertise in airway management is very dependent on context and setting so assessment of competence requires a range of scenarios in different settings. Simple additions or modifications can be made to patient simulators to increase the degree of challenge or complexity.

◆ Video-feedback is routinely used during 'full mission' simulation. Video-feedback of procedures and interventions attempted by novices on simple part-task trainers is also effective and enhances learning.

6.1 Introduction: changing the way airway management is taught

Good airway care is essential in anaesthesia, resuscitation and many other medical emergencies. All medical, nursing and paramedic training programs require their graduates to be proficient in basic airway management and postgraduate training programmes of acute care disciplines require acquisition of more advanced airway interventions. Airway management has been taught in many settings but many have ethical or logistical constraints and some have created their own adverse events. Mason's recommendation that all teaching hospitals develop an airway care training facility[1] was mostly ignored until recently when many clinical skills and simulation facilities have been created and most include an element of airway management.

It is now expected that a synthetic training environment will be used for teaching clinical skills and the management of complications associated with them. In surgery, residents need to demonstrate proficiency in basic techniques before operating on patients[2]. In acute care

Table 6.1 Settings and materials used for teaching and training airway interventions

Humans

- Cadavers
- Newly deceased (in the ER)
- In coma (in ICU)
- Undergoing routine anaesthesia (in the OR)
- Manufactured difficulties or simulated complications (in the OR) – this has given rise to adverse outcome
- Recovering from anaesthesia (in the PACU)

Animals

- Large live animals (e.g. dogs)
- Small live animals (e.g. kittens)
- Dead animals (e.g. white deer)

Simulators

- Part-task trainers (e.g. bench models, desktop/small simulators, medical phantoms)
- Whole-body mannequins
- Computer-controlled patient simulators
- Virtual reality (VR) simulators

disciplines, practitioners should have demonstrated competence in the skills they will use before the transition to delivering patient care without immediate supervision.

Airway skills have been taught in a range of settings (Table 6.1) including some unethical use of patients in the past[3]. Consent must be obtained from patients (or their responsible agent if they are unable to provide consent) before they are used for training. Most patients will give consent for students or trainees to undertake procedures on them as long as the risk of harm is not increased. In the case of patients who have died in the ER, if asked next-of-kin will generally agree to the deceased being used for teaching intubation. Teaching in this setting is opportunistic and a structured training programme will require patient simulators.

In some aspects of airway management there is quite a difference between teaching and training. Teaching is based on understanding and concepts (e.g. the consequences of not ventilating a patient for an extended time while trying to secure the airway) and training, which is based on operational requirements (e.g. if the airway cannot be secured by intubation in 30 seconds attempts will be abandoned and the patient will be ventilated by other means). Simulation can assist with both but for educational purposes only one or a small number of simulations can assist learning but for consistent care training requires many hours of practise.

The sections of this chapter outline basic airway training devices useful for all health professionals and airway training devices that support learning advanced airway interventions. Ideally teaching airway devices use is matched to current guidelines and recent recommendations and these should be readily available for trainers and trainees to refer to. Regular review of training is necessary because guidelines do change in both content and emphasis. For example, the recommendations on endotracheal intubation in resuscitation were changed when it became apparent that attempts to intubate the trachea could themselves contribute to mortality[4].

6.2 **Education in airway care**

Teaching using simulation requires a different mindset among trainers as well as trainees. Our teaching methods have been strongly influenced by theories of the way that motor skills are learnt and how expertise is developed. The three-stage theory of motor skill acquisition proposed by Fitts and Posner[5] is widely accepted as the basis for acquisition of psychomotor skills. The three stages provide a sound basis for designing airway skill teaching that accommodates the transition from novice to expert.

6.2.1 Cognitive stage (novice)

In this stage, the novice learns the sub-tasks (steps) needed to perform the skill/complete the task. Understanding and mastering individual steps or sub-tasks occurs at different rates so performance will appear halting and erratic. This stage has been referred to as being 'consciously incompetent'. Part-task trainers are ideal at this stage providing a low-cost platform for repetitive practice of particular steps and sequences.

Demonstration of steps by the trainer, videos, posters and display models enhance learning. Systems and devices that facilitate observation and recording of elements of the learner's performance help the trainers provide specific feedback.

'Practice makes permanent' so part-task trainers used at this stage must provide an accurate representation of real life to ensure only correct behaviour patterns are laid down. More detail on this is provided below.

6.2.2 Integrative stage (advanced beginner/trainee)

Practise and feedback facilitates progress to this stage where the learner must still think about performance but can move between steps more 'fluidly' and can cope with minor variations. Practitioners in this stage can be thought of as being 'consciously competent'. Whole body mannequins are good to use at this stage because they require clinically appropriate actions and positioning. Non-anatomical models (e.g. Dexter[6]) can also be used to provide variation and challenges to enhance the range of important psychomotor skills.

6.2.3 Autonomous stage (competent)

The practitioner no longer needs to think about the steps, readily adapts to different conditions, can accommodate interruptions and can divide attention with other tasks. This is the stage of being unconsciously competent but this can lead to lapses and other errors. High fidelity simulators and a system to record performance and replay it for review are most appropriate at this stage. Additional challenges may be needed to encourage competent practitioners to continue improving[7].

6.3 Aids for teaching and learning airway management

6.3.1 Basic life support

Key skills in basic life support (BLS) are assessment of consciousness, identifying and removing airway obstruction, opening the airway using head tilt/chin lift or jaw thrust manoeuvres, insertion of an oropharyngeal airway, and artificial ventilation using expired air techniques or a self-inflating resuscitator.

6.3.1.1 Basic airway manoeuvres

A comparison of basic airway trainers revealed that many had shortcomings. Some design features that made it easy to make and clean the models or to open the airway impacted on realism and meant that only stylised psychomotor skills were used by learner[8]. This may limit transfer of skills and contribute to poor performance in an actual emergency. Also, most

Table 6.2 Useful features for a model for teaching and assessing basic airway management

- Realistic size and appearance
- Head tilt and chin lift can open airway (needs a chin that lifts and a head that tilts)
- Has a palpable mandible that can be felt to move with a 'jaw thrust'
- Can feel expired air
- Stomach insufflation with overzealous ventilation
- Range of difficulties (e.g. obesity, beard)
- Cleanable between students

models appear young, fit looking and have good teeth whereas most people requiring resuscitation are old and overweight and many have poor dentition or dentures. The better models have soft features, articulation between head and neck and a palpable mandibular angle (Table 6.2).

6.3.1.2 Artificial ventilation

While ventilation by first responders at sudden cardiac arrest may be less important than once thought there will always be a need for this in trauma care, resuscitation from drowning and after return of spontaneous circulation. Basic training models must have a visible chest rise but models for healthcare professional training should be able to indicate volume and flow to provide feedback on performance.

Using different shaped face masks and adding a beard to models are good ways of increasing difficulty with mask ventilation. The models need to be disinfected when mouth-to-mouth or mouth-to-mask techniques are being taught. The risk of student to student spread of infection is very low but students with a respiratory illness or open sores should be taught separately from the rest of the group.

The authors recommend two inexpensive devices, both from O-Two Medical Technologies, that can help improve training in artificial ventilation. The Mini Ventilation Training Analyzer® (http://www.otwo.com/prod_tv.htm) is a system that demonstrates the impact of too rapid lung inflation during artificial ventilation. The device has a stylised lung and stomach and while appropriate ventilation causes only lung inflation, overzealous ventilation causes progressive filling of the stomach bag. The other device is the SmartBag®, a self-inflating resuscitator that has a spring-loaded mechanism that operates to limit pressure and flow when the bag is squeezed to fast (http://www.otwo.com/prod_bmv.htm). The auditory and tactile feedback it gives makes it an excellent training tool.

All peak resuscitation organisations recommended cricoid pressure during bag and mask ventilation in resuscitation as well as in emergency intubation. If the cricoid pressure is applied in the wrong place, wrong direction, wrong amount of force or at the wrong time the technique cannot be relied on to contribute usefully to patient care. There is a large body of research indicating that cricoid pressure is poorly applied and that experience does not automatically lead to good performance[9]. Cricoid pressure can be learnt using a model larynx on weighing scales or using a purpose designed trainer (Fig. 6.1). Using the trainer allows the airway care provider and assistant to practise working together[10,11] and for the location and direction of applied force to be learnt as well as the amount of force. Team building activities need to be included in training whenever possible and not just in scenarios using a high fidelity patient simulator.

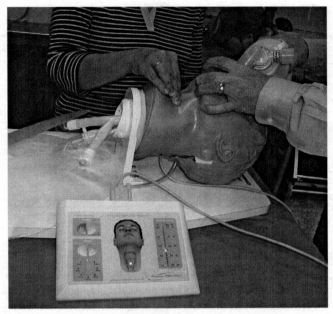

Fig. 6.1 The Cricoid Pressure Trainer from Flinders Meditech allows cricoid pressure and airway management to be practised separately or together.

6.4 **Advanced airway interventions**

6.4.1 **Supraglottic airway devices**

The original Laryngeal Mask Airway (now known as the LMA Classic®) has a related range of reusable and single-use devices, and several manufacturers have brought out their own versions. The original Combitube is still widely available and also has competitors that use similar features to facilitate artificial ventilation. Most airway models and patient simulators have limitations that make many if not most supraglottic airway devices function poorly when used in them[12].

Typically it is not easy to insert a correctly sized LMA in airway training models and when the cuff of the LMA is inflated the device does not rise up as it does in patients. This may encourage trainees to use a smaller LMA than ideal. The CPaRlene® model (http://www.eNasco.com) is just an adequate model for teaching LMA use but has a useful feature arising from the shape of the pharynx and larynx. If the LMA used is smaller than recommended some air often passes into the stomach providing a good demonstration of why following the manufacturer's guidelines on sizing is important. The C-Trac® from the LMA Company is a video-enabled intubating LMA that can also help demonstrate issues associated with using an LMA of the wrong size.

There is continuous innovation in design of supraglottic airway devices and new devices are regularly introduced. New airway devices may not perform well in the current airway trainers – this was (and still is) a problem with the SLIPA (Streamlined Liner in the Pharynx Airway). Potential users should be given adequate opportunity to experiment using a new device in an airway skills area and ideally in simulated patient care or before using it on patients. New device manufacturers should be encouraged to sponsor development of training models to support their product.

Table 6.3 Features to look for in a simulator for teaching endotracheal intubation

- Dimensions similar to human anatomy – including distance from teeth to vocal cords and vocal cords to carina
- Epiglottis moves realistically during laryngoscopy
- Has realistic looking vocal cords
- Has palpable upper airway cartilages (thyroid and cricoid)
- Shape of upper airway changes with external force applied to airway cartilages
- Allows practise of additional measures to confirm intratracheal placement, such as ODD (see Table 6.4) and intra-tracheal ridges
- Can see chest rise with lung inflation
- Lung auscultation in axillae (not apices)
- Epigastric auscultation
- Allows capnometry
- Range of difficulties (e.g. limited mouth opening, limited neck movement, prominent upper incisors)

6.4.2 **Endotracheal intubation**

Endotracheal intubation (ETI) is widely considered to be the ultimate airway intervention and is sometimes referred to as the gold standard. There are several elements to consider in education on ETI – basic skill training, ETI in the difficult airway, and rescue from the failed intubation. There is much information on harm from pre-hospital intubation[13] so ETI teaching must include supraglottic rescue airway devices[14] and trans-tracheal techniques to secure airway access. A list of features to look for in simulators for teaching endotracheal intubation is shown in Table 6.3.

Observation of the trainee's actions can assist the trainer provide specific feedback on technique. Video feedback on technique provides insight into technique that assists learning[15]. Some technique traits are easy to see and record (e.g. rotating the laryngoscope and levering on the teeth, and poor posture during intubation, which can have a big influence on success)[16,17]. Without special aids, the view the trainee or student has of the larynx can only be guessed by the teacher. Ambu make an intubation trainer with an open side for visualising intubation and there is an inferior Chinese copy of this (Fig. 6.2).

Other ways of viewing the larynx during intubation include placing a fibreoptic scope in the nasopharynx to view intubation or a small camera that can be installed in the nasopharynx of an airway trainer. Miniature cameras are cheap but the short distance between camera and glottic opening means that a 'close-up' lens is required for focus and this can cost more than the camera. A propriety training aid, the ET-View®, is an endotracheal tube with a miniature USB camera at its tip (http://www.etview.com/products_2.asp). It must be connected to a PC but it is easy to use the system and it does provide a large and clear image on the screen. Unfortunately, the ET-View® trainer is both expensive and available only in an 8.0 mm ET-tube when a 7.0 mm ETT is the largest size recommended for many airway models.

A number of systems designed to facilitate intubation of patients can be used to assist ETI training through demonstrating laryngeal anatomy. We have used the Glidescope (http://www.saturnbiomedical.com), the Truphatek EVO2® (http://www.truphatek.com), the C-Trac® (http://www.lmana.com) and the AirTraq® (http://www.airtraq.com) to demonstrate airway anatomy of patient simulators. Video imaging has been reported to improve initial success rate of novices learning intubation[18]. Some new video-laryngoscope systems are currently being introduced into anaesthesia, for example McGrath® laryngoscope (http://www.aircraftmedical.com/index.htm) and the Pentax AWS-S100 Airway Scope® (http://www.pentax.co.jp/english), and they may be useful training aids.

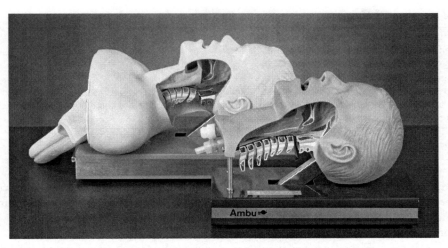

Fig. 6.2 A tale of two airway trainers. One device is from a Scandinavian medical equipment manufacturer and has been refined over several years. The other is made in China and appears to be a copy with some modifications and rough edges – *caveat emptor*!

The AirwayCam® is a unique system for demonstrating conventional laryngoscopy and intubation on a simulator and in clinical care, but it is relatively expensive and has an appreciable learning curve of its own. In theory the AirwayCam® would give the trainer a trainee's eye view of the airway. The head needs to be kept quite still for a good view of the larynx with the AirwayCam® and the area of interest to be kept in the optical centre of the viewing system but novices move their heads and eyes a lot as they try to visualize the larynx. At the time of writing, a new version of the AirwayCam® is about to be released (see http://www.airwaycam.com).

Some airway devices function differently in simulators to the way they perform in patients. The maker of the McCoy laryngoscope, for example, has specifically warned against using it in simulators. Also, when the airway anatomy of a model departs from the normal range performance of airway devices based on patient size can be a problem. The upper airway of the SimMan® UPS has been reported to be unrealistically short[19] so recurrent training on this simulator only could lead to unintended and unwanted clinical behaviours.

Some features to look for in a simulator for teaching endotracheal intubation are shown in Table 6.3

There is some evidence that learning intubation is more efficient if models that are easier to intubate are presented before more difficult airways[20]. Novices learn more from a successful intubation that an unsuccessful attempt. Once a particular airway has been mastered little is gained from repeated successful intubations so as experienced is gained, health professionals need to be presented with more challenging airway simulations. Some models incorporate features that can make intubation more difficult but this needs to reflect the area the trainee is training to work in. Trismus is a common cause of difficulty in the pre-hospital setting so models that have this feature are useful for paramedic student training. In the operating room (OR), anatomy and pathology are more likely to be a cause of airway difficulty.

6.4.2.1 Confirmation of intubation

Endotracheal intubation is supposed to improve patient outcome; however, recent evidence suggests that there is an unacceptably high incidence of errors in airway management in pre-hospital

Table 6.4 Methods of confirming correct intubation

- Visualize ETT passing through the vocal cords
- Can feel the clicks of a bougie on tracheal cartilages
- Use an oesophageal detector device (ODD)
- Visualize bilateral chest expansion
- Auscultate the epigastrium ('breath sounds' should not be heard)
- Auscultate over lung fields bilaterally in axillae to determine adequate and equal breath sounds
- Observe ETCO$_2$ by either waveform or colorimetry

settings and emergency departments even after training[21]. The results of such an error such as unrecognized oesophageal intubations is very serious but even a relatively minor error during intubation can cause problems (e.g. mild hypoxaemia from main stem bronchus can give rise to major injury in a trauma patient with head injury).

There are many methods of confirming correct endotracheal intubation and students should use those listed within resuscitation council guidelines but be aware that no one method is 100% fail proof. Not all guidelines list the same methods but a comprehensive list from the Australian Resuscitation Council[22], American Heart Association Inc.[23] and the European Resuscitation Council[24], can be created (see below) and used during training of ETI (Table 6.4 and Fig. 6.3).

When training in endotracheal intubation skills, confirmation methods must be practised and become second nature. However, there is no one part-task trainer available today that allows all of the methods listed to be performed. High fidelity simulators (e.g. METI-HPS®) come close but are very expensive and certainly not widely available for basic training. Students and trainees can be informed of limitations of the simulators (e.g. the LMA doesn't rise up on inflation of the cuff) but this then reduces the value of the training.

Looking for chest rise is an important sign after intubation but for novices a model without a chest can have some value, seeing one lung lying limp whilst the other inflates provides a good lesson on the need to control how far the tube is advanced beyond the cords. Once this is understood further practise requires a model with a thorax and epigastrium that makes the trainee go through confirmation of successful intubation in the correct manner. Chest rise is not always readily apparent so at this stage a model with a fixed chest (e.g. the CLA range of airway trainers can be useful). Beware of models that encourage poor practice like the Laerdal Adult Airway Trainer that has auscultation points only over lung apices. Once this has been mastered a model that allows the difficulty of intubation to be increased is very desirable (e.g. the Trucorp AirSim Multi®). In our unit we use at least five models in basic ETI training including the simulators mentioned above and some in which 'BURP' is and isn't helpful[25] and in which the ODD provides a false positive result[26]. Recurrent practise in recognizing signs of correct intubation makes it more likely that oesophageal intubation will be identified[27].

When a misplaced ETI occurs in training, it should be recognized quickly and the 'patient' extubated immediately and if a second attempt to intubate also fails, the 'patient' should be ventilated by other means (e.g. face mask, supraglottic airway device [SAD], cricothyrotomy). This ensures that skill learning incorporates use of alternative skills that would be used in clinical practice. Students should also be aware that in some circumstances, methods of confirming correct intubation can produce false-negative results such as in the case of pulseless or poorly perfused patients with little or no ETCO$_2$ being detected. This error (referred to as a type II error) may lead to an ETT that is properly placed, being unnecessarily removed.

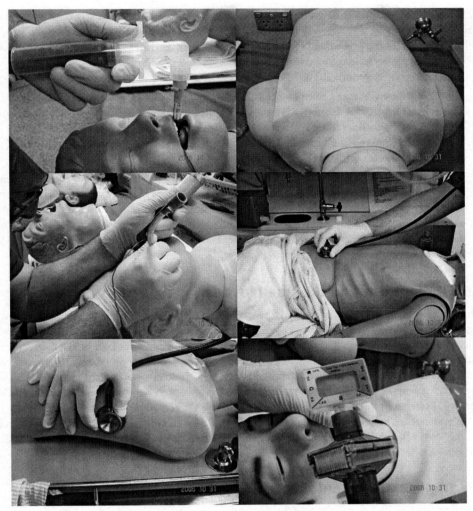

Fig. 6.3 This sequence of images shows the sequence of steps used to confirm endotracheal intubation. The ODD is typically used during resuscitation from cardiac arrest and must be used before artificial ventilation.

6.4.2.2 Difficult extubation

Difficult intubation is generally followed by extubation and so training in the use of airway exchange catheters should be a part of difficult intubation training. Nursing staff from the post-anaesthesia care units, high dependency units and critical care units will also need to receive training on caring for patients with airway exchange catheters, etc *in situ*.

6.4.2.3 How much intubation practice is needed?

The rate of learning ETI can be quite different between trainees and some may never become competent. Published studies suggest between 50 and 100 intubations are required but it would be better to track the acquisition of skills of individual practitioners than rely on a particular number of attempts[28,29]. Recently introduced IT makes personal audit relatively easy to adopt but it does require the practitioner to be able to assess their performance and self-reporting of deficiencies in airway management are frequently inaccurate[30].

There are several questions about ETI that need to be asked.

◆ Can practitioners become competent in ETI through practise on patient simulators alone? This is most important for non-anaesthesia healthcare professionals who do not have good access to patients undergoing ETI as part of their clinical care. Simulator training in ETI is excellent preparation for a controlled environment[31] but there is still no data on how well it actually prepares for difficult clinical settings.

◆ For practitioners who need to maintain a very high level of expertise in airway management techniques, is there an optimal mix of simulator training and clinical exposure? This is very relevant to anaesthesia providers who will be presented with some very difficult airways that must be managed quickly and correctly to avoid morbidity and mortality. Techniques learnt during simulation need to reflect local policies because they will quickly be extinguished if they are not reinforced by clinical experience[32].

6.5 Fibreoptic intubation training aids

Fibreoptic intubation (FOI) is a core skill for securing the anticipated difficult airway in the operating theatre. Sophisticated cognitive and psychomotor skills are required for FOI and providing sufficient training opportunities has always been an issue[33]. Any airway simulator can be used for this and probably every one of them should be used as a part of deliberate practise. Non-anatomical models are also useful for honing scope skills. Physical models do not replicate the give of real tissue or the movements of a patient but virtual reality models have been very successful in creating these illusions. Research indicates that training received using a VR FOI simulator can be effective[34].

VR systems are not easily modified to include aids used in clinical practice (e.g. the Aintree catheter or the Bermann guide) so there will always be a role for physical models for demonstration and practice.

6.6 Trans-tracheal ventilation

Occasionally ventilation cannot be achieved without bypassing the upper airway and using a trans-tracheal ventilation (TTV) technique to access the airway. In an emergency this is best achieved by cricothyrotomy (cricothyroidotomy) and there are several training aids and models made specifically for this purpose. It is certainly possible to make a training aid from discarded items or inexpensive components from a hardware store and there is much to recommend this approach for familiarization with equipment for TTV and the steps of the procedure. Part-task trainers and whole-body patient simulators are needed when the task is being practised in context and 'when' is being learnt as well as 'how'. All the models have limitations but some have a more life-like feel than others, an example of this is the Portex TTV trainer that has 'skin' that moves, wrinkles and stretches. The models we have available for TTV training are shown in Fig. 4. Neck skins and tracheas need regular replacement but the cost of cricothyrotomy kits is the major expense.

The use of locally assembled parts to make an oxygen delivery system should be discouraged, particularly in a simulation facility or teaching hospital. These systems may appear to work in the skills laboratory but cannot be relied on in an emergency. We teach needle cricothyrotomy with the inexpensive Enk oxygen flow modulator system and do not use 14g IV cannulae for access.

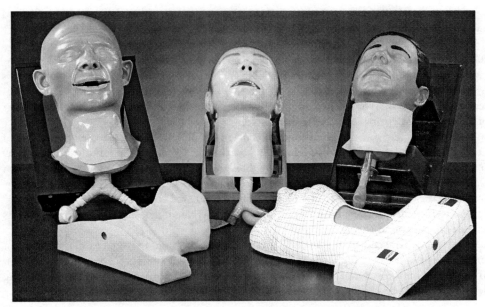

Fig. 6.4. Several small simulators from the USA and Europe for learning and practising emergency transtracheal ventilation.

Once the technique has been mastered it can be incorporated in scenarios but it is easy to give inappropriate signs to participants in a simulation. If reduced mouth opening of a simulator is used to make intubation impossible then whenever that feature is used in a scenario it will signal need for TTV. We have other less obvious methods to make intubation more difficult in our SimMan simulators including a series of modified upper dentures.

Training in emergency TTV has only been studied from a number or different perspectives[35]. Anaesthetists are generally more used to needle-based technique and may be reluctant to resort to a surgical approach. Percutaneous techniques can provide as good access as a surgical technique sometimes in a shorter time[35]. Older practitioners tend to have worse vision and more hand tremor and this can seriously affect cricothyrotomy performance and we have moved away from using systems that require wires to be inserted through a needle because of this. It is essential to be able to perform cricothyrotomy in a very short time and Wong *et al.*[35] recommend at least five attempts or until it can be achieved with 40 s or less. We also use more than one simulator to be more confident that patients of different size and shape can be managed.

6.7 The challenge of airway competence

There have recently been several publications from indicating that specialists and trainees in acute care disciplines do not have the skills needed for difficult airway management[36]. Deaths due to airway mismanagement have prompted official recommendations for teaching and maintaining skills to avoid patient injury from hypoxia[37]. It is clear that repeated attempts at intubation are dangerous[38] and training needs to reflect this. If trainees are allowed to make multiple attempts at intubation in a skills lab then they are being set up to transfer this undesirable behaviour to the OR or emergency department (ED). Difficult airway management guidelines have been developed by many organizations and every hospital with trainees should have a range of part task trainers that can be used to teach DAM. Teaching should be based on national guidelines and include medical and nursing staff. Local variations of DAM guidelines should be avoided.

Video-feedback can help identify errors and provide insight into improving performance[30] so should be a routine part simulation training to gain the most from training time. To take advantage of the range of airway simulators available and to use them most effectively requires this training to be embedded in a clinical curriculum[39]. Assessment of training needs several presentations of airway scenarios in a number of different settings and probably needs in the order of ten separate or distinct exercises to be reliable[40].

Management (and sometimes mismanagement) of the difficult airway has been the subject of Coronial inquiry. Infections and operations in and close to the airway can quickly lead to airway compromise. Several publications have highlighted that training in airway management is often lacking[41] but concerted action often requires a trigger such as an unanticipated fatality. Following the death of a patient after an operation for a dental abscess a number of recommendations were made including the level of training and equipment that should be available in areas where such patients are being cared for[37].

There are a several courses that include airway care teaching (e.g. advanced cardiac life support and advanced trauma life support). The airway training in these courses is quite short in relation to the desired outcome. Simulation has been used to identify training gaps[21] and there is growing debate over what changes might be needed to the content and delivery of these courses.

6.8 Airway training devices in the future

Training using simulators will become essential in the near future and airway management training is falling into three distinct categories. One is teaching basic airway management to all health professionals and automated systems that provide feedback will be developed for this in the same way that systems have been developed to guide external cardiac compression during CPR. Another is providing a way of developing skills in advanced airway interventions for anaesthetists and Virtual reality (VR) become increasingly used for this. We have sophisticated (VR) airway simulators that can effectively prepare trainees for clinical procedures on patients now[43] but VR simulators for ETI[44] and cricothyrotomy[45] are still relatively crude.

The third category includes health professionals who need to provide effective airway care occasionally and often in difficult settings. Pre-hospital and emergency intubation has such a high failure rate[46] that the 'occasional intubator' will increasingly be expected to undertake simulation for skills maintenance and simulation for assessment of proficiency will probably be mandated in certain settings. Laryngoscopic skills decay rapidly and it is possible that another device or intubating system that has less skill decay over time will become more widely used[47]. Improved airway training devices are needed and research on intubation has given clear pointers towards what features will be included in them[48].

Augmented reality systems offer novel techniques to help teach airway management. A prototype system that displays airway anatomy of a patient simulator to a trainee emergency care provider has been developed[49].

6.9 Conclusion

Airway skills teaching has to be designed to cater for all adult learning styles and to adapt to the rate of learning by participants. Content has to be relevant to engage learners so their background and achievements must be ascertained when the teaching is being planned. Most healthcare practitioners want to provide better care so relevant links that can be made to actual clinical care can be helpful. Training that may lead to negative transfer must be avoided.

Teaching should be based on published guidelines rather than personal opinions and use the best available equipment rather than local 'fixes'. Outcome of patient care is dependent on the 'weakest link' so all steps need to be included in teaching. For example, teaching intubation should include teaching how to apply safe and effective cricoid pressure.

Deliberate repeated skills practise is important to develop 'unconscious competence' so that working memory is freed up for other tasks. There is no one device that provides everything needed for airway skills teaching so quality education and training will require airway teaching facilities to have several different part-task trainers and patient simulators.

There are many aids for teaching airway skills and choice should be determined by the learning objectives of the teaching or training. There is no one model or device that can be recommended over another and some that are useful for one group may not be as useful for another. Budgets for airway skills and simulation training facilities will need to reflect this now and in the future.

References

1. Mason RA (1998). Education and training in airway management. *Br J Anaesth* **81**: 305–7.
2. Reznick RK, MacRae H (2006). Teaching Surgical Skills – Changes in the Wind. *N Engl J Med* **355**: 2664–9.
3. Ginifer C, Kelly A (1996). Teaching resuscitation skills using the newly deceased. *Med J Australia* **165**: 445–7.
4. Cummins RO, Hazinski MF (2000). Guidelines Based on the Principle "First, Do No Harm": New guidelines on tracheal tube confirmation and prevention of dislodgment. *Circulation* **102**: I-380–4.
5. Fitts PM, Posner MI (1967). *Human Performance*. Belmont, CA: Brooks/Cole.
6. Martin KM, Larsen PD, Segal R, Marsland CP (2004). Effective nonanatomical endoscopy training produces clinical airway endoscopy proficiency. *Anesth Analg* **99**: 938–44.
7. Ericsson KA (2004). Deliberate practice and the acquisition and maintenance of expert performance in medicine and related domains. *Acad Med* **79**: S70–S8.1
8. Rosenthal E, Owen H (2004). An assessment of small simulators used to teach basic airway management. *Anaesth Intensive Care* **32**: 87–92.
9. Owen H, Follows V, Reynolds K, Burgess G, Plummer J (2002). Learning to apply effective cricoid pressure using a part task trainer. *Anaesthesia* **57**: 1098–111.
10. Morey JC, Simon R, Jay GD, *et al.* (2002). Error reduction and performance improvement in the emergency department through formal teamwork training: evaluation results of the MedTeams project. *Health Services Research* **37**: 1553–81.
11. Salas E, Wilson KA, Burke CS, Wightman DC (2006). Does crew resource management training work? An update, and extension, and some critical needs. *Human Factors* **48**: 392–412.
12. Parry K, Owen H (2004). Small simulators for teaching procedural skills in a difficult airway algorithm. *Anaesth and Intensive Care* **32**: 401–9.
13. Gausche-Hill M (2003). Ensuring quality prehospital airway management. *Curr Opin Anaesth* **16**: 173–81.
14. Ander DS, Hanson A, Pitts S (2004). Assessing resident skills in the use of rescue airway devices. *Ann Emer Med* **44**: 314–9.
15. Kardash K, Tessler MJ (1997). Videotape feedback in teaching laryngoscopy. *Can J Anaesth* **44**: 54–8.
16. Matthews AJ, Johnson CJ, Goodman NW (1998). Body posture during simulated tracheal intubation. *Anaesth* **53**: 331–4.
17. Walker JD (2002). Posture used by anaesthetists during laryngoscopy. *Br J Anaesth* **89**: 772–4.
18. Levitan RM, Goldman TS, Bryan DA, Shofer F, Herlich A (2001). Training with video imaging improves the initial intubation success rates of paramedic trainees in an operating room setting. *Ann Emerg Med* **37**: 46–50.

19. Hesselfeldt R, Kristensen MS, Rasmussen LS. Evaluation of the airway of the SimManTM full-scale patient simulator. *Acta Anaesthesiol Scand* 2005; 49: 1339–1345

20. Plummer JL, Owen H (2001). Learning endotracheal intubation in a clinical learning center: A Quantitative Study. *Anesth Analg* 93: 656–62.

21. Barsuk D, Ziv A, Lin G, *et al.* (2005). Using advanced simulation for recognition and correction of gaps in airway and breathing management skills in prehospital trauma care. *Anesth Analg* 100: 803–9.

22. Australian Resuscitation Council (2006). *Equipment and Techniques in Adult Life Support. (Guideline 11.7)*, Feb 2006; http://www.resus.org.au

23. American Heart Association Inc (2005). Part 7.1: Adjunct for airway control and ventilation. Guidelines for cardiopulmonary resuscitation and emergency cardiovascular care. *Circulation* 112 (Suppl.); IV51–5.7

24. Nolan JP, Deakin CD, Soar J, Bottiger BW, Smith GB (2005). *European Resuscitation Council Guidelines for Resuscitation* 67 (Suppl. 1): S39–S86.

25. Takahata O, Kubota M, Mamiya K, *et al.* (1997). The Efficacy of the "BURP" Maneuver During a Difficult Laryngoscopy. *Anesth Analg* 84: 419–21.

26. Owen H, Plummer JL (2002). Improving learning of a clinical skill: the first year's experience of teaching endotracheal intubation in a clinical simulation facility. *Med Educ* 36: 635–42.

27. Gordon RD (2006). Selective attention during scene perception: evidence from negative priming. *Memory & Cognition* 34: 1484–94.

28. Bolsin S, Colson M (2000). The use of the Cusum technique in the assessment of trainee competence in new procedures. *Int J for Qual in Health Care* 12: 433–8.

29. de Oliveira Filho GR (2002). The construction of learning curves for basic skills in anesthetic procedures: An Application for the Cumulative Sum Method. *Anesth Analg* 95: 411–16.

30. Mackenzie CF, Jefferies NJ, Hunter A, *et al.* (1996). Comparison of self reporting of deficiencies in airway management with video analyses of actual performance. *Human Factors* 38: 623–35.

31. Hall RE, Plant JR, Bands CJ, Wall AR, Kang J, Hall CA (2005). Human patient simulation is effective for teaching paramedic students endotracheal intubation. *Acad Emerg Med* 12: 850–5.

32. Olympio MA, Whelan R, Ford RP, Saunders IC (2003). Failure of simulation training to change residents' management of oesophageal intubation. *Br J Anaesth* 91: 312–8.

33. Goldmann K, Steinfeldt T (2006). Acquisition of basic fiberoptic intubation skills with a virtual reality airway simulator. *J Clin Anesth* 18: 173–8.

34. Goldmann K, Braun U (2006). Airway management practices at German university and university-affiliated teaching hospitals – equipment, techniques and training: results of a nationwide survey. *Acta Anaesthesiol Scand* 50: 298–305.

35. Wong D, Prabhu A, Coloma M, Imasogie N, Chung F (2003). What is the minimum training required for successful cricothyroidotomy?: A study in mannequins. *Anesthesiology* 98: 349–53.

36. Mulcaster JT, Mills J, Hung OR, *et al.* (2003). Laryngoscopic Intubation: Learning and Performance. *Anesthesiology* 98: 23–7.

37. Department of Health, Government of Western Australia. Operational Circular. 16/9/2004 www.health.wa.gov.au/criticalcare/docs/Management%20of%20the%20Difficult%20Airway.pdf.

38. Mort TC (2004). Emergency Tracheal Intubation: Complications Associated with Repeated Laryngoscopic Attempts. *Anesth Analg* 99: 607–13.

39. Schaefer III JJ (2004). Simulators and difficult airway management skills. *Pediatric Anesthesia* 14: 28–37.

40. Epstein RM (2007). Assessment in medical education. *N Engl J Med* 356: 387–96.

41. Rosenstock C, Østergaard D, Kristensen MS, Lippert A, Ruhnau B, Rasmussen LS (2004). Residents lack knowledge and practical skills in handling the difficult airway. *Acta Anaesthesiol Scand* 48: 1014–18.

42. Rowe R, Cohen RA (2002). An evaluation of a virtual reality airway simulator. *Anesth Analg* 95: 62–6.

43. Blum MG, Powers TW, Sundaresan S. Bronchoscopy simulator effectively prepares junior residents to competently perform basic clinical bronchoscopy. Ann Thorac Surg 2004; **78**: 287–291.

44. Mayrose J, Kesavadas T, Chugh K, Joshi D, Ellis DG (2003). Utilization of virtual reality for endotracheal intubation training. *Resuscitation* **59**: 133–8.

45. Liu A, Bhasin Y, Acosta E, Bowyer M (2005). A haptic-enabled simulator for cricothyroidotomy *Medicine Meets Virtual Reality 13*. Westwood DJ *et al.*, Eds. IOS Press.

46. ILCOR (2005). International Liaison Committee on Resuscitation (ILCOR). Part 4: Advanced Life Support. *Resuscitation* **67**: 213–47.

47. Maharaj CH, Costello J, Higgins BD, Harte BH, Laffey JG (2007). Retention of tracheal intubation skills by novice personnel: a comparison of the Airtraq and Macintosh laryngoscopes. *Anaesthesia* **62**: 272–8.

48. Noh Y, Nagahiro K, Ogura Y, Solis J, *et al.*(2006). Design of airway management training system. itab2006 proceedings http://medlab.cs.uoi.gr/itab2006/proceedings/Education%20&%20Training/104.pdf

49. Rolland JP, Biocca F, Hamza-Lup F, Ha Y, Martins R (2005). Development of head-mounted projection displays for distributed, collaborative, augmented reality applications presence: *Teleoperators & Virtual Environments* **14**(5): 528–49.

Chapter 7

Equipment

Gary Hope and Chris Chin

Overview

◆ Effective clinical simulation requires learners to suspend disbelief and interact with the human patient simulator and the simulation environment as if they were real.

◆ The simulator mannequin is often considered the mainstay of simulation training and an increasing range from low to high fidelity mannequins are available

◆ The presence of medical equipment is also essential for providing a sense of realism and a vast array from the less expensive (stethoscopes, intravenous, and airway equipment) to the more costly (endoscopes, ventilators, anaesthetic machines) may be required.

◆ The use of props can be invaluable if they help or enhance the perception of reality of the scenario being created.

◆ Local health and safety policies should be followed in regards to equipment used in the simulation environment.

◆ Video playback can be a powerful teaching tool and audiovisual equipment plays and important role in enhancing simulation training.

7.1 Introduction

As with any tool, the effectiveness of simulation technology depends on how it is used. For clinical simulation training to be most effective, learners must 'suspend disbelief' and interact with the simulator and the simulation environment as if they were real[1]. While other types of simulation such as case studies, part-task trainers and role-play are also an effective way of training, a complete clinical simulation facility will also provide access to mannequins that reliably duplicate patient signs and symptoms[2]. In addition to these mannequins such a centre also provides the sights, sounds, and other sensations associated with a real clinical environment. A simulation centre therefore attempts to recreate characteristics of the real world, with the term simulation fidelity traditionally used to define the degree to which reality is replicated. Setting up a high fidelity clinical simulation scenario can be likened to a good theatrical production. The simulation room and human patient simulator, the actors/trainers, the equipment and the props support the illusion of reality and allow the trainee to become fully immersed in the experience. Designing, developing, and maintaining a simulation centre that reproduces the patient-care environment with high fidelity is a costly, challenging task which includes the provision of appropriate equipment and the development and use of props to create an appropriately realistic environment. To increase the effectiveness of the training, the simulator setting will also include audiovisual equipment to allow clear observation of the scenario and, as importantly, to allow objective feedback to the participants[3,4,5].

Within the simulator environment the terms 'equipment' and 'prop' can actually be considered to have a spectrum of uses. A piece of equipment might be any fully functioning machine, tool or object that could be used in the real clinical world. However, the presence of medical equipment in the simulator environment is also essential for providing a sense of realism whether being used in any particular scenario or not. When equipment is used purely to create a sense of realism it might therefore more appropriately be considered to be a prop. While a prop would normally be considered as anything which has the aim of mimicking the real world but which itself is not functional, as alluded to above, a functioning piece of equipment might also be usefully placed in any appropriate scenario to increase the sense of realism. In addition, in the current safety conscious training environment, many training devices (e.g. a deactivated training defibrillator), are now used in the simulator or training setting in exactly the same way as the real equipment, but as they are not active, cannot be used in the real clinical setting[6]. For the purpose of this chapter, the term 'equipment' will be used for any device or tool that could be used in the clinical setting.

7.2 Human patient simulators

The simulator mannequin can be considered the mainstay of simulation training. A screen-based computer system linked to a patient monitor to display physiological parameters such as the ACCESS® system developed by Byrne *et al.* from Cardiff combined with an advanced life support mannequin has been used to provide anaesthetic simulator scenario training[7]. In such low fidelity systems there is no direct link between the computer and the mannequin. Several commercial human patient simulators (HPS) (e.g. METI-HPS®) are now available varying in their degree of complexity. These more sophisticated HPS have a controlling computer workstation which generates realistic physiological signals (ECG, pulse oximetry, blood pressure, $PECO_2$ and invasive parameters) for display on a standard patient monitor. Many of the physical parameters can also be changed such as ease of intubation, breath sounds and respiratory movements, heart sounds and pulses. In addition these whole body mannequins can be instrumented (venous cannulation, intubation and ventilation, cricothyroidotomy, chest tube insertion). The development of these mannequins with realistic responses allows different types of patients to be simulated as real entities.

With Gaumard 3000Hal® and Laerdal SimMan®, the computer operator or preprogrammed trends adjust physiological variables in response to clinical events[8,9]. The METI Emergency Care Simulator® also has pharmacological and physiological modelling built into the software providing increased automaticity of the device[10]. The most sophisticated mannequin, the METI-HPS® takes this a step further with the inclusion of servocontrol mechanisms such that action or inaction of participants will lead to automatic changes in the vital signs of the mannequin brought about through the physiological and pharmacological modelling[10]. This is particularly relevant to ventilation such that the lung simulates gaseous exchange with addition of appropriate amounts of relevant gases to the lung for exhalation. Adult HPS systems have been available for some time, but high fidelity and mid fidelity paediatric HPS in child and infant models are now also on the market[8,9,10].

7.3 Creating a realistic environment

Hospitals use a vast array of medical equipment that can range from less expensive items, such as stethoscopes, intravenous and airway equipment, to more costly medical equipment such as ventilators. In order to provide an appropriate and realistic environment, a typical anaesthetic course might include the following: anaesthetic machine with all the peripherals including breathing circuits and vaporizers, patient monitor including electrocardiogram (ECG) leads, non-invasive blood pressure cuff, pulse oximetry probe, intubation equipment, patient trolley, operating table, syringe drivers. For anaesthesia scenarios based around surgical operations the relevant equipment and props might also include appropriate surgical instruments, a diathermy machine, suction bottles, endoscopic or arthroscopic instruments with television monitors and appropriate videotapes, surgical drapes, sutures, swabs and dressings. For other specialist courses the list would likely become extensive, for instance obstetric courses would have to include items related to the care of the expectant mother and the new born child: babytherm, CTG machine, epidural and spinal equipment, patient bed.

7.3.1 Real equipment

Wherever possible real equipment should be used; however, in many situations it will be necessary to use props. Props have a place in simulation only if they enhance or help the perception of the reality of the scenario being created and give the outward appearance of being real and useful. Such use of props may include the modification of the mannequins as of the process for improving the realism of the scenario[11,12]. The use of poor, unconvincing props, which might handicap the realism of the scenario, should be avoided if this could diminish the impact of the training. A prop should be considered successful if it convinces the participant that it is real and or persuades the participant to perform as they would in real life. The way in which a prop is used can also influence the success of that item. For example, using surgical instruments in a convincing manner, although they may not be intended for that purpose, may be sufficient to convince the participant that a surgical procedure is occurring.

7.3.2 Fluids, medications, and body fluids

Medications, blood products, and bodily fluids can provide interesting challenges. While water can often be used for intravenous medications, if special colouring is required, appropriate food dye can be used. The cost of using several bags intravenous fluids during courses can also be greatly reduced by refilling used bags with water between courses or between scenarios. Drugs that take a powder form can be replaced with baking soda/flour. Pills and tablets, if required, can be replicated with sweets that come in all sizes and colours. All participants must be made aware at the beginning of the course that no medications are intended for human use. Also it must be stressed that no controlled substances are on the premises.

Blood, blood products, and body fluids are props that can be created, simulated or bought. There are countless variations of recipes in use and these can be found on the internet through many acting and theatrical sites.

The main problem with making blood-like products is that they can involve the use of thickening agents (such as corn syrup) that are sugar based. These products can be difficult or time consuming to cleanup. As an alternative, blood concentrate can also be purchased from theatrical or joke shops and diluted to requirements. Platelets, fresh frozen plasma and cryoprecipitate can be reproduced using pineapple or pear juice at various dilutions.

Other body fluids include urine (apple juice with added water to lessen concentrate) and melaena (Weetabix®, coffee granules, orange flavour Fybogel® and black food colouring). The latter should be made fresh before use for a distinctive smell. Another distinctive smell is ketotic breath that can be created by the use of nail varnish remover. Vomit can be created quite easily and almost anything can be used; however, chunky vegetable soup is a good option. Finally, hair gel is very good for sputum, while glycerine is great for sweat.

7.4 **Acquiring equipment and props**

The scope and diversity in medical simulation is continually widening, which also increases the need for equipment and resources. A complete list of equipment is unfeasible within the scope of this chapter and will also vary depending on the training undertaken by the simulation center. However, as there will usually be a limit to the equipment and props budget available, various sources should be considered for the acquisition of the required equipment. While purchase of new equipment may be necessary, it is generally not the cheapest way. Acquiring equipment and props therefore requires a degree of resourcefulness, imagination and help. As might be expected hospitals can be a very useful source of equipment and/or props. Many healthcare simulation training centres will be affiliated to a hospital, or through training staff will have links to hospitals. As hospitals can often purchase equipment in bulk for a discounted rate it might be cost effective to purchase a piece of equipment at the same time as the hospital. In addition, hospital equipment that is no longer being used or that is being upgraded, and broken equipment that is unsuitable for clinical use might be donated to the centre or purchased at a much cheaper price than a new piece of equipment. Operating departments are a good hunting ground for surgical and anaesthetic sundries. There are too many to mention all but items range from Abbott catheters, epidural needles, swabs, breathing filters, suction catheters all of which can still be used safely in simulation after the expiry date has passed.

Use of drugs plays a large part in clinical scenarios immensely and while techniques for creating 'drugs' have already been suggested, provision of labelled ampoules will increase the realism. In some scenarios reconstituting intravenous drugs from the powdered form may play an important role and in such circumstances, the use of appropriate drug bottles is essential for this. Many simulator centres will rely on donation of expired drugs, and operating theatres, wards, hospital departments, and the hospital pharmacy as a useful source of these.

Equipment loans and donations from health related companies are a potential source of equipment and are a useful means of providing new and up-to-date products as well as any training required. In addition to the obvious benefits for the simulator centre, such arrangements can also be useful for companies as it provides an opportunity for any participants attending a simulator course to become familiar with equipment they might not otherwise have encountered.

Eventually after exhausting all other channels the department may have to purchase equipment, which could be used or obtained at a discount from a company offering exposure for said brand. In addition to the purchase cost, some equipment will also require substantial ongoing revenue fees that will need to be factored into the appropriate budget.

7.5 **Health and safety**

Potentially the simulation centre can be a dangerous environment. Local health and safety policies must be followed in regards to equipment used in the department, which include anything from the storage and disposable of sharps to the use and storage of medical gases. All equipment received from any clinical area will also need to be decontaminated before use and any electrical equipment should be subject to an annual audit. Regular safety checks should be carried out by the medical or clinical engineering department at which time the equipment can be certified safe for use. In some cases adjustments to equipment may be needed such as alarms and monitoring on the anaesthetic machine or making a decommissioned defibrillator safe for use. Candidates should be familiarized with the simulator setting and the equipment before commencing a course and this time can also be used to highlight any issues and adjustments made to equipment that may affect candidate safety.

7.6 **Audiovisual equipment**

Audiovisual (AV) equipment plays an important role in successful high fidelity simulation training. While not all simulation training will require video debriefing playback, this can be a very powerful teaching tool and should not be relegated to full-scale simulations only[3,4,5]. It has two distinct purposes:

- To allow the operator, people in the console room and participants observing from the seminar room to see clearly the patient monitor and simulation room from all angles.
- To record and provide the participants with a video feedback of the simulation.

The equipment design and camera and monitor placements should maximize the amount of information gathered. Information recorded can include vital signs in addition to audio and video from multiple angles. In addition, when considering what AV system to install, it is important to remember that unless dedicated staff is continuously available to operate it, the AV equipment must be simple and straightforward to use. Many simulator centres will rely on visiting instructor staff to run training courses and most of these will not be expert with AV equipment. These instructors will often choose not to use complicated AV equipment.

Systems may be as basic as single camera set-ups or may become more complex. Laerdal SimMan® and SimBaby®, for example, include the potential to use a simple videocamera connected to a laptop for the AV recording of a simulation scenario. Other entry-level equipment is available which can allow basic recording and mixing of signals (e.g. overlaying the patient monitor output with that of the video action) for eventual playback. AV products are constantly evolving and beyond these more basic options, centre designers have a wide range of options to choose from and the budget and scope of the project will be significant dictating factors. More sophisticated professional equipment is widely available but might be prohibitively expensive.

Recording and storage of audio and video presents special challenges for any centre. While VHS might still be used, optical media such as DVD is increasingly replacing these systems. The advantages include improved AV quality, and playback of digital video during debriefings is also easier and quicker. Additional benefits include ease of storage with a reduction in space required for storage, and increased life span of media (when compared with VHS). When using digital media, it is important to choose digital storage formats that are well-established standards and are widely accepted. Using standardized formats will increase the likelihood of forward portability of the media. A variety of media are also available for storing the large amount of compressed data. One popular option might be to record directly onto a commercial DVD recorder with a built in hard drive, but recording AV material direct to a computer hard drive is also a possibility[13,14].

Recorded material (and discussion) in simulation training must remain confidential and should be protected to assure the full participation of the participant. The establishment of this trust-bond with the participant is important. While there are circumstances where the use of recorded material outside of the centre is permitted, specific permission must be granted by all members of the simulation (including actors).

Additional AV equipment that may be of use are radio headsets. These may be worn by trainers and actors within the simulation room and allows them be in voice contact with the simulator operator. This contact is useful for allowing the simulator operator to confirm actions by the participant(s) that were not seen on camera. It also allows the simulator operator to feed appropriate prompts (via the actors), such as physical signs that cannot be portrayed on the mannequin (e.g. cyanosis, peripheral perfusion) to the participant.

References

1. Steadman RH, Coates WC, Huang YM, *et al.* (2006). Simulation-based training is superior to problem-based learning for the acquisition of critical assessment and management skills. *Critical Care Medicine* **34**(1): 151–7.

2. Maran NJ, Glavin RJ (2003). Low- to high-fidelity simulation – A continuum of medical education? *Medical Education* **37**(Suppl.1): 22–8.

3. Birnbach DJ, Santos AC, Bourlier RA, *et al.* (2002). The effectiveness of video technology as an adjunct to teach and evaluate epidural anesthesia performance skills. *Anesthesiology* **96**(1): 5–9.

4. Gaba DM, Howard SK, Flanagan B, Smith B, Fish KJ, Botney R (1998). Assessment of clinical performance during simulated crises using both technical and behavioral ratings. *Anesthesiology* **89**(1): 8–18.

5. Savoldelli GL, Naik VN, Park J, Joo HS, Chow R, Hamstra SJ (2006). Value of debriefing during simulated crisis management: oral versus video-assisted oral feedback. *Anesthesiology* **105**(2): 279–85.

6. http://www.aedsuperstore.com

7. Byrne AJ, Hilton PJ, Lunn JN (1994). Basic simulations for anaesthetists: a pilot study of the ACCESS system. *Anaesthesia* **49**: 376–81.

8. http://www.gaumard.com

9. http://www.laerdal.com

10. http://www.meti.com

11. http://www.patientsimulation.co.uk

12. http://www.limbsandthings.com

13. http://www.blinemedical.com

14. http://www.smots.org

Chapter 8

Cardiopulmonary resuscitation and training devices

Sheena Ferguson

Overview

- The availability of passive and low fidelity tools for a simulation lab is extensive and varied.
- Factors that influence your selection include course frequency, course size (number of mannequins needed), durability, cost, portability, and level of functionality.
- Assess the needs of the lab, know what you are getting in advance, and understand that there is usually a balance among several factors that are specific to a particular centre.
- Provide a variety of devices and stretch the learning and practice of effective interventions; consider having several different mannequins.
- Rotate learners through several stations to practise different mannequins; each can add something different to the learning experience.
- Select the right tool for the learning objective.

8.1 Introduction

There are a myriad of passive mannequins and partial task trainers that are available on the market (e.g. Ambu, Armstrong, Gaumard, Laerdal, Limbs & Things, Lifeform, Nasco, Simulaids) to augment or 'accessorize' the range of low to high fidelity full-body human simulators on today's market. Some of these catalogue giants are retailers for several smaller companies and may include their own unique products. The numbers of products are much larger than most simulation lab directors realize and it is worth shopping around and checking with colleagues to see what the experience of other centres has been with a product. Customer service and post-purchase assistance varies tremendously. The end of this chapter includes a resource section; this information is provided as a service, not an endorsement of any particular product. The B*A*T*C*A*V*E* (University of New Mexico) is a multidisciplinary simulation and skills centre that purchases the best tool for the task at hand.

The routine training of the healthcare professions and the community training of the public have given rise to the widespread use of basic cardiopulmonary (CPR) mannequins over the past 40 or more years. Mannequins are now so affordable, portable, and low-tech (e.g. the Styrofoam versions); community instructors are able to purchase their personal sets for CPR training. As additional courses were developed in first aid, intermediate and advanced life support, additional passive trainers have become more and more available. It is also true that the attempt has been made to develop greater fidelity, allow more interventions, and increase features to become more lifelike. However, by their very nature such trainers are passive and automation is negligible. The basic level task trainers are specifically useful for the acquisition of psychomotor skills, rather than focusing on any comprehensive simulated physical response for the student to interpret.

Decisions about the best tools for a particular simulation centre must be made with consideration of many factors.

8.2 **Cardiopulmonary resuscitation**

CPR mannequins that accept ventilation and allow compressions run the gamut in terms of simulation options. On the high end of the spectrum are the high fidelity, full-body simulators that provide one of the highest degrees of realism for CPR situations, in that they demonstrate chest rise, return breath, generate pulses, are defibrillatable, as well as other features. For a large numbers of learners (e.g. 'stadium days' for community CPR training), this is not the best use of these high-end simulators as the instructor: student ratio is shifted to a non-efficient ratio. Additionally, portability and the wear and tear on the simulators are also generally not considered as being acceptable. For large groups of students or routine courses, the passive trainers or low fidelity systems can be optimal. Early on at the inception of CPR training, the passive mannequins who provided the greatest student and instructor feedback were the 'Annies' by Laerdal in the early 1960s. In 25 years of training, the author doesn't recall being at a single healthcare facility to train staff where these highly prevalent originals were not the mannequin of choice. When CPR training became more stringent, the electronically recording 'Annies' that recorded the number and depth of compressions and the number and depth of ventilations became the mannequin of choice. This same version also had an audible 'tick-tock' tone so that the novice could have a reference for how quickly to compress. In other words they would compress at the same rate as the ticking tone. These mannequins did provide the student with a more lifelike physical work-out for simulating CPR at that time since they were state-of-the-art, but as the philosophical approach to education has changed over the years, the rigidity of this type of exercise fell out of favour. A review of the recall and implementation of CPR by the public identified that the layperson believed pulses being felt when there was not one and not feeling a pulse when there was a pulse actually present. A reduction in the complexity of the sequence and the number of steps was needed. The 'perfect' recorded strips model was retired, and the performance standards were simplified. Since actual people needing CPR did not have recorders, the emphasis was on compressing as fast as the provider could compress while generating an adequate pulse as the new standard for performer feedback. These 'Annies' are still very common as they are virtually indestructible and in fact make excellent rescue victims when they are no longer needed for CPR, because of their weight, which more closely simulates an actual victim and the sturdiness of the material with which they are made.

Simulation of compressions and ventilations during CPR, specifically in terms of difficulty and rigour, can be a complex and perplexing dilemma. Novices do not know what to compare the simulation to in terms of life experience. The other points on the range all have various perspectives or experiences. Seasoned providers either feel that the more substantial mannequins are close to a real-life situation or not similar at all. The variety of mannequins on the market and the inter-mannequin differences can be looked at as being like the variations in patients themselves, that there are variations that mimic the particulars of the situation or the pathologies that can be encountered clinically. The B*A*T*C*A*V*E staff believe that these variances in mannequins serve to teach a variety of interventions that may useful in a variety of clinical situations.

At the lower end of the spectrum, though quite functional, are the Styrofoam or pillow models. These are lightweight and highly portable and affordable, though being somewhat featureless in terms of anatomical landmarks and providing any feedback to the student. This requires additional emphasis by the instructor to demonstrate or simulate anatomical features on students or use alternate methodologies.

In summary, there is a wide variety of mannequins on the market. Looking at the gamut of vendor catalogues for 2007, there are 47 different types and models of devices for CPR training.

8.3 **Mannequin selection**

There are many factors to consider when purchasing CPR mannequins for a simulation lab. The director will need to identify what portion of the budget will be directed towards these items. The determining factors in this assessment will include the focus of the simulation lab ('simlab') itself. If the simlab will be supporting community activities such as public programs for training car, then a larger number of mannequins will be needed. Recent guidelines from the national organizations that have developed CPR training programmes is for each student to have their own mannequin, this is very different than previous decades where the mannequin student ratios were 6:1.

The selection of a mannequin should also include a clear plan for maintaining the infection control process. While some centres may still provide each student with their own mannequin face (to swap out between testing), this requires an area for decontamination onsite or decontamination (sterile processing) plan to an offsite location. Most simlabs avoid this time and expense by using a disposable airway or shield of some sort. The complexity and time to replace a disposable airway, as well as the actual cost of these disposable airways should play a factor in the selection process.

Additional considerations may extend to portability issues, mannequin weights (wanting more for some simulation exercises if rescue is involved, less weight if routine toting to external venues is planned). The size of the mannequins, the size and weight of the cases are all important when mobility is a part of the simlab scope.

Next, the durability of the device should be considered. Styrofoam or lightweight plastics will not endure high-use situations. Alternatively, the sturdier and heavier weight mannequins can hold up with many thousands of hours of use. Some of the mannequins in the B*A*T*C*A*V*E* are still very usable a decade later and were in the moderate price range when purchased. And though this may go without saying, you should have an equipment log of the date purchased and monitor what complications and/or problems you have with any of these mannequins as well as your expensive items.

Another consideration is the ability to repair a mannequin and the cost of the repair. In some mannequins the cost of the repair approaches the cost of the mannequin. In assessing this, look at the number of movable parts and the materials of which the mannequin is made. Inquire with the sales representative about the warranty, a list of replaceable parts, labour charges, and note where the mannequin needs to be shipped to for a repair. It will save you 'sticker shock' at a later date. If your mannequins are going to be portable, assess the storage case for costs, weight, and functionality. Lastly, inquire about the composition of the mannequins to identify latex-allergy risk. This is important and should be a consideration in the selection process.

Mannequin diversity on the market today allows the educator to tailor their purchases to the needs of their students. Mannequins are available in a wide-range of sizes and colours (Fig. 8.1). The paediatric sizes include 'premie' (premature baby) (e.g. Gaumard), newborn, toddler, child, adolescent as well as adult ranges. Creativity can enhance the simulation level. For in-hospital settings, many of the mannequins can be altered to include tracheostomy tubes, gastric tubes, casts, and a variety of other devices. Mannequins can also be ordered in a variety of skin colours,

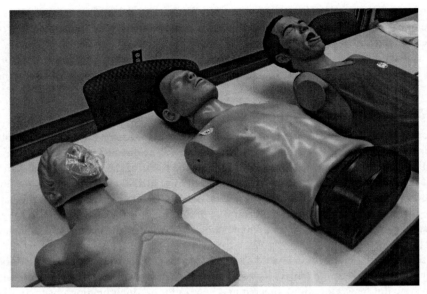

Fig. 8.1 Mannequins have various types of airways for sanitation: washable faces, disposable plastics or face shields.

and with ethnic skin features (Fig. 8.2). Mannequins are available that simulate a variety of patient conditions, including a series that simulates obese patients.

One other element mannequin selection in CPR would be the basic life support situations, such as choking. mannequins with physical obstructions are also available on the market. These mannequins can also be obese or pregnant, and come in a variety of age ranges as well. An object is connected around the mannequins' neck by a barely visible nylon thread to prevent them from getting lost or separated from the mannequin. A properly delivered abdominal thrust relieves the obstruction and the student has a visual cue of the airway obstruction being relieved (Fig. 8.3).

In summary, considerations of the type of device to be incorporated into any simulation lab should include the following:

◆ Budget allowance and mannequin cost
◆ Course frequency and size
◆ Types of learners (layperson, healthcare professions)
◆ Specialty situations or care
◆ Infection control components
◆ Ease of disposable airway/shield use
◆ Cost of the disposable airway/shield
◆ Durability of the mannequin (latex-free)

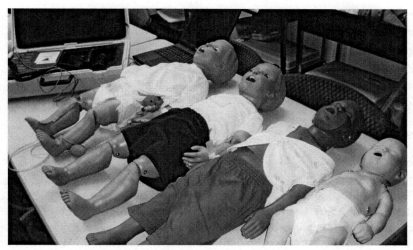

Fig. 8.2 Mannequins come in various ages, sizes, colours, and ethnic features to simulate a diverse culture.

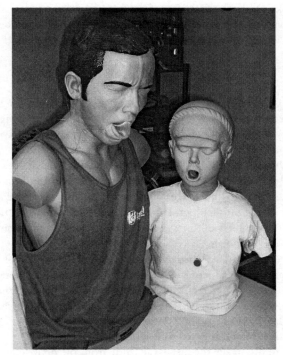

Fig. 8.3 Mannequins go beyond those used for cardiopulmonary resuscitation and can enhance basic life support skills, such as practise in relieving airway obstructions with actual obstructive devices.

- Portability (mannequin cases)
- Repair ability and cost
- Diversity and ranges
- Additional BLS features.

The order of importance of these factors will vary with the simlab's mission, customer base and budget.

8.4 Defibrillators

8.4.1 Devices

CPR training has traditionally included the A-B-C or airway-breathing-circulation. D has traditionally been defibrillation. The Gaumard virtual series includes a virtual defibrillator in their low fidelity computer interface based systems. Many simlabs have had substantial difficulty obtaining either enough numbers of defibrillators for training, or the current version. To begin, assess what your lab needs. Novices becoming familiar with defibrillation may not need the newest version, whereas rapid response or code teams will benefit from the same models they will encounter in a clinical situation. Assess your simlabs affiliations: an academic medical centre may present different opportunities than a smaller school. Be aware of changes in healthcare organizations in your community that are downsizing or expanding as these often present opportunities for acquiring equipment. Do not fail to check out the basement or storage facility for the hospital and ask for a donation. It is surprising what is available to be pressed into service when one looks or asks. Often, the sheer size of the institution's purchases can assist in negotiating a stripped-down version of a newer model, the trade-in of an older model for a newer one, a shifting of resources within the organization for a low use area swap-out for an older but still functional unit.

8.4.2 Safety

The second question is safety. The simlab gets a defibrillator, but should the defibrillator be fully functional? There are several schools of thought on this topic, neither is right or wrong. Some simlabs use full energy at the recommended levels of joules. Arguments in favour are that the students know that 300 joules (higher settings) takes longer to reach than 2 joules (lower settings). The student has the benefit of audible (the energy whine) and visual cues (red lights) on the defibrillator. They learn to look for these when troubleshooting in a clinical situation. Disadvantages include the potential danger of an accidental discharge and a student or faculty injury. The responsibility of the faculty is enormous and there must be little room for student misadventure. Given the numbers of times defibrillators are used in many simlabs, the wear and tear on the defibrillator is very high.

Other labs use live energy but at a vastly reduced load, usually the lowest setting. Favourable arguments include a safer environment, and the ability to have audible (though the time to a full charge is very short and this may result in learning incorrect procedures) and visual cues. Disadvantages include the student (later the practitioner) not expecting a charge to take as long as they can take and then he or she believes the machine to be dysfunctional. Newer defibrillators may have reduced charge times compared with earlier models.

A third solution is to disengage the discharge route from the defibrillator. The audible and visual cues are intact but there is no electrical discharge. Clinical engineering at the hospital will be able to assist with this modification. This preserves all of the arguments in favour previously discussed, but with none of the disadvantages. The caution in this scenario is that a disabled defibrillator must not find its way into a clinical situation. It should have appropriate labels affixed. There may be a few simlabs where the defibrillators are never turned on or charged, and the student loses many of the opportunities for learning in this situation.

8.4.3 Semi-automatic external defibrillators

The widespread implementation of semi-automatic external defibrillators (SAED) in public areas is also intertwined into the CPR curriculum. The devices which are widely known as automatic external devices are actually misnamed, because they are not automatic and require operator initiation of the electrical discharge based upon a system prompt. However, the mislabel notwithstanding, they are in wide use, with virtually every airport and large shopping centre, sports venue or industrial facility. In CPR training, most vendors which produce these devices for use in the community, also produce and sell training versions of their SAED (Fig. 8.4).

Organizations which are responsible for the state-of-the science (e.g. American Heart Association, European Heart Association) alter their recommendations on heart care, first aid or emergency care based on the latest research findings. The early versions of SAEDs were often not easily altered. Their thrifty cost and limited alterability necessitated a re-purchase of newer models to allow instructors to use them in training with the more recent guidelines. Hence programmability and the ability to update via a chip or other method are important. If the parent organization is planning a large purchase of SAEDs, discussions with the vendor should include the trainers being included in the training package. The ability to change or select different scenarios assists the instructor with having to take out the 'verbal staging' and allows the student to respond to the situation. The durability of the casing is important for good value in length of service. The padded cases that come with some of the SAEDs really prevent damage as some of the plastic cases do not hold up well. The ability to use either AC or DC assists with the variability of having long sessions or the need for portability to areas without electrical outlets. Consider if the device uses an unusual or particularly expensive battery type. The warranty, access to repairs, and again up grade ability should also be evaluated. If the community has selected a standard public vendor,

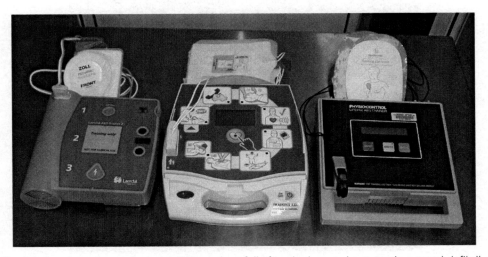

Fig. 8.4 A variety of manufacturers that produce fully functioning semi-automatic external defibrillators (AED) also produce low-cost trainers for education.

for familiarity and training effectiveness, this also plays a part in the selection of a product if community training is part of the simlab mission. Otherwise, the model that the organization is using internally is the obvious choice. Finally, the importance of assessing the cost, durability and functionality of the SAED training pads cannot be overstated. Some training pads are very flimsy and not repairable. Others are much more robust. The costs can vary considerably. The stickiness or ability to clean the mannequins after use is also a factor. Simlabs that use a large number of these training pads should consider using velcro tabs to apply the pads to the mannequin. Such skin tone velcro packets are inexpensive and barely visible (Fig. 8.5).

In summary, factors to consider when purchasing these devices include:

◆ Upgradeability with algorithm guidelines
◆ Cost per unit
◆ Programmability with different scenarios
◆ Carrying case type and cost
◆ Durability of the material
◆ Electrical and/or battery powered
◆ Warranty and repair ability
◆ SAED brand used internally and/or in the community
◆ SAED training pad cost and durability.

The order of importance of these factors will vary with the simlab's mission, customer base and budget.

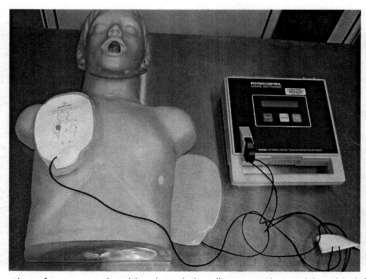

Fig. 8.5 Alteration of a mannequin with velcro circles allows practise applying the defibrillator pads without the sticky residue.

Resource websites: a partial list of vendors

Ambu: http://www.ambu.com
Armstrong: http://www.armstrong.com
Boundtree Medical: http://www.boundtree.com
Childbirth: http://www.childbirthgraphics.com
CPR prompt: http://www.cpr-prompt.com
Gaumard: http://www.gaumard.com
Laerdal: http://www.laerdal.com
Limbs & Things: http://www.limbsandthings.com
Nasco: http://www.enasco.com/healthcare
Simulaids: http://www.simulaids.com

Disclaimer

The author has no affiliation with any industrial partner and has never received remuneration from any. Selection of mannequins and trainers should be based upon the needs of the simlab after a careful assessment.

Part 3

Education components

Chapter 9

Teaching and learning through the simulated environment

Iris Vardi

Overview

- ◆ Teaching for learning in the simulated environment requires sound planning, good teaching, and evaluation that supports improvement.
- ◆ Planning involves the development of learning objectives, tasks, activities and assessments.
- ◆ Good teaching in the simulated environment focuses on learning through doing, and involves sound management of sessions, clear delivery of information, and attention to students' needs and styles of learning.
- ◆ When evaluating to improve, it is important to draw from various perspectives including those of the teachers, the students, experts in the field and educational experts.

9.1 Introduction

The simulated environment offers many opportunities to learners that extend far beyond the traditional lecture, classroom, tutorial or laboratory setting. It has the potential to provide learners with an opportunity to take on a new role, to learn by doing, to experiment, to take risks, to solve problems, and to make decisions within a safe context that is as close as we can get to the 'authentic' workplace.

In the real-life context, we have no control over the nature of the problems or conditions that present. This sometimes leaves learners to deal with situations when they have not yet developed the necessary skills. With simulation, this can be overcome. It is the educators, rather than the presenting patients, who determine the nature of the learning experience including the difficulty and complexity of the task. In such a controlled environment, learners can be given the time and space to learn from the actions they took and the decisions they made without the pressure of the daily work environment and its associated accountabilities.

However, in order to fully realise the potential of simulation, we need to do more than simply place learners within a simulated environment and provide them with varied experiences. Realising the full potential of the simulation lies in the planning, execution and follow-up to the learning experience.

9.2 Planning for learning in the simulated environment

Planning is an essential part of the teaching process. The better you plan, the better the learning will be. There are many things you need to decide in order to achieve a successful course with sound learning experiences. At the most basic level, you need to know how many sessions or lessons you need to run, what will be covered in each session, and how long they should run for. However, there is much more to plan. You need to determine what needs to be taught, the best ways to teach for maximum learning, how to best sequence activities, how and when feedback should be provided, how you will determine what the participants have learnt (and what they have misunderstood), and how to support appropriate transference to the workplace.

9.2.1 Determining the learning objectives

In order to plan properly, your first task is to determine what the participants need to learn. There are so many different types of skills and abilities that can be learnt through simulation. Students could increase their core knowledge, develop practical manual skills, improve their abilities to read, analyse and interpret clinical signs and symptoms, solve problems, make decisions and work effectively in a team – to name but a few.

Deciding which skills and abilities to develop is, to a large degree, dependant upon your audience and the reasons for providing the learning experience in the first place. Neophytes in any given area may well need to start with core knowledge and practical manual skills. But experienced practitioners probably need something different. For instance, they may have the manual skills, but need to develop their team work or decision making skills.

Clearly articulating what your participants will be able to do as a result of your course provides a set of parameters for your planning. These are usually expressed in the form of learning objectives, also known as learning outcomes (Table 9.1).

Table 9.1 Examples of learning objectives / outcomes for a course

By the end of this course, the student will be able to:
◆ Recognize and appropriately manage an unconscious patient
◆ Recognize and appropriately manage VF, VT and asystole

You can see that these learning objectives focus on both the content that will be covered (unconscious patients, VF, VT and asystole) and the behaviours that learners will be able to demonstrate with that content within a workplace context (recognize and appropriately manage). Matching learner behaviours with content is the key to providing your students with active learning experiences which make use of the simulated environment. It will also help you to design activities in which the students think and act through practising, evaluating what they have done, analysing situations and making decisions. This is in stark contrast to simply listening to others telling them about good practice.

When putting your learning objectives together for your course, try to progress beyond basic skill development to more challenging outcomes. The learning experience could also focus on, for instance:

◆ Following protocols

◆ Differential diagnosis and appropriate selection of treatment

◆ Evaluation of critical incidents

◆ Working effectively as a team during a crisis.

9.2.2 Tasks and activities for learning

Your learning objectives set the scene for determining what will occur in the course. Start by designing real-life complex tasks that your students could do in the simulated environment which would demonstrate their achievement of the learning objectives. We will refer to these as the learning objective tasks. Let us have a look at some complex simulation tasks that would demonstrate the learning objectives given previously (Table 9.2).

Table 9.2 Examples of complex tasks that demonstrate learning objectives

Learning objective	Learning objective task
Recognize and appropriately manage an unconscious patient	Initial team management of an unconscious patient using ABC in a number of different scenarios with differing patient histories.
Recognize and appropriately manage VF, VT and asystole	Team assessment and management of life threatening arrhythmias in a number of different scenarios with differing patient histories.

As these examples show, the learning objective tasks will generally be too difficult for your students to achieve at the start of the course. These become the **summative tasks** – the ones that allow you to evaluate the sum of knowledge and skills that the students have gained by the end of the course. To successfully achieve these summative tasks, you need to think about the types of prerequisite knowledge and skills that the students would need. For example, to be able to manage an unconscious patient in a team setting, each of your students will first need to be able to:

◆ establish an airway and commence breathing

◆ check pulse and establish circulation

◆ work effectively as part of a team.

This prerequisite knowledge can be taught first, often in smaller, less complex support tasks. These are often referred to as the **formative tasks** – those tasks in which the students learn and practise using the underlying skills and knowledge required for the summative task.

Formative support tasks are extremely important in ensuring that your students will be successful when they finally attempt the more complex summative learning objective task. There are so many different types of support tasks that you could design. For instance, in addition to practising manual skills, your students could make and justify differential diagnoses based on evidence/ data they collect, design and trial safe protocols or working environments, or even trial and evaluate different treatment procedures. Whatever you decide, these tasks will need to be sequenced so that knowledge and understanding is built and reinforced.

To get the most out of your tasks, each one needs to be carefully thought through and developed. Remember, people learn in different ways. Some are listeners and watchers, some learn by doing, some like to work on their own and others like to work in groups. Often, people like a little bit of each. You can cater for different learners by building in listening, speaking, doing, reading, writing, working alone and working together into each task. Since students rarely learn everything the first time, building in these different types of activities into each task also supports and reinforces learning as they provide the learner with a means for engaging with the same information in different ways.

You can plan to support learning through building in a variety of activities to be completed before, during and after each task.

9.2.2.1 Before the task

Prior to any task, there is usually background information that each participant needs to be aware of. This could include understanding how the simulators operate, how the environment works, and the essential medical knowledge for completing the task. Such background information could be developed in a variety of ways. First, there are the activities that you could do. You may decide to give a short talk, lecture or practical demonstration. These types of activities provide learners with an opportunity to listen and watch. It has been found that most people can listen effectively for about 20 minutes. So plan to keep these types of activities within that time frame.

However, there are also activities that your students could do before the task. Your students come with a range of experiences and knowledge that you can draw out, use and build upon. This is a good opportunity for your participants to think and talk. Thinking and talking activities could include, for example, brainstorming, short multiple-choice quizzes to attempt and then discuss, and asking participants to share practices within their particular medical context. Some of these activities could be done individually, some in pairs and others with the group as a whole. As the aim is to prepare for the task, design these activities to be quick and short; 10–15 minutes would be a good time frame to aim for.

As these examples show, even before you begin the task, you can incorporate listening, watching, speaking and thinking. Many educators actually find starting with the thinking and speaking activities first to be highly successful. Not only do these get the students engaged from the start, they also provide the teacher with an idea of the knowledge and understandings that the participants bring. The teacher can then follow these with a talk and/or demonstration which can be used to confirm and build on understandings, as well as correct any misunderstandings that may have been revealed earlier.

9.2.2.2 During the task

The task provides the opportunity for the participants to actually do activities that simulate what is done in the work environment. This also requires careful detailed planning. Think about:

- what the students are required to do
- why they are required to do this
- the context or the patient history that requires this action
- the information that the students will need in order to successfully complete the task
- whether the students will work alone or in groups
- what role each member of the group will take
- how all participants will have an opportunity to take on each of the roles
- whether the students will need a practical demonstration first
- whether a checklist would be helpful for the students when they practise.

Addressing the mechanics of the task in this way will provide you with the basis for developing a set of steps and materials that will support the students in their learning. Remember to build in plenty of opportunities for the students to practise and to design materials that will support students to make decisions on their own and to check how they and their fellow participants are progressing.

9.2.2.3 After the task

Designing the simulated task is not, however, the end of the planning. You also need to plan post-task activities. The aim of these activities is to provide the students with an opportunity to reflect on the actions they took in the simulation, explore other options and possibilities, and extend their learning. Reflecting on actions requires a framework, or set of standards or behaviours against which students can evaluate and discuss. Design activities in which students recall what happened, rate or examine their actions and discuss how they could improve. This could occur through the completion of self-evaluation checklists, small group discussion and/or large group discussion.

These after-task activities are critical and can result in the most learning. Through these activities students can learn from own another, and set their own goals for improvement. Opportunities for discussion also provide a time for the teacher to confirm and reiterate the important 'take home' messages. In addition, they allow the teacher to make sure that no-one leaves with any misconceptions or misunderstandings.

9.2.3 Assessments

The teaching and learning tasks and activities discussed thus far allow you to assess or evaluate your students' learning in an informal manner through observation. Based on these informal observations you can intervene and teach as required to improve learning. Some courses, however, require formal assessment of students' skills and knowledge. Within the simulated setting, assessment is usually either competency based or grade based.

In competency based assessment, you are assessing a set of skills, each of which the student must demonstrate to the necessary level (Table 9.3).

Table 9.3 Examples of competencies

- Correctly relieves foreign body airway obstruction in both a conscious and unconscious adult according to the established guidelines
- Demonstrates rescue breathing on an adult using a self-inflating bag-mask with supplemental oxygen as per the established guidelines

---

Competency-based assessment can be a very useful form of assessment when it is important to ensure that the participants can execute each skill correctly and safely.

A competency-based assessment simply requires a checklist for each student. As each skill is demonstrated by the student, so it is checked off by the instructor. With this type of assessment, you can run a special assessment task or simply use the tasks and activities that you have already designed and add the checklist for the instructor to use once the students have demonstrated that they have mastered the skills.

In a grade-based assessment, a student receives a mark (e.g. 50%, 65%) or a grade (e.g. A, B+ or pass, distinction). This type of assessment is used to demonstrate the level of knowledge or skill a student demonstrated through a test or set assessment task usually run under test conditions. These types of assessments can include paper-based tests with multiple-choice, short answer or essay type questions as well as practical assessment tasks. With these types of assessments, it is important that you design a marking key so that marks are awarded on the same basis to all students.

9.2.4 Documenting your planning

This detailed planning is usually documented in a teaching plan. Teaching within a simulated environment often requires extensive co-ordination between the teachers in the course, the technicians and the administrative staff. A well constructed teaching plan provides all concerned with a clear understanding of how the course is to proceed.

Teaching plans often include:

- the tasks and their associated learning activities
- any assessments that will be run

- how long each assessment, task and activity will take
- what equipment is needed, including medical equipment, models, multimedia devices, cadaveric material, handouts, worksheets, checklists.

Appendix A shows a sample teaching plan based on the learning objective 'Recognize and appropriately manage an unconscious patient'. It incorporates the learning objective task as well as the support tasks which develop the prerequisite knowledge and understandings required. It also shows how pre and post activities for each task can be incorporated.

As you look through the sample teaching plan in Appendix A, take note of a number of features important for good teaching and learning. Firstly, note how the plan is focussed on student activity: talking, thinking and doing. Teacher talk is limited to the essentials that wrap around the learning activities: introductions, explanations and demonstrations, clarification, and summing up of important points.

Next, note how information is recycled, checked and reinforced. This is carefully built into the plan through the use of the formative support tasks, pre-task activities and quick revision activities. In this plan, teaching starts from the students' own knowledge base by probing what they already know. It then moves to teaching and practising first AB and later C. As you look carefully through the plan, you will see that knowledge and skills are recycled, checked and reinforced through the systematic incorporation of:

- modelling
- practice
- use of checklists for peer feedback and evaluation
- use of self-evaluation forms
- group discussion
- a quick revision activity.

All of this formative activity occurs before the students attempt the complex summative task that reflects the learning objective for the course. Designing a course in this way, supports your students in their learning and helps them to be successful.

9.3 **Facilitating learning**

While a solid plan lays the foundation for good teaching and sound learning experiences, it is the teachers who bring the plan to life and create the learning experience for each student. Teachers take on many roles for students. They are session organizers and managers, mentors, guides, sources of expertise and knowledge, motivators, and confidence builders. Each of these roles reveals itself in different ways as teachers and students interact. The manner in which this interaction proceeds determines whether learning occurs at all, is impeded or is progressed.

9.3.1 **Managing the session**

Students will only be able to complete all the activities and tasks, and meet the learning objectives for the course if you manage the session well. This involves sound management of tasks, activities, time and participants. The teaching plan lays out the nature of the tasks and activities, and the time frame in which they need to be completed. It is important that you adhere to these times, so that students can engage with and recycle information and skills as planned.

There are many ways to successfully manage the session and your students.

- Be succinct in your explanations and instructions.
- Explain the need to keep to time so that everyone has an opportunity to 'have a go'.

- Prior to starting a task or activity, let students know how much time they have for completion, (e.g. *"You have five minutes to ..."*).
- Explain what needs to be accomplished in that time frame (e.g. *"By the end of this activity you should have 8 examples of ..."*).
- Before the end of the task, let students know how much time they have left (e.g. *"You have just one more minute before you need to swap over"*).
- Circulate between groups, resolving any problems and keeping your participants on task.
- Thank talkative participants for their input and let everyone know that due to time constraints you may need to limit discussion time.
- Have a back-up plan for the participant who needs more time to learn such as a spare station or model that they can practise on at their own rate.

9.3.2 Conveying information clearly

To be a good manager of a session and developer of knowledge, it is important to convey instructions and knowledge in a clear, logical and succinct manner. Not only does clarity make it easier for the students to understand, it also provides students with a sense of safety and trust in the instructor: safety that the teacher clearly knows what s/he is doing and trust in their ability to guide the learning. In fact, in surveys of what adult learners value in their teachers, 'clear explanations' rate very highly indeed.

Within the simulated environment, students need to be clear about many things:

- The key knowledge they need to have 'under their belt' in order to be successful
- The task or activity they are to complete
- How the simulated experience relates to the participants' own working lives
- How to use the equipment
- Which skills and abilities they need to demonstrate
- How to demonstrate these skills and abilities
- How skills and abilities will be evaluated
- The important points they can take into their practice in the 'real world'.

9.3.2.1 Clarity when speaking

Being clear about the points you want to make often requires planning and practice. It can easily take as long, if not longer, to prepare for teaching as it does to actually teach. Good teachers spend a substantial amount of time planning what they are going to say in their talks, in their introductions to activities and tasks, and in their summing up of activities and tasks.

Before teaching, examine the teaching plan carefully, identifying where you need to convey information. Wherever you need to speak, prepare the main points you want to make and organize them in a logical order. Remember that you will often have limited time to speak and won't be able to tell your participants everything you know. So pick out and concentrate on the most important points. Illustrate these with real-life examples, models, graphs, photos and the like. This will help keep your audience engaged. The notes, overheads or slides and supporting written material that you develop will help you to feel confident and clear in your own mind about what you need to cover and how you will go about this.

Once prepared, it can also be useful to practise your delivery. Try to do this without reading. When practising, take note of your pace of delivery: too fast and your participants may not have a chance to absorb the points you are making; too slow and you may lose your audience. Also, listen to what you say and how you say it. Are you being clear? Are there points that need repeating? Are you too repetitive? This type of practise and self-evaluation will help you to improve and to feel confident. If you are confident and enthusiastic about your topic and your delivery, then your students will be too.

9.3.2.2 Clear modelling

Sometimes, actions speak louder than words and it can be far easier to show how something is done rather than just explain it. This also requires careful thought and planning. Often, when we are expert at carrying out a procedure or executing a skill, we do it automatically without thinking about how we actually accomplished the task. It can be useful during the planning stage to deconstruct the steps you take in a task before you try to teach it to others. Think about why you do it in this way. Now you have a set of steps or points to make along with explanations that you can take your group through. As before, you will only have a limited time to model, so highlight the most important aspects that your participants should know. The finer details can come later as you work with your students while they practise.

Whenever you are modelling, make sure that everyone can see what you are doing. This may require you to limit the size of the group. Also be aware that different students will be seeing things from different angles as they group around you. When students are observing, they may not all attend to the details that you want them to focus on or notice. Make sure you direct their attention as you go. For example, *"See how I am ..."* and *"Notice the way that ..."*

9.3.3 Focussing on the student

Imparting knowledge in a clear and enthusiastic way is important, but gives us no idea how much the student has actually learnt. In fact, whenever we simply impart information, no matter how clearly, we do not really know whether that information was new to the student, whether it covered all that they needed to know, whether they understood it correctly or even whether they could use it effectively within the work environment. Asking "Do you understand?" may also not yield sufficient information, particularly when students are too embarrassed to confess their lack of understanding or when they mistakenly believe that they have understood.

To guide, mentor and progress student learning, you need to go beyond imparting information to focussing on the students, their needs and their understanding. A good teaching plan should provide you with multiple opportunities to check student understanding and ascertain their needs as knowledge and skills are repeatedly brought to bear in different student activities. As you work with students through the various activities, you need to be alert to student strengths, weaknesses, gaps and misconceptions. With this information in hand, you can tailor your teaching to both group and individual needs.

9.3.3.1 Facilitating learning

The different tasks and activities in the teaching plan require more than your organization. They also require you to actively facilitate the learning. How to do this, however, will vary from student to student. Different students bring different approaches to learning. For instance, some students like to work independently and to try things out for themselves. Others like or need more guidance and direction. Some get frustrated if they do not succeed the first time, while others are prepared to give it a go and to learn from their mistakes. In order to meet individual student needs, it is important that you and everyone in the teaching team circulate and attend to each and every student. This individual attention allows you to tailor your teaching to match the different styles of learning. This requires you to do more listening and watching, and less talking and directing. You can then determine when to step in and guide learning, and when to let the participants be.

As you observe your students engage in tasks and activities, to be alert to these types of differences and provide support, input and advice as required.

Sometimes it can be difficult to judge what students need and how to help them, particularly when they come from different academic, cultural, religious and linguistic backgrounds. Try to be respectful of individuals, the knowledge and experiences they possess, and the questions and comments they make, no matter how strange, unusual or ill-informed you think they may be. Try to understand where these questions and comments are coming from and respond in a supportive manner.

Be particularly aware of students for whom English is a foreign language. Not only may they have difficulty tuning in to your accent, they may also have difficulty with the high level of English and technical language that you may be using. To help these students:

- Provide notes that summarize what you have said.
- Put your instructions for tasks and activities in writing (e.g. in a handout or up on the whiteboard).
- Be aware that nodding or saying "yes" may mean that they are attending to what you are saying, not that they are understanding.
- Provide them with time to gather their thoughts in English before they speak.
- Keep your sentences short and clear; do not speak too rapidly.
- Spend some one-to-one time with them on their tasks and activities.

9.3.3.2 Providing feedback

Guiding learning requires the ability to give good quality feedback at the right time. The students are reliant on you as the expert to provide them with feedback that they can use and learn from. Both positive and corrective feedback are important. Positive feedback lets students know what they are doing correctly and how well they are doing it, for example, "*Your use of the ... is extremely good. Keep it up.*"

Corrective feedback helps students to improve and develop their knowledge and skills. When providing corrective feedback, make sure that you focus on only one or two main points at a time. Don't try to correct everything at once. You can focus on other areas for improvement later. As you work with individual participants on their activities or tasks, make sure that your corrective feedback is direct and unambiguous. You could ask your students to recall something that was taught earlier, for example "*Do you remember ...* ", and use their response as basis for guiding or correcting what they are doing. Or, you could simply tell the student what to do and how to do it, for example, "*Pull the ... back*". Provide praise as they get it right "*Yes, that's it!*"

Whenever providing feedback, or in fact whenever you are teaching, you also need to be aware of your students' state of mind. This is where your role as a confidence builder and motivator comes into play. Students will come to your course with various levels of confidence. Some may be concerned about revealing a lack of knowledge, failure or mistakes in front of their colleagues, and see it as a loss of face. This requires sensitivity on your part in where, when and how you speak to your students. Look out for the quiet students. They may prefer to chat separately with you about their learning, whereas others may be happy to speak up, learn and receive feedback in front of others. It is important that you create a safe environment for all students to discuss how they are going, where they need help and how to improve.

In group discussions, it is also important to provide feedback. In this context, feedback goes beyond positive and corrective feedback to building on students' ideas. In order to do this effectively, it can be useful to display group contributions on a board. This allows you to make connections between the ideas proffered, highlight the ideas that are important, add extra information, and correct (in a sensitive manner) any misconceptions or inaccuracies brought up by the group. It is important to ensure, that your students do not leave a group discussion with any misconceptions or incorrect information.

No matter what the context, or for what purpose you are providing feedback, always strive to be encouraging, respectful and supportive to your students. This will help them to participate, try things out for the first time and to remain motivated.

9.4 Evaluating for improvement

Once a course is over, it is important to evaluate how it went. Evaluation should provide you with the information needed to determine what went well and how to improve. Evaluations for improvement can range from participant perceptions of the course to comprehensive evaluations that gain the insights of others such as experts in the field, the teaching staff and educational experts. The depth of evaluation you need to conduct depends upon the context. If you are running a course for the first time, you will need different types of information than if you are running or reviewing an established course. Remember, it usually takes a few iterations to get a course to the stage where you will be satisfied with how it runs. It is very rare indeed that everything goes so well the first time that no improvement is needed.

Evaluating for improvement can cover a number of different areas including quality of the course, the teaching and the learning.

9.4.1 Quality of the course

An important aspect to examine when looking to improve is the course itself. This includes examination of the content, the learning objectives, the tasks, the activities and the assessments.

+ Was the course complete and up-to-date? Were there any gaps in the knowledge and skills being taught?
+ Were the activities and activities well structured and sequenced? Did they result in the intended learning?
+ Did everyone have sufficient opportunity to participate and practice?
+ Did the assessments accurately capture student learning? Were they given sufficient time to complete the assessments and demonstrate their knowledge and abilities?
+ Was the equipment appropriate?
+ Did the set-up of the room and the equipment allow for sound observation and learning?

As you consider these types of questions, think about what needs to be modified for improvement.

9.4.2 Quality of the teaching

No matter how good the planning and set-up are, without good teaching it all goes to waste. Hence evaluation of the teaching is enormously important.

+ Were sufficient teaching staff available?
+ Did they have the necessary skills and expertise?
+ Were they clear in their explanations?
+ Were they focussed on the students, circulating and providing useful feedback?

- Were they respectful to the students and sensitive to their feelings?
- Were they encouraging to the students?

Think about improvements, and the types of teacher or facilitator training might be of benefit to you and other staff.

9.4.3 Quality of learning

Of course, student learning and student reaction to the teaching and the course should lie at the heart of your evaluation. There is no point in running a simulation course if students leave without being positive about what they learnt and without being able to take away safe practical skills and abilities that they can apply in the workplace. So it is important to ascertain what students learnt, what they didn't learn, and how they felt about it. There are a number of aspects to consider:

- How did the students change in their skill and knowledge set from the start of the course to the end of the course?
- What were their reactions to instructions, activities, tasks and the amount of time given?
- What were their reactions to the styles of the different teaching staff?
- Did all the students participate and were they engaged?

As you examine the student learning experience, consider what you would have liked for them to have learnt, whether or not this was achieved, and what you would do differently next time.

9.4.4 What and how to evaluate

As shown above, evaluation can take quite a bit of time and effort. Determining what to evaluate depends upon the context. A first time course which you intend to run again needs a comprehensive analysis covering the learning, the course and the teaching in depth. If you are monitoring an ongoing and successful course, you may only need to examine the quality of the teaching. On the other hand, if the course is not going to be run again, you might be satisfied with a more superficial evaluation.

Once you have decided what you need to find out, you need to determine how you will gather the information. It is important to gather information from a variety of different sources to ensure reliability and accuracy of your findings. The first place to gather information is from the participants themselves. Their perceptions of their own learning and the quality of the activities, tasks and teaching can be gathered through questionnaires and/or focus groups.

Student perceptions will provide you with an indication of how well you were able to focus on the student. Student perceptions can be gained on a range of matters including:

- how well the course addressed their needs in the workplace
- how well the course and teaching suited the way they learn
- the amount of content covered
- their motivation
- the amount of time they had for the activities
- what they liked
- what they didn't like
- their overall levels of satisfaction.

Student perceptions can be extremely important and helpful when thinking about how to improve the course, the teaching and the learning from the students' point of view.

Another important source of information is from the assessments you ran. How well did they perform on these assessments? Did they learn the knowledge and skills you set out for them to learn at the start of the course? How well did they achieve the learning objectives?

Assessments, however, are not the only sources of information about learning. Structured observations also can provide important information. Observations can be collected from the teaching staff themselves and/or external observers. To help teaching staff in their observations, it can be useful to develop observation forms or checklists to use during a course that allow documentation of student learning and progress. These can provide objective measures for judging student learning and can provide insights that teachers can act on during the course as well as after the course when you consider the improvements that need to be made.

Also of importance are your discussions with other teaching staff. A debrief at the end of a course allows teachers to share their general observations and put together suggestions for improvement. These could cover a range of matters including:

+ the content of the course
+ the support materials used
+ the organization and layout of equipment
+ the nature and design of the tasks and activities
+ how student learning progressed
+ the roles the teachers are meant to take in each task.

These sessions are also useful for sharing and discussing your findings on the participants' perceptions of the course, their learning and the teaching that they received.

9.5 **Where to from here?**

Evaluation is not the end of the process. Often, it takes you right back to the beginning with planning, execution and re-evaluation. Teaching and learning is a complex process with so many different variables which come together in differing ways. First, there are the students with different needs, work contexts, experiences and styles of learning. Then there is the context for the course with its distinctive content and set of learning objectives to be achieved. And finally, there are the teachers with different backgrounds, ways of working and teaching styles. This introductory chapter has attempted to provide you with a framework and a basis from within which you can view teaching and learning. From here you can only learn more. The following chapters will provide you with more techniques, insights and ideas. Practise and experiment with these. With sound planning, implementation and evaluation, your course, your teaching and your students' learning can only improve and grow.

Useful resources

Biggs J (1999). *Teaching for quality learning at university: What the student does.* Buckingham: Society for Research into Higher Education and Open University Press.

Cannon R (1992.) *Lecturing.* Campbelltown, NSW: Higher Education Research and Development Society of Australasia.

Chalmers D, Fuller R (1996). Teaching for learning at university: Theory and Practice. London: Kogan Page.

Fraser K (1996). *Student centred teaching: the development and use of conceptual frameworks.* Campbelltown, NSW: Higher Education Research and Development Society of Australasia.

Kember D, Kelly M (1993). *Improving teaching through action research.* Campbelltown, NSW: Higher Education Research and Development Society of Australasia.

Ladyshewsky R (1995). *Clinical Teaching.* Campbelltown, NSW: Higher Education Research and Development Society of Australasia.

MacDonald R (1997). *Teaching and learning in small groups.* Birmingham: SEDA

Ramsden P (1992). Learning to teach in higher education. London: Routledge.

Appendix A: Sample teaching plan

Course Name:

Session Name: ABC and the unconscious patient   **Session Time: 8.30 am – 12 noon**

No. of participants: 20 Learning Objective: recognize and appropriately manage an unconscious patient

Start	Task/activity	Equipment	Time
8.30 am	◆ Teacher introduces course ◆ Students brainstorm – what needs to be done when you Find an unconscious patient?	◆ Whiteboard and markers ◆ Electronic slide presentation	15 mins
8.45 am	**Support Task 1: Establish an airway and commence breathing**		**45 mins in total**
8.45 am	**Before task 1** ◆ 5 groups of 4 ◆ Teachers explain and demonstrate AB	◆ 5 Mannequins/models for demonstration ◆ 20 handouts on ABC ◆ 5 pocket masks	15 mins
9.00 am	**Task 1** ◆ In pairs students practise AB ◆ One student practises, while other marks the checklist and provides feedback ◆ Students then swap roles ◆ 5 – 6 minutes practice each	◆ Electronic slide with task details ◆ 10 mannequins/models for practice ◆ 20 checklists with AB behaviours to demonstrate ◆ 20 pocket masks	15 mins
9.15 am	**After task 1** ◆ Students each fill out a self-evaluation form ◆ Teacher facilitates group discussion, discusses implications for the workplace and summarizes main 'take home' messages	◆ 20 self-evaluation forms ◆ Electronic slides ◆ Whiteboard and markers	15 mins
9.30 am	**Support Task 2: Check pulse and establish circulation**		**35 mins in total**
9.30 am	**Before task 2** ◆ 5 groups of 4 ◆ Teachers explain and demonstrate C	◆ 5 mannequins/models ◆ 5 backboards	10 mins

Time	Activity	Resources	Duration
9.40 am	**Task 2** ◆ In pairs students practise C ◆ One student practises, while other marks the checklist and provides feedback ◆ Students then swap roles ◆ 5–6 minutes practice each	◆ 10 mannequins/models for practice (10 pairs) ◆ 20 checklists with C behaviours to demonstrate ◆ 10 backboards	15 mins
9.55 am	**After task 2** ◆ Teacher facilitates group discussion ◆ Students write personal goals for improvement in the workplace	◆ Electronic slides ◆ Whiteboard and markers	10 mins
10.05 am	**Break**		**20 mins**
10.25 am	**Learning Objective Task 3: Initial team management of the unconscious patient**		
10.25 am	◆ Revision – ABC multiple choice quiz for individuals to complete (3 mins) ◆ In pairs students compare and discuss answers (4 mins) ◆ Group shares and discusses answers (8 mins).	◆ 20 ABC multiple choice quizzes ◆ Whiteboard and markers	15 mins
10.40 am	**Before task 3** ◆ Teacher introduces task ◆ Students brainstorm the characteristics of good team work. ◆ Teacher shows slides covering good team work	◆ Whiteboard and markers ◆ Electronic slides	15 mins
10.55 am	**Task 3 Part 1** ◆ 5 groups of 4 ◆ Each group has a different scenario.	◆ 5 different scenarios (blocked / unblocked airway, adequate / inadequate breathing, with / without pulse) ◆ 5 copies of each ◆ 5 mannequins/models prepared as per scenarios ◆ 5 rooms/cubicles	15 mins
11.10 am	**After task 3 Part 1 – debrief** ◆ Students each complete a group evaluation checklist ◆ In their separate groups & rooms, students discuss with teacher their clinical and group skills in the scenario ◆ Students write individual goals for improvement	◆ 20 group evaluation checklists covering ABC and group behaviours ◆ Whiteboard and markers ◆ 5 separate rooms/cubicles	20 mins

Continued

Appendix A: (continued) Sample teaching plan

Time	Activity	Resources	Duration
11.30 am	**Task 3: Part 2** ♦ Same groups, students swap rooms and scenarios	♦ 5 scenarios as before. 5 copies of each ♦ 5 mannequins/models each prepared as per scenarios ♦ 5 rooms/cubicles	15 mins
11.45	**After Task 3 – debrief** ♦ All groups together ♦ Teacher facilitates whole group discussion on what learnt and important take home points	♦ Whiteboard and markers	15 mins
12 noon	**Lunch**		

Chapter 10

Developing your teaching role in a simulation centre

Ronnie Glavin

Overview

- The core component of teaching has been described as the arrangements of environments within which the student can interact.
- This core component is actually a lot more complex than first appears and requires that the teacher fulfil a variety of different roles.
- Each of these roles, in turn, requires a set of skills.
- There is more to teaching than just the face-to-face encounter between teacher and learner.
- Teachers have to prepare and plan so that the interaction of the student with the environment will be productive and promote the educational goals that the teacher is promoting.
- The above applies to nearly all forms of teaching. However, simulation-based teaching carries its own challenges.
- The psychological risks to the learner may be greater than occurs with more conventional forms of teaching.
- Effective learning will not occur when psychological safety disappears.
- Simulation-based teaching therefore carries its own set of skills that are not seen in other forms of teaching.

10.1 Introduction

This chapter aims to give an overview of the different roles of the teacher within the context of simulation-based teaching. It will overlap in content with some of the other chapters but that is inevitable in a chapter that intends to give a broad overview of this area. A chapter in a textbook can help make explicit some of the theory that underpins practice and can elaborate on the skills that are required for each of the roles described but there are limits as to how far reading about skills can take a learner. Very few people successfully learn to play musical instruments solely by reading about playing an instrument. They learn by practising under the guidance of a teacher who will fulfil many of the roles described in this chapter. The conditions are not so different for those who find themselves using simulation-based courses as a teaching tool. The best way to learn is to practice under the supervision of someone with greater expertise. I hope that this chapter will provide some assistance to those using simulation but no chapter can provide all of the solutions. Practice is based on theory and so I shall refer to theoretical models where relevant. However, the emphasis is on providing a framework and structure that someone new to simulation-based teaching can adapt to his or her own needs.

Table 10.1 List of features of adult learners

- In children, readiness to learn is a function of biological development and academic pressure. In adults, in contrast, readiness to learn is a function of the need to perform social roles
- Children have subject-centred orientation to learning, whereas adults have a problem-centred orientation to learning
- Adults need to know why they need to learn something before commencing their learning
- Adults have a psychological need to be treated by others as capable of self-direction
- Adults have accumulated experiences and these can be a rich resource for learning
- For adults the more potent motivators are internal

10.2 **Teachers and teaching**

The core of the process of teaching was described by the American educator and philosopher John Dewey as 'the arrangements of environments within which the student can interact'[1]. Simulation provides excellent opportunities for arranging environments and encouraging interaction. However, the interaction can only be considered educational if it is intended to lead to a set of desirable outcomes on the part of the learner. Although Dewey's description may give the impression that there is one role for a teacher the reality is that many roles are required to make those interactions educational. The skills of the teacher will require to be wide ranging and as in any other sphere of human action different skills will come into play at different times. What I want to do in this chapter is provide a framework of teaching skills that are necessary to ensure that simulator-based courses are effective educational experiences for the learners who participate in them. The advantages of a framework are that you can use it as a skeleton on which to hang your own practices and by so doing review and come to better understand those practices. Many of you are already involved in teaching, whether simulation-based or not. Some of the skills will also have been covered in other chapters in this book but by providing a framework you can use your existing knowledge and experience to better effect.

The active role of the teacher that is being promoted in this chapter may give the impression of the learner as a somewhat passive contributor to this process. We all know from our own experience that this is not the case. Learners come with their own needs and agendas and a lot of the work on adult learners that appears in the educational literature reflects the importance of taking into account those needs (see Table 10.1 for a list of key features of adult learners[2]).

Fish and Coles[3] describe the interaction with the environment as one that affects both teacher and learner, each gaining something from the other, in a process that is much more organic than the original description may have implied.

The different roles of the teacher are listed in Table 10.2. I shall explore each role and in doing so expand on some of the concepts referred to above in the context of simulation.

Table 10.2 Roles and duties of teachers in simulation-based teaching

- Identify the needs of the learner
- Create learning objectives
- Transform learning objectives into clinical scenarios
- Prepare the clinical scenarios
- Create an appropriate learning environment
- Tailor general learning outcomes to the needs of the individual learner
- Help the learner reflect on the experience of the clinical scenario
- Provide appropriate feedback
- Review the session

10.3 Identify the needs of the learner

This may not seem to be a role that springs to mind when thinking about teaching but it is crucial. Remember, Table 1 points out that adults want to learn what they perceive as being relevant. If they can't see a use for it then they will not be interested. Some of this section will overlap with the chapter on designing courses and so I shall not dwell on the specific skills in too much depth. Some readers will have experience of simulation from being either candidates or instructors on courses such as advanced cardiac life support or advanced trauma and life support. The triad of 'set', 'dialogue' and 'closure' may be familiar to you. In the world of education 'set' or preparation is of crucial importance. What am I going to teach? What does the learner want or need to learn? The first stage is to address these questions.

So, how do we find out what the learners need? We can ask them. One of the skills for this role is being able to formulate the appropriate questions. Another is identifying whom you are going to ask so that we can confirm or triangulate the information that we get.

As some examples of this approach we can ask different groups. We can ask the learners:

◆ For which clinical areas did your course give adequate preparation?

◆ For which of the following clinical scenarios did you feel under prepared?

We can ask those people who supervise the graduates or participants who have completed a course:

◆ "Which aspects of practice do your graduates manage well?"

◆ "With which aspects of practice do your graduates struggle?"

Not all of these areas may be best suited to simulation-based teaching. Someone at the centre has to make a decision of which aspects of a curriculum are best suited to simulation-based teaching. Not every teacher in a simulation centre may require this skill but to get the best investment from the input of resources someone has to be able to do so. Further reading on conducting a needs assessment exercise is provided by Hesketh and Laidlaw[4].

10.4 Create learning objectives

In the previous section we considered which aspects of a curriculum were best suited to simulation-based teaching. In this section the key teaching skills are those of identifying which behaviours we wish to promote in the learners. Let us take a clinical example. Suppose that a clinical colleague had approached us and asked if we could develop a course on 'the management of major haemorrhage in pregnant women around the time of delivery' then we have to break that down into some behaviours. What does that involve? Well, we could begin by discussing a range of possible behaviours such as ability to recognize major haemorrhage, ability to follow a protocol, ability to perform certain practical skills such as intravenous cannulation or setting up and using rapid intravenous infusion devices. We would also want to know whether this was for a particular group of health care professionals – obstetricians alone – or for a multidisciplinary group – obstetricians, anaesthetists, midwives etc. The key question we are beginning to formulate is what do you want these learners to be able to do by the end of the course that they cannot already do? We may only wish to confirm that they can do these actions, in which case we are moving into the realm of assessment rather than teaching. There will be a lot of possible learning objectives even in a fairly specific topic such as major obstetric haemorrhage and this is where the organizational skills of the teacher will come into play as he or she refines which of these many behaviours should be converted into learning objectives. Teachers with experience of simulation-based teaching should also be able to explain which behaviours are more suited to simulation based teaching. For example, the curriculum in which 'major obstetric haemorrhage' is embedded may include 'an understanding of the coagulation cascade pathways'. This, clearly, is not an area that plays to simulation-based teaching's strengths. Whereas 'the ability to interpret coagulation screen results and use that information to manage a patient' would be much more suited to simulation-based teaching.

10.5 **Transform learning objectives into clinical scenarios**

The description of teaching that we are using is promotion of constructive interaction between the learner (participant) and the environment. The clinical scenario is that environment. An effective clinical scenario should therefore encourage interactions that will bring about the learning objectives. As teachers we already do this in non-simulated environments but may not be aware of doing so. Our environment may be a room with chairs and a flip chart. The interaction may be in the form of a teacher asking the learners some questions – about the coagulation cascade, for example. The same principles apply in such an environment. We should have some idea of the needs of the learners, we should have some idea of the desired learning outcomes and we should be structuring our environment and interaction (e.g. lesson, tutorial, seminar, small group teaching session) to achieve our learning goals.

One of the potential dangers in simulation is that we remember an interesting clinical scenario and decide to try and replicate it in the simulated environment solely because it was interesting. Participants on a course with such scenarios may learn a lot but they may not be achieving the learning outcomes that are most useful or necessary for their own needs. So, instead of beginning with a clinical scenario we should begin with our learning objectives. The skill that we are invoking at this stage of the process is the ability to create an environment (scenario) that will promote interaction between scenario and learner and that will lead to our learning objectives. Such an interaction may promote other learning objectives that we had not intended; this should not matter so long as the major ones are achieved.

As an example, let us think about a case in which in which a woman with pre-eclampsia (high blood pressure in pregnancy) was being managed with labetalol and so did not increase her heart rate when she had some bleeding after delivery. This unusual case of failure to show the normal physiological response to bleeding was a challenging case. We may wish to recreate the events as a major haemorrhage scenario but will it help our learners achieve their goals? If they are very experienced professionals working in this setting then the atypical features may be useful in promoting factors to consider in the recognition of major haemorrhage. If our participants are at a much more junior stage then this may confuse them. The danger is that this could become a scenario on the management of a patient with pre-eclampsia rather than the management of major obstetric haemorrhage.

We often have to work backwards from the learning objectives. What sort of clinical events would move a learner towards such management? What sort of clinical events would discourage a learner from moving towards our goals? By using this process we create a story board and from those outlines we can write a script. Unlike scripts for Hollywood films our scripts have to be capable of responding to learners who may not choose to go where we want them to. We shall return to this theme in a later section.

10.6 **Prepare the clinical scenarios**

In the previous section we concentrated on the storyboard and script. In this stage we concentrate on the physical aspects of the environment. Many people describe this as making the scenario realistic. No amount of physical equipment can compensate for a poorly designed scenario but equally the environment we attempt to recreate must allow and indeed encourage the learner to interact. This takes us into the realm of props, equipment etc. For example, if the protocol for major obstetric haemorrhage states that the team should use blood warmers or rapid infusion devices then that equipment needs to be available. The appropriate methods of interacting with haematology and blood transfusion services should also be available (forms, blood specimen bottles, telephone access etc). We do not need to recreate every possible component from the real clinical environment but we must provide that which allows the interactions that we have designed to promote the attainment of learning goals. The key teaching skill that requires to be developed is learning what props and equipment must be present and which ones need not be. For example, an operating theatre in an obstetric unit would have neonatal resuscitation facilities available. If the intended outcomes of the scenario relate to the mother then a fetus like doll can be handed to a member of the supporting cast, who in turn can take it away from the clinical environment. This will not impact on the learning outcomes if they relate solely to the mother. However, if the staff were unable to gown and glove and did not have any surgical instruments then it becomes more difficult to get into the role of someone participating in a caesarean section. We are not recreating a scene to resemble accurately in every detail what would happen, we are attempting to provide enough stimuli to help promote the types of interaction that will lead to the attainment of the learning objectives.

10.7 Create an appropriate learning environment

Teaching is all about creating environments that promote interaction with the learner. We want that interaction to be a positive experience. Simulation based teaching can appear very threatening to learners. Learners may worry that they will expose their shortcomings to themselves and their peers. In the context of professional practice this is a serious consideration. A professional's sense of self-identity is tied up with his or her professional role. If we diminish that role by inappropriate experiences then we may diminish that person's self esteem and even sense of self. So far we have concentrated on the type of clinical experience we are attempting to recreate to help bring about learning objectives. In this section the emphasis is now on setting up an environment that is 'intellectually safe'. We want to create an environment that will stretch the learners but will not break them; an environment that will be conducive to learning. This requires a set of skills that many teachers will not have had to develop. As teachers we prepare an environment but usually those preparations address the physical and intellectual needs of the learners. For example, if we are to give a lecture on a particular topic to a group of undergraduates then we would do some preparation beforehand. What is the topic? Where does it fit into the curriculum? Will it overlap with the topics to be covered by other lecturers? When we have addressed those questions then we can address the next set of issues. How many will attend? What audiovisual materials shall I need? Will the room be of an adequate size, appropriate temperature, appropriate lighting etc? How will the learners know where to go? At the start of the lecture most lecturers present an overview of what they are going to cover – "Today, I am going to cover major obstetric haemorrhage. I shall begin with the aetiology of the more common causes and then go onto the principles of recognition and management. I shall end with some current and possible future developments." There may not appear be much interaction in this type of teaching but learners have the option of comparing what they already know in this area with the information and material presented by the lecturer. The challenges for the lecturer are often along the lines of how to engage the learners. This involves addressing such questions as "Why is this relevant?" "Why should you be interested in this topic?"

But very few learners will feel unsafe during such an experience. They may not interact very much at all. They may be daydreaming about meeting friends or what they are going to do next weekend etc. They are not very likely to feel psychologically threatened.

10.7.1 How do we create a safe environment?

We do this by being explicit about what is permissible and what is not. We give our learners rules. If the course is formative, that is, it is intended to help the learners find out something about their existing strengths and weaknesses then we can begin by insisting on confidentiality. We can also make it very explicit that we do not expect perfection but want to use the interaction with the environment as an opportunity for further reflection. Many of you who have been involved with small group teaching will be familiar with the concept of introducing rules to allow smooth functioning of the group. Many of these skills can be used and developed in simulation-based teaching. Learners must be reassured that they will not be humiliated or held up to ridicule by the faculty or peers if they do not perform well.

As many groups of learners have become more used to simulator-based teaching the use of these skills has probably become less challenging. However, there are plenty of groups of learners who do not have experience of simulator-based learning and will require that the teacher exercise these skills. The more senior in their respective professions the participants have become the greater the need for the establishment of a safe environment.

Participants will not interact effectively unless they feel that it is safe to do so.

10.8 Tailor general learning outcomes to the needs of the individual learner

This set of skills will be more familiar to anyone who has been involved in teaching. In the context of simulation-based teaching we can regard it as modifying the experience with which the learner is interacting. In principle this is the same as with small group teaching in a classroom setting. If a teacher finds that the subject being discussed is difficult because the learners do not have the necessary knowledge or understanding then the nature of the lesson is changed in an attempt to bring the learners up to the required level of knowledge or understanding. When a learner in a simulation-based course is struggling then we are faced with similar choices. For how long do we let the learner struggle? Do we provide support? We may not wish to make the experience so easy that the learner is unaware of his/her difficulties. On the other hand we do not want to make the experience so threatening that the participant feels overwhelmed and his/her sense of professional well being threatened. In that respect we are carrying on from the last section.

The main teaching skills that are required are the ability to recognize that the participant is struggling and the ability to decide how much support to give. Recognition of a struggling participant is usually straightforward because the learner may ask for help or appear unable to make appropriate decisions etc. The scenario can be modified by either providing help (a member of faculty can come in and make some suggestions) or some clues can be provided. For example, if the participant in a major obstetric haemorrhage course has not declared a major obstetric haemorrhage then a faculty member playing a role in the scenario may ask "How much blood do you think the patient has lost?" Escalation of support can be provided.

Equally, we may wish to make the scenario more challenging if the learner is seen to be coping easily. The educational justification for this is that we want participants to learn something about themselves, in particular their own strengths and weaknesses. We can think of this section as being about fine tuning to get the experience to a level consistent with each learner's limits.

The design of the course and selection of the target group of learners will help but we may need to make further interventions as described.

So far, I have described the modification of the experience as beginning during the scenario i.e. modifying the experience during the interaction. However, we can begin the process before the learners participate in the scenario. At the beginning of the course we can ask the learners to give us an account of their previous experience and we can use this information to help decide who should participate in which scenario and whether we should modify the scenarios before the learners participate. Exercising the judgment required to do so is part of the set of teaching skills.

10.9 Help the learner reflect on the experience of the clinical scenario

The teaching skills that are relevant for this section include those that apply to debriefing, which has been covered in another topic. In this section I shall not go into the process of debriefing in any detail but confine discussion to the major educational headings.

It is easy to think of Dewey's model of organizing the environment to promote interactions that will in turn help bring about learning objectives in terms of the clinical scenarios of a simulation-based teaching course. However, the environment and interaction also include the process of review and reflection (debriefing).

The main educational purpose of the simulation-based course is to promote specified learning objectives. As we have seen in the previous sections this may be supplemented by learning objectives specific to each learner. The primary task of debriefing is to help the learner achieve those aims. The process of reflection should help the learner make the most effective use of the experience of the clinical scenario. The learner should be able to make some sort of sense of the experience that he/she has just undergone. A very powerful tool that can help learning is cognitive dissonance. This term refers to that state where what happens is not what the learner expects to happen. Simulation-based teaching can be a very powerful tool in demonstrating this situation. Review of the performance, especially if supported by an audiovisual recording, shows the learner what he or she actually did. There is no room for escape. The evidence is there in front of their eyes. This has to be handled appropriately so that the principles of adult learning come into play. The learner will be more likely to make lasting change if he/she comes to accept the need for that change by themselves rather than being told how to change. The teacher can help the learner in this process by encouraging the learner to explore behaviours that would help manage the clinical situation and by helping the learner appraise his or her performance realistically. For example, the teacher could ask the learner to list the components in a protocol for management of major obstetric haemorrhage and then ask how these components could be effectively translated into clinical practice. If the teacher then helps the learner review his/her performance in the clinical scenario by encouraging the learner to highlight the difference between what he/she thinks can be done and what was actually done then the learner is more likely to change behaviour towards the learning objectives.

In the previous paragraph I have made the assumption that the learner was one individual. However, the course may not have been intended for one learner but for groups of learners. The skills are essentially the same but a greater sensitivity may be required when moving between the performance of the group as a whole and the performance of the individual members of the group. Remember, if an individual feels that he/she is being singled out for individual attention, especially negative attention, then we risk losing the climate of intellectual safety and in turn reduce the likelihood of achieving our educational goals for the session.

Another resource for the teacher is making use of the experience of the other participants. By asking questions such as "How would you have managed that case?" we invite peer opinion, which may have a very persuasive effect on the learner at the focus of attention. We can also use the experience by asking if anyone has actually managed such a case and asking them to describe the events and the management. This helps to set the performance of the individual learner, or the group, into a wider context.

Although the learning objectives have been formulated by the course organizers the main educational purpose of the debriefing period is to help and encourage the learner to formulate his/her own learning objectives. Learning objectives developed by the learner are more likely to be taken seriously by that learner and followed up.

10.10 **Provide appropriate feedback**

We have already begun the process of delivering feedback in the previous section. I have described this in terms of helping the learner review his/her performance. The emphasis was on identifying the gap between what the learner thought should have been done and what the learner actually did. The emphasis was on the negative side of the performance. Feedback should reward positive actions by the learner. The learner may not feel that there have been many positive points. Giving positive feedback may not seem to very difficult but learners appreciate structured feedback[5]. Can a simulation centre based teacher give structured feedback in an area in which he or she may not have any clinical expertise? Work from problem based learning style teaching suggests that those who have had facilitator training are more effective than those who are subject matter experts but have not had facilitator training. However, the best is someone with subject matter expertise and facilitator train. This is not often possible in simulation based teaching because it can be difficult to train someone to carry out all of the roles mentioned above. The usual compromise is to share the duties by having someone with subject matter expertise attend as faculty in addition to someone from the simulation centre. The subject matter expert brings credibility and the simulator based teacher brings the teaching and simulation expertise. Subject matter experts can also use that credibility to confirm standards and make explicit codes of practice etc.

So far we have also concentrated on providing feedback at the level of the individual learner. Important as this is there is also the skill of giving feedback at the level of the whole group. There are many lessons that can be gained from reviewing the performance of all of the learners. We can highlight common areas where the learners were challenged and we can also highlight areas where performance was of a consistently high standard.

The educational goal of feedback is to help the learner set realistic educational goals to help them develop in their professional roles. How successful or otherwise we were as teachers in achieving those goals leads us into the final set of skills in this chapter.

10.11 **Review the session**

I have described simulation based teaching in terms of environments that encourage interaction with learners that in turn promote learning outcomes; some specified in advance, some acquired on the day. We encourage the learners to reflect on their performance and simulation-based teaching offers plenty of opportunities for doing that. It would seem contradictory and even illogical if we did not carry out such an exercise ourselves. We can review the roles described above. Were our learning outcomes appropriate? Did the scenarios promote the type of interaction we wanted? Were they promoting the learning outcomes?

The key skills for this section require us to be able to exercise judgment over the whole course and then have the diagnostic capabilities to identify which areas require amendment and which ones do not.

This is not an exercise confined to the end of the course. During the introduction, during the briefings, during the individual scenarios and during the debriefing we may encounter difficulties that require us to change our approach. Donald Schön[6] describes this as reflection-in-action. This is the ability to seek out solutions while carrying out one or more of the teaching skills described above.

Schön also describes reflection-on-action. This is the reflective process that is often initiated by encountering a challenging set of circumstances. We know something that normally worked didn't. Why was that? What would we do differently if we came across such a set of circumstances again? The process does not end there. If we recognize that some of our skills are not so well developed then what can we do to improve them?

These skills in principle are no different from those that we use in other aspects of our professional lives. Reflection is as much a part of being a teacher as being a doctor or a nurse.

We can also think of this phase as resembling the audit cycle. Where do we want our course participants to be? How close or how far are they from that place? If there is a gap then what are we going to do to minimize the gap between where they are and where they should be?

We need to be able to find out where the learners are (end of course evaluation, post course follow up etc) and then we need to use that information to modify subsequent courses.

10.12 Conclusion

I have attempted to provide a framework against which teachers in simulation centres can compare their own performance. It is not exhaustive. There are other teaching skills such as coaching, instructing, supporting and mentoring that may feature in other contexts, especially hands-on practical skill courses, but are less relevant in high fidelity simulation-based courses. Each teacher will have to decide which parts are relevant and which not.

References

1. Dewey J (1916). *Democracy in Education*. New York, Macmillan Inc.
2. Knowles M (1990). *The Adult Learner: A Neglected Species*. Houston (TX), Gulf Publishing Company.
3. Fish D, Coles C (2005). *Medical Education: Developing a Curriculum for Practice*. Maidenhead (England), Open University Press.
4. Hesketh EA, Laidlaw JM (2002). Developing the teaching instinct, 4: Needs assessment. *Medical Teacher* 24: 594–8.
5. Kurtz S, Silverman J, Draper J (2005). *Teaching and Learning Communication Skills in Medicine*. Oxford (England), Radcliffe Publishing.
6. Schön DA (1987). *Educating the Reflective Practitioner*. San Francisco (CA), Jossey-Bass Publishers.

Chapter 11

Teaching in clinical settings

Fiona Lake

Overview

- The clinical setting, when trainees care for patients, is very important for learning and offers opportunities to integrate the various domains necessary for a practice as a competent clinician.

- Many clinicians find themselves teaching in both simulated and clinical settings, the latter bringing challenges of needing to facilitate learning whilst providing quality care, dealing with unpredictable availability of learning material and the need to teach trainees at different levels.

- Effective clinical teachers need to combine being a competent clinician, supportive supervisor and interested mentor with being a teacher.

- Adult learning principles, useful guides to consider when teaching, require understanding the learner's motivation, ensuring the learning is meaningful, experience centred, set at the appropriate level, has clearly set goals, involves the learners, and provides feedback and time for reflection.

- Teaching, or facilitating learning whether in a discrete session done 'on the run' in a clinical (e.g. inpatients, outpatients, handover meetings) or tutorial setting, or across a clinical attachment, requires planning.

- The learning cycle provides a useful framework for considering learning, both from the teachers and learners viewpoint and moves from defining outcomes, through to planning learning/teaching, doing it, providing assessment, appraisal and feedback which then allows revisiting of the outcomes the trainee needs to address.

- Outcomes should be clear, achievable and measurable and cover all aspects of competence including clinical management, communication and professionalism.

- A framework for planning an educational encounter should include *set* (what are the outcomes, the methods and environment), *dialogue* (using a variety of teaching methods and questions to engage, consider the patient) and *closure* (provide a summary, link to future learning).

- In the clinical setting, frameworks such as the one minute teacher, and SNAPPS (where the learner probes the teacher on areas they do not understand), are useful.

- Assessment (a judgement whether performance reaches a certain level, against defined criteria, usually external) and appraisal (educational and developmental process, with judgment about current performance used to develop a plans addressing the learning needs)

> **Overview** (continued)
>
> are part of the learning cycle but to be done well require observation on many occasions by many members of the team.
>
> ◆ Feedback should use the positive critique, by first asking the trainee and then providing your feedback on firstly what is going well and secondly what could be improved. Feedback should be specific, incorporate a plan for improvement, occur frequently, and in sufficient time for trainees to try to improve.
>
> ◆ Evaluation of the learning experience should happen after all encounters and is key to improving teaching and learning. A variety of methods including reflection on what went well and what could be improved, gathering verbal or written feedback from trainees, or asking for peer review on discrete sessions or clinical attachments should be used.

11.1 Introduction

Learning in the simulation setting offers the opportunity to closely plan educational encounters, provides a safe environment, can ensure trainees receive detailed feedback and provides repetition allowing consolidating of skills. Trainees learn from making mistakes, and in the simulation setting, such mistakes when combined with reflection are powerful learning opportunities. However, the point of the learning is to take it back to the real life setting and apply the skills and knowledge to patient care. Clinicians, be they doctors, nurses or clinical educators, usually find themselves teaching in both simulated settings and in the clinical setting, in the latter often both teaching and supervising students and trainees while caring for patients[1]. Unless some thought is put into how skills are taken from simulated to clinical settings, there is some evidence that learning is not transferred[2]. Learning in the clinical setting is often chaotic; patients need care, other tasks need to be completed, the clinical team consist of different people with different needs. In the clinical setting mistakes need to be anticipated and minimized but when they do occur, a supportive no-blame environment where trainees can reflect on their practice is important. Often in this clinical environment, teaching and learning need to be done 'on the run'.

A good teacher must not only be a good doctor but have educational knowledge and skills and the flexibility to apply them under varying circumstances which may arise. Although this unpredictability may occur more commonly in the clinical setting, such flexibility may also be required in the simulation setting, when a trainee unexpectedly performs at a different level to the rest of the trainees, or equipment fails. Being able to teach on the run requires significant planning, with stored 'scripts' that can be grabbed at the right moment, and the confidence to use educational knowledge and skills to suit the circumstances. This chapter will detail key steps in learning from a teacher's perspective, namely planning, teaching, assessing, and appraising and evaluating, which are important for a good learning environment. It will focus on a teacher who is responsible for both facilitating learning on the job and running discrete teaching sessions for trainees they are responsible for. The term 'trainee' is used to cover anyone from undergraduate, prevocational through to vocational levels.

11.2 Teachers, learners, the educational environment, and the learning cycle

11.2.1 Clinical teachers

Clinical teachers, namely clinicians who are expected to teach in the clinical environment in which they work, facilitate learning in a variety of settings, for example:

- while providing clinical care – inpatient or outpatient settings, on clinical rounds, when performing procedures, with the Consultant and trainee either jointly or separately seeing patients
- in clinical meetings or handover
- in small group interactive tutorials
- in large group (lecture) sessions.

A clinical teacher needs to consider not only the effectiveness of a session (such as how much learning occurred during a ward round or clinic), but a complete attachment, such as the 3 months or 6 months a trainee spends on a unit. As will be detailed, the same cycle of planning, teaching, assessment and evaluation can be applied to short sessions or long attachments.

An effective clinical teacher needs to be all of the following[1]:

- Clinician – competent, caring and professional, a role model.
- Supervisor – who can ensure support is given when caring for patients and who provides feedback.
- Mentor – who shows interest and provides career and personal advice.
- Teacher – understands the learner and their needs and plans and ensures effective learning.

The relationship one has with the learner, such as knowing their name, their needs and their abilities, is key to whether the learning experience is effective. In some studies the interpersonal factors can account for up to 50% of the variance in teaching effectiveness. Although this chapter focuses on the skills required of the teacher, ensuring adequate support is given, role modelling clinical care and behaviour and so forth requires thought.

11.2.2 Learners

Trainees are adults who want to learn and want to have input into that learning. They come with a whole range of prior skills and knowledge that must be built upon. The features of an adult learner have been explored as principles (Table 11.1) and are useful 'models of assumption about learning', even if not evidence based. They are sensible and should be considered when planning to teach or a starting point for reflecting on sessions that haven't gone well[3].

Table 11.1 Adult learning principles

- Learner's motivation – do they want to improve care or pass an exam?
- Meaningful – the topic should be relevant to the trainee's current or future work
- Experience centred – simulation, by definition, is experience centred. In the clinical setting, trainees want learning to be linked to work they are doing or to patient care
- Set at the appropriate level – for their stage of training, rather than too high or too low
- Clear goals are articulated – with the outcomes for the session or attachment defined
- Involvement of the learner – so they are actively involved in the learning process through being questioned, seeing patients or performing procedures
- Feedback provided – so trainee knows how they are performing
- Reflection – allow time to reflect and encourage reflection on the learning
---

Shifting from thinking about what needs to be taught to what learners need to know, or are learning, shifts from a teacher-centred to learner-centred approach. It is important to consider what this requires. A learner-centred approach requires the teacher to have a clear concept about what needs to be learnt (outcomes) and what knowledge or skills the learner comes with or lacks (what is their prior knowledge level). The learning is facilitated with this information in mind. Finally, it requires review of what learning is occurring (what are they still confused about?). Built into the teaching strategy has to be a way to find out about the knowledge level of the learner or their needs, through for example, observing and questioning, as will be expanded on later.

11.2.3 Teaching and learning styles[4]

Learning is about creating gaining new knowledge and skills by integrating new information with old, an active process which challenges the learner's prior knowledge. As learners progress, there is often a shift from being dependant (the learner needs significant input and direction), to interest, where the learner needs some guidance, to someone who is self directed, taking personal responsibility for their own learning. In addition, learners come with their own learning style (i.e. deep, superficial) and instructional preference (written, verbal, visual, interactive, didactic).

The strategies used by a teacher needs to take into account their own teaching preferences and abilities (an authority, a motivator or facilitator, a delegator), as well as the learner stage and learner preference. Expecting a struggling junior doctor to define their own needs, or presenting a mini-lecture to a mature and enquiring registrar will de-motivate both. Some mismatch can be a good thing and challenge the learners. Shifting teaching styles from authoritarian (telling them) to delegating (getting them to tell us) shifts the workload away from the teacher and can make it more fun. Flexibility however is key, as everyone likes to learn, and teach, in different ways at different times.

11.2.4 Educational environment

The simulated environment if done well provide training for some areas which need to be covered by a trainee. However simulation cannot cover all areas, either because they cannot be well simulated or because of resource constraints. Additionally, there is some evidence that skills learnt in a simulated environment are not automatically taken back to clinical practice, but may require a specific programme of clinical supervision to ensure they are applied[2]. The clinical environment discussed here relates to health care settings, where patients are being cared for and the learning is with the aim of becoming a competent clinician, in terms of clinical management, communication and professional behaviour. In becoming a clinical expert, recent reviews suggest it is not only how much experience trainees get (by seeing many patients) but how this exposure occurs (what is the emphasis, what feedback occurs) which contributes to efficiency in learning[5,6]. As opposed to the apprenticeship model of learning, which is often unstructured, so called 'deliberate practice' details what needs to be focussed on during learning. In the clinical setting deliberate practice means:

- having good supervision and feedback
- defining tasks which are important to focus on that will improve practice
- having an opportunity to repeat tasks and improve.

This is more than reflective practice. Rather than presuming by immersing trainees in clinical work they will optimally learn, consideration of elements of deliberate practice (Is feedback occurring?, Are they getting enough exposure?) should inform teaching[5,6].

Two other aspects about the educational environment are important. Firstly, one learns more from what one doesn't know, than from reinforcing what one does know. Encouraging problem

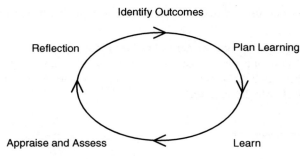

Fig. 11.1 The Learning Cycle – the learner's viewpoint. (Adapted from Peyton JWR. *Teaching and Learning in Medical Practice*(1998). Rickmansworth, UK: Manticore Europe Limited: 13–19.)

solving, rather than focussing on factual recall can facilitate the learner working out what they don't know. You then want to inspire (or cajole) them into doing something about that lack of knowledge. Secondly, this will only occur if an environment where it is acceptable to demonstrate a lack of knowledge and not feel embarrassed and inadequate, is fostered. So a supportive and safe environment is key.

> The three most important words in education are "I don't know",* either from the teacher or learner.
>
> *Modified from David Pencheon, UK Public Health Physician[7]

11.2.5 **The learning cycle**

A framework for thinking about how trainees learn, and how teachers can facilitate learning is embodied in the learning cycle (Fig. 11.1)[1,8]. The cycle involves planning, teaching, assessing/appraising and providing feedback, and finally an evaluation of the process. Although these processes usually occur continuously and simultaneously, (a trainee should receive feedback throughout the term), it is helpful to deconstruct them into parts. The framework applies not only to running a learning 'session' (ward round, tutorial or lecture) but a clinical rotation. In the next section, the components in the cycle will be addressed for complete attachments as well as single teaching sessions, which may be part of an educational programme.

11.3 **Teaching and learning in clinical attachments**

11.3.1 **Planning**

Whether planning for a 3-month clinical attachment or a 1-hour session, the first stage of planning requires definition of what outcomes are expected; what the teacher wants the learner to achieve[9]. Outcomes may be provided by the course coordinator, University or College and will be developed by you as the teacher. For clinical attachments, often little is provided to guide clinicians as to what is expected to be achieved. For single sessions, often little more than the title of a session is provided. However, experienced clinicians often have a good idea as to what we think is important but need to consider how that links with the rest of the training programme, to avoid repetition or gaps and ensure the outcomes are appropriate.

Outcomes should be:

- specific, so they can be described and addressed
- achievable during that attachment or session

♦ measurable, in that the learner can be assessed to determine whether they have achieved that outcome.

Outcomes should be relevant and important for the learner and pitched at the right level.

There are a range of domains that a training doctor needs to address to ensure competent practice. The broad categories, such as those used in the Australian Curriculum Framework for Junior Doctors (http://cpmec.org.au/curriculum/index.cfm) are:

♦ Clinical management
  • Clinical assessment and patient management
  • Procedural skills
  • Emergency management
  • Patient safety, quality in healthcare and risk management

♦ Communication
  • Interpersonal skills with patients
  • Team work/interpersonal skills with other members of the health team
  • Written communication/record keeping

♦ Professionalism
  • Professional behaviour
  • Scholarly practice
  • Doctor's role in society

Outcomes for an attachment or session usually cover a number of these domains in different ways, through explicit teaching or role modelling. A fault of teachers is to try and cover too much, so focussing on a manageable number of important outcomes is better than trying to address all important areas. Additional outcomes can be used to guide further learning. In addition to set outcomes, in clinical attachments in particular, trainees will have their own personal learning needs, based on their interests or weaknesses. These need to be aired and addressed.

The second consideration is how these outcomes are going to be achieved. As previously discussed, the apprenticeship model of training is the tradition, where an unstructured attachment with plenty of exposure and a bright interested trainee allows the outcomes to be gradually met. Using an approach of *deliberate practice*, focussing on both how much a trainee sees as well as what else is happening when the trainee is seeing patients is important[5,6]. Consideration of having well defined tasks (which match to the outcomes), such as from a history and examination, formulating a problem list or writing relevant discharge summaries, having opportunities to practice whilst receiving good supervision and feedback, and being encouraged to do self reflection on how well they are being done should be part of the planning. This means the clinician teacher has to add structure to ensure this happens. It becomes evident then, learning can occur when trainees are alone with patients, are working with more senior clinicians or are in separate 'sessions' such as a tutorial.

An *orientation*[10] at the beginning of the attachment is important for detailing what outcomes they would be expected to cover and how, as well as covering basic issues such as what is expected of the trainee in the job, administrative arrangements, what teaching they can expect from you and their clinical and other responsibilities. How they are going to be assessed and when feedback will be provided (appraisal) should be defined. Trainees should be directed to resources (websites, handbooks, people).

11.3.2 **Teaching and learning**

When trainees are busy caring for patients, it is hard for them to recognise what learning is occurring. As outlined with the concept of deliberate practice, emphasizing learning by providing feedback and encouraging self reflection are important.

In thinking about specific learning opportunities, in the clinical setting trainees value informal and formal registrar teaching, formal and informal consultant teaching (although this occurs less frequently), simulation, clinical skills sessions and tutorials[10,11]. Ward rounds and clinics in the community or hospitals when patients are discussed are valued whereas Unit meetings, Grand Rounds and computer programmes were not found to be valuable[10]. Although not shown to be the best method to stimulate thinking and knowledge transfer, trainees like tutorials, perhaps a reflection of the need to have a break and meet with friends and colleagues.

In teaching in these clinical settings, over time clinical teachers build up 'teaching scripts' related to diagnosis, management, ethics and so forth (i.e. management of pneumonia or interpretation of an electrocardiogram). Using the patient as the starting point, teachers can draw on these scripts to ensure they teach essential points. Even though much of the teaching is 'on the run', it needs to be planned and by knowing the topics that recurrently come up, teachers can be ready for a 5-minute grabbed moment, a 30-minute interactive tutorial or a 1-hour lecture, as required.

In any teaching session, from 5 to 60 minutes, a framework consisting of *set* (what you need to be considered before), *dialogue* (what happens during) and *closure* (how you finish off) is useful[12].

The essentials of *set* include:

◆ Outcomes: as noted above, what the learners need to learn should be achievable in the time, relevant and important for the learner, and set at the right level. Trainees like frameworks rather than facts and often the attempt is to cover too many facts.

◆ Environment: whether the seating, the room (not busy, noisy, public or uncomfortable), the patient or the teaching 'props' are adequate. Not all 'moments' are good if you or the learners are tired or hungry or have other pressing duties.

The *dialogue* involves interaction between the learner and the teacher and this could appropriately be one way (didactic), interactive or a mixture. The attention span of an adult is short (10–15 minutes) and varying methods of delivery to break up a session can significantly increase factual recall in learners. Using questions, eye contact and names can engage learners, keep them all involved and allow checking of understanding.

The *closure* should provide a summary, suggest further learning and be an opportunity for clarifying what is not understood. The session should finish on time. This is also the time to evaluate the session by asking what went well and what should be changed.

In applying this to learning around patients, the structure can ensure the focus is not just on what is wrong with the patient or what needs to be organized, but can check knowledge and encourage thinking. The aim is to make the trainee's knowledge and reasoning transparent, ensure feedback is given and further learning planned. Models which are based around discussions of clinical cases include the one minute teacher[13], where after reviewing a patient, the teacher:

◆ questions the trainee for their reasoning

◆ teaches on general important points

◆ provides feedback on what was done well

◆ corrects faults.

Another approach is SNAPPS[14], where the trainee:

+ **S**ummarizes the case
+ **N**arrows the differential diagnosis
+ **A**nalyses the differential diagnosis
+ **P**robes (the learner asks the teacher about areas they don't understand)
+ **P**lans management
+ **S**elects an issue for self directed learning.

The probing is a change from usual teaching, where by getting the trainee to ask the questions they can focus on what they don't know, rather than the teacher reinforcing what they do know. This structure can also allow teachers to look for one of the commonest diagnostic error; premature closure – that is the failure to consider alternate diagnoses.

A focus on where common errors occur, such as with premature closure, patient instructions, medication charts and communication with other doctors, can encourage reflection and prevent mistakes. Despite that mistakes may occur or care could be better. Medical error rarely is a result of a single error, but multiple errors which stack up. An environment that is safe and encourages reflection and not blame, so all can learn, is important.

Patients are frequently part of teaching encounters and evidence shows they like being involved[15]. It increases the time doctors spend with patients and studies have shown they are more satisfied with their inpatient stay. Frequently it is an opportunity to educate patients and have their concerns addressed, as well as allow teachers to observe how trainees interact with patients. Problems arise when patient's rights are not recognized, when they have medical or psychiatric conditions not appropriate to discuss in front of a group, or the discussion is upsetting or confusing. Essentials are asking for the patient's consent before the session, introducing everyone to the patient, being approachable, asking for questions and providing clear explanations. Trainees perform many basic and complex procedures on patients, depending on their level of training. These are frequently unsupervised. The supervising doctor needs to ensure a certain level of competence to ensure patient safety by observing and teaching in the early stages. Simulation can play an important role in providing basic skills and testing for a level of competency, in a safe environment.

Applying set, dialogue and closure to more formal sessions[15] such as tutorials is relatively easy. The most common mistake made is to try and cover too much in a session, with too many outcomes or too many facts. A framework is valued more. In keeping in mind the attention span of an adult learner (10–15 minutes), variation in pace or method (didactic *versus* interactive, video *versus* paper-based stimulus) has been shown to improve retention. With easy access to electronic presentation, this medium is frequently allowed to overwhelm the message, with significant loss of value. As with any other aspect of a teaching session, it is essential to consider the purpose of visual aids being used and make sure they are simple, clear and add to the session.

The use of questions[10] can provide a stimulus for learners, promote their thinking and allow the teacher to assess the knowledge level of the learner. Simple yes/no questions or closed questions (looking for a single answer or fact) may not be as powerful as open questions (where there is not one correct answer, but reasoning can be probed) in determining the knowledge level of a trainee and encouraging thinking. Questions starting "What do you think....?, or "What are you uncertain about?" are useful. Providing an environment where trainees feel comfortable to explore their thinking and demonstrate a lack of knowledge is essential.

In working in a small group, group dynamics need to be addressed, in particular making sure all are involved (by keeping an eye on who hasn't spoken, by directing questions to all), dealing with different levels of learners (redirect basic questions to more senior trainees), that disruptors are re-engaged (by sitting or standing near them, directing a question to them), and ensuring the topic is relevant and they are not getting confused (check by asking them).

11.4 Assessment and appraisal in clinical attachments

11.4.1 Assessment and appraisal[16]

Determining how a trainee is going and whether they are learning in the programme should be reviewed continuously as it is critical for allowing trainees to reflect on and plan further learning and for teachers to adjust their teaching programme. Additionally, clinicians are frequently involved in assessment for external bodies in the work setting, at undergraduate, prevocational and vocational levels. The terms assessment and appraisal are often confused and used interchangeably, but it is important to have a working understanding of the terms as there are potential conflicts between the different roles. Evaluation is another terms which may confuse and is discussed later.

Assessment is a judgement about whether someone's performance reaches a certain level, measured against defined criteria, usually external. Importantly, it can affect the progress of trainees in their career. This is also termed *summative* assessment. *Formative* assessment mimics the summative but the purpose is to 'inform' the learner, so they can determine how prepared they are for their summative assessment. Assessment tools may include written assessment (essay, multichoice), structured clinical assessment (OSCEs – Objective, Structured Clinical Examination, mini-CEX – structured short case reviews) or multiple pieces of evidence, including a 360° assessment from colleagues and patients, gathered into a portfolio. All have their own profile of reliability, validity and feasibility. In the work setting, so call 'in-training assessment' based on observation by a more senior clinician is the most common form of assessment used.

Appraisal is a process that is primarily educational and developmental, in that it makes a judgment about current performance and then develops plans addressing the learning needs of an individual. Although similar to formative assessment in that it informs the trainee on progress, it is viewed as much wider than just preparing for a specific assessment, but preparing for future practice. Appraisal involves both the trainer and trainee who provide input to the judgement and the development of the plan. Appraisal should be confidential and non-threatening. Tools that can inform the process include all of those noted under assessment, and additional material such as the trainees self appraisal, publications and so forth. Information from an assessment can be used to inform an appraisal.

In the clinical setting, the information gathered for both assessment and appraisal is from the same source. Thus, both in-training assessment and appraisal generally involve a senior clinician's impression of the clinical competence, communication skills and professional behaviour of the trainee. There is a potential conflict between in-training assessment and appraisal as the supervising consultant is usually both the assessor and appraiser. Appraisal is designed to help. Poor performance needs to be addressed in a confidential way, allowing trust to develop. However, if the trainee understands the information gathered may at a later date be used against them in an assessment, they are unlikely to fully participate in the process. Most of the time it does not matter as trainees are good and willing to improve. With poor performance the conflict may be important and one of the roles should be handed over to an independent party.

A perception that assessment is 'independent', reproducible and reliable, but appraisal is subjective and less robust is not always justified. An ideal assessment should be reliable, valid, have an impact on learning and practice and be feasible (acceptable in method and cost). Although there

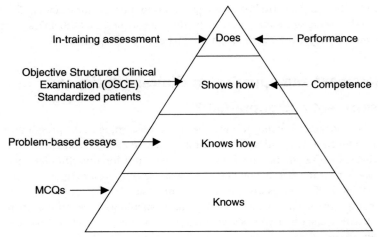

Fig. 11.2 Framework for clinical assessment. (Adapted from Millar GE (1990). The assessment of clinical skills/competence/performance. *Acad Med* **65** (9 Suppl): S63–67.)

is better understanding of strengths and weaknesses of current tools, for many, a key is doing the assessment a sufficient number of times. There are real challenges with getting sufficient observation in the busy clinical setting, but clinical teachers can improve the way they assess or appraise by:

♦ understanding the outcomes the trainees are expected to achieve

♦ understanding to what level the trainees should be performing, as shown in Millar's Pyramid[17]: knows, knows how, shows how, does (Fig. 11.2)

♦ finding 'assessable' moments – actually observe the trainee

♦ building in observations on multiple occasions

♦ collecting observations by multiple people.

11.4.2 **Feedback**

A mark of a good supervisor is they are supportive and provide regular appraisal, which must, by definition, involve feedback. Receiving feedback on how they are doing and helping plan ways to address concerns makes it more likely trainees will pass their assessment or be fulfilled in professional life. However there is evidence that feedback is often not provided, is given too late or given in such a fashion that it is useless. In a study where medical students had to solicit written feedback once every two weeks from a senior and junior clinicians (instead of the usual setting where students wait for seniors to say something), more feedback was received than usual. However, only 10% of the feedback was determined to be effective as most was too general to allow the students to understand what they did well or what they should change. Feedback should be positive (allows the trainee to understand what they did well and what they need to improve) and constructive (gives guidance as to how they can address areas where they are performing poorly). As shown in Table 11.2, ineffective feedback is too nonspecific to allow the trainee to understand what area they need to focus on or what strategy they can use to overcome the deficiency. More thinking about and analysing what has gone well and what needs to change should occur before a feedback session.

Table 11.2 Effective and ineffective feedback

Poor quality feedback

- "You did a great job."
- "Excellent, have you thought about doing respiratory medicine?"
- "That was hopeless, you really need to do more work on this."
- "Poor case history."

Effective feedback

- "You need to learn about sterile technique when putting in an IV cannula."
- "Your history taking was very good, you were organized, you were clearly think about what was happening and your questions led to your diagnosis."
- "Your physical examination revealed the main finding, which was good. It was disorganized, however, and was stressful for the patient as you had them sitting up and down all the time. Best to start in the front and move to the back. Look at the proforma in the *Core Clinical Methods* book, and practice that on family members till you can do it without thinking. Let us check your technique at the next tutorial."

In providing that feedback, teachers should use the framework of *positive feedback*[18]:

- Ask the learner what they did well.
- You discuss what they did well.
- Ask the learner what they could improve.
- You discuss what they could improve (and how).

This encourages both self appraisal and balances good and poor. Positive feedback is not about avoiding the issues that need to be addressed. It is about providing that information in a constructive manner. Discussing what and how they could improve rather than what they did badly implies a plan of action to guide their efforts

The feedback should be *specific* and achievable, for example on a particular area or topic rather than a broad learning topic (Table 11.2). So for letters to general practitioners, the feedback may provide a framework for covering important areas a GP is interested in, as a basis for writing letters next time. Feedback should be provided at the time the observation has been made, on an almost daily basis. An overall review should occur at formal times during the term (mid-term), which should be set during the orientation. Feedback must be provided in time for trainees to address concerns before the end of the attachment,

11.4.3 **Self-appraisal**[10]

Good doctors underestimate their abilities, poor doctors overestimate their abilities. We can get better at self-appraisal by benchmarking with feedback from experienced clinicians. Challenges arise when doctors do not accept a view of their deficiencies. A marker of professional misconduct is an inability to accept or act on any advice from supervisors. When faced with this challenge, patience is required. The teacher should focus not on the person but the issues and provide clear examples. If the issues are important, they need to addressed and not avoided, which may mean seeking help from more senior supervisors or directors of educational programmes in the area.

11.5 **Evaluation**[1,19]

Evaluation as a term is often used interchangeably with assessment or appraisal. Evaluation usually focuses more on the teacher or the programme, and is the trainees judgement of how well the session or programme was delivered and met their needs. It should be an integral part of any teaching programme. Teachers should gather information, usually in a variety of ways, so they can review and revise as required. Information could focus on both the teaching (content, session organisation and format) and learning (did they learn what they were meant to learn, what is still causing confusion). Methods for gathering data could include:

- verbal feedback – asking what went well and what should be changed
- written feedback – from complex surveys to a quick jot on a scrap of paper
- peer observation of teaching with feedback.

Just as there can be conflict between assessment and appraisal, there can be conflict between evaluation and either assessment or appraisal. A trainee is unlikely to give an honest but negative opinion of teaching, if they know the assessment will be completed by the same person. Separating the two processes or gathering the information in an anonymous form may be important.

11.6 Flexibility

Flexibility in teaching in clinical settings is required to cope with the varied needs of learners at different levels, the broad outcomes which need to be met including clinical competence, communication and professionalism, and the fluid nature of the clinical environment. However, planning which takes into consideration what needs to be covered, the many ways it can be covered and how appraisal and assessment will occur puts some structure in this environment. Finally it is worth considering what are the responsibilities of the learner and what part they will play in allowing the educational programme to be implemented. By sharing the load, it is far more likely to be successful.

References

1. Lake FR (2004). Teaching on the run tips Teaching on the run tips: doctors as teachers. *Med J Aust* **180**(8): 415–6.
2. Heaven C, Clegg J, Maguire P (2006). Transfer of communication skills training from workshop to workplace: The impact of clinical supervision. *Patient Educ Coun* **60**: 313–25.
3. Kaufman DM (2003). ABC of learning and teaching in medicine: Applying educational theory in practice. *BMJ* **326**: 213–16.
4. Vaughn L, Baker R (2001). Teaching in the medical setting: Balancing teaching styles, learning styles and teaching methods. *Med Teacher* **23**: 610–12.
5. Peyton JWR (1998). The learning cycle. In: Peyton JWR, Ed. *Teaching and learning in medical practice*. Rickmansworth, UK: Manticore Europe Limited: 13–19.
6. Schuwirth LWT, van der Vleuten CPM (2006). Challenges for educationalists. *BMJ* **333**: 544–6.
7. Smith R (2003). Thoughts for new medical students at a new medical school. *BMJ* **327**: 1430–3.
8. Ericsson KA (2004). Deliberate Practice and the acquisition and maintenance of expert performance in medicine and related domains. *Acad Med* **79**(Suppl. 10): S70–81.
9. Prideaux D (2000). The emperor's new clothes: from objectives to outcomes. *Med Educ* **34**: 168–9.
10. Gordon J (2003). ABC of learning and teaching in medicine: One to one teaching and feedback. *BMJ* **326**: 543–8
11. Dent AW, Crotty B, Cuddihy HL, *et al.* (2006) Learning opportunities for Australian prevocational hospital doctors: exposure, perceived quality and desired methods of learning. *Med J A* **184**: 436–40.
12. Lake FR, Ryan G (2004). Teaching on the run tips 3: planning a teaching episode. *Med J Aust* **180**(12): 643–4.
13. Furney SL, Orsini AL, Orsetti KE, *et al.* (2001) Teaching the one minute preceptor. A randomised controlled trial. *J Gen Intern Med* **16**: 620–4.

14. Wolpaw TM, Wolpaw DR, Papp KK (2003). SNAPPS: A learner centred approach for outpatient education. *Acad Med* **78**: 893–8.

15. Howe A, Anderson J (2003). Involving patients in medical education. *BMJ* **327**: 326–8.

16. Lake FR, Ryan G (2005). Teaching on the run tips 8: Assessment and Appraisal. *Med J Aust* **182**: 580–1.

17. Millar GE (1990). The assessment of clinical skills/competence/performance. *Acad Med* **65** (Suppl. 9): S63–67.

18. Pendelton D, Schofield T, Havelock P, Tate P (1984). *The consultation: an approach to learning and teaching*. Oxford: Oxford University Press.

19. Morrison J (2003). ABC of teaching and learning in medicine. *BMJ* **326**: 385–387.

Chapter 12

Scenario design: theory to delivery

Chris Holland, Chris Sadler, and Angie Nunn

Overview

- The aviation industry has guidelines for designing flight simulation scenarios; these guidelines are also applicable to medical simulation scenario design.

- The object of good scenario design should be to provide students with a scenario or short course that is integrated with their whole curriculum and which they will have no problem seeing the relevance of to their learning needs.

- The initial definition of clear and unambiguous learning objectives, with the involvement of all stakeholders in the intended student audience's education is imperative.

- Cognitive task analysis techniques can prove useful in breaking complex tasks performed by task experts into their constituent parts and therefore determining what some learning objectives should be.

- Scenarios should be written with the intention of allowing students to display the skills and behaviours that would indicate that the learning objectives have been achieved. The events that will trigger the performance of these actions must be written into the scenario in a credible fashion.

- Credibility is further enhanced by teaching students using evidence-based practice, and this should be written into the scenario from the outset.

- The actual scenario script should be as detailed, comprehensive, and unambiguous as possible. It represents the scenario lesson plan and should enable all competent simulator faculty to consistently provide the scenario to high standards.

- Once written, scenarios should be practised and modified as required. This process should continue, even after the scenario enters the student curriculum.

12.1 Introduction

The scenarios used in simulation teaching are equivalent to a classroom teacher's lesson plan. Just as a high school teacher would not start teaching for a new curriculum without creating new lesson plans, so scenario scripting should be accorded the attention it requires. In addition, the high school teacher will want to ensure that their lessons fit into the whole student curriculum in a logical way that will make their lessons seem relevant and necessary to the student.

If written well, a scenario will consistently provide students with multiple opportunities to practice technical and non-technical skills in a believable clinical situation, in which the student will have no hesitation in participating. The better a scenario is the easier the students will find it to suspend disbelief and immerse themselves in the learning opportunity being afforded to them.

In this chapter we discuss some educational theory and best practice for scenario design and the evidence supporting the process we advocate. We also offer suggestions for approaches and some considerations based on our own experience of many years of scenario design. We provide a worked example of scenario design drawn from our most recent experiences of creating a 1-day, made-to-order course completely from scratch. Finally, we present a completed scenario as used in our simulation centre (Appendix 12.1).

If the concepts and tools described below are used, then scenario design can be an intellectually stimulating and immensely creative exercise. The satisfaction of seeing a student benefit from well written and stimulating scenario designed with their precise needs in mind should not be underestimated.

12.2 **Theory**

As discussed in the chapter *Lessons from Aviation Simulation* (chapter 4) the aviation simulation industry has much to inform medical simulation, and so it is for scenario design. Federal Aviation Administration (FAA) Advisory Circular AC120–35C[1] describes the five stages of flight scenario design:

- Identification of primary crew resource management/technical training objectives.
- Identification of possible incidents that will produce the training/learning objectives.
- Specification and development of scenario event sets (the trigger event, reactions, and the consequences of those actions is called an event set).
- Evaluation and modification of the scenario as required.
- Instructor training implementation and ongoing evaluation of scenarios.

Applying a similar evolutionary approach to medical simulation scenario design will ensure that students experience a carefully planned scenario which has been created with specific learning objectives in mind and has content validity. Students will gain more from a learning opportunity they recognize as being relevant to them.

When embarking on designing a scenario consideration should be given to whether the scenario is to be part of a larger course that will, in part, occur external to the simulator and be delivered by other teachers, or if the whole course is to be provided by the simulator faculty. If it is to be the former then the learning objectives should be written jointly by simulator and non-simulator faculty. The scenarios must also sit comfortably within the objectives of the student's overarching curriculum. Examination of a pre-existing formal curriculum can prove invaluable at this stage of the design process and members of the wider teaching faculty will also be able to advise if the proposed scenarios complement the rest of the course.

If simulator faculty are not proficient in the subject matter to be taught then task experts should also be involved in the scenario design process from the outset. These are practitioners who have performed the tasks many times, to the point that they can perform the uncomplicated task semi-automatically with little conscious thought and perform the task in more complex circumstances with obvious proficiency[2]. Involvement of proficient or expert practitioners may also raise the validity of scenarios from face to content validity. Task experts are sometimes so unaware of their precise actions and thought processes whilst performing the task that they need careful interrogation to identify the skills that a novice must acquire to perform the task. If this interrogation is difficult, or the environment or task to be simulated is highly complex, one way of identifying precisely what the learning objectives should be is by using *cognitive task analysis* techniques (see below). Spending time and effort at these early stages goes a long way to making the scenario as credible as possible. This collaboration between task expert and simulator expert also helps to ensure that learning environment fidelity is matched to the desired learning outcomes and what is achievable with available facilities. Higher fidelity does not automatically result in better real-world task performance and some complex skills can be taught using surprisingly low fidelity teaching methods[3].

Scenario content should be written, not only with the input of task experts, but also using a defensible evidence base. Technical skills required, clinical practice guidelines used and the overall education programme should be based on evidence of clinical effectiveness[4]. Additionally, consideration should be given to providing teaching on this evidence based practice either before or after the course or during the feedback session following the relevant scenario[5]. It is our practice to provide candidates with a list of the references we have used in our scenario design at the end of each course. This also provides reflective and self-directed learners with some foundations for further learning, building on our initial teaching.

Issenberg and colleagues, suggest several features of scenario and course design that lead to effective learning in their Best Evidence Medical Education (BEME) Guide Number 4[6]. Scenarios primarily offer the opportunity for experiential learning and practising of skills, many centres (ourselves included) do not perform instructional teaching during the running of a scenario. As discussed below, we script simulator faculty into the scenario to act as discrete guides and facilitators only. Issenberg *et al.* found that one of the aspects of simulator training most valued by students is the provision of feedback. Thus, the learning opportunities do not end with the students simply performing the desired observed behaviours but extend beyond individual scenarios and into the debriefing session that should follow every scenario. The aims and objectives of this debriefing will be suggested by those of the scenario. The results of Issenberg *et al.'s* systematic review also suggest that repeated practice of required skills, integrating learning objectives with the learner's curriculum, using scenarios with different levels of difficulty, using different learning strategies and capturing a wide variety of clinical variation all contribute to effective learning in medical simulators. If the scenario is being written as one of several that candidates will observe and/or participate in as part of a short course then this allows for repetition of skills in the scenarios and repeated discussion in the debriefing sessions, both reinforcing learning. The programme for the debriefing sessions, must strike a compromise between ensuring that students are provided the opportunity to not only acquire new knowledge and fill in gaps exposed by their experience of the scenario but also discuss behaviours and non-technical skills required to participate in the scenario.

12.3 Cognitive task analysis

Hopefully the need for a clear conceptualization of the requirements of the learners and precisely what it is the simulation will teach them is now apparent. The less open to interpretation this concept is the easier it is to write scenarios which will enable the students to achieve the desired objectives. Cognitive task analysis (CTA) is a set of methods used for identifying cognitive skills, or mental demands, needed to perform a task proficiently. Militello and Hutton describe the rationale of using CTA and offer advice on how to perform the analysis[7]. When an individual performs an action required for their job they are completing a task. Task analysis techniques were initially developed to facilitate the improvement of physical working environments in order to make them safer, more ergonomic and more efficient. However, in industries such as healthcare, aviation and nuclear power which are highly safety critical, advances in technology have increased the mental demands placed on workers. While task analysis attempts to describe the series of physical actions required to perform a task, CTA attempts to discern the cognitive skills and processes of task performance as well. CTA is especially applicable when the analysed tasks are complex and it becomes important to understand the reasons behind experts observed behaviours. The analysis frequently requires the input of task experts. There exists an extensive body of literature about CTA containing a large variety of techniques that can be used [8].

Cognitive task analysis results in three subsets of information about how the task is performed by an expert:

- The knowledge required in performing the task.
- The skills used to perform the task.
- The congnitive processes and behaviours that can be observed during performance of the task.

12.4 Stages of scenario design

12.4.1 Identification of primary crew resource management/technical training objectives

Crew resource management skills can obviously be compared to crisis resource management skills or anaesthetic non-technical skills[9]. Technical training objectives are concerned with training students in the performance of a task using specific equipment. The explicit identification of technical and non-technical learning objectives means that all simulator faculty are likely to conduct the scenario and subsequent feedback with the same set of learning objectives and desirable observed behaviours as set endpoints. Salas and Burke[3] describe how simulation is most effective when scenarios are written with the required learning objectives embedded from the outset.

12.4.2 Identification of possible incidents that will produce the training/learning objectives

This can usually be achieved by a formal or informal faculty meeting or review of the literature aimed at identifying a critical incident, or clinical near-miss event, which will lend itself to creating the desired learning opportunities for students. Credibility is easier to ensure if scenarios are designed using real events as templates.

12.4.3 Specification and development of scenario event sets

By stage three of the scenario planning process we have used multiple sources of information to evolve a detailed concept of precisely what it is we want to teach, who our target audience is and what the credible clinical background to the scenario will be. Task experts have also helped to identify the triggers we will incorporate within the scenario which should induce our students to display the desired behaviours. In other words, we have the raw material to script the event sets embedded within the scenario. Hamman[10] suggests a framework for conceptualizing each event set: topic, subtopic, skill and observable behaviour.

As the scenario is created using the learning objectives and storyboarding process as outlined, overarching topics will be identified. Each topic will have multiple subtopics and each subtopic will require the exercising of specific skills. Each skill is demonstrated by the observation of certain behaviours. The data from any CTA already performed will naturally lend itself to this method of categorization.

For example, a scenario may be required to teach emergency airway management. One of the topics for that scenario will be patient safety. The topic would have multiple subtopics, one of which would be reduction of aspiration risk. This would require skills and knowledge involving the anatomy of the upper airway. An observable behaviour demonstrating this skill would be utilisation of cricoid pressure. This framework can be applied to non-technical as well as technical skills.

It is helpful to consider the many different ways in which students could respond to each trigger event and determine how the scenario will respond to each student reaction. A member of faculty trained in scenario facilitation should be scripted into the scenario at all times to allow the learning experience to be guided in the desired direction should students deviate from the planned storyboard. This facilitator can then interject with suggestions, in a credible fashion, if the students are struggling or remain in the background providing technical support as required. Skilled facilitators within the scenario who have received instruction in the learning objectives intended for the scenario will be able to fade in and out of the background as required and keep the students largely following the desired path. When scripting for this facilitator we try to consider how the scenario will respond to as many conceivable student responses as possible. It is also useful to decide if there are to be any limits on how far certain situations will be allowed to deviate from the planned storyboard (e.g. will the mannequin be allowed 'to die' or how will instructors respond if students behave in a truly unanticipated manner). We usually ask participating faculty to intervene, in a credible way, to prevent 'death' and with experience our instructors have become immensely skilful at guiding students away from unanticipated outcomes. Assuming that the scenario will be used on repeated occasions, different groups of students will naturally display different levels of competencies. Some will require a lot of guidance from the simulator instructor participating in the scenario to achieve the desired outcomes, others will rapidly respond to the trigger event and display the desired behaviours. In our centre we do not advocate prolonging scenarios once the desired outcomes have been reached as this then means the scenario is progressing to areas which have not been subjected to the rigorous design process outlined above and therefore will have lesser degrees of validity.

12.4.4 Evaluation and modification of the scenario as required

The FAA and others[10] recommend that once a scenario is written the script should explicitly describe the event sets, event trigger and the related topics, subtopics, skills and observed behaviours for the benefit of those that will administrate the scenario. Once scripted in such a fashion it should undergo a 'dry-run' using at least two different groups of experts as candidates and involving the instructors who will administer the scenario. This will hopefully expose flaws in the scenario script and allow required modifications to be made.

12.4.5 Instructor training implementation and ongoing evaluation of scenarios

An unambiguous version of the scenario that is to be used for teaching students can be published and the instructors can be trained in its administration. It is our experience that even when the scenario is in actual use as a teaching tool, unexpected student behaviours are observed which require the scenario to be modified further to enhance the learning opportunities provided.

12.5 Worked example

So how does all this happen in reality? Recently our simulation centre has been involved in the creation of a 1-day simulation course for Foundation Year 2 (FY2) doctors. These are pre-registration doctors in their second year post graduation from a UK medical school. They have a very detailed formal curriculum[11] which covers six generic competencies required of them as well as 16 competencies related to the care of the acutely unwell patient. When a simulation based course was proposed this document provided explicit learning objectives and details of the knowledge, skills and behaviours required of this group of doctors.

We began by using a collaborative process involving simulator faculty, representatives from the organisations which regulate training schemes for these doctors, college tutors, educationalists and clinicians with responsibility for teaching FY2 doctors to seek and reach consensus on eight credible clinical events that could be used as storyboards into which the required event sets could be embedded. From the outset we sought a wide range of clinical problems and aimed to produce a set of eight scenarios of varying degrees of difficulty.

The FY2 curriculum core competencies were then reviewed and appropriate trigger events in each of the clinical episodes identified. Once this was done storyboards were scripted in more detail. In the case of the FY2 core competencies each competency required at least one event set covering one topic. It was clear from the text of the formal curriculum document what the relevant subtopics should be. Experienced simulator faculty and experts in acute medicine contributed to the identification of the skills associated with the subtopics and what explicit behaviours would provide evidence for possession of these skills. Each scenario script had more detail inserted as the various layers of design were built up.

Once a script of sufficient detail was drafted its component event sets were then mapped back onto a matrix, or grid. As all eight scenarios took shape we were able to ensure that every topic was embedded into more than one scenario. This process allowed us to create opportunities for repetition of each competency over the duration of the course and therefore to observe each behaviour in more than one clinical situation. A systematic review by Issenberg[6] identified that focused repetition of skills in a manner designed to engage the student was the second most important feature of effective learning in a high fidelity simulation.

Our clinical scenarios covered acute medical emergencies ranging from cardiac arrest to epileptic seizure. As each scenario was scripted literature searches for current evidence based guidelines were performed. These guidelines were then used to inform the scripting of the scenarios in such a fashion as to guide the students towards current standards of best practice. All eight scenarios were scripted to include at least one facilitator playing the role of a health care professional acting as an assistant to the student who would be the main source of guidance for the candidate, should guidance be required during the running of the scenario. Scenarios we have designed for other courses have used students to play the roles of other healthcare professionals, such as theatre nursing staff. These roles are used to exploit opportunities to teach the importance of non-technical skills such as interdisciplinary communication.

Our centre uses a template for scripting scenarios at this stage of development. The template acts as a standard layout that all simulator faculty can become familiar with. To continue the initial analogy of a lesson plan, this document represents an unambiguous guide for running the lesson which would allow different teachers to conduct the lesson and achieve the same learning objectives. It contains all the required information to run the scenario from set-up to debrief and can also be used to quickly orientate faculty members, not regularly involved with that particular scenario, to their required roles. The template is organized under the following headings (with some examples in italics):

1. Course Title; Patient Details; Clinical Diagnosis

   Anaesthetic Crisis Resource Management Course; Mr John Smith; Anaphylaxis

2. Synopsis

   Mr Smith is a 56-year-old man undergoing GA for elective inguinal hernia repair. He has reflux and has been intubated. He has an anaphylactic reaction to the muscle relaxant.

3. Learning objectives

   In this section we list the event sets and topics, sub-topics, skills and desired observed behaviours which the authors of the scenario had in mind when writing it. One event set might be:

   - Patient becomes unwell while under anaesthesia (event set)
   - Maintains vigilance (topic)
   - Monitors heart rate (one subtopic under this topic)
   - Uses all means of monitoring heart rate (skill)
   - Observes heart rate on monitor and confirms with pulse check (observed behaviour)

4. Environment set-up

   These are the instructions for the 'stage-hands', those members of faculty who are setting up for the scenario. It describes where the scenario is set, what props are required, what is happening as the scenario begins and a cast list of characters required for the scenario.

   Operating theatre, general anaesthetic and surgery in progress, male manikin, IV access, IV Fluids running, intubated and ventilated, surgical set, radio playing, hospital notes, anaesthetic chart, prescription and fluid chart.

   Faculty: Anaesthetist, Anaesthetic Assistant, Surgeon, Surgical Assistant

5. Console initial set-up and changes to variables required throughout the scenario

   This is the most important section, for those in the control room, during the actual running of the scenario. Here we specify the initial settings required for manikin, anaesthetic machine etc. The actual variables stated will vary according to simulator fidelity, but should be as detailed as possible.

   This section also explains all the parameter changes required as the scenario progresses, with the corresponding triggering observed behaviours. It is important that this section in particular is concise, clear and unambiguous so that faculty can run the scenario in a smooth and credible way with no interruptions, no matter how frenetic the pace of the scenario becomes.

   We restate here if the scenario is not intended to progress to certain events such as cardiac arrest in order to remind faculty not to ad lib.

6. Event trigger

   Patient becomes tachycardic and hypotensive with bilateral wheeze.

   Airway pressures on ventilator rise, tidal volumes fall.

   (We specify actual values for such variables)

   If candidate asks anaesthetic assistant – the patient has a rash

7. Scenario progression

   If candidate gives bronchodilators wheeze improves slightly but heart rate and blood pressure do not.

   If adrenaline given IV blood pressure improves but tachycardia worsens.

   If adrenaline given IM both blood pressure and tachycardia improve.

   If no active or incorrect intervention by candidate, faculty will suggest calling for help and physiological parameters will worsen.

   Again we specify actual parameter values in this section.

   Patient does not arrest before help arrives.

   Surgeon only becomes aware of problem if candidate tells them directly.

   Surgeon will have to be asked to stop surgery, otherwise will continue.

Surgeon asks to send for next patient and does not recognise need to find high dependency bed for current patient.

8. Patient history; Past medical history; Drug history; Investigation results

This is a précis of all the information available to the candidate in the notes and charts available to them in the scenario, including the results of any blood tests they might reasonably ask for. It is important that all faculty are aware of this information as different candidates may seek information in different ways; some ask the surgeon and ignore the nursing staff, others do not communicate with the surgeon at all but direct all information gathering activity at the anaesthetic assistant. In scenarios involving an awake patient with whom the candidates must interact then faculty need to know the facts of the patient's situation in order to answer the candidate's questions.

9. Candidate Information / Handover

This is the information the candidate is given just prior to going into the scenario and in the patient handover. This will vary in detail from scenario to scenario; some scenarios require detailed handovers designed to direct the candidate to a certain course of action, others may have as an event trigger a poor quality handover. Others may have no handover at all but simply require the candidate to respond to a crisis situation already in progress, an example of this is given in Appendix 12.1.

10. Faculty characterizations

We describe here how we want our faculty to behave whilst in character. Some of our scenarios contain roles that are written to intentionally display challenging behaviours. The management of these behaviours will be one of the learning objectives for the scenario. We do not put candidates into scenarios where everyone is 'against them' and always have at least one member of faculty who will provide moral support if needed.

For example, in Appendix 12.1, one of the learning opportunities is the management of poor performance in colleagues. We have written the scenario to include a member of faculty acting the role of a ward nurse who has recently completed basic life support (BLS) training. This faculty member is instructed to bolster the student's confidence in challenging the incorrect management of VF arrest by the surgical trainee, but only if the students are hesitant about doing so.

11. Scenario endpoints

This section describes the desired observed behaviours that indicate a candidate has successfully negotiated all the scripted event sets.

e.g. in the scenario requiring the management of anaphylaxis while under anaesthesia.

Candidate has stopped administration of muscle relaxants, antibiotics, blood and any other possible trigger agents.

Patient is being ventilated on 100% oxygen and anaesthesia is being maintained.

Candidate has called for help

Candidate has given two doses of at least 100 micrograms of IM adrenaline.

Candidate has begun process of moving patient to place of safety, usually by making phone call to ITU to request bed.

12. Suggested debriefing topics

We write these with a certain degree of flexibility as we strongly believe that each debriefing must primarily deal with the behaviours actually observed and learning needs identified by those observations. If the scenario has been well designed and has run as expected then these will be exactly as planned and should be outlined at this point. Broadly speaking there will be some technical skills and knowledge specific to the clinical scenario (e.g. management of anaphylaxis and then a whole range of possible non-technical skills and behaviours that could potentially be discussed). As discussed elsewhere in this chapter candidates may achieve all, some or none of the desired learning outcomes and should be debriefed according to their individual needs. In addition, we do not advocate using just one scenario to cover all possible debriefing points. Instead, we try to write several scenarios per course that will facilitate discussion of a few points with a degree of repetition built into the whole course to allow for flexibility should one debriefing session become devoted to fewer topics for discussion than expected.

Once a scenario has been formatted to this template we keep a secure master copy and a working copy for further development, updating the master copy as required. At this stage we start to circulate the scenario to a wider group of members of faculty who will act as instructors and facilitators for the scenario in an attempt to solicit feedback and evaluation of the proposed script. As the script reaches an ever wider audience there has to be an agreed process of discussion and reaching consensus before changes to the script can be made, otherwise the careful embedding of planned learning objectives can become undone.

Once consensus has been reached the scenario is reviewed and the required props and accessories identified, for example if patient notes are required to add to scenario fidelity then these must be written at this stage, credible investigation results must be sourced including blood, ECG and X-ray examinations. This also applies to requirements for appropriate manikin fidelity such as wounded limbs or other findings on examination and ability to catheterise or perform other practical procedures necessitated by the scripted clinical scenario.

Scenarios at this stage are now ready to be trialled. We try to run scenarios first as a rehearsal with stops whenever necessary to identify and resolve issues followed by a dress rehearsal with no interruptions to ensure that the scenario actually unfolds in the intended fashion. This process needs to be repeated as often as required until the scenario runs smoothly along a credible path. Once required changes have been made the final version of the scenario has to be distributed to simulator faculty in a timely fashion so that all participants can become familiar with their required roles and any faculty training requirements can be identified.

Now the scenarios are ready to be used for teaching purposes. The first few performances with students frequently result in further scenario refinements to either enhance or reduce the impact of specific characteristics of the learning opportunities. We are constantly surprised that even with the development process outlined above, watching the intended students participate in the scenarios still reveals unexpected learning opportunities. Before making changes however, faculty must decide if these unexpected events should be enhanced or suppressed. The decision is often dependent on time constraints for the scenario and faculty must not loose sight of the original learning objectives they set out to achieve. It may be to the overall detriment of the course if other objectives are enhanced at the expense of the original ones. We have also learnt from experience that, occasionally, a scenario has to be simplified for its intended audience because the students do not have the skills or knowledge expected of them by the authors. If a scenario needs to be significantly edited to satisfy such learning needs then careful consideration has to be given as to whether the whole scenario is fit for purpose or if modification or embedding of additional event sets will be sufficient. Such insights can also arise from the feedback sessions following the scenario or from student evaluation forms at the end of each course. Over time experience in scenario writing is accumulated and major rewrites become less and less frequent. In addition it is best educational practice to review all scenarios frequently to ensure they remain fit for purpose.

Over the course of several years we have built up a library of scenarios sufficiently large that we frequently have 'off-the-shelf' solutions if asked to participate in *ad hoc* courses. We have also developed and maintain links with other simulator centres which have, on occasion, allowed us to source scenarios designed using the benefit of others' experiences.

12.6 **Conclusion**

The aviation simulation industry has a recommended procedure for scenario design and implementation. Planning scenarios in this way requires the initial, unambiguous definition of desired learning objectives. We advocate an inclusive process involving contributors with expertise in simulation, the skills and tasks being taught and the overall requirements of the intended student audience. Students will expect to be taught to use evidence-based clinical practices and, if such evidence exists, it should also be incorporated into the scenario. If this approach is applied it ensures that scenarios are produced which are likely to have significant content validity. We have written many scenarios following this action plan and feel that it results in scenarios of excellent quality which stand up to rigorous scrutiny, are credible and utilise the appropriate level of simulator fidelity. We have devised a template for scenario scripting so that every one of our scenarios is presented with the same degree of clarity. This adds to consistency of scenario provision when running different courses or when different faculty teach specific scenarios. An example of a completed scenario following this template can be seen in Appendix 12.1. We use test runs, or dress rehearsals, using task experts as scenario candidates with subsequent modifications as required. These need to be run at a timely stage prior to course dates so that provision can be made for instructor training using the finished scenario before the scenario begins to be used as an educational tool.

Finally, evaluation data from students should be used in an iterative fashion and may uncover unanticipated learning needs requiring ongoing updating of a scenario library. In addition, scenarios should be regularly reviewed to ensure they continue to teach best evidence-based practice and the learning objectives of the target audience.

References

1. US Department of Transportation (2004). Advisory Circular 120–35c. *Line Operational Simulations: Line Oriented Flight Training, Special Purpose Operational Training, Line Operational Evaluation*. Washington DC: US Department of Transportation, Federal Aviation Authority.
2. Dreyfus HL, Dreyfus SE (1986). *Mind over Machine: The Power of Human Intuition and Expertise in the Era of the Computer*. New York: Free Press.
3. Salas E, Burke CS (2002). Simulation for training is effective when... *Qual Saf Health Care* **11**(2): 119–20.
4. Grol R, Grimshaw J (2003). From best evidence to best practice: effective implementation of change in patients' care. *Lancet* **362**(9391): 1225–30.
5. Lockyer J, Ward R, Toews J (2005). Twelve tips for effective short course design. *Med Teach* **27**(5): 392–5.
6. Issenberg SB, McGaghie WC, Petrusa ER, Lee Gordon D, Scalese RJ (2005). Features and uses of high-fidelity medical simulations that lead to effective learning: a BEME systematic review. *Med Teach* **27**(1): 10–28.
7. Militello LG, Hutton RJ (1998). Applied cognitive task analysis (ACTA): a practitioner's toolkit for understanding cognitive task demands. *Ergonomics* **41**(11): 1618– 41.
8. Crandall B, Klein G, Hoffman RR (2006). *Working minds: A practitioner's guide to cognitive task analysis*. 1st ed. Cambridge, Boston: MIT Press.
9. Flin R, Glavin R, Maran N, Patey R (2003). *Anaesthetists' Non-Technical Skills (ANTS) System Handbook v1.0*. Aberdeen, UK: University of Aberdeen.

10. Hamman WR (2004). The complexity of team training: what we have learned from aviation and its applications to medicine. *Qual Saf Health Care* 13 (Suppl. 1): i72–9.

11. The Foundation Programme Committee of the Academy of Medical Royal Colleges (2005). *Curriculum for the Foundation Years in Postgraduate Education and Training*. UK: Departments of Health, UK.

Appendix 12.1 Example scenario

Harry Barlow; SC 48372; 21/09/1938

Scenario: Cardiac Arrest and Maintaining Good Medical Practice

Synopsis

This scenario needs careful choreographing to run as intended.

Harry is 68-year-old man with previous IHD and bypass 15 years ago. He was admitted for an elective inguinal hernia repair 3 days ago. He had an episode of chest pain in recovery post op and was kept in for cardiology follow-up. Troponins were negative and he is due for discharge today. Has VF arrest on ward. Surgical trainee attempts to lead arrest team but does so badly and using out of date guidelines.

Learning objectives

Candidates are expected to:

1. Know 2005 ALS guidelines

    a. Ventilate at 30:2 BVM ratio
    b. Shock at 360 Joules from initial shock when using a monophasic defibrillator
    c. Shock is primary to giving adrenaline

2. Participate in cardiac arrest team

    a. Follow initial directions from team leader
    b. Effective BVM ventilation
    c. Attach monitoring
    d. Assess rhythm (VF)

3. Take over leadership of arrest team

    a. Recognize poor leadership
    b. Manage surgical doctor's poor leadership

4. Communicate with surgical SHO

Ward set-up

Male mannequin, ward staff nurse, surgical SHO

	In situ	Monitored
Arterial line	NO	
NIBP	NO	
Peripheral line	YES	
ECG	YES	YES VF
SATS	NO	

In room: cardiac arrest trolley, defibrillator, 2005 ALS guidelines on wall.

Dressing over right inguinal area. Right inguinal drain with old blood minimal volume.

Investigations

Hb	12.2	**Na**	136
WCC	8.0	**K**	4.7
Platelets	575	**Urea**	12
Glucose	4.5	**Creat**	50
ECG	Old ECG Q-waves	**Troponin**	<0.1

Appendix 12.1 (continued) Example scenario

___

Drugs on prescription chart

___

- Simvastatin 10 mg
- Aspirin 75 mg OD (stopped for surgery)
- Losartan 50 mg OD
- Enoxaparin 20 mg BD changed to 60 mg BD post chest pain
- Temazepam 10 mg nocte
- Paracetamol 1 g QID
- Ibuprofen 200 mg 8-hourly
- Oromorph 20 mg 2–4-hourly

No known allergies

___

Console

___

Initial observations:

- Make the amplitude of the VF as coarse as possible on **both** the laptop and the touchscreen monitor.
- **The candidates must not confuse this for fine VF**

HR	VF
BP	unrecordable
SaO$_2$	unrecordable
RR	apnoea
ECG	VF

- **After first shock at 200 joules if candidates have still not recognized that SHO does not know new guidelines then rhythm becomes VT and surgical SHO gives atropine to treat it.**

Once one cycle is completed correctly then:

HR	68b/m
BP	94/56
SaO$_2$	92
ECG	Sinus with ST depression

___

Event triggers

___

- Initial call for help from ward
- Instruction to perform incorrect compression ratio
- Administration of atropine for VT

___

Scenario progression

___

- The ward round has just left the ward. Mr Barlow is having his sheets tucked in by a junior ward nurse. The nurse notices that Mr Barlow is unresponsive, shakes him and calls for help.
- The surgical SHO calls in the two candidates and tells them he is running the cardiac arrest and one must take the head and one must get the defib.
- He does not tell them to put out a cardiac arrest call – the candidates must initiate that.
- **Candidate is instructed to do synchronized BVM at ratio 15:2.**

Continued

Appendix 12.1 (continued) Example scenario

- Candidate is given history as they are following these instructions:

  Previous MI over 10 years ago and he had a bypass then. Since then no chest pain has stopped smoking and walks his dog every day. He was admitted for an elective right inguinal hernia repair 3 days ago. Surgery was uneventful but in recovery he was cold, clammy, hypotensive and had some chest pain. ECG unchanged but has been kept in for cardiology review and serial troponins. Cardiology due to come round and discharge this morning. The ward round had just left his bed when he became unresponsive.

- If candidates do not challenge BVM ratio of 15:2 the nurse says to candidate that when they were at BLS training last week there was talk of new guidelines.
- SpR will continue at 15:2 ratio and give 200/200/360 J shocks and adrenaline every cycle.

After first shock if candidates have still not recognized that SHO does not know new guidelines then rhythm becomes VT and surgical SHO gives atropine to treat it.

Patient history

Past medical history

- IHD for 16 years. Presented with acute MI and had single vessel bypass same year. Since then no angina.
- Risk factors:
  Hypercholesterolaemia
  Hypertension
  Family Hx brother died MI aged 59 years
  Ex-smoker stopped after MI.

Drug history

- Simvastatin 10 mg
- Aspirin 75 mg OD (stopped for surgery)
- Losaartan 50 mg OD
- Enoxaparin 20 mg BD
- Temazepam 10 mg nocte

Allergies

- Nil known

Social

- Lives at home with wife and dog
- Retired undertaker

Candidates information

You are just starting your shift on a general surgical ward. The morning ward round has happened early and is just finishing.

Nurse instructions

You are friendly to candidate and enthusiastic at chest compressions. You vaguely heard at your BLS training that there were some new guidelines and as the candidate voices concerns you will back them up.

Surgical SHO instructions

- You lead the arrest confidently following old protocol.
- You initially are dubious about new guidelines having never heard of them but if candidate and nurse are sure you'll ask what you should be doing.
- If poster of new guidelines is pointed out to you then you have to accept their word.

Appendix 12.1 (continued) Example scenario

After one shock of 200 joules, if candidates have still not recognized that you do not know new guidelines then rhythm will become VT and you give atropine to treat it. As you do this say loudly:

"One MiniJET of atropine for the VT"

Scenario aims

Technical skills

♦ Perform simple airway manoeuvres (with adjuncts)
♦ Manage cardiac arrest following ALS 2006 guidelines

Non-technical skills

♦ New ALS guidelines
♦ Effective communication
♦ Leadership

Debriefing

♦ 2006 ALS guidelines
♦ How does a junior member tell a senior team member they should do things differently?

Chapter 13

Debriefing: theory and techniques

Brendan Flanagan

Overview

- Debriefing is the term used to describe the period of structured reflection and feedback after a simulation exercise and is considered to be an essential element of simulation-based education.
- Despite this there is surprisingly little published research about the benefits of debriefing, effective models of debriefing or comparison with other educational techniques.
- Current theory underpinning the role of debriefing draws heavily on work in relation to experiential learning and reflective practice.
- Debriefing has both emotional support and educational benefits for learners.
- While effective debriefing is important to maximise learning, performed badly debriefing may be a source of harm to the learner.
- Establishing a safe and supportive learning environment is one of the fundamental tenets of an effective debriefing.
- Although the actual style of the debriefing may vary somewhat, there are recognized phases that should be considered in the conduct of any debriefing.
- The expertise of the debriefer is arguably the most important element of effective simulation-based education, yet many of the skills required remain ill defined.
- Opportunities for formal faculty development with respect to debriefing skills are increasingly available

13.1 Introduction

In this chapter the term debriefing refers to the purposeful, structured period of reflection, discussion and feedback undertaken by learners and teachers usually immediately after a scenario-based simulation exercise involving standardised patients and/or mannequins. Usually this involves a group of learners, rather than an individual and there may be video playback capability available to stimulate recall of the actual events.

A distinction is made between debriefing as a technique to stimulate reflective learning in which all the discussion occurs after the scenario (reflection 'on' action) and the use of simulation in which a scenario may be intermittently paused (frozen) on one or more occasions during the conduct of the scenario to explore immediate impressions and/or help (usually novice) participants who are struggling to proceed with the management of the situation. This latter 'pause and discuss' format captures the participants' understanding of the situation in the moment (reflection 'in' action) but is not discussed further here.

This chapter will briefly outline the theory underpinning debriefing as well as describing some currently used debriefing techniques in the hope of providing some assistance to novices and experienced workers in this field. There is still surprisingly little research to support much of what occurs during the debriefing process, so much of the material presented here is the product of the author's own reflections after fourteen years of involvement in simulation-based teaching, including participation in and conduct of Train the Trainer courses in this field. Any text in italics represents an example of some actual words that might be useful to use in the related section of a debriefing.

13.2 The theory

13.2.1 Purpose

There are two principal reasons for undertaking debriefing after simulation scenarios.

- One is for emotional support, that is to manage any untoward psychological after effects by providing supportive feedback for any responses that if left unchecked could create distress for an individual.
- The other is educational, to provide an opportunity for the learners to explore their own and others' practice with respect to medical/technical knowledge and skill base and/or non-technical skills, depending on the goals of the session.

Well-planned debriefings 'can allow for reflection-on-action and planning for different ways of handling the event next time'[1]. One of the aims of formal debriefing should be to stimulate participants so they will continue reflecting upon the experience after the formal debriefing period has ended. This informal reflection may occur individually or with others afterwards.

13.2.2 Educational theory

The theory underpinning the role of debriefing in reinforcing the learning associated with an experiential exercise is drawn from many sources. The two most significant involve Kolb's theory of learning[2] – in particular that learning is facilitated through experience – and Schon's work on reflective practice[3]. Readers are referred to Dunn[4] for a succinct summary of the five accepted major learning theories in relation to simulation-based education.

Gaba's group at Stanford were the first to describe a simulation-based curriculum in healthcare that incorporated video-assisted debriefing (see Howard)[5]. They developed their debriefing techniques based on guidelines for debriefing in crew resource management training in aviation[6], and termed the training crisis resource management (CRM) in part to reflect this lineage. The goal during CRM debriefing was (and is) to discuss what happened during the simulation scenario in the context of sound medical practice, to explore alternatives and to consider the events in the context of a non-technical framework of CRM key points (Table 13.1). The participants are encouraged to link their observations to behaviours and events in the real world and to extrapolate to analogous situations they may encounter in the future. Ideally the debriefer 'facilitates' the

Table 13.1 Key points of crisis resource management (modified after Gaba)[8]

- Know and optimize your environment
- Anticipate and plan
- Call for help early enough
- Communicate effectively
- Ensure leadership and role clarity
- Allocate attention wisely and use all available information
- Distribute the workload and use all available resources

process of the group debriefing itself though there are invariably elements of traditional content-expert 'instruction' in regard to medical/technical issues and in terms of the CRM principles. Data from participants in both aviation and healthcare support the view that the debriefing sessions are the most important aspect of simulation-based training[7,8].

13.2.3 Challenges

Debriefing provides a powerful learning opportunity but it continues to be considered one of the hardest aspects of simulation-based education for clinician educators to master. This should not be surprising as the skills required are neither clearly defined[9] nor has the technique formed a traditional part of the training of healthcare practitioners, be they teacher or learner[10]. All too often in the real world, a structured debriefing session only happens after an adverse outcome and is often associated with a tendency to attribute blame – this represents a challenge in terms of acceptance of debriefing in the simulation environment as participants may well be expecting the same approach. However in simulation the debriefing process is structured, genuinely reflective and conducted in a manner that is promoting of a positive culture.

Each of the players in the simulation environment – teacher and learner – bring some 'baggage' with them to the interaction:

- The learners bring baggage in the form of the anxiety based on their (hopefully) erroneous expectation of what is going to happen – namely a 'test' followed by video playback of their failings in the company of their peers.
- The teacher brings the master/novice role modelling that they themselves encountered as learners, often unconstrained by any formal educational instruction. A truly learner-centred approach involves a letting go of control of the agenda in the debriefing – this is a source of anxiety for the debriefer.

Hence the temptation for the debriefers and learners to conduct themselves in a 'traditional' manner during the debriefing – in which the debriefer as 'teacher' controls the agenda and the learners sit passively, too timid to speak – is strong. It must be resisted!

13.3 The practice

13.3.1 Conceptual phases

Although the actual structure of the debriefing may vary somewhat, it is generally agreed that there are three phases to the process[8,11,12,13].

Descriptive phase attempts to elicit the participants' feelings, as well as having them explain the 'story' of the scenario in which they have been involved. Group discussion then elicits the main issues for subsequent reflection, which can be stimulated by video playback if available.

Understanding and analogy phase in which the issues discussed are explored for their underlying meaning in the context of sound medical practice (and in relation to a non-technical skills framework if relevant) – what was done well and how might things be done differently next time?

Generalization and implication/application phase in which the learning from this particular scenario and debriefing is reviewed and extrapolated into a real-world context with a view to consideration of how to implement any new learning into the participants' daily practice.

13.3.2 A suggested structure

Each debriefing usually follows immediately after the corresponding simulation scenario. Several scenarios and debriefings may occur in the context of a single simulation-based course and there is much overlap between planning the debriefings and planning the course as a whole. Likewise many of the important issues for successful debriefing are similar to those for any small group learning exercise.

The following section outlines one possible structure for conducting a debriefing session.

13.3.2.1 Plan

As with any educational activity, adequate planning is essential to ensure the session achieves its objectives. Important practical considerations for the session as a whole and for the debriefings are: Who are the learners? What are the learners' – and the teachers' – expectations of the session? What is the group size? Is there one or more than one healthcare discipline involved (medical, nursing, both)? What are the learning objectives of the particular scenario and debriefing? Is the purpose of the debriefing predominantly for the participants to explore, discuss and learn about medical/technical issues, non-technical issues or both? What are the roles of the respective debriefers, if there is more than one (see later)?

Effective debriefing requires time, so part of the planning is to ensure that adequate time is available. As a general rule, the length of time for debriefing should not be less than the time taken for the scenario itself: usually more time is ideal.

13.3.2.2 Establishing a safe and supportive learning environment: setting the scene

So much of the success of the debriefing process is determined well before the start of the first debriefing. It is essential that every effort be made throughout the course as a whole to establish a safe and supportive learning environment for the participants and to help them realize that this is the case.

Participant expectations vary enormously hence their expectations are worth exploring during the introduction to the course. Some participants may be quite anxious. This should be acknowledged with a view to striking an emotional balance between the extreme of having the learners being so anxious as to compromise learning, versus explicit acknowledgement of the positive impact of some level of emotional engagement on learning.

Despite suggestions regarding its importance, there is little information in the literature regarding strategies to assist in establishing a safe and supportive learning environment. In the author's experience the following steps may be helpful:

- Send out pre-course material to the participants well before their session to help explain the purpose and format of the day.
- Plan social interaction with course participants at the time they arrive for the session as part of the introductions of staff and participants to each other ('meet and greet')
- Take an interest in the learners' clinical (real) work.
- Explain the format and objectives of the session at the start of the session.
- Openly discuss the expectations of learners and teachers:
    "Why have you come?"
    "What do you hope to get out of the day?"
- Clarify confidentiality issues, including the process for deleting the videos.
- Explain any research considerations.

13.3.2.3 Priming for the scenarios

An important way of reassuring the participants is to be explicit about the efforts you are going to, to prepare them for the scenarios. For medical/technical aspects of the upcoming scenarios this is often best done by conducting procedural workshops on the topic at hand (e.g. airway management, advanced cardiac life support). For non-technical subject matter, lectures, videos, games, and case-based discussions are useful ways of introducing and exploring these topics (e.g. communication, teamwork, leadership).

During this introduction/priming period, it is important to foster an environment where 'not knowing' is OK. Do so by:

- adopting a learner-centered approach

  Ask learners what their experience/level of comfort is with the topic at the outset

  Ask learners what they would most like to cover

  Show an interest in the learner's understanding

- acknowledging the difficulty of the subject

  "The reason we are all here is because resuscitations are difficult"

- as a teacher, admitting your own uncertainty when appropriate

  "Actually I'm not too sure about that – would someone else like to comment?"

- avoiding putting learners on the spot

- being careful with questioning techniques.

13.3.2.4 Familiarization with the simulation environment

The process of familiarizing the participants with the simulation environment is crucial in terms of increasing the prospect of 'suspension of disbelief', whereby the participants can immerse themselves in the situation, as though it was real. The familiarization needs to be systematic and clearly acknowledge what is real and not real about the environment and the mannequin, how this may impact on performance and clarify ways to get around the elements that aren't real.

13.3.2.5 Briefing

Brief the learners on what is expected of them in the scenario:

"For this scenario we would like you to do everything you would do if it was real"
while at the same time acknowledging that this can be difficult for some:

"Some folks find it easier than others to get into the scenario. We all know the patient is just plastic and metal, but we would like you to try your best to imagine it's real"
Be very careful about the use of humour – although the intention is well meaning, the wrong choice of words might make the learners feel even more uncomfortable.

13.3.2.6 Set

In terms of the actual debriefings, it is important to ensure the environment is conducive to learning as follows:

- If using video playback, a horseshoe arrangement of seating works well with the debriefer/s at the (either) end – avoid gaps in the horseshoe.
- Check that the equipment is functioning: TVs, computer etc.
- A whiteboard should be available for documenting discussion points.
- Have relevant cognitive aids at hand or on the wall in hardcopy or *via* a data projector (e.g. algorithms, non-technical skills frameworks).
- Avoid the presence of 'over the shoulder' observers in the debriefing – their presence can be distracting to the participants and may be a source of disruption by unsolicited comments from outside the learner group.

13.3.2.7 **Foundation**

One of the aims of the scenario is to get the participants into a heightened state of emotional arousal. Creating psychological challenges that trigger emotional engagement gets to the affective component of learning[2], and sets the scene for a more meaningful debriefing, provided it is managed appropriately.

Participants need to discharge some of this emotion before they are able to objectively debrief the scenario. This process is known as venting and it begins as soon as the scenario ends. Therefore getting the participants out of the simulation room and into the debriefing room needs to be managed as quickly as possible. There should be no break in proceedings at this stage – the important thing is to capture the learners' immediate feelings to gain an insight into their emotional state. The general level of conversation may be an indicator of the collective mood of the group who have just been in the scenario. A lot of noise is typical and reflects normal emotional release. A quiet or sombre feel may indicate a general perception that the situation wasn't handled well.

A useful opening question at this stage is: *How are all of you who were in the scenario feeling right now?* Ask this as a general question, but make sure that each participant answers in turn. Impress upon the participants that this question is distinct from how they felt *during* the scenario and is not about the *technical* aspects of the scenario – it is not "how do you think you managed the situation?" Recognize that identifying and raising vulnerable feelings may be difficult for participants – most won't answer the question, or will indeed answer the question as though it was "how do you think you managed the situation?" It is a good idea to record any points raised in answer to this question on the whiteboard to capture the vented issues – it may help assist future discussion. It is important once you have asked this question to acknowledge the range of emotions – stress, relief, embarrassment, frustration, anger – that this is normal and that it is actually helpful to have some element of adrenaline rush to maximise the learning potential of the debriefing.

A separate but similarly important question is: *"How did it feel when you were in there?" Was it real for you?* It is useful to get some sense of the level of immersion achieved by the participants: again this is likely to vary from individual to individual. If the level of realism was high, this is an excellent opportunity to reinforce the power of the learning opportunity that the debriefing affords: *"Great, you are now in for a unique learning opportunity – you are going to get a chance to do something you just can't normally do, namely watch yourself in action dealing with a situation that felt real for you at the time"*. Likewise it is informative to get an indication early on of those participants for whom the feeling of realism was not very high. Be aware that some participants will cite a lack of realism as a defence for their actions if they feel they have performed poorly, but also that some learners will genuinely struggle to achieve the level of immersion in the scenario that is hoped for[14]. While this is not ideal, it is easier to address having been discussed explicitly. A helpful strategy in such situations is to discuss the situation asking the participant to consider the scenario 'as though it was real'.

De-roleing The participants need to realize that they have been participating in a role-play – albeit an unusual one in that they have been playing themselves. Because the conflict between what is real and what is not can be difficult to assimilate in a dynamically evolving situation, the scenario may distort the way the participants play themselves. This may produce a strange emotional reaction in participants because it may not be easy for them to identify the boundaries between 'self' and 'acting'. So it is important to acknowledge that there are reasons the way they conducted themselves in the scenario may not reflect how they might behave in real life (issues of buy-in with no real patient, lack of some clinical cues, awareness of being videotaped, confusion about ability to call for help). Deroleing is the process of shedding the role taken on for the purpose of an activity and resuming one's usual persona[15,16]. If deroleing does not take place, participants in the debriefing may still react in the context of the role they had assumed in the scenario, which can hinder their ability to make the most of the debriefing session. This is similar to actors being 'stuck in role' who are left with feelings which do not belong to them.

An example of some words to use is as follows:

It is important to recognize that because this situation wasn't actually real, you have been undertaking a role-play. Even if you have done role-plays before, this situation is unusual in that the role that you have been playing is you, albeit in an artificial situation. So that you don't have any lingering concerns about what you did or didn't do in the scenario, and so that we can make the most of the available discussion time, we need you now to step out of those roles. Is that OK? Is everyone OK with that?

Clarifying the purpose and format of the debriefing and roles and expectations Having allowed time for venting and de-roleing it is now time to get started on the debriefing proper. The participants need to know the format of the debriefing, the objectives of the particular debriefing, what is expected of them, the debriefers' roles, and any 'ground rules'.

Remind the participants that while some learning occurs by experiencing the situation in the scenario, added learning occurs by discussing the situation in more detail. Considering the implications of how things unfolded cannot only fill in knowledge gaps about important aspects of medical care, it can also provide a stimulus to alter or influence our future practice in the workplace – this is the purpose of the debriefing. The scenario is only a starting point for discussion and other real life experiences of similar events/situations may be raised by participants to explore relevant issues.

Ideally the group debriefs themselves, but as they may not be familiar with such a process, the debriefer/s will need to generate the discussion from time to time. The primary debriefer's role is to facilitate discussion, direct the flow of discussion topics, where possible link the discussion topics back to a particular medical protocol or non-technical framework, depending on the aim of the debriefing and summarize what has been said. Facilitation involves allowing the group to figure things out for themselves and encouraging them to do most of the talking. If there is a secondary debriefer, their role is to assist the primary debriefer as necessary, for example by providing the role of medical content expert, documenting relevant discussion points on the whiteboard, and observing group dynamics.

If video playback capability exists, inform the participants that it can be used to stimulate collective recall of the actual sequence of events: video provides a unique perspective that is not usually available in clinical practice. There will not be time to show the entire video but some segments may be instructive in the context of the discussion.

Some example words to preface the commencement of the debriefing are:

The format of the debriefing is that we have about 30 minutes to talk about what happened in the context of current best medical practice. Did you know what needed to be done and if so how did you go about getting it done?

The objectives for this particular debriefing are (for example):

◆ *to review what happened with respect to the current cardiac arrest protocol in our hospital*

◆ *to discuss aspects of teamwork in association with managing a cardiac arrest.*

The intention is that you will do most of the talking, using the following questions as a framework to provide some structure to the discussion:

◆ *What happened?*

◆ *What went well and why?*

- *What was difficult and why?*
- *What if anything would you do differently in a similar situation in the future?*
- *What you have learned from this experience and how you will put what you have learned into practice?*

We (the debriefers) will:

- *write down on the whiteboard some of the issues you raise for further discussion*
- *intermittently ask some questions of you*
- *show some video footage to remind us of how some aspects of the situation actually played out*
- *try to tie this discussion back to any relevant framework:*
  - *algorithms or protocols for the medical issues (GREAT[17])*
  - *non-technical frameworks as relevant (ANTS[18], NOTSS[19], CRM).*

This explanation of the format should be outlined in detail for the first debriefing. A more succinct reminder can introduce the subsequent debriefings.

Some other points (ground rules) that can be helpful

- Everyone should feel free to contribute, though it is usual for the discussion to start with those who were actually in the scenario, moving on later to the observations of those who were watching.
- For some of the things that are discussed there will be quite clear guidelines for what is supposed to happen in such clinical situations.
- For some there will be no right or wrong answer or scripted solution.
- Criticisms should be constructive and specific and be sensitive to the feelings of others: one way to manage this is to remember to critique the perform*ance* not the perform*er*

13.3.2.8 Body

Events Get the participants to discuss the events in the scenario. 'What happened?' A non-judgemental discussion of the sequence of events helps clarify things in the participants' minds. If participants enter the scenario at different stages then this process is useful to fill in the story for those who did not see the beginning of the scenario. This process also provides a starting point for discussion regarding clinical handover.

Experience Explore participants' real life experiences in this type of situation *"Has anyone been in this situation in real life? Can you tell us about it"* This is less confronting and involves all members of the group rather than focussing on the primary participants. Ask what was difficult and what went well in the real life situation (this can also be recorded on whiteboard) and why. Then bring this back to the 1° participants in the scenario: *"Did you have a similar experience in the scenario?"* (if the difficulties are similar in the scenario it provides an opportunity to reinforce the value of the simulation experience) and explore the scenario from there.

What do the participants' want to talk about? Reinforce again the idea that the participants should do most of the talking. You may need to give the group examples of possible starting points for discussion. Then start with a general statement to open the discussion, such as: *"So what do you want to talk about?"*

In this way discussion then goes in the direction of medical/technical or non-technical issues according to what is important to the group. If the group fails to engage in this process, ask them more specific questions. One of the challenges is determining the appropriate level of facilitation required to initiate and maintain discussion within the group[6]. Some groups require minimal assistance from the debriefers to initiate discussion. More often though groups need a lot of assistance from the debriefers to get started, especially if they are new to this type of learning environment and/or the participants don't know each other particularly well beforehand. Once participants have raised/exhausted an issue the facilitator asks follow up questions to encourage deeper discussion[12].

If you need to help them start talking, *are there specific medical/technical issues to address?* This is a useful to suggest early on as participants may be unable to address non-technical issues if they are preoccupied with a medical or technical issue: first and foremost they will want to know if they did the 'right' thing/s. Or you may want to find out if they know what they were meant to do, even if they didn't do it.

Other ways to get the group talking are to use the feedback questions outlined earlier as follows:

- *What needed to happen for optimal management of the situation?*

- *What did you do to manage situation and why?*

- Having agreed on what did happen, this discussion can be a starting point eventually leading back to strategies to bridge the gap between 'actual' and optimal. Was the gap (if any) due to knowledge gaps or due to non-technical issues (lack of clear leadership, ineffective communication)?

- *What went well?* Participants often find this a difficult question to answer. It is important to give them time to reflect on this question, and for them and you to acknowledge sound management practices.

    Why did things go well? Was there use of an algorithm or protocol, or sound non-technical skills in evidence?

- *What was difficult?* Question counter-productive behaviours.

    Why was it difficult? Why was it hard to get done the things that you knew needed to be done?

- *What would you do differently next time?*

- *What have you learned?* How would you reproduce these behaviours next time?

What do the debriefers want to talk about? The debriefers' challenge is to have a plan for how to proceed with the debriefing, but not too rigid a plan, as the ideal is that the learners decide what the topics of discussion will be in the early part of the debriefing.

Even if the group manages to generate discussion without much input from the debriefers, there is still much to do:

- Keeping everyone engaged/involved, not just the outspoken participants

- Raising important medical/technical or non-technical issues not covered by participants in their discussion. Failing to address an oversight or misconception may be interpreted as validation of a particular form of medical management by the participants. Participants need to be made aware of inappropriate decisions and actions or inactions, and be made aware of the consequences of such if translated into the workplace. This may involve periods of instruction within the debriefing that aims to enhance the knowledge base of the group and highlight issues the group may have overlooked.

- Stressing that inappropriate actions (or inaction) does not necessarily imply that the participants would have handled the situation the same way if the situation was actually real – or that they are 'below standard'. But it is important to question them as to why they did what they did and to ensure they realize such management would be inappropriate in a real situation. It is situations such as these in which learning occurs.

Use of video The use of video in the debriefing session provides a powerful trigger for reflection and discussion as it allows replay of the actual sequence of events in the scenario, revealing what actually happened, rather than participants' recollections/perceptions, which are sometimes flawed.

Another advantage is that it provides objective feedback of the actual performance, including positive aspects of performance that participants often struggle to articulate. The use of video may help foster a reflective approach to learning.

Use of video can be problematic in that:

- it can be expensive
- the actual system available may not be entirely user-friendly
- the technology can be fragile, leading to failures at inopportune times
- tt can be anxiety-provoking and even threatening for the participants, especially if they are unclear on the purpose of the video – and the fate of the video!

Preparatory work is essential for this to succeed in terms of reassuring the participants and gaining their trust through appropriate confidentiality measures, explaining that the video is not being used for any assessment purposes and clarifying the process by which the video will be erased after the session.

If a piece of video is played it is very important to preface the segment with a description of where it takes place in the chronology of the scenario and what issues you are wanting participants to think about in the context of this particular video clip. This focuses all the participants on one aspect of the tape and leads to more meaningful discussion – to not do this leads to as many issues for discussion as there are people in the group! If the video illustrates aspects of management of the scenario that were problematic, it can be reassuring for the participants to have them also acknowledge things that went well in that section of tape before moving on. Try to avoid showing a large number of segments or very long segments. If any discussion starts up while you are showing the video, pause the tape and pursue the discussion.

A useful sequence is:

- Preface the video.
- Look at the video.
- Discuss the issue in question in relation to the video.
- Discuss the issue in question in a broader context as a whiteboard discussion (e.g. safe defibrillation practice, ventilation:compression ratios, elements of effective communication, leadership, fixation error).

> *Let's have a look at this piece of video. It's at the point in the scenario when .....*
>
> *I'd like you to pay particular attention to the communication.*

Then show the video clip.

> *What aspects of the communication were effective? Why? Ineffective? Why?*
>
> *What are the features of effective communication?*

13.3.2.9 Closure

An important reason staying on schedule is to ensure adequate time is available to close out the debriefing appropriately. Make it clear that the debriefing session is ending e.g.: "*It's time to wrap up the debriefing session*". This involves summarizing the topics covered and lessons learned, emphasising their importance in relation to the workplace. Ask each of the participants in turn to state the most important thing they have learned from the discussion and how this will influence their future practice. "*What will you take away to your daily practice? How will you do it?*"

Remind the participants that the system in which they work tacitly supports their current behaviour. If they have learnt something today that needs to change, how are they going to make it happen? Some strategies include:

◆ Mental 'rehearsals' in the workplace.

◆ Discussions with staff during 'downtime'.

◆ Actually checking/exploring protocols and equipment in their work environment.

At the end of the course, make sure to provide the participants with options for further discussion/counselling should they so desire, including a method of contact.

13.3.3 Debriefing with good judgement

Recently Rudolph[20] has outlined a theory and method for debriefing 'with good judgement'. This approach helps debriefers manage on the one hand the need for critical inquiry without being overly confrontational with learners, and on the other the temptation to avoid or 'sugar-coat' errors so as to avoid being anything other than non-judgemental. The method has three elements. First they propose a conceptual model whereby people's (participants') actions are shaped by how they interpret the situation they are in – that is their 'mental model' or 'cognitive frame' of the situation. Second is that an important role of the debriefer is therefore to uncover the learners' underlying frames that determined their actions, through a process of genuine inquiry. Finally the debriefer states (advocates) their own view of the situation as a means to explore the learners' views in more depth. This process provides an environment in which the debriefer can work with the learners to develop alternative frames and actions for the future. Rudolph's group has extensive experience both using and teaching this technique. Readers are strongly encouraged to read Rudolph's account of this approach to gain a clearer understanding of this method.

13.4 Some other considerations

13.4.1 Things to do

◆ Be familiar with the event you will debrief – annotate important events from the scenario as they occur.

◆ Use open-ended questions (*what, how, why*?) to initiate discussion. Once participants have finished discussing a topic, use follow up questions to acknowledge the importance of group ideas and encourage deeper discussion.

◆ Reflect questions asked to you by participants back to the group for an answer, rather than giving your own opinion too prematurely (if at all).

◆ Get used to using silence as a technique to encourage participant input to the discussion, rather than answering your own questions (this can be really hard). If you don't speak, someone else usually will. Try counting to 20 after you ask a question if necessary before speaking again.

◆ Body language is important

   Leaning forward with open hands facing outwards and an interested, enthusiastic facial expression is far more engaging than gestures that indicate boredom, frustration or negativity (such as folded arms, hands behind head)

13.4.2 Things to avoid

◆ Instructor centred discussions

◆ Lecturing

- Giving the impression that only your opinion is important
- Giving personal evaluation before the trainees have completed their analysis
- Interrupting participants
- Interrogation: be careful how you ask questions
- A rigid agenda: you need to have an agenda, but be prepared to be flexible with it
- Linking patient outcome with performance
- Patient death, unless issues surrounding death and dying form part of the objectives of the session.

13.4.3 **Debriefing style**

Although this has not been formally studied in relation to simulation-based education, it is unlikely that there is a single debriefing style appropriate for every situation. Different personalities will feel more comfortable with varying degrees of control and structure in terms of their individual style and how to modify their style depending on other factors, such as:

- One debriefer or two
- Group size – may vary from 1 up to 12 or more
- Experience level of the participants

    Novice or experienced: note that novices need more rules to support their learning[21]. In general they respond less well to open-ended questioning and are more likely to need to be guided through the debriefing with an emphasis on clarifying what they needed to do in the scenario

- Single craft group or an inter-professional group
- Participants' prior experience with simulation-based education

    Is it the same or is the extent of previous exposures mixed?

- Objectives of the session

    Medical knowledge: the debriefer's predominant role is likely to be more as an instructional teacher.

    Non-technical issues: the debriefer's predominant role is likely to include both an instructional role and as a facilitator.

- Participants who present challenges during the debriefing:

    Quiet participants

    Talkers

    Participants who are resistant to or negative about the process

    Satellite discussions between individuals participants rather than with the group as a whole.

13.5 **Debriefing instructor training**

Issenberg[9] has recently reminded us of the pivotal role of the healthcare educator in ensuring effective simulation-based healthcare education, but that the many and complex skills required of the simulation educator are ill defined. This is certainly true of the development of expertise as a debriefer, an issue that has received surprisingly little attention despite the explosion of interest in the use of simulation in healthcare.

Rall et al.[22] surveyed a number of European simulation centres in an attempt to define the key elements of debriefing. Although the numbers surveyed were small, many of the findings are echoed by established centres around the world, namely that not only is effective debriefing crucial to maximise learning, but that performed badly it can be a source of harm to the learner. Therefore training of the instructor should be emphasized.

Debriefing exposes the debriefer at times to challenging questioning, to uncontrolled emotions, and to divergent and even irrelevant ideas and viewpoints. Debriefers need to have organising skills, group process skills, communication skills, conflict resolution skills, and counselling skills[15]. A common finding is that debriefers initially seek and need control over the debriefing process, often related to their own anxiety about loss of control, reflecting a lack of confidence in their skills. However true learner-centredness requires the debriefer to have respect for the participants as co-learners to allow them to share control of the process – as the participants, their needs and expectations are extremely important factors in any debriefing. The ideal is an open and flexible style, based upon mutual negotiation and collaborative learning – meaning that the needs and expectations of all members of the group can be made explicit and shared. Openness, warmth and flexibility are likely to be important characteristics for debriefers.

Although there is no formally accredited postgraduate course yet, many of the more-established centres around the world, recognizing the challenge of developing and maintaining accomplished faculty, are making training opportunities available (see Issenberg[9] for a list of these centres). These programmes devote a portion of time to debriefing training in the form of interactive workshops outlining the theory underpinning simulation debriefing as well as the opportunity to actually practice debriefing. While these courses provide a useful introduction to the concept, a lengthy apprenticeship process is required to develop a degree of mastery[23].

The principles involved in optimising the effectiveness of simulation-based training apply also to the process of instructor debriefing training, in particular the need for systematic and repetitive practice with timely feedback on performance. As a minimum this should involve routine discussion at the end of the course as to the conduct of the debriefings, asking of the debriefers the standard feedback questions of: 'What went well and why?'; 'What was difficult and why?'; 'What have I/we learned that I/we should ensure happens next time?

Just as video is a powerful tool to stimulate reflection after a simulation scenario for course participants, so too is video of the debriefing to assist in honing the skills of the instructor. Use of video enables feedback on a number of important debriefing skills such as: body language of the debriefer/s; amount of time that the talking is done by the debriefer/s rather than the participants; the debriefer/s question style; the use of silence; and, attention to group dynamics.

If a simulation centre's staff does not consist of a multiprofessional group including educationalists and psychologists to support the clinician educators, then consideration should be given to ensuring ongoing intermittent access to such expertise to promote ongoing reflective practice amongst the debriefers[22].

13.6 **What does a successful debriefing 'look' like?**

- There was spirited discussion within the group.
- The debriefers didn't talk too much and facilitated discussion rather than lectured.
- Everyone in the group was involved in the discussion.
- Everyone including quiet participants, felt safe contributing.
- Vocal participants were managed courteously.

- The discussion focused more on what the participants were interested in rather than the debriefer's agenda.
- Participants learnt from each other: when relevant the discussion helped promote inter-professional understanding.
- Video was prefaced and used appropriately.
- There was discussion of both effective and ineffective medical/technical management – points of knowledge were clarified for the whole group.
- Discussion occurred around both effective and ineffective non-technical skills and strategies to improve.
- By the end, no one was unduly disappointed in themselves.
- All participants learnt at least one thing about themselves and/or the way they practice and left the session inclined to reflect on this new learning in an ongoing fashion with the intention of incorporating change into their work practice.

13.7 **Debriefing research**

The debriefing process during simulation-based education has been poorly studied despite its educational importance. Some of the areas in urgent need of rigorous research include the following:

- What are the techniques to establish and maintain a safe supportive learning environment?
- How important is the use of video? What is the return on investment? What are the downsides?
- What is the optimum number of instructors? How does this relate to the group size?
- Is craft group equity important in relation to debriefing? Do inter-professional participant groups benefit more from inter-professional debriefers?
- What is the place of humour in debriefing? Is it helpful or harmful?
- What verbal/non-verbal debriefer techniques optimise/compromise the debriefing process?
- What is the impact of stress on learning? Who learns better by doing and who learns better by observing?
- What are the attributes of the 'ideal' debriefer?
- What constitutes optimal instructor training for attainment and maintenance of debriefing competence?
- What techniques maximise transfer of learning to the real world?
- Does debriefing have a role as a means to learn and develop cognitive decision-making skills?[24]

13.8 **Conclusion**

Most of what individual participants will take away from a simulation session is predicated upon their view of their performance in their simulation scenario/s – how the debriefing is conducted will have implications for whether this is a positive or a negative experience. The debriefer's task is to guide participants to new perspectives by turning a challenging, albeit artificial, clinical situation into a positive learning experience.

Debriefing requires lots of practice to develop expertise: it can't be learnt from a book – not even this one! The good news is that increasing attention is being paid to the development of models and theories of debriefing and the skillset required of expert debriefers[25,26]. Debriefers owe it to their learners to make the most of the increasingly available opportunities to maximize their expertise in this regard.

References

1. Dannefer EF, Henson LC (2004). Refocusing the role of simulation in medical education: training reflective practitioners. In: Dunn WF Ed. *Simulators in Critical Care and Beyond*. Des Plaines IL, Society of Critical Care Medicine: 25–8.

2. Kolb D (1984). *Experiential learning. Experience as the source of learning and development*. Englewood Cliffs, New Jersey: Prentice-Hall.

3. Schon D (1983). *The Reflective Practitioner*. New York: Basic Books.

4. Dunn WF (2004). Education Theory: Does Simulation Really Fit. In: Dunn WF, Ed. *Simulators in Critical Care and Beyond*. Des Plaines IL, Society of Critical Care Medicine: 15–19.

5. Howard SK, Fish K, Yang G, Sarnquist F (1992). Anesthesia Crisis Resource Management: Teaching anesthesiologists to handle critical incidents. *Aviation Space and Environmental Medicine* 63(9): 763–70.

6. McDonnell L, Jobe K, Dismukes R (1997). *Facilitating LOS Debriefings: A Training Manual (NASA Technical Memorandum 112192 DOT/FAA/AR-97/6)*. Ames Research Center Moffett Field, CA: National Aeronautics and Space Administration.

7. Dismukes RK, Smith GM (2000). *Facilitation and debriefing in aviation training and operations*. Aldershot, UK: Ashgate.

8. Gaba D, Howard S, Fish K, *et al.* (2001). Simulation-based training in anesthesia crisis resource management (ACRM): a decade of experience. *Simulat Gaming* 32: 175–93.

9. Issenberg SB (2006). The Scope of Simulation-based Healthcare Education. *Simul Healthcare* 1: 203–8.

10. Dismukes RK, Gaba DM, Howard SK (2006). So many roads; facilitated debriefing in healthcare. *Simul Healthcare* 1: 23–5.

11. Lederman LC (1992). Debriefing: Toward a systematic assessment of theory and practice. *Simulat Gaming* 23: 145–60.

12. Raemer D (2005). Improving Instructors' Debriefing Skills. Pre-conference workshop to the SimTecT 2005 Healthcare Simulation Conference Brisbane, Australia. October 31, 2005.

13. Steinwachs B (1992). How to facilitate a debriefing. *Simulat Gaming* 23: 186–95.

14. Beaubien JM, Baker DP (2004). The use of simulation for training teamwork skills in health care: how low can you go? *Qual Saf Health Care* 13(Suppl. 1): i51-i56.

15. Pearson M Smith D (1986). Debriefing in experience-based learning. *Simulat Gaming* 16(4): 155–71

16 Stafford F (. The significance of de-roleing and debriefing in training medical students using simulation to train medical students. *Med Educ* 39 (11): 1083–5.

17. Owen H, Follows V (2005). GREAT simulation debriefing. *Med Educ* 40(5): 488–9.

18. Fletcher G, Flin R, McGeorge P, Glavin R, Maran N, Patey R (2003). Anaesthetists' Non-Technical Skills (ANTS): evaluation of a behavioural marker system *Br J Anaesth* 90: 580–8.

19. Yule S, Flin R, Paterson-Brown S, Maran N, Rowley D (2006). Development of a rating system for surgeons' non-technical skills. *Medical Education* 40(11): 1098–104.

20. Rudolph JW (2006). There's no such thing as "nonjudgmental" debriefing: a theory and method for debriefing with good judgment. *Simul Healthcare* 1: 49–55.

21. Dreyfus H, Dreyfus S (1985). *Mind over machine: The power of human intuition and expertise in the era of the computer*. New York: Free Press.

22. Rall M, Manser T, Howard S (2000). Key elements of debriefing for simulator training. *EJA* 17(8): 516–7

23. Mort TC, Donahue SP (2004). Debriefing: the basics. In: Dunn WF (ed). *Simulators in Critical Care and Beyond*. Des Plaines IL, Society of Critical Care Medicine: 76–83.

24. Bond WF, Deitrick LM, Eberhardt M, *et al.* (2006). Cognitive versus technical debriefing after simulation training. *Acad Emerg Med* **13**(3): 276–83.

25. Fanning RM, Gaba DM (2007). The role of debriefing in simulation-based learning. *Simul Healthcare* **2**(2): 115–25.

26. Yule S, Flin R, Maran N, Paterson–Brow S, Rowley D, Youngson G (2007). Observe one, rate one, debrief one. Using the NOTSS system to discuss non-technical skills with trainee surgeons. Cognition, Technology and Work (in press).

Chapter 14

Teaching a clinical skill

Jeff Hamdorf and Robert Davies

Overview

- Successful adult learning requires the identification of clear goals, relevance to clinical practice and the opportunity for reflection.
- Many senior clinicians will recall their learning was very much an apprenticeship model, today's doctors are expecting a structured learning programme.
- The teaching of technical and procedural skills is readily adaptable to simulated learning environments.
- The challenge for the teacher is to remain mindful that he/she has achieved unconscious competence whereas the learner is working from first principles.
- The four-step approach to teaching a skill is an excellent technique, which ensures that learners develop an appropriate level of awareness before attempting a skill.
- When designing a skills teaching episode, establishing learning objectives defines a learning pathway that guides the learner and the teacher.
- A successful skills teaching episode will embrace elements of positive critiquing, allow formative and summative assessment and will be subject to evaluative scrutiny to determine that it has met its objectives.

14.1 Adult learning

The teachers who have had the greatest impact on us achieved that effect not necessarily because they were the best surgeons or physicians in their fields. Rather they were good teachers because they may have made a difficult concept seems straightforward, a boring subject interesting or relevant, or may even have imparted a level of inspiration to those they were teaching.

Adult learning is substantially different from childhood education for a variety of reasons. The following key aspects of adult learning should be taken into account when teaching an adult a new clinical skill:

- Adult learners retain 90% of skills learnt by **doing rather than by watching.**
- Adult learning needs to be **immediately relevant.**
- Adults need to be **actively involved.**
- Adult learners have a surprisingly **short concentration span.**
- Adult learners need **clear goals and objectives.**
- Adult learners need **feedback.**
- Adult learners need an opportunity for **reflection.**

> The most important features of successful adult learning include the identification of clear goals, relevance to practice and the opportunity for reflection.

14.2 **Apprenticeship model**

The teaching of clinical skills has of recent times undergone somewhat of a paradigm shift. Historically the model has followed the traditional master–apprentice relationship and at times has been akin to 'learning by osmosis'. The concept of 'see one, do one, teach one', though, can no longer be argued as adequate. There have been a number of factors influencing this change. Strong drivers include an increasingly focussed student and junior doctor body demanding teaching and a consequent alignment towards student-centred learning versus the historical teacher-centred approach. Accordingly this has necessitated a somewhat different approach to teaching skills.

> Picture the historical vignette of the teaching ward round. The white coat resplendent senior consultant and his entourage sweep through the ward. The patient has been brought into the hospital 2 days before her operation in order for there to be an adequate exposure for the team's medical students. The students might clerk the patient, the consultant attends for the teaching ward round and examines the patient, demonstrating the signs to the students before proceeding to discuss the case over the patient at the bedside.
>
> Student: "Sir why is the potassium level raised in renal failure?"
> Consultant: "Because it always has been, and always will be"

There is a move towards reducing the length of training programmes and with this attention needs to be drawn towards ensuring that trainees are adequately exposed to appropriate learning opportunities allowing them to achieve the broad competencies required at graduation. The essential differences between the time-honoured apprentice model and the structured programme approach are summarized in Table 14.1.

Table 14.1 Apprenticeship *versus* structured programme participation[1]

Apprenticeship	Structured programme
Art and craft	Science and craft
Long working hours	Shift work
Low technology, low cost	High technology, high cost
See and do	Formal skills training
Problem-driven accountability	Evidence-based accountability
Moderated by peer pressure	Moderated by peer pressure
Mentor evaluation	Objective evaluation
Assessment based upon traits	Competency-based assessment

14.3 **Simulated learning environments**

The teaching of technical and procedural skills are readily adaptable to simulation using inanimate substrates such as knot tying jigs, silicone co-polymer skin substitutes, torso trainers for laparoscopy, etc. Yet synthetic substitutes are relatively expensive and may not simulate human tissue as reliably as animal tissue. The aims of using simulations in such training situations are firstly to allow trainees to learn a skill without the need to expose a patient to the increased risk of the novice operator and secondly to allow for the teaching of skills in a planned and timely fashion without having to wait until a patient arrives with a particular pathological process.

Simulation based training should employ a reproducible systematized approach to demonstration and teaching. This allows for courses to be repeated in the future and in different venues with a minimum of further effort. It also provides a framework on which other skills courses may be based. The other advantage is that a robust reproducible process will allow the supervision of the course to be undertaken by others, perhaps less senior, whilst ensuring that the same learning objectives and teaching methods are embraced.

14.4 **Unconscious competence**

Teaching a skill is undoubtedly more challenging than one considers at first glance. The teacher is an expert, having achieved mastery in his/her craft, and performs such skills on a daily basis as a part of his/her professional practice. Where this is a complex technical skill like surgical anastomosis or interpreting an ECG, the skilled clinician will display 'unconscious competence' in performing the task. Senior clinicians carry with them significant past experience and this is borne out by a high level of pattern recognition. The novice on the other hand is clearly not competent and perhaps may really not be aware of this – 'unconscious incompetence'. The learning cycle (Fig. 14.1) reminds us of the stages the novice needs to negotiate in order to achieve competence.

The challenge for the teacher is to remain mindful that he/she has achieved unconscious competence whereas the learner is working from first principles.

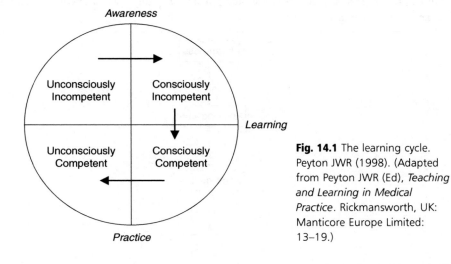

Fig. 14.1 The learning cycle. Peyton JWR (1998). (Adapted from Peyton JWR (Ed), *Teaching and Learning in Medical Practice*. Rickmansworth, UK: Manticore Europe Limited: 13–19.)

Table 14.2 Four-step approach to teaching a skill[2]

1. Demonstration	Trainer demonstrates at normal speed without commentary
2. Deconstruction	The task is broken down into its component steps and the trainer demonstrates while describing these steps
3. Comprehension	Trainer demonstrates while learner describes steps
4. Performance	Learner demonstrates while learner describes steps

14.5 **Teaching a skill in four easy steps**

Consider the last time you taught someone a new skill outside of the medical field. It may have been relatively simple like changing a tap washer or it may have been a more complex task. When new skills are taught we innately break the skill down into a series of steps. You might have demonstrated the skill in real time first and then demonstrated the skill in slow motion while commenting on the important steps before allowing the person that you are teaching an opportunity to try it themselves. An analogous approach can be applied to teaching a clinical skill.

Peyton[2] has formalized and popularized this into a four-step approach to teaching a skill (Table 14.2).

This process ensures that the learner has first observed the skill at a level of competence, then comprehends the component steps and finally is able to perform the skill under supervision. This fulfils the learning paradigm shown in Fig. 14.2.

The process allows for steps which are not successfully completed to be reviewed and repeated before proceeding to the next step. Another aspect that is frequently not considered is providing the opportunity for the trainee to practice the skill learnt, and certainly teaching hospitals and jurisdictions need to remain mindful of the obligation to ensure that the newly acquired skill must be used lest it be lost.

This approach takes a little practice in real life and the tendency may be for the teacher to talk themselves through the first demonstration. This should be avoided.

> Before presenting a skills course you should practice breaking down both complex and simple tasks into their component steps.

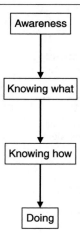

Fig. 14.2 Learning paradigm

14.6 Designing a skills teaching episode

14.6.1 Learning objectives

When designing a teaching episode consider addressing the three broad aspects of planning, content and closure[3].

14.6.1.1 Is it clear what the learners are going to learn?

Establishing learning objectives defines a learning pathway which guides both the learner and the teacher. In particular the context and goals of the teaching programme need to be considered. Learning objectives for a bowel anastomosis workshop might then include:

- To employ previously learnt safe surgical techniques.
- To understand the principles of handling tissues and employ optimal suture placement in the formation of an intestinal anastomosis.
- Further objectives might include the ability to form specific suture placements such as mucosal-inverting vertical mattress sutures, extramucosal techniques versus full thickness anastomoses, etc.

14.6.1.2 Am I designing this lesson at the right level?

A learner embarking on a bowel anastomosis workshop should have previously achieved competence in a number of skills prior to presentation such as safe handling of instruments and sharps, suture placement, formation of surgical knots by hand and using an instrument tie technique, etc.

14.6.1.3 Is there immediate relevance to the learners' current clinical practice?

As noted previously, effective adult learning needs to be immediately relevant.

14.6.1.4 Will they be able to put the new skill into action in the near future?

Timely practice under supervision allows trainees to reinforce motor pathways and establish durable neural networks that ultimately allows them to become independently competent.

14.6.2 Learning environments

14.6.2.1 Is the environment conducive to the learning experience?

Many hospitals now have specific training workshops and access to larger dedicated skills facilities. Accordingly the environment will generally be adequate for the workshop's purpose. There does need to be adequate lighting and the bench or table height needs to allow for a safe and comfortable posture for the learners. If learners are to spend a half or whole day learning a new technical skill then they will need to be comfortable so matters such as heating/cooling of the workshop and avoidance of work distractions need to be considered. Have they arranged for someone else to carry their bleeper/pager? Have mobile phones been turned to silent?

14.6.2.2 What simulation will be used for the workshop?

Animal parts will often be readily available and relatively cost effective for use in technical skills courses. Examples which are frequently used include pig bellies for suturing and trotters for tendon repair (Fig. 14.3), legs of lamb or turkey for debridement of contaminated wounds, lamb thoraces for tube thoracostomy, etc. In addition to the advantage of availability, the tissue handling characteristics are often most akin to the human form.

Special considerations apply to the use of animal parts or viscera. Planning needs to be given to surface protection from contamination and for the disposal of tissue. Some participants may

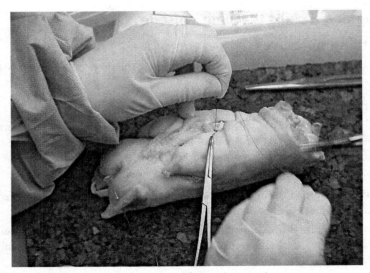

Fig. 14.3 Pig's trotters provide an excellent model for tendon repair.

express conscientious or religious objection to the use of animal tissues and synthetic substrates may need to be available. Participants handling animal tissues will need to be provided with adequate contamination barriers, a minimum of which would include gloves, plastic apron and protective spectacles. In addition, the supply of the tissues should be reliable.

14.6.2.3 Are instruments and consumables available for the course?

Many training workshop facilities have relied on the goodwill of recently retired Surgeons to supply their instruments. Other sources include replaced instruments from the operating theatres. Often instruments may be purchased on the receipt of seed funding from health services and private benefactors. Whatever the source of supply of the instruments used it is important that the instruments are at least in good working order and they are size matched (Fig. 14.4).

Sutures and ligatures should match those that the learners will use in practice.

14.6.2.4 Are there any foreseeable barriers to the course proceeding successfully?

Barriers to running a successful course fall into a variety of categories. Junior doctors may face challenges in being released from their service commitments although there has been an encouraging recent trend towards quarantined training time for junior doctors. Equally a junior doctor who has 'swapped into' a night shift in order to be able to attend a workshop is unlikely to perform and learn at his/her best. Heavy clinical commitments, as well as concern for, or preoccupation with, sick patients may impact on the attendance and commitment of faculty members.

Course participant and teacher numbers need to carefully planned to ensure that there is an optimal teacher: learner ratio. Basic courses in which the learners are embracing fundamental skills should be planned with a ratio of 1:4, whereas this may be eased to 1:6 or 1:8 where the learners are acting more independently.

14.6.2.5 Is the programme achievable?

Can I take this group of surgical trainees from a pre-task level of basic suture placement to anastomosis formation in this session? The determination as to whether the learning objectives can

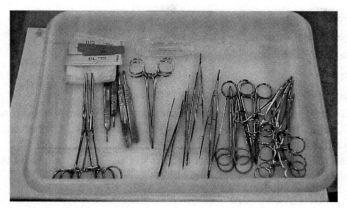

Fig. 14.4 An open surgery instrument set.

be achieved in the allotted time is one which can be challenging. One way of helping to ensure that the learner is ready to 'hit the ground running' might be to make arrangements for pre-learning of the cognitive aspects pertinent to the skills to be taught. There will always be a spectrum of performance among learners and accordingly the teachers will need to monitor the progress of their learners and be prepared to offer more assistance to those whose progress does not meet the programme expectations. To that end use of continuous formative assessment can be very valuable in this situation. Whether there is a need for a summative assessment is dependent on programme objectives and will be discussed a little later in this chapter.

Formative assessment is of immediate benefit to the learner providing the critiquing is performed in a positive manner and is timely.

14.7 Critiquing, assessment, and evaluation

14.7.1 Positive critiquing

Critiquing a student's performance of a task is a skill in itself. Positive critiquing is very valuable to a trainee's outcome whilst arguably a negative critique may markedly reduce the value of an educational experience. Critiquing using a participant-driven method described here will allow the learner to reflect on performance. After the participant has completed the skill the following four-step approach to critiquing is applied:

1. What the student thought went well.
2. What the other learners, or teacher, thought went well.
3. Opportunities for improvement identified by the learner.
4. Opportunities for improvement identified by the teacher.

Naturally if opportunities for improvement have been identified then ideally these will be exploited during the course.

14.7.2 Assessment

14.7.2.1 Formative assessment

An example of the use of formative assessment might include a simple score as to how well a learner is able to complete a new task:

- No errors observed.
- Occasional errors but corrected by participant.
- Occasional errors uncorrected by the participant.
- Frequent errors.
- Unable to proceed without step-by-step instructions.

The most important aspect of formative assessment using a model such as this is that the learner's performance is judged against his/her own progress, not against an external standard or peer performance standard.

Careful and considerate assessment of the learners will allow identification of those requiring remedial attention and directly benefit the learner.

14.7.2.2 Summative assessment

Summative assessment is quite different from formative assessment. Summative assessment is where the learner's performance is judged against a standard set as part of the learning programme (e.g. in the case of bowel anastomosis the standard might include the distance between adjacent sutures, a judgement as to the tension of the knots formed, and even the watertightness of the anastomosis) (Fig. 14.5).

The following points should be taken into account when we consider fair summative assessment of learners in the workshop environment.

- The purpose and manner of assessment should be well stated (transparency of assessment).
- The assessment should be clinically relevant (e.g. a bowel anastomosis that will be used again in practice).
- There should be an adequate time allowed for the assessment to take place.
- The assessment should be a multiple level process – previous knowledge should be included as well as material from the current course and perhaps from extended experience. This allows the excellent students to excel.
- Student expectations should be met by the assessment process.
- Provision of assessor checklists or a defined way of identifying how the assessment is to proceed.

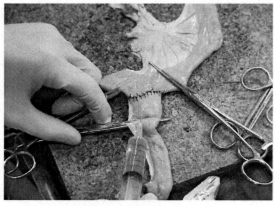

Fig. 14.5 Benchtop testing of an intestinal anastomosis.

◆ Assessment may be competency-based and therefore a decision needs to be made about what to do by way of remediation.

◆ Consider global assessment *versus* an objective structured approach.

14.7.3 Evaluation

Evaluation is an assessment of an educational programme. It is the process of determining the value of a course to its participants and offers an opportunity for reflection on the merit of the education or training episode. The evaluation process should address the following considerations:

◆ The course meets its aims and objectives.

◆ The needs of the target group are met (i.e. the course is 'pitched' at the right level).

◆ There is a mechanism for implementation of changes suggested by the evaluation process.

Methods of evaluation include:

◆ observation

◆ written.

14.7.3.1 Observation

Observation of faculty and participants by trained observers (educators) can be distracting.

14.7.3.2 Written

Written observation is the most common method. This uses entry and exit questionnaires with space for free text comments. Questions are aimed to gauge the participants' opinion of the extent to which a workshop has met their expectations. A Likert scale is usually used to allow comparative grading between different courses. The Likert scale seeks for the respondent to identify their level of agreement with a statement, for example:

The links between basic science and clinical practice have been highlighted in the course:

1. *Strongly disagree*

2. *Disagree*

3. *Neither agree nor disagree*

4. *Agree*

5. *Strongly agree*

While there are some limitations, Likert scale scores may be analysed to inform further course development and enhancement.

References

1. Hamdorf JM, Hall JC (2000). Acquiring surgical skills. *British Journal of Surgery* **87**: 28–37.
2. Peyton JWR (1998). The learning cycle. In: Peyton JWR, Ed. *Teaching and learning in medical practice*. Rickmansworth, UK: Manticore Europe Limited: 13–19.
3. Lake FR, Hamdorf JM (2004). Teaching on the run tips 5: teaching a skill. *Med J Aust* **181**: 327–8.

Chapter 15

Training and assessment with standardized patients

John R Boulet and Anthony Errichetti

Overview

♦ The use of standardized patients, lay people trained to model the medical conditions and mannerisms of 'real' patients, for training and assessing medical personnel is widespread.

♦ Although standardized patients are used primarily for formative assessment purposes, they have recently been included in high-stakes certification and licensure examinations.

♦ Developing standardized patient programmes can be complex and special attention should be paid to centre design, case development, and standardized patient recruitment and training.

♦ Based on over 30 years of research, standardized patient assessments can yield valid and reproducible scores as long as there are sufficient numbers of encounters, the evaluation rubrics are properly designed, and the assessors and standardized patients are well trained.

♦ The lessons learned from administering and validating standardized patient assessments can be used to help develop and improve other healthcare simulation modalities, including those employing part-task trainers and full-body mannequins.

♦ For all healthcare simulations, including those that use standardized patients, additional research efforts focusing on refining the scoring models, developing integrated assessments, and identifying potential threats to the validity of score interpretations are warranted.

15.1 Introduction

Although simulation in healthcare can take many forms, the use of standardized patients (SPs), lay people trained to model the mannerisms and complaints of real patients, is prevalent throughout the world[1,2,3,4,5]. Starting with their employment for medical student training[6], SP-based evaluation methods have evolved to be of sufficient quality to become part of high-stakes certification and licensure examinations[7]. Standardized patients have also been used in many disciplines outside of medicine, including dentistry and nursing[8,9,10]. Along the way, numerous research studies have been published covering diverse topics ranging from case development to training methods to equating performance scores[11,12]. These research endeavors, while extremely valuable for the advancement of SP-based evaluation and training methods, also provide some lessons to help guide other performance-based simulation activities in medicine and related healthcare disciplines. As a result, it will be informative for those individuals involved in simulation activities, not necessarily only those that are SP-based, to have some understanding of how SPs have been employed to train and evaluate healthcare practitioners. Moreover, knowing how SP-based training and evaluation programmes are set up, including the development of case materials and the layout physical facility, can help guide future, potentially more complex and integrated, simulation activities.

The purpose of this chapter is to present a wide-ranging overview of the use of SPs in medical education and assessment. To provide a broad context, general information will be provided on the typical structure of SP-based simulations and the history of SP-based assessment. This will be followed by particulars on setting up SP programmes, the basic layout of the physical facility, administering assessments, using the evaluation data, and judging the quality of the assessments. In addition, the role of SP-based methods in other simulation venues will be briefly discussed. Not only can SP methodology (e.g. scoring mechanisms, validation research) be exported to other simulation environments, but, from a practitioner competence perspective, integrating the knowledge that currently exists in this particular field with the plethora of other emerging simulation-based evaluation methods should lead to more comprehensive, defensible, assessments.

15.2 Typical structure of SP-based simulations

Although much more detailed information on SPs and SP-based assessments will be provided later in this chapter, it is important to first be familiar with the general structure of simulations that employ SPs. While there can be much variation in the way that SP encounters are configured, some commonalities exist, especially for those assessments designed to train and assess medical students and physicians. Typically, trainees receive a brief orientation covering assessment protocols (e.g. use of available equipment, restricted physical examination manoeuvres, timing) prior to beginning any simulated clinical encounters. On the door outside the examination room, the trainee may be provided with some background information about the SP, including vital signs and the reason, or reasons, for the visit. Once this information is reviewed, the trainee enters the examination room and proceeds to take a relevant history and/or perform a focused physical examination. Depending on the nature of assessment, these encounters normally last from 15 to 45 minutes. The SP, having been trained to model the mannerisms and affect of a 'real' patient, provides semi-scripted answers to the trainee's queries and reacts appropriately to physical examination maneuvers. In some encounters, SPs can be trained simulate physical findings (e.g. absent breath sounds on one side); in others, SPs with stable physical findings (e.g. heart murmur, chronic arthritis) are employed. Once the allocated time is spent, or the interview/examination is finished, the trainee leaves the room. Most often, reentry is not allowed since the SP is typically involved in evaluation activities such as rating communication skills or documenting history taking questions asked. For some assessment designs, the trainee will complete a timed post-encounter exercise after the SP encounter (e.g. writing a progress note or completing a multiple-choice quiz). If the assessment includes multiple encounters, the trainee then rotates to the next station, starting again with a review of the background (doorway) information for the upcoming SP interaction.

15.3 History of SP-based assessment

The use of SPs goes back almost 40 years[6,13]. Initially, their use was directed primarily at formative educational activities. By and large, a medical student would interact with one or more trained patients, some of whom may have had real physical findings, and then be provided with qualitative feedback concerning his/or her performance. This feedback was generally unstructured, and often did not reference any quantitative measure of performance. Over time, these

SP-based encounters became more formalized; SPs were provided with more training, objective scoring systems were developed, multiple-station assessments were created, administration conditions were standardized, relevant post-encounter exercises were added (e.g. reading EKGs, writing progress notes), feedback techniques were enhanced, and so forth. Nevertheless, for the most part, the SP-based assessments, commonly referred to as objective structured clinical examinations (OSCEs), were primarily used for formative purposes – providing medical students with feedback so that they could improve their clinical skills.

Beginning in the 1980s, there was general recognition that SP-based evaluation methods might well be used for summative purposes, including credentialing and certification[14,15]. Numerous studies, conducted by both medical school personnel and licensing/certification bodies, suggested that if there are sufficient numbers of simulated encounters, and they are sampled appropriately from the practice domain, reliable and valid assessment decisions could be made[16,17]. In 1992, the Medical Council of Canada (MCC) initiated the Qualifying Examination Part II, a licensure requirement for Canadian medical school graduates[18]. This examination, which continues to be offered at various sites throughout Canada, uses a series of SP encounters to evaluate clinical skills. Since the start of the MCC exam, other certification and licensure organizations have developed and administered 'high-stakes' multistation OSCEs. Most notably, these include the General Medical Council (GMC) of the UK[2], the Educational Commission for Foreign Medical Graduates (ECFMG)[19], and the United States Medical Licensing Examination (USMLE)[20,7]. In addition, many medical schools now demand that students successfully complete a SP-based clinical skills assessment to be eligible to graduate[21]. Although the movement of SPs from the formative to the summative arena has taken place rather quickly, it has been supported by a large number of studies, many of which provide guidance in the areas of assessment programme development, SP training, scoring, quality assurance, rater calibration, and psychometrics[22,23,24]. Going forward, the lessons learned and information gained in the SP arena over the past 30 years will certainly provide some much needed direction for other simulation-based assessment activities.

15.4 Setting up a standardized patient programme

Setting up a SP programme involves many interconnected steps, including designing the physical facility, developing simulation content and measurement tools, faculty development, and recruiting and training staff and SPs[25,26]. While this process will vary as a function of the purpose of the programme and the available resources, there are a number of important factors that should be considered. In the following sections, we provide a general overview of some of the issues that should be addressed when setting up an SP programme. This is not, however, meant to be a 'how to' manual. The interested reader should consult some of the available references for more detail on programme implementation, architecture, logistics, and costs[11,27,28,29,30,31,32,33].

15.4.1 Physical facility

Historically, SP-based training and evaluation centres were modeled after real clinics. Typically, there were a few rooms, sometimes only one, constructed and equipped to look like a 'real' patient examination venue. In many instances, existing hospital or clinic facilities were used, after hours, to host evaluation activities. Over the past several years, however, SP programmes have gradually evolved into multifaceted simulation centres, specifically designed and constructed to host an array of simulation activities[34,35,36,37]. These centres can incorporate many simulation technologies, including SPs (warm simulators), mannequins (e.g. full-size electromechanical models, part-task/ body trainers, surgical trainers), and virtual reality programs (cool simulators).

However, regardless of the scope of simulation activities, the simulation centre should be built, or modeled, to allow for a smooth integration of SP and patient simulator exercises and for the efficient training of allied health professionals, both individually and together. The following section will focus specifically on the basic set-up and use of the SP facility, highlighting some recent technological advances that can simplify various administrative and logistical tasks.

15.4.1.1 Training/assessment area

The typical SP facility contains a number of identical examination rooms and some peripheral office space for training and teaching, computer and video resources, staff offices, and storage. The SP training and assessment area must be realistic (simulating a multidisciplinary clinical working environment) and versatile (able to provide experiential and didactic sessions for student, faculty and standardized patients). When considering a site, one must weigh the cost of new construction *versus* the logistical constraints of retrofitting existing space. There are obvious advantages to building a new centre. The ability, for example, to wire, plumb and design hallways and corridors to better accommodate student-SP traffic flow, on the surface, make this the preferred option. Locating SP training labs in hospital or clinic environments, when in close proximity to a medical school or health sciences facility, will certainly appeal to students who want to learn in a more realistic environment. In general, simulations, regardless of fidelity, seem to have more relevance when they take place within an actual working environment populated by actual patients and family members, physicians, nurses, and other allied health professionals.

Exam rooms are commonly equipped with basic diagnostic equipment (e.g. sphynomamometer, otoscope, ophthalmoscope), a working sink, and other peripheral equipment normally found in 'real' exam rooms. Where possible, it is advisable to have separate entrance and exit for students (examinees) and SPs. This will help facilitate traffic flow, especially when numerous people are being assessed at the same time in different examination rooms. Outside of the exam rooms, equipping stations (carrels or pull-down desks) with wireless internet connectivity will allow for both pre-encounter (e.g. viewing lab results or reviewing patient information) and post-encounter exercises (e.g. completing a progress note or answering a quiz based on the patient's complaint).

In the North America, SP programmes most often concentrate on training first and second year medical students, preparing them for the clinical clerkship years through a series of clinical exercises and formative evaluations[21]. Training programmes often include case-based encounters (e.g. a student encountering a simulated patient presenting with an identified illness or condition such as asthma or headache). In some special programmes designed to teach and evaluate communication skills, the student may also encounter a SP and various family members[38]. Often, in the role of physical examination teaching associates, SPs are used to train students to correctly perform certain physical examination manoeuvres[39]. In these exercises, the teaching associates typically work with one to three students, reviewing physical examination techniques. As a result, the training/exam rooms must often be large enough to accommodate several people.

If multiple simulation platforms are being used (SPs and mannequin-based patient simulators), they should be located in close proximity. This will not only make some scenarios more realistic and practical, but will also simplify the logistics of exam administration. For example, in a 'bad news' practice scenario, a medical team works with a dying patient (patient simulator) and then counsels family members (SPs) in a simulated waiting area, located close by, about possible treatment options[40]. Realism can be enhanced with an audio system playing ambient hospital or emergency room sounds. The general point is that the training/assessment area must be as flexible as possible. Although the layouts of centres used for high-stakes credentialing purposes often serve as templates for other programmes, their 'one use' assessment function makes them less desirable as models for the more dynamic medical school or residency training programmes.

15.4.1.2 Other functional space

Ideally, the SP centre or laboratory includes a student (examinee) reception area; this provides space for a pre-encounter orientation or post-encounter debriefing session. If it includes a personal computer and a large flat screen to view various media, this area can serve as a general purpose classroom. By furnishing this area with moveable tables and chairs, and basic diagnostic equipment, training sessions can be held there. Trainers can conduct didactic sessions, demonstrate physical examination maneuvers, and role play with SPs in front of the entire group. Individual SP training can also occur in the trainer's office or any of the available exam rooms. If exam video technology is available, exam room training allows for recording and reviewing of practice sessions.

15.4.2 Simulation connectivity systems

Today's state-of-the-art centres are typically equipped with advanced simulation connectivity systems. These systems include hardware and software for managing and distributing simulation activities. They tie together the various simulations activities through digital audiovideo systems, performance data collection capabilities, scoring and reporting modules, and programme management algorithms.

If possible, exam rooms should be equipped with two digital pan-tilt-zoom cameras managed by a technician in a control room. All training and assessment sessions can be recorded and stored on a server and access given according to defined security protocols. Live or previously recorded videos can be used by students and clinical faculty to review students' work, by SPs and trainers to conduct quality assurance activities, and by SPs to review their own work or to learn how to portray a case more accurately[41]. For certain types of assessments, including research projects, clinical faculty may want to rate students using live or recorded video[42]. Faculty and students can view work live or recorded at the training site or, provided the web-based infrastructure is adequate, remotely from other locations. This 'anytime, anywhere' feature of web-based digital systems effectively solves many logistical issues associated with training and scoring. Training videos can be produced as needed or culled from existing video recorded during teaching sessions.

To generate scores, provide feedback, or assign outcomes (e.g. pass/fail), the SP-based performance assessment requires a system to gather, analyse and report data. Historically, this was accomplished with paper-based forms, manual data entry, and basic statistical analysis. Today, the preferred approach for data collection is a personal computer (PC) placed in an exam room, or other area, for the SP, or any other evaluator, to assess each performance. If external raters are used (e.g. faculty), they can view videos and enter ratings wherever there is an available computer. To produce individual or group score reports, 'canned' statistical programmes, capable of summarizing and analysing the performance data, are usually included as part of the connectivity software.

Simulation centres are busy operations that can be made more efficient and cost effective through the use of programme management software and hardware. Examples include automated announcements that time programmes and move trainees between rooms, automated video recording that switches cameras on and off, email notification system for scheduling trainees and SPs, room scheduling software, and an inventory control system for allocating and tracking simulation equipment.

15.5 Developing the simulation content

Standardized patient cases and performance checklists are typically developed by case development committees or teams[11,43]. In general, the committees are composed of clinical faculty and

SP trainers. Within the group, it is preferable to have a mix of medical specialties and some first-hand knowledge of the skill level of those individuals who are going to be evaluated using the simulated cases.

15.5.1 Case development

The basis of SP encounters is the case. The case is not a medical record but rather a training document used by the SP to learn how to simulate, or present, a clinical problem. The case is normally generated from a template that lists the important scenario facets, including clinical classification (e.g. setting for the encounter, SP hiring criteria, differential diagnosis) and the patient characteristics (e.g. chief complaint and its history, past medical history, psychosocial information, body mass, ethnicity). Template information is generated and discussed by clinical faculty, and then edited into a training document by the SP trainer. A web-based case template enables committee members to develop the content on the 'paperless' case efficiently; edits can be made instantaneously and SPs can also give input into the case over the web. In medical schools where meeting frequently is not practical, web-based tools can greatly facilitate the case writing process.

After completing the case, the committee typically reviews the subject matter before it becomes part of any assessment activities. As a step toward content validation, a faculty member or a student surrogate can examine a SP trained to the case. The development team can then critique the case as well as the verisimilitude of the patient simulation with respect to demeanor, symptoms, affect, and response to the physical examination.

15.5.2 Constructing performance measures

Presently, most SP-based assessment and evaluation activities involve some sort of data collection activity[44]. Historically, analytical tools (e.g. checklists) have been used to gather data related to history taking and physical examination. The checklist items are usually developed by expert committees and can be weighted to reflect clinical importance[45,46]. Most often, the checklists are constructed with the SP's specific medical condition in mind. For example, a modeled encounter that covers 'atypical pneumonia' may incorporate history taking checklist items such as 'asks about muscle or body aches' or 'pain when taking a deep breath'. Similarly, in term of physical examination, the candidate might be expected to 'examine the throat' or 'palpate the anterior cervical lymph nodes'. The creation of case checklists should also take into account the expected skill level of the person to be evaluated. For example, a history checklist constructed for a first year student may include mastery questions (i.e. basic data the student must gather from all patients). More advanced history checklists should include discriminatory questions, ones that test for advanced clinical judgment or problem solving.

Although checklist scoring is common, at least for data gathering activities, holistic rating scales are also incorporated in SP-based assessments[47,42,48]. For some traits such as doctor–patient communication, rating scales provide a means to assess multifaceted behaviours that may not be amenable to checklist-type decomposition. Although these types of rating scales can be difficult to construct, and have often been criticized as being 'subjective', there is ample psychometric evidence to support their use[49,50]. Furthermore, cases can be constructed to foster certain types of interactions (e.g. interplay between patient physician when breaking bad news), providing more opportunities to measure relevant constructs. Overall, provided the rubrics are defined, the raters are well chosen (e.g. are intimately familiar with the trait being assessed), and their training is appropriate, reliable and valid ratings can be procured[51,52,53]. Ultimately, the choice of scoring modality (analytical – checklists; holistic – rating scales) will be dependent on a number of factors, including what is being measured, the expertise level of those who are being assessed, the availability of 'experts' to serve as raters, logistics, and cost[54].

15.6 **SP recruiting and training**

Standardized patients are lay people trained to simulate patient problems, document skills, and give feedback. Although SPs can be trained to simulate various physical conditions, there are many clinical abnormalities that cannot be imitated, at least realistically. For these situations, it is sometimes possible to recruit SPs with stable physical findings. Regrettably, while this may be an effective strategy for low-stakes formative assessments, questions concerning the constancy of the 'real' physical findings, comorbidity, and potential patient harm from repeated physical assessments usually dissuade credentialing organizations from employing these types of SPs. Fortunately, as technology improves, other simulation modalities (e.g. full-body mannequins) are likely to be used to fill gaps in the assessment practice domain.

15.6.1 **Recruitment**

The SP recruitment challenge is finding individuals who are intelligent, literate, who exhibit good will toward the learner and enjoy learning themselves, and who have basic acting skills[28]. Screening of individuals can involve basic tests of literacy and memory. For example, potential SPs can be asked to review selected student–patient encounters and complete rudimentary checklists. Viewing videos also informs them what to expect when a doctor takes a history and performs a physical examination.

15.6.2 **Training**

In case-based encounters, where students demonstrate or practice patient examination skills, the SP training process usually involves learning to simulate medical illnesses and conditions, to document abilities, to rate certain skills such as doctor–patient communication, and to debrief students[27]. These instructional activities are typically completed by SP trainers using a variety of educational methodologies[55,56]. Since the encounters typically last from 15 to 45 minutes, SPs are often taught memory enhancing techniques. A new innovation in SP training involves the use of computers to deliver case content. In this self-training model, SPs work through a series of modules alone where they learn how to portray a case and document skills using a checklist. Such training uses text, graphics and videos to deliver the content, and has been shown to be effective[57]. When these computer-based modules are delivered over the web, training can take place anywhere the SP has access to a high-speed internet connection.

15.6.3 **Debriefing candidate performance**

For many formative assessments, in addition to portraying the case and documenting what transpired in the encounter, SPs provide candidates with feedback concerning their performance. Here, SPs are best employed for giving information about strengths and weaknesses in interpersonal communication and physical examination technique. Feedback on history-taking should be confined to quality of questioning and to specific topics, for example discussing psychosocial issues or health maintenance/risk factors that are pertinent to the case. For communication debriefing, SPs can complete a rating scale after the encounter and then discuss these ratings with the student or trainee. This is best accomplished through an observation-comment approach whereby the SP offers an observation about a communication issue and asks the students to comment. Normally, SPs are trained to avoid a didactic approach during this debriefing process and students/trainees are encouraged to reflect upon SP observations. Debriefing and feedback is greatly enhanced through a video review process, for example, where the SP shows a video of the encounter and asks the student for comments. Giving feedback about the physical examination is more straightforward; using a physical examination checklist as a guide, SPs can ask students to perform the skills done incorrectly or incompletely and then correct errors (e.g. demonstrating how to place a blood pressure cuff correctly). Debriefing and giving feedback is a specialized skill, and may be one of the most difficult tasks for SPs. Screening SPs for this pedagogical responsibility is essential.

15.6.4 Performance fidelity

One method of working toward patient accuracy and consistency in performance and documentation (checklist completion) is to involve SPs in quality assurance activities[41]. Protocols include getting patients to observe each other and give feedback, or to observe their own performance. In both cases they can observe either live or recorded sessions and complete a performance fidelity or accuracy checklist in which salient performance points are listed, such as giving the correct opening line, giving correct information, and not volunteering information that wasn't asked for.

15.7 Using the evaluation data

As mentioned in previous sections, various clinical skills can be measured via SP-based evaluations, including data gathering (history taking and physical examination), doctor–patient communication, interpersonal skills, clinical reasoning, and patient management. These skills can be measured *via* both analytical (e.g. checklist) and holistic (e.g. rating scale) tools[58]. For some elements, the scoring/rating can be completed by the SP (after the clinical encounter) or by an observer (e.g. faculty) who can be inside or outside the room. Where the technology is available, videotape scoring can also be accomplished. If a post-encounter exercise is included in the assessment, ratings, or scores, can be procured from individuals who are specifically trained to evaluate the targeted performance domain[59].

For history taking and physical examination, case-specific checklists are the norm for documenting performance. More often than not, the performances for each checklist item (completed, not completed) are simply added together to generate an encounter or case score. This can be done separately for history taking and physical examination, or combined. If the SP-based assessment has multiple stations, the data gathering scores can be averaged. Although the use of checklists is rather simplistic, and they have been criticized for rewarding thoroughness as opposed to efficiency[60], they provide a reasonably reliable documentation of what the candidate did and did not do. From a formative assessment viewpoint, they can serve as a reference point for providing meaningful performance feedback.

When an SP-based assessment is being used for summative purposes, and not all students/candidates encounter the same cases or SPs, it is often necessary to equate individual scores. Fairness issues arise if one set of candidates sees less (or more) challenging test content (mixes of cases), or is evaluated by less (or more) stringent raters. Although the process of equating can be technically complex, it involves collecting data to be able to establish the difficulty of specific cases and leniency/stringency of particular raters[12]. These data are then used to adjust individual scores based on particular test form (SPs, cases, raters) that the examinee encountered. Basically, if a candidate encounters a particularly difficult set of cases, or more stringent evaluators, a few points are added to his/her score. The converse would be true for someone has a less challenging assessment form. Regrettably, score equating, even for high stakes assessments, is often ignored, potentially compromising the reliability and validity of the assessment scores.

Whenever numerical scores are gathered as part of an SP assessment, especially if the stakes are high, it is important to gather quantitative quality assurance data. This usually takes the form of double scoring based on some sampling of performances. If these secondary scores can be obtained, various statistical measures can be used to identify discrepant scorers or raters[41]. Even if only the 'live' scores are available, potential scoring problems can be identified fairly easily by looking at basic statistical summaries. For example, if clinical skills domains such as doctor–patient communication are being evaluated, one would expect that an examinee's ability would not vary considerable from one encounter to the next. Therefore, within a given test session, where all examinees see the same SPs, the mean SP ratings, calculated for all encounters, should be close. For larger scale operations, where there may be more than one SP for a given clinical encounter, it can also be useful to look at mean scores. If all SPs are consistently trained, both for scoring and portrayal, and they encounter examinees of approximately equivalent ability, then one would anticipate that their mean scores (e.g. checklist documentation of history taking and physical examination) would be comparable.

15.8 Assessing the quality of the evaluation

Regardless of whether the purpose of the SP-based evaluation is formative or summative, some attention needs to be paid to the psychometric properties of the scores. Ultimately, it is important to know how the assessment results can be extrapolated to other situations and whether the results generalize to similar evaluations[61,62,63,64]. The answers to these queries can be obtained by gathering evidence to support the validity and reliability of the assessment scores.

15.8.1 Validity

For SP-based assessments, numerous studies have been conducted to provide evidence that the scores are valid; that is, they provide a sound scientific basis for the proposed score interpretations[65,66,67]. While there are many potential sources of validity evidence, they can be categorized into five general areas: test content, response processes, internal structure, relations to other variables, consequences of testing. For test content on SP assessments, one wants to make sure that the types of cases are reflective of the practice domain and that the skills being measured are important for healthcare delivery. This is often accomplished by referencing local or national databases to see what types of patients healthcare workers normally see[68]. Cases can then be developed with reference to the 'true' practice domain. In terms of determining the important skills, efforts are usually made to solicit the opinions of experts and to explore the curricular materials that are used to train practitioners. By crossing the skill domain with the practice domain, and constructing the SP assessment with this in mind, content validity is assured[61].

Validity evidence from response processes can take many forms, including the documentation of how examinees proceed through the examination[69], the investigation of whether the evaluators use the score scale as intended[42,70], and questioning test takers about their performance strategies[71]. For example, if checklists are used for scoring, and there is no penalty for irrelevant inquiries, it would be useful to know whether examinees are purposefully asking more history taking questions and performing additional physical examination manoeuvres, even though the patient's condition does not necessarily warrant these types of queries. If so, this could be a threat to the validity of the test scores. The realism of the clinical scenarios, and how trainees interact with SPs in the simulated environment, can also raise some validity concerns. To the extent that trainees cannot 'suspend disbelief', their interaction with the SP may be somewhat artificial. Here, it is important to gather evidence to support the verisimilitude of simulated clinical scenarios and the fidelity of the SP portrayals. This can be accomplished through normal quality assurance activities and/or targeted surveys of trainees who have participated in the assessment.

Investigating the internal structure of assessment can also yield validity evidence. If the SP assessment includes both history taking and physical examination elements, it would be reasonable to hypothesize that performance in one of these domains would be related to the other. Likewise, individuals with better communication skills should be able to gather more relevant data from the SP. More important, it is essential to know whether particular items function differently for identifiable subgroups of examinees. On SP assessments, the item could be the case, the SP, or the associated combination. For example, where communication ratings are used in the evaluation, one would not expect that examinee scores would differ meaningfully as a function of gender of the SP or the type of case[52]. If they do, this may indicate some form of bias or, equivalently, threat to the interpretation of the test scores.

Analysing the relationship between the SP assessment scores and other variables is another way of procuring validity evidence[72,73]. External variables can be other test scores (e.g. knowledge examination) or even group membership (e.g. experts, novices). For example, one would expect that, in terms of clinical skills, practicing physicians would outperform medical students. Here, it would also be useful to investigate whether coached and uncoached groups perform differently. If clinical skills performance can be elevated substantially via short-term coaching, this may be a threat to validity. Finally, from a test-criterion relationship viewpoint, one would anticipate that scores obtained in the simulated environment will, to some extent, predict performance with 'real' patients[74]. Unfortunately, these types of investigations often yield only moderate associations. Like a driver's test, the SP assessment provides information on what a candidate can do, not necessarily what he or she will do in the future. Nevertheless, it is still very important to gather data to help establish that performance with simulated patients translates to real-world situations[58].

The final, frequently ignored, source of validity evidence is based on the consequences of testing. Often, there are both intended and unintended consequences of test use; these should be investigated and acknowledged. Based on the historical use of SPs, especially for assessment-related purposes, many benefits appear, including, amongst others, the fact that the students get better clinical training, there is an increased emphasis on doctor-patient communication in the curriculum and, because of standardization, the perceived fairness of the assessment is enhanced[75]. Ultimately, albeit difficult to establish cause and effect, one would expect, for example, practising doctors to be better trained, patient satisfaction to increase, and there to be fewer malpractice claims or referrals to licensing boards. For countries with national SP-based clinical examinations, the validation process would involve gathering evidence to support the fact that these potential benefits of testing are actually happening.

15.8.2 Reliability

To establishing the quality of SP-based assessment, one also needs to provide some evidence that the scores are consistent and relatively free of error[76]. Traditionally, this has been accomplished by providing measures of internal consistency (how well performance on one case is related to the next) and inter- and intra-rater reliability (how consistent are evaluators in their provision of ratings or scores). These reliability estimates can be provided for the whole exam, if total scores are calculated, or individual parts (e.g. history taking). While this strategy is effective, it may be conceptually easier to think about reliability in terms of specific error sources.

For SP-based examinations, the decomposition of sources of error has been reported in numerous studies[67,77,16,12]. In general, regardless of the scoring methodology employed, task sampling variability is the key facet that impacts the reproducibility of scores[78]. For multistation performance assessments in general, and SP-based models in particular, the content of individual exercises tends to drive performance, at least to some degree[79]. That is, even though specific skills are being measured across cases, individuals will perform better, or worse, as a function of their familiarity/experience with the content. As a result, if the content (mix of cases) is different from one test form to another, an examinee's score may not be generalizable, especially if the number of encounters is small. Therefore, if score reproducibility is an issue, it is usually advisable to increase testing time (number of encounters). This will help ensure that estimates of an examinee's ability will not be overly dependent on the choice of particular cases.

Although other sources of score variability exist for SP assessments, namely those associated with the rater, they usually do not play a significant role if proper training is provided[80,59]. Here, whether SPs or external observers are scoring, it is important to establish specific criteria that pertain to the assignment of ratings or the crediting of checklist items. Furthermore, as part of the training regime, it is useful to provide benchmarked performances so that individual scorers will know why their ratings are discrepant and make appropriate corrections. By doing this, inter-rater and intra-rater reliability can be enhanced.

15.9 Applicability of SP-based methodology to mannequin-based simulation

Although SP-based methods have been around for over three decades, their use in high-stakes certification and licensure examinations has come only recently. This movement from primarily formative teaching to summative assessment spurred numerous research efforts, many of which were designed to address methodological shortcomings and psychometric concerns[38]. The resultant literature can be of much assistance to those individuals who are, or are considering, employing simulations as part of the training and/or evaluation of healthcare workers.

To date, very few, if any, high-stakes clinical skills assessments employ part-task trainers or electromechanical mannequins. However, given the practice domains that are covered, and the clinical skills that are measured, it would seem useful to integrate these models, where possible, into the assessments[81]. For many SP-based clinical scenarios, it is difficult to simulate abnormal physical findings. Furthermore, certain physical examination maneuvers are often banned (e.g. pelvic examination, breast examination) because it would be too difficult, and expensive, to recruit willing SPs. Therefore, provided the logistical and measurement considerations can be worked out, it would seem prudent to embrace integrated models – those that employ both SPs and mannequins in the evaluation framework. Recently, this has been accomplished in a number of clinical areas, albeit most often within the context of low-stakes formative assessments[82,83,84].

Even though SP-based research has been extensive, and provides many answers related to logistics and measurement, there are certainly some issues that will still need to be addressed as simulation technology expands. Some of these issues are briefly outlined below.

15.9.1 New scoring models

As noted in a previous section, SP-based assessments often employ checklists and/or rating scales. These rubrics could easily be used for mannequin-based scenarios[85]. However, unlike basic clinical abilities (e.g. interviewing a patient, performing routine physical examination manoeuvres), measured most efficiently via SPs, mannequins allow for the assessment of more complex procedural skills (e.g. airway management) under more acute and stressful conditions. As a result, issues such as sequencing and timing come into play. Although some success in scoring has been achieved with holistic and key action methods, additional work is certainly needed[86,87,88]. Going forward, provided that the physiological reactions of the mannequin accurately model those of a real patient, it may be possible to derive a valid score based on how the simulated patient (mannequin) reacts to management strategies that are employed.

15.9.2 Validation work

Much has been written concerning the validity of SP-based methods. In contrast, likely due to their novelty, relatively little has been published concerning assessments that employ mannequins or part-task trainers[89,90,91]. Like SPs, it is important to know whether performance in the simulated environment extends to the real world, with real patients. Moreover, as different simulation models are introduced, research efforts should be focused on determining which methods, or combinations, work best and under what specific conditions. Finally, like SP-based scenarios, the focus of evaluations using mannequins generally concerns the interaction between the patient and the provider. In this type of model, many important facets of effective healthcare delivery go unmeasured. Simulations scenarios, whether they employ SPs, mannequins, part-tasks trainers, or some combination, need to be developed to effectively tap other domains such as teamwork, interdisciplinary communication, professionalism, and patient safety.

15.9.3 Task specificity

In general, SP-based assessments are used to measure basic clinical skills such as history taking, physical examination, and doctor–patient communication. Therefore, it is possible to generate a reasonably reproducible measure of someone's ability as long as multiple scenarios (usually 10 or more) are employed and effective training methods, both for the SPs and any evaluators, are employed[92]. As the cases become more specific, perhaps demanding higher-level skills (e.g. breaking bad news), the overall reliability of the skill scores in a multistation evaluation tends to diminish. An examinee may do extremely well on one scenario yet, because of lack of familiarity with the medical content, perform poorly on the next.

The problem of content specificity is even more pervasive when mannequins or part-task trainers are employed in the assessment. Here, the modeled scenarios tend to be more content driven. For example, mannequins can be used to simulate a wide range of clinical conditions, including acute haemorrhage, anaphylaxis, and myocardial ischaemia. If an assessment was designed to measure patient management skills, an individual's performance may fluctuate quite dramatically as a function of specific experience with these types of conditions. Therefore, to get a reasonably precise measure of patient management ability, several scenarios, purposefully sampled from the practice domain, are required. Unfortunately, while the reproducibility of SP-based clinical skills scores has been studied, and documented in numerous articles, the same cannot be said for evaluations that employ part-task trainers or mannequins. Here, generalizability studies should be employed to determine the optimal measurement designs[93,94]. These studies can inform test length (number of stations), timing, the selection of content (scenarios to be modeled), and choice and number of raters.

15.10 Conclusion

Training and evaluating with SPs, although often expensive and logistically challenging to implement, is commonplace. From an assessment perspective, unlike other evaluation modalities (e.g. real patients), trainees can be exposed to the same clinical content, ensuring fairness, and allowing for valid comparisons of performance. Advancements in the field are coming in many areas, namely computer-based SP training modules, more sophisticated scoring models, better designed physical facilities, defensible standard setting protocols, and more efficient feedback methods. As a result, there is likely to be a further expansion of the use of SPs, especially as part of summative assessment activities.

The experience gained over the past three decades of SP use will be invaluable to those who are embracing other simulation platforms. Whether part-task trainers or full-body mannequins are being used, knowledge of centre design, case development, scoring, and validation research are all needed to establish effective training and/or evaluation programmes.

References

1. Reznick RK, Blackmore D, Dauphinee WD, Rothman AI, Smee S (1996). Large-scale high-stakes testing with an OSCE: report from the Medical Council of Canada. *Acad Med* **71**(1 Suppl.): S19–S21.

2. Tombleson P, Fox RA, Dacre JA (2000). Defining the content for the objective structured clinical examination component of the professional and linguistic assessments board examination: development of a blueprint. *Med Educ* **34**(7): 566–72.

3. Lawson DM (2006). Applying generalizability theory to high-stakes objective structured clinical examinations in a naturalistic environment. *J Manipulative Physiol Ther* **29**(6): 463–7.

4. Barrows HS (1993). An overview of the uses of standardized patients for teaching and evaluating clinical skills. AAMC. *Acad Med* **68**(6): 443–51.

5. Glassman PA, Luck J, O'Gara EM, Peabody JW (2000). Using standardized patients to measure quality: evidence from the literature and a prospective study. *J Comm J Qual Improv* **26**(11): 644–53.

6. Harden RM, Stevenson M, Downie WW, Wilson GU (1975). Assessment of clinical competence using objective structured examination. *BMJ* **1**: 447–51.

7. Dillon GF, Boulet JR, Hawkins RE, Swanson DB (2004). Simulations in the United States Medical Licensing Examination (USMLE). *Qual Saf Health Care* **13** (Suppl. 1): i41-i45.

8. Broder HL, Janal M (2006). Promoting interpersonal skills and cultural sensitivity among dental students. *J Dent Educ* **70**(4): 409–16.

9. Wilson L, Gallagher GM, Cornelius F, *et al.* (2006). The standardized patient experience in undergraduate nursing education. *Stud Health Technol Inform* **122**: 830.

10. Rushforth HE (2006). Objective structured clinical examination (OSCE): Review of literature and implications for nursing education. *Nurse Educ Today* 2006 Oct 26.

11. King AM, Pohl H, Perkowski-Rogers LC (1994). Planning standardized patient programmemes: case development, patient training, and costs. *Teach Learn Med* **6**(1): 6–14.

12. Swanson DB, Clauser BE, Case SM (1999). Clinical Skills Assessment with Standardized Patients in High-Stakes Tests: A Framework for Thinking about Score Precision, Equating, and Security. *Adv Health Sci Educ Theory Pract* **4**(1): 67–106.

13. Harden RM, Gleeson FA (1979). Assessment of clinical competence using an objective structured clinical examination (OSCE). *Med Educ* **13**(1): 41–54.

14. Vu NV, Steward DE, Marcy M (1987). An assessment of the consistency and accuracy of standardized patients' simulations. *J Med Educ* **62**(12): 1000–2.

15. Taylor A, Rymer J (2001). The new MRCOG Objective Structured Clinical Examination–the examiners evaluation. *J Obstet Gynaecol* **21**(2): 103–6.

16. Newble DI, Swanson DB (1988). Psychometric characteristics of the objective structured clinical examination. *Med Educ* **22**(4): 325–34.

17. Robb KV, Rothman AI (1985). The assessment of clinical skills in general medical residents – comparison of the objective strucured clinical examination to a conventional oral examination. *Annals RCPSC* **18**(3): 235–8.

18. Medical Council of Canada (2002). Qualifying Examination Part II, Information Pamphlet. Ottawa, Ontario, Canada, Medical Council of Canada.

19. Whelan G (2000). High-stakes medical performance testing: the Clinical Skills Assessment program. *JAMA* **283**(13): 1748.

20. Federation of State Medical Boards and National Board of Medical Examiners (2003). 2004 USMLE Step 2 CS Content Description and General Information Booklet. Philadelphia: FSMB and NBME.

21. Hauer KE, Hodgson CS, Kerr KM, Teherani A, Irby DM (2005). A national study of medical student clinical skills assessment. *Acad Med* **80**(10 Suppl.): S25–S29.

22. Whelan GP, Boulet JR, McKinley DW, *et al.* (2005). Scoring standardized patient examinations: lessons learned from the development and administration of the ECFMG Clinical Skills Assessment (CSA). *Med Teach* **27**(3): 200–6.

23. Stillman PL, Swanson DB, Smee S, *et al.* (1986). Assessing clinical skills of residents with standardized patients. *Ann Intern Med* **105**(5): 762–71.

24. Vu N, Baroffio A, Huber P, Layat C, Gerbase M, Nendaz M (2006). Assessing clinical competence: a pilot project to evaluate the feasibility of a standardized patient – based practical examination as a component of the Swiss certification process. *Swiss Med Wkly* **136**(25–26): 392–9.

25. Boursicot K, Roberts T (2005). How to set up an OSCE. *The Clinical Teacher* **2**(1): 16–20.

26. Jain SS, Nadler S, Eyles M, Kirshblum S, DeLisa JA, Smith A (1997). Development of an objective structured clinical examination (OSCE) for physical medicine and rehabilitation residents. *Am J Phys Med Rehabil* **76**(2): 102–6.

27. Ainsworth MA, Rogers LP, Markus JF, Dorsey NK, Blackwell TA, Petrusa ER (1991). Standardized patient encounters. A method for teaching and evaluation. *JAMA* **266**(10): 1390–6.

28. Adamo G (2003). Simulated and standardized patients in OSCEs: achievements and challenges 1992–2003. *Med Teach* **25**(3): 262–70.

29. Reznick RK, Smee S, Baumber JS, *et al.* (1993). Guidelines for estimating the real cost of an objective structured clinical examination. *Acad Med* **68**(7): 513–7.

30. Stillman PL (1993). Technical issues: logistics. AAMC. *Acad Med* **68**(6): 464–8.

31. Kelly M, Murphy A (2004). An evaluation of the cost of designing, delivering and assessing an undergraduate communication skills module. *Med Teach* **26**(7): 610–4.

32. Wilkinson TJ, Newble DI, Wilson PD, Carter JM, Helms RM (2000). Development of a three-centre simultaneous objective structured clinical examination. *Med Educ* **34**(10): 798–807.

33. Cusimano MD, Cohen R, Tucker W, Murnaghan J, Kodama R, Reznick R (1994). A comparative analysis of the costs of administration of an OSCE (objective structured clinical examination). *Acad Med* **69**(7): 571–6.

34. Parr MB, Sweeney NM (2006). Use of human patient simulation in an undergraduate critical care course. *Crit Care Nurs Q* **29**(3): 188–98.

35. Earle D (2006). Surgical training and simulation laboratory at Baystate Medical Centre. *Surg Innov* **13**(1): 53–60.

36. Magee JH (2003). Validation of medical modeling & simulation training devices and systems. *Stud Health Technol Inform* **94**: 196–8.

37. Kurrek MM, Devitt JH (1997). The cost for construction and operation of a simulation centre. *Can J Anaesth* **44**(11): 1191–5.

38. Petrusa ER (2004). Taking standardized patient-based examinations to the next level. *Teach Learn Med* **16**(1): 98–110.

39. Davidson R, Duerson M, Rathe R, Pauly R, Watson RT (2001). Using standardized patients as teachers: a concurrent controlled trial. *Acad Med* **76**(8): 840–3.

40. Bowyer MW, Rawn L, Hanson J, *et al.* (2006). Combining high-fidelity human patient simulators with a standardized family member: a novel approach to teaching breaking bad news. *Stud Health Technol Inform* **119**: 67–72.

41. Boulet JR, McKinley DW, Whelan GP, Hambleton RK (2003). Quality assurance methods for performance-based assessments. *Adv Health Sci Educ Theory Pract* **8**(1): 27–47.

42. Boulet JR, McKinley DW, Norcini JJ, Whelan GP (2002). Assessing the comparability of standardized patient and physician evaluations of clinical skills. *Adv Health Sci Educ Theory Pract* 2002; **7**(2): 85–97.

43. Gorter S, Rethans JJ, Scherpbier A, *et al.* (2000). Developing case-specific checklists for standardized-patient-based assessments in internal medicine: A review of the literature. *Acad Med* **75**(11): 1130–7.

44. O'Connor HM, McGraw RC (1997). Clinical skills training: developing objective assessment instruments. *Med Educ* **31**(5): 359–63.

45. Gorter S, Rethans JJ, Scherpbier A, *et al.* (2000). Developing case-specific checklists for standardized-patient-based assessments in internal medicine: A review of the literature. *Acad Med* **75**(11): 1130–7.

46. Boulet JR, van ZM, De CA, Hawkins RE, Peitzman S (2006). Checklist content on standardized patient assessment: an ex post facto review. *Adv Health Sci Educ Theory Pract* **13**(1): 59–69.

47. Solomon DJ, Szauter K, Rosebraugh CJ, Callaway MR (2000). Global ratings of student performance in a standardized patient examination: Is the whole more than the sum of the parts? *Adv Health Sci Educ Theory Pract* **5**: 131–40.

48. Cohen DS, Colliver JA, Marcy MS, Fried ED, Swartz MH (1996). Psychometric properties of a standardized-patient checklist and rating- scale form used to assess interpersonal and communication skills. *Acad Med* **71**(1 Suppl.): S87–S89.

49. Guiton G, Hodgson CS, Delandshere G, Wilkerson L (2004). Communication skills in standardized-patient assessment of final-year medical students: a psychometric study. *Adv Health Sci Educ Theory Pract* **9**(3): 179–87.

50. Hobgood CD, Riviello RJ, Jouriles N, Hamilton G (2002). Assessment of communication and interpersonal skills competencies. *Acad Emerg Med* **9**(11): 1257–69.

51. Hodges B, Turnbull J, Cohen R, Bienenstock A, Norman G (1996). Evaluating communication skills in the OSCE format: reliability and generalizability. *Med Educ* **30**(1): 38–43.

52. Chambers KA, Boulet JR, Furman GE (2001). Are interpersonal skills ratings influenced by gender in a clinical skills assessment using standardized patients? *Adv Health Sci Educ Theory Pract* **6**(3): 231–41.

53. Boulet JR, Ben David MF, Ziv A, *et al.*(1998) Using standardized patients to assess the interpersonal skills of physicians. *Acad Med* **73**(10 Suppl.): S94–S96.

54. Hodges B, McNaughton N, Regehr G, Tiberius R, Hanson M (2002). The challenge of creating new OSCE measures to capture the characteristics of expertise. *Med Educ* **36**(8): 742–8.

55. Amano H, Sano T, Gotoh K, *et al.*(2004). Strategies for training standardized patient instructors for a competency exam. *J Dent Educ* **68**(10): 1104–11.

56. Foley KL, George G, Crandall SJ, Walker KH, Marion GS, Spangler JG (2006). Training and evaluating tobacco-specific standardized patient instructors. *Fam Med* **38**(1): 28–37.

57. Errichetti A, Boulet JR (2006). Comparing traditional and computer-based training methods for standardized patients. *Acad Med* **81**(10 Suppl.): S91–S94.

58. Norcini J, Boulet J (2003). Methodological issues in the use of standardized patients for assessment. *Teach Learn Med* **15**(4): 293–7.

59. Boulet JR, Rebbecchi TA, Denton EC, McKinley DW, Whelan GP (2004). Assessing the written communication skills of medical school graduates. *Adv Health Sci Educ Theory Pract* **9**(1): 47–60.

60. Cunnington JPW, Neville AJ, Norman GR (1997). The risks of thoroughness: reliability and validity of global ratings and checklists in an OSCE. *Adv Health Sci Educ Theory Pract* **1**: 227–33.

61. LaDuca A (1994). Validation of professional licensure examinations. Professions theory, test design, and construct validity. *Eval Health Prof* **17**(2): 178–97.

62. Schuwirth LW, van der Vleuten CP (2003). The use of clinical simulations in assessment. *Med Educ* **37** (Suppl. 1): 65–71.

63. Roberts C, Newble D, Jolly B, Reed M, Hampton K (2006). Assuring the quality of high-stakes undergraduate assessments of clinical competence. *Med Teach* **28**(6): 535–43.

64. Boulet J, Swanson D (2004). Psychometric challenges of using simulations for high-stakes assessment. In: Dunn W, editor. Simulations in Critical Care and Beyond. Des Plains, IL: *Society of Critical Care Medicine*: 119–30.

65. Brailovsky CA, Grand'Maison P, Lescop J (1997). Construct validity of the Quebec licensing examination SP-based OSCE. *Teach Learn Med* **9**(1): 44–50.

66. Pangaro LN, Worth-Dickstein H, Macmillan MK, Klass DJ, Shatzer JH (1997). Performance of "standardized examinees" in a standardized-patient examination of clinical skills. *Acad Med* **72**(11): 1008–11.

67. Vu NV, Barrows HS (1994). Use of standardized patients in clinical assessments: Recent developments and measurement findings. *Educational Researcher* **23**(3): 23–30.

68. Boulet JR, Gimpel JR, Errichetti AM, Meoli FG (2003). Using National Medical Care Survey data to validate examination content on a performance-based clinical skills assessment for osteopathic physicians. *J Am Osteopath Assoc* **103**(5): 225–31.

69. Chambers KA, Boulet JR, Gary NE (2000). The management of patient encounter time in a high-stakes assessment using standardized patients. *Med Educ* **34**(10): 813–7.

70. McKinley DW, Boulet JR (2004). The effects of task sequence on examinee performance. *Teach Learn Med* **16**(1): 18–22.

71. Gimpel JR, Boulet JR, Errichetti AM (2003). Evaluating the clinical skills of osteopathic medical students. *J Am Osteopath Assoc* **103**(6): 267–79.

72. Ayers WR, Boulet JR (2001). Establishing the validity of test score inferences: performance of 4th- year U.S. medical students on the ECFMG Clinical Skills Assessment. *Teach Learn Med* **13**(4): 214–20.

73. Boulet JR, McKinley DW, Whelan GP, van Zanten M, Hambleton RK (2002). Clinical skills deficiencies among first-year residents: utility of the ECFMG clinical skills assessment. *Acad Med* **77**(10 Suppl.): S33–S35.

74. Whelan GP, McKinley DW, Boulet JR, Macrae J, Kamholz S (2001). Validation of the doctor-patient communication component of the Educational Commission for Foreign Medical Graduates Clinical Skills Assessment. *Med Educ* **35**(8): 757–61.

75. Errichetti AM, Gimpel JR, Boulet JR (2002). State of the art in standardized patient programmemes: a survey of osteopathic medical schools. *J Am Osteopath Assoc* **102**(11): 627–31.

76. Crossley J, Davies H, Humphris G, Jolly B (2002). Generalisability: a key to unlock professional assessment. *Med Educ* **36**(10): 972–8.

77. Shatzer JH, Wardrop JL, Williams RG, Hatch TF (1994). Generalizability of performance on different-station-length standardized patient cases. *Teach Learn Med* **6**(1): 54–8.

78. Swanson DB, Norcini JJ (1989). Factors influencing reproducibility of tests using standardized patients. *Teach Learn Med* **1**(3): 158–66.

79. Norman GR, van der Vleuten CP, De Graaff E (1991). Pitfalls in the pursuit of objectivity: issues of validity, efficiency and acceptability. *Med Educ* **25**(2): 119–26.

80. Boulet JR, Gimpel JR, Dowling DJ, Finley M (2004). Assessing the ability of medical students to perform osteopathic manipulative treatment techniques. *J Am Osteopath Assoc* **104**(5): 203–11.

81. Berkenstadt H, Ziv A, Gafni N, Sidi A (2006). Incorporating simulation-based objective structured clinical examination into the Israeli National Board Examination in Anesthesiology. *Anesth Analg* **102**(3): 853–8.

82. Nestel D, Kneebone R, Black S (2006). Simulated patients and the development of procedural and operative skills. *Med Teach* **28**(4): 390–1.

83. Kneebone RL, Kidd J, Nestel D, *et al.* (2005). Blurring the boundaries: scenario-based simulation in a clinical setting. *Med Educ* **39**(6): 580–7.

84. McKenzie FD, Hubbard TW, Ullian JA, Garcia HM, Castelino RJ, Gliva GA (2006). Medical student evaluation using augmented standardized patients: preliminary results. *Stud Health Technol Inform* **119**: 379–84.

85. Boulet JR, Murray D, Kras J, Woodhouse J, McAllister J, Ziv A (2003). Reliability and validity of a simulation-based acute care skills assessment for medical students and residents. *Anesthesiology* **99**(6): 1270–80.

86. Murray D, Boulet J, Ziv A, Woodhouse J, Kras J, McAllister J (2002). An acute care skills evaluation for graduating medical students: a pilot study using clinical simulation. *Med Educ* **36**(9): 833–41.

87. Devitt JH, Rapanos T, Kurrek M, Cohen MM, Shaw M (1999). The anesthetic record: accuracy and completeness. *Can J Anaesth* **46**(2): 122–8.

88. Devitt JH, Kurrek MM, Cohen MM, *et al.* (1998). Testing internal consistency and construct validity during evaluation of performance in a patient simulator. *Anesth Analg* **86**(6): 1160–4.

89. Devitt JH, Kurrek MM, Cohen MM, Cleave-Hogg D (2001). The validity of performance assessments using simulation. *Anesthesiology* **95**(1): 36–42.

90. Morgan PJ, Cleave-Hogg DM, Guest CB, Herold J (2001). Validity and reliability of undergraduate performance assessments in an anesthesia simulator. *Can J Anaesth* **48**(3): 225–33.

91. Pugh CM, Youngblood P (2002). Development and validation of assessment measures for a newly developed physical examination simulator. *J Am Med Inform Assoc* **9**(5): 448–60.

92. Wind LA, Van DJ, Muijtjens AM, Rethans JJ (2004). Assessing simulated patients in an educational setting: the MaSP (Maastricht Assessment of Simulated Patients). *Med Educ* **38**(1): 39–44.

93. Boulet JR (2005). Generalizability theory: Basics. In: Everitt BS, Howell DC, editors. Encyclopedia of Statistics in Behavioral Science. Chichester: John Wiley & Sons, Ltd, 704–11.

94. Keller LA, Mazor KM, Swaminathan H, Pugnaire MP (2000). An investigation of the impacts of different generalizability study designs on estimates of variance components and generalizability coefficients. *Acad Med* **75**(10 Suppl.): S21–S24.

Chapter 16

Team building and simulation

Andrew Anderson

Overview

- Team building and the associated communication skills are now recognized as a vital element in doctor and nurse training.
- The use of simulation in team training is so far limited largely to anaesthesia and emergency care.
- The use of assessment tools and a move to competency measures provides potential for measuring outcomes of team and communication training.
- We can borrow techniques and training programmes from other industries such as aviation and use them for team building in medicine.
- The use of personality profiling can greatly enhance team building.
- By using ice breakers and non-medical-based team building games training can become fun and team building more effective.
- By integrating actors with high fidelity simulators very realistic scenarios can be generated to allow combined training in technical and team skills.

16.1 Background and team building theories

16.1.1 Introduction

The advantages of simulators in enhancing the objectivity and efficiency of training are clear, and the increased emphasis placed upon the ability to perform a task (rather than simply having knowledge of it) is now an accepted advantage of such systems. Anaesthesia is one of the few areas of medicine which has embraced the use of simulator technology, and a network of high fidelity simulator centres has been developed in the UK since 1997. There are now over 20 such centres across the country and most offer some sort of team building training course. Despite the wealth of positive experience and peer-reviewed papers emanating from these centres, in 2006 simulator-based assessment had not been incorporated into the anaesthesia curriculum.[1] The higher the fidelity designed into the simulator the more expensive it is and this has been a barrier to their more widespread use and adoption.

There is, however, a new assessment-based culture in medicine. The move from a time-based to competency-based curriculum has driven a need for improved assessment techniques. It has also shifted the measurement of competence from being based upon purely technical skills onto a more rounded assessment based upon specified areas of Good Medical Practice. In the UK the GMP Guidance[2] identifies the skills necessary for working with colleagues (Table 16.1).

Table 16.1 UK guidance for Good Medical Practice – working with colleagues

- Respect the skills and contributions of your colleagues
- Communicate effectively with colleagues within and outside the team
- Make sure that your patients and colleagues understand your role and responsibilities in the team, and who is responsible for each aspect of patient care
- Participate in regular reviews and audits of the standards and performance of the team, taking steps to remedy any deficiencies
- Support colleagues who have problems with performance, conduct or health

As a result of the assumption that assessment drives learning, interest in the use of simulators for assessment has grown in recent years as their capability has increased and the relative cost of obtaining some of the higher fidelity systems has fallen. If simulation is to take its proper place in medical training it needs to embrace two things:

- a broader, more relevant applicability to the curriculum
- assessment criteria that provide better measures of the effects of simulated training.

Team building training (TBT) offers an application that has the potential to fulfil both requirements and could enable training and simulation centres the opportunity to widen their appeal to all areas of healthcare.

A team can be defined as:

'a small number of people with complementary skills who are committed to a common purpose, performance goals, and approach, for which they are mutually accountable.'

Katzenbach JR, Smith DK (1993). *The wisdom of teams: creating the high-performance organization.* Boston: Harvard Business School: 45.

Team building can be defined as: 'a planned effort made in order to improve communications and working relationships by managed change involving a group of people'. Team building is most effective when used as part of a curriculum strategy that identifies the types of teams and their interactions with patients. Simulation has a major role to play in effective team building by offering the opportunity to analyse and practise team skills in realistic patient-based environments and to improve patient care as a result. This chapter explores the reasons why team building is important and offers suggestions about how simulation can be used as a platform for change in the way we train and manage team working in healthcare.

16.1.2 **Measurement of outcomes**

Before embarking upon any training initiative, it is imperative that those attending the courses are going to benefit from them and that there is some measure of positive behavioural change. The foundation programme in the UK is a 2-year general training programme that forms the bridge between medical school and specialist/general practice training. It is pioneering the measurement of competence by using a range of assessment instruments to provide objective measures of skills, knowledge and attitudes. Early data suggest the most useful of these tools is multi-source feedback (MSF) – a means of assessment based upon collated questionnaires that ask co-workers to rate skills and attitudes of colleagues, including communication and team

Table 16.2 Working with colleagues – SPRAT© factors

- Verbal communications with colleagues
- Written communications with colleagues
- Ability to recognize and value the contribution of others
- Accessibility/reliability
- Leadership skills
- Management skills

working (Table 16. 2). One of the few validated MSF tools is named SPRAT© (Sheffield Peer Review Assessment Tool). A shortened version (entitled mini-PAT) is being used as part of the foundation assessment programme in the UK. SPRAT, and other tools such as Case Base Discussion (CBD) and DOPS (Direct Observation of Procedural Skills), may suggest areas of communication or team work where performance is below standard. By conducting these assessments before and after training some measure of effectiveness can be demonstrated.

The performance issues identified by assessments can be corrected in team building exercises in the simulation arena. Behavioural markers can be used to clearly direct areas of improvement such as 'exchanging information' or 'assessing the capabilities of others'[3]. By measuring these skills before and after training objective measures of improvement and associated benefits of using simulation could be derived.

Team performance is reduced when members fail to share unique information with other members of the team. Stasser[4] showed that team members who have some common and some unique information tend to spend time discussing the common information and fail to share enough of the unique information, and therefore make poor decisions. Real-world studies of high-level political decisions and airline crashes demonstrate that groups make poor decisions when members fail to speak assertively. Blum et al[5] showed that anaesthesiology faculty OR residents participating in 1-day training programmes in a simulated operating room (OR) setting did not share vital clinical information due to a variety of factors. Individual team members were given 'probes' or pieces of specific, potentially important, information for patient management, and how and when these probes were shared were observed. This study offers another example of the importance of effective communication in medicine and a way of highlighting them in a simulated setting.

16.1.3 Why team building is important and types of teams

West et al.[6] examined the relationship between the people management practices in hospitals and patient mortality and found that the higher the percentage of staff working in teams the lower the patient mortality. On average, in hospitals where over 60% of staff worked in formal teams, mortality was around 5% lower than expected. Two major studies found that adverse events caused by poor medical management and miscommunication occurred in 2.9% and 3.7% of patients respectively.[7]

The same report made several notable recommendations that training institutions should adopt with regard to medical education, the main one being for them to 'establish interdisciplinary team training programmes, such as simulation, that incorporate proven methods of team management.'

There are many types of teams found within the healthcare environment, including:

- primary healthcare
- secondary healthcare

- emergency
- management
- clinical
- OR.

For the purpose of planning team training using simulated environments, teams can be divided into two categories:

- semi-permanent teams, such as clinical firms and OR teams
- *ad hoc* teams, such as those dealing with emergencies or cardiac arrests.

For permanent teams who have to work together on a regular basis, the *One Minute Manager* series offers an insight into successful techniques used in large corporations. The *One Minute Manager Builds High Performing Teams*[8] has several useful techniques and insights that can be applied to medical training. These include:

- The stages of team development – orientation, dissatisfaction, production and integration.
- Things to observe in teams – participation, decision making, conflict, problem solving, etc.
- Leadership styles – validating, collaborating, resolving and structuring.

For those situations where healthcare workers come together to deal with short-term situations, the requirements for effective team performance (see section 16.1.5) are even more relevant. The aviation industry has managed to build selection and training programmes that allow flight crew members who have never met to perform effectively, eliminating barriers to communication such as status, personality clashes and hidden agendas. Simulation is critical in providing effective training for pilots and so medical training should copy this paradigm.

16.1.4 What can we learn from other industries about team dynamics and simulation?

Robert Katz identified three managerial skills that are essential to successful management: technical, human, and conceptual (Table 16.3). Medical training has focused on providing students with the technical knowledge required to perform effectively but there is an increasing recognition that it needs to incorporate the other attributes described by Katz. The study of the way in which an individual performs within a system, and hence the potential reasons for failure of that system, is often referred to as human factors or non-technical skills (NTS).

Medicine has incorporated this style of training, usually centred around simulator-based courses, but as yet in a piecemeal, episodic fashion which relies on participants volunteering to attend courses. Unlike in other industries, there is no systematic approach to linking the content of this teaching with a more conventional range of topics. As a consequence it is difficult to assess the impact of human factors training in medicine. This is partly because very little work has been done to date in identifying the key NTS required in medicine, and the overall experience of workplace-based assessment is limited, although as referred to above, MSF does provide at least some data in this area. Lessons from other high reliability organizations may help to address

Table 16.3 Skills portfolio

Technical skills:	Process, knowledge, experience
Human skills:	People management, communication skills
Conceptual skills:	Formulation of ideas, entrepreneurship, strategic planning

Katz R (1974). *Skills of an effective administrator*. Harvard Business Review September–October: 90–101.

the main challenges of developing the content, integrating it into the curriculum, reinforcing the concepts in the workplace through staff development and establishing its role in summative assessment.

In aviation, human factors training is known as crew resource management (CRM). CRM can be taught to individuals from a single discipline (using instructors and retired personnel to play other team roles), which makes it possible to focus on the behaviour skills most needed in that discipline. CRM can also be taught to combined teams of individuals from different disciplines in one work unit. This approach facilitates cross-training and building cohesion of real working teams. These two techniques are complementary, and both can be pursued to achieve greater impact.

Challenging situations happen much more often in healthcare than in commercial flights. For example, 20% of anaesthesia cases involve an unexpected incident. The principles of CRM apply not just to anaesthesia or surgery, but also to a wide range of clinical domains and practitioners. A CRM-based approach focuses on the integration of behavioural skills with technical and conceptual skills. Simulation is a key component of a CRM-based approach in healthcare, because it lets teams and team members actually practise these skills in the context of plausible, time-critical scenarios.

Modern high-fidelity simulators based around virtual reality can provide many of the features of real patients, including eye blinks, active pupils, breath sounds and the look and feel of surgical procedures. Participants can be presented with scenarios that are very challenging not only medically and technically, but also in terms of the principles of decision making and teamwork. After the simulation, participants can take part in a detailed debriefing where they can see a video of what actually happened and discuss the pros and cons of their actions. This approach has worked well in aviation and it works well in medical simulation.

16.1.5 What makes an effective team?

The basic requirements for a team to be effective are:

- **Communication and negotiation** – team members need the ability to state ideas or questions clearly, listen to others attentively, and to resolve disagreements in a non-confrontational manner. These are skills that many students may lack.

- **Analytic and creative skills** – team members need to evaluate information and propose creative solutions. Many students have these skills but may not be able to effectively communicate their views or concerns.

- **Organization** – the team needs to be able to track and complete all of its tasks on time. Tensions can often arise if deadlines are missed.

For a team to function effectively there must be a clarity of purpose for what the team will achieve and the interpersonal relationships of the team must not be hampered by hidden agendas or personality clashes. Members must have a chance to contribute and learn from and work with others. In medicine a team can often be made up of members who have never met and the importance of leadership, clear roles and absence of conflict is even greater in these situations. Simulated exercises are extremely useful in throwing together multidisciplinary groups and observing how they interact.

Team members have a responsibility to become involved in the working of the team and should:

- contribute ideas and solutions
- recognize and respect differences in others

- value the ideas and contributions of others
- listen and share information
- ask questions and get clarification
- care about the team and the outcomes

16.1.6 **Understanding personality types and team dynamics**

Multidisciplinary team working has become an in-vogue approach over recent years. The use of simulation to put teams together in semi-realistic situations and film their interactions for formative assessment has been one of the major factors in the increased adoption of simulated patient systems worldwide. Anecdotal evidence suggests that the success of these courses in making teams more effective is limited. This is due, in my opinion, to two factors:

- the status issues and clashes between healthcare professionals, especially between doctors and nurses
- the lack of understanding of personality types and their impact on human interactions

Only by focusing on the clinical outcomes can we overcome the inherent status issues exacerbated by the differences in medical and nurse training. The use of psychometric profiles such as Myers Briggs® or Belbin® has become more widespread in healthcare but their use in analysing team dynamics is limited. Dr Meredith Belbin, a UK academic and consultant, developed the Belbin team roles model in the late 1970s. Belbin's work at Henley Management College demonstrated that balanced teams comprising people with different capabilities performed better than teams that are less well balanced.

A simple and easy source of information about how team members will interact is the DISC approach. The 1970s work by Dr John Geier brought the DISC system into practical application with substantive research and, while this isn't a full 'personality test' in the strict technical sense, it provides an insight into an individual style that is more than adequate to predict the likely trends of the subject's behaviour in the future and in particular in team building situations. It has a major advantage in that it can be completed quickly and can be interpreted easily. The system evaluates four key factors in an individual style, rather than the sixteen or more that are often seen in full personality tests (for example, DISC makes no attempt to measure such factors as intelligence).

The tests classify four aspects of personality by testing a person's preferences in word associations. DISC is an acronym for:

- **D**ominance – relating to control, power and assertiveness
- **I**nfluence – relating to social situations and communication
- **S**teadiness – relating to patience, persistence, and thoughtfulness
- **C**ompliance (or conscientiousness or caution) – relating to structure and organization

These four dimensions can be grouped in a grid with D and I sharing the top row and representing extroverted aspects of the personality, and C and S below representing introverted aspects. D and C then share the left column and represent task-focused aspects, and I and S share the right column and represent social aspects (Table 16.4).

- **Dominance**: People who score high in the intensity of the D styles factor are very active in dealing with problems and challenges, while low D scores denote people who want to do more research before committing to a decision. High D people are described as demanding, forceful, egocentric, strong-willed, driving, determined, ambitious, aggressive, and pioneer-

Table 16.4 DISC factor relationships

	Task focused	Social focused
Extrovert	Dominance	Influence
Introvert	Conscientious	Steadiness

ing. Low D scores describe those who are conservative, low-key, cooperative, calculating, undemanding, cautious, mild, agreeable, modest and peaceful.

◆ **Influence**: People with high I scores influence others through talking and activity and tend to be emotional. They are described as convincing, magnetic, political, enthusiastic, persuasive, warm, demonstrative, trusting, and optimistic. Those with low I scores influence more by data and facts, and not with feelings. They are described as reflective, factual, calculating, sceptical, logical, suspicious, matter-of-fact, pessimistic, and critical.

◆ **Steadiness**: People with high S styles scores want a steady pace and security, and don't like sudden change. Low S intensity scores are those who like change and variety. High S persons are calm, relaxed, patient, possessive, predictable, deliberate, stable, consistent, and tend to be unemotional and poker-faced. People with low S scores are described as restless, demonstrative, impatient, eager, or even impulsive.

◆ **Conscientious**: Persons with high C styles adhere to rules, regulations, and structure. They like to do quality work and do it right the first time. High C people are careful, cautious, exacting, neat, systematic, diplomatic, accurate, tactful. Those with low C scores challenge the rules, want independence and are described as self-willed, stubborn, opinionated, unsystematic, arbitrary, and careless with details.

Prior to building teams or training a group of people who have never worked together before, it is very helpful for the trainer, but even more important for the team members, to understand their personality types and how they will feel when interacting with other types. For example, a high D personality can find a high S person frustrating because they make slow decisions. The high S or high C personalities are not generally assertive and can therefore not contribute what could be vital information to the team if they feel dominated. I would recommend the use of such analysis in any team building scenario.

16.1.7 **Simulator technologies**

Simulator facilities are used in undergraduate, graduate, and continuing medical education. The increasing number of simulation systems for procedures such as endoscopy, laparoscopy and other complex or high-risk procedures such as epidural injections offers the simulation community the chance to move away from a focus on anaesthesia and trauma training. Multidisciplinary sessions allow participants to improve their leadership, communication, and team resource management skills, which are key components needed in managing medical crises. The use of role plays can be very valuable in exploring communication skills but add a trained actor and plastic training models and the engagement of participants improves markedly. Identify the training objectives and choose the appropriate training tools and scenario. For example, the use of an actor combined with the monitor output from a high-fidelity mannequin for non-invasive scenarios can allow sophisticated communication scenarios to be developed that are very realistic.

16.2 **Practical aspects**

16.2.1 **Running a team building day**

As for all training, the key to success is in the planning. In preparation, trainers should:

- Practise the team building exercise yourself first to check that it works: check timings and materials, and ensure you have all the answers. Anticipation and planning are vital.
- Make sure all team building games' instructions are clear and complete – essential for keeping control and credibility.
- Become proficient yourself first with any team building games or equipment that you use.

For the day itself, an outline plan is shown in Table 16.5. Given time, you can bring in many of the techniques described below to make the day more effective, including:

- Distribute Post-it notes and ask each attendee to write one thing they wish to achieve from the training. Use these notes to review what was achieved at the end of the course.
- Use ice-breaking exercises to open discussion and team dynamics (see below).
- Either in advance or on the day, conduct psychometric profiles to facilitate understanding of how team members interact.
- Once these dynamics are understood, review the purpose of the team and what makes teams effective. Ask delegates to engage with each other and expose any hidden agendas or status issues.
- Use video and verbal feedback from the simulator sessions to explore team and communication issues.

16.2.2 **Exercises for opening communication and breaking down barriers**

16.2.2.1 Ice breakers

The first aim of any course is to facilitate learning, and in a team building programme or course this cannot be done without effective communication within the team. To break down barriers and improve mutual understanding and respect, I would suggest using ice-breaking techniques at the start of any training day or programme. These tasks are designed to get the individuals in the group talking to each other and communicating in a non-threatening way. They also allow the facilitator to begin to understand the group make up and identify different personality types, a useful basis for team exercises later. Some examples are:

- Break the participants into groups of three or four and ask each member to tell the others a major like and dislike, either work-related or not. The group, having heard from each member, chooses one like and one dislike they are willing to share with the whole class.

Table 16.5 Outline of a team building day

- Objectives, personal and for the day
- Ice-breaking exercises
- Team building games/scenarios
- Discussion on what the team needs to achieve
- Simulated exercises
- Review and de-brief

◆ Ask each participant to pick out three events, challenges or moments of recognition from their career so far (include any prior to medicine) they are willing to share. Again, ask each group to share the most interesting with the whole class.

◆ Tell the newly formed groups that their assignment is to find ten things they have in common, with every other person in the group, that have nothing to do with work. Exclude body parts or clothing items as this helps the group explore shared interests more broadly. Tell the groups that one person must take notes and be ready to read their list to the whole group upon completion of the assignment. Ask for a volunteer to read their whole list of things in common first. Then, ask each group to share their whole list with the whole group. Because people are your best source for laughter and fun, the reading of the lists always generates a lot of laughter and discussion.

16.2.2.2 Interactive team games[9]

If you have time, examples of more interactive exercises that generate a lot of communication and feedback are:

Skills, knowledge and attitudes exercise First, using a flip chart, brainstorm with the team their ideas of great managers and leaders – can be real and fictional: famous, celebrity, local business personalities ... whatever. Allow a few minutes to collect a selection of names. Tack this sheet to the wall. Then ask the team to call out what they think are the attributes most associated with the various names on the list, that make them good at what they do. In any order, doesn't matter. Write these attributes on the flip chart. Then ask one of the more dominant delegates to come to the front and circle all the 'skills' on the sheet, with the help of the team, and the facilitator if necessary. There will be hardly any. Next ask a quiet team member to come to the front and circle all the 'attitudes' on the sheet. It will be most of them.

The point for discussion is that while a certain **skill** level is necessary to do a job, the fact is that **attitude** determines whether the job is done well, and whether the job holder makes a real difference to their organization, colleagues and environment. People commonly believe that skills are the most important attributes and the biggest training priorities. Often they are not. Usually lifting beliefs and changing attitudes have a far greater impact on individual performance and organizational effectiveness. This simple exercise helps to explain the differences between skills and attitude, and why attitude is so much more important than skill. The activity is for groups of any size, although you can split large groups into smaller teams with appointed team leaders to run the exercise in syndicates, and then review the different teams' findings afterwards as a whole group.

Personal goal setting exercise[9] The exercise is then to ask the team members to think about one aspect of their own personal character (how many is up to the facilitator) that they would like to develop, change, or improve. For example, this might be to develop greater confidence; to manage their time better; to deal with stress better; to be more creative; to be more accurate; to finish tasks on time; to take more exercise; to spend more time with their children; to achieve a qualification; or anything about themselves and their lives, at home or work, that it is reasonable to want to change. Depending on the group, you can give extra guidance as to particular areas to focus on or avoid. Be mindful of the group's comfort zone and keep within it in terms of the personal nature of weaknesses and sensitivities that you expect people to think about, and if appropriate, to divulge to others. If you wish to ask the team members to think of more than one aspect for change, you can guide them to select different types of change, for example, one for work and one for home; or one for now, one for the next month and one for the next three months.

Use your imagination and refine your instructions to fit the situation. Bear in mind that certain changes that people seek to make will contain more than one element, which is relevant to the next stage of the exercise.

When people have thought and decided on their aspect(s) for change, you can ask them to discuss their ideas and feelings in pairs, so as to validate, confirm, and reassess their thoughts. Alternatively you can ask people to keep their thoughts to themselves. It depends on the group as to whether you make the exercise 'open' or 'secret'. Next, ask the team members to translate each desired change into a **specific positive statement**, which (in keeping with the technique), should be in the **present tense**. If a desired personal change contains more than one behaviour then it can help to break it down into two or more statements. Broadly, the more ambitious and complex the desired change then the more likely it will be to need to break it down into separate statements, which could be different behaviours or steps.

The facilitator should decide and agree with the delegates whether they wish to share their aims and statements with others. It is helpful to share, because people can then work in pairs to give and receive feedback as to the changes and positive statements which represent the changes desired. There are various ways to review the exercise, the process, the feelings and the outputs, and various ways to agree follow-up actions and commitments if appropriate, all of which depend on the group and the situation, and especially the wishes of the individuals involved. This activity can be varied to suit the situation. It is a simple and yet potent exercise to encourage and help team members to think about and hopefully commit to personal change and development, especially if linked to a commitment to take action after the exercise. The exercise will also encourage self-analysis and goal-setting.

Mnemonic exercise[9] This is a simple and very flexible activity to help a team of people (or children) to learn and remember key facts and information – about anything, and certainly relating to the particular theme or subject of the team meeting or training session. The exercise is based on the method of memorizing through association. Examples of mnemonics using association are:

- Richard Of York Gave Battle In Vain (the initial letters match those of the colours of the rainbow, Red Orange Yellow Green Blue Indigo Violet)
- Every Armpit Does Get Body Odour Eventually (Notes of the strings on a guitar)
- SWALK (Sealed with a loving kiss)
- The word 'stalagmites' contains an 'M' for mountain (which points up, as opposed to stalactites, which point down)
- The word 'stationery' (relating to paper) contains an 'er', as does 'paper' (as opposed to the word stationary = 'not moving')
- Numbers can be remembered by association with similarly shaped images, for example: 1 = wand, 2 = swan, 3 = flying bird, 4 = yacht, 5 = hook, 6 = elephant (trunk), 7 = cliff, 8 = spectacles, 9 = balloon on a stick, 0 = beach ball, 10 = stick and a hoop. There are many other alternatives. This memory method enables long numbers to be remembered by creating a story linking the respective images.

The exercise itself is simply to ask team members, individually or in pairs, to create their own mnemonic for a given piece of important information, facts or figures. The information could be related to the theme of the meeting or not, depending on the situation. Examples of types of information that are useful to support with mnemonics are: a process, a theory or model, a formula, technical data, a product range, codes and numbers, procedures and policies, document references, etc. Mnemonics should then be presented back to the group and discussed as to their effectiveness. Sharing ideas for memorizing key data helps teams on a number of levels: it improves retention of the particular subject matter used in the exercise; it teaches people how to improve their memory, and it gets people working together in a creative way. There is also always the likelihood that some particularly good ideas will come out of the exercise, which can then be conveyed and used to reinforce key information across the wider organization.

Life raft scenario[9] The scenario is that the team is stranded in a life raft that is too small to hold everyone without sinking. Someone (or you could say two or three people – it's flexible) must be thrown overboard (or eaten, if you prefer the really macabre version) – the group must decide who is/are to be the unfortunate victim(s). First delegates have the opportunity to present their reasons why they should stay (the facilitator can decide what media is to be used, but watch out for the time – this part needs to be reasonably brief). Delegates can be directed either to base their presentations on their own real selves or, if a less emotive approach is required, to adopt the personality of a character from history or, a TV soap, etc. The facilitator must decide how best to instruct the team on this aspect. After presenting their own cases, the group then debates people's relative values and strengths. Within this debate individuals can continue to argue their own cases if they wish, after which the group makes its decision. Set a time limit for each presentation, the debate and the decision, for example 2 minutes per presentation; 20–30 minutes for the debate; 5 minutes for the decision or vote. The facilitator can guide the group as to the decision method, for example secret ballot or show of hands, or preferably, leave the group to decide the decision process, as this highlights other interesting behaviours and capabilities within the team. This is also an interesting exercise to use in group selection recruitment as an interaction game.

◆ Decide on who you are – yourself or another personality

◆ List qualities to support why you should not be thrown overboard

◆ 1 minute for each person to make their case

◆ Debate each one

◆ 5 minutes to decide voting method (can be secret or open)

◆ Vote

◆ Discussion

Points to review if used in other than a group selection context:

◆ Quality and effect of individual presentations

◆ How individuals behave and respond to threat and possible rejection

◆ How different personality types within the group react in different ways to the debating and decision process

◆ How the group organized itself to manage the difficult discussion process

◆ The different perceptions among the team of relative strengths, weaknesses, values, etc.

◆ The way the group decided on how to make the decision (unless told how by the facilitator)

◆ The reaction of the team members and colleagues of the victim(s) after the vote – balance between relief and sympathy

For more ideas and a wealth of business-related ideas about team building I would recommend the following websites:

http://www.humanresources.about.com/od/icebreakers/
http://www.businessballs.com/

16.2.3 **Examples of team building and communication skills training using simulation from the UK**

16.2.3.1 Operating or emergency room

Courses such as Anaesthesia Crisis Resource Management (ACRM)[10] and The Anaesthetists' Non-Technical Skills system (ANTS)[3] identified a number of key elements for a successful team and simulated team building scenarios. The team building elements they identified are listed in Table 16.6. Using high-fidelity centres or more portable equipment such as METI-ECS® or Laerdal SimMan®, it is possible to build a scenario around a procedure, such as difficult intubations, involving different grades of staff. By introducing pieces of key information to lower grade staff you can see how more senior members interact with them.

16.2.3.2 Recognizing risk and improving patient safety R²IPS™

Queens Hospital, Burton has in the UK has been using a high-fidelity simulator in a number of team building scenarios. Nicole Stewart, the non-clinical skills and simulation coordinator, is a former pilot with British Midland Airways and has no medical background. Nicole comments "because of my flight training background, we have used the simulator to develop a number of courses and scenarios using CRM principles. We have observed situations where junior members of staff do not challenge more senior members even though they have superior knowledge." Nicole and her colleagues have developed a specific course based around human factors, R²IPS™ (Recognising Risk and Improving Patient Safety), which draws upon the experience of patients within healthcare settings. This takes delegates through a simulated patient journey through a hospital focusing on the non-clinical issues that cause errors and potential harm to the patient.

16.2.3.3 Flexible sigmoidoscopy training using a VR simulator

Linking technical and communication skills has been pioneered by Roger Kneeebone and his colleagues at Imperial College London. In 2003 they published work[11] using the Accutouch® Endoscopy Simulator (Immersion Medical Inc.) that used scenario-based assessments linking the simulator to simulated patients. By positioning the SP next to the simulator and arranging the room to resemble an outpatient endoscopy room, a very realistic and engaging environment was created to allow practice and assessment of how technical and communication skills interrelate.

16.2.3.4 Integrated procedural performance instrument

The work of Roger Kneebone has continued and in a recently published paper[12] an integrated procedural performance instrument (IPPI) is described. In IPPI clinicians are assessed on 12 clinical procedures in a simulated setting which combines simulated patients with inanimate models or items of medical equipment. Candidates are observed remotely by assessors and feedback is provided to the trainee within 24 hours. This type of training and assessment complements the DOPS process (where real patient procedures are observed and rated) and by

---

Table 16.6 Elements of the non-technical skill system[3]

- ◆ Co-ordinating activities with other team members
- ◆ Exchanging information
- ◆ Using authority and assertiveness
- ◆ Assessing capabilities
- ◆ Supporting others

using the two in tandem it should be possible for simulated training to influence real-world skills and measure such effects objectively.

16.3 **Summary**

The techniques of team building and communication training are vital to improving patient care and safety. The use of realistic exercises based around new simulator technologies and in controlled environments offers the simulation community the chance to educate a wide variety of healthcare professionals in the benefits of simulated training. By using assessment instruments and follow-up skills evaluation, the investment made in simulation technologies can be justified by demonstrating observable improvements in patient safety. Simulation can then take its rightful place as a platform for improving and measuring all aspects of doctor performance.

References

1. Galvin R (2006). Simulation and anaesthetic training: a personal viewpoint. *Bulletin of the Royal College of Anaesthetists* **35:** 1746–8.
2. General Medical Council (GMC) (2001). *Good Medical Practice*. http://www.gmc-uk.org
3. Fletcher G, Flin R, McGeorge P, *et al.* (2003). Anaesthetists' Non-Technical Skills (ANTS) development and evaluation of a behavioural marker system. *Br J Anaesth* **90:** 580–8.
4. Stasser G (1992). Pooling of unshared information during group discussion. In: Worchel S, Wood W, Simpson JA, Eds. Group process and productivity. Newbury Park, CA: Sage: 48–67.
5. Blum RH, *et al.* (2005). A Method for Measuring the Effectiveness of Simulation-Based Team Training for Improving Communication Skills. *Anesthesia & Analgesia* **100**(5): 1375.
6. West MA, *et al.* (2002). The link between management of employees and patient mortality in acute hospitals. *International Journal of Human Resource Management* **13**(8): 1299–310.
7. Quoted in Institute of Medicine (2000). *To Err is Human: Building A Safer Health System*. Washington DC: National Academy Press.
8. Blanchard KH, Carew D, and Parisi-Carew E (2004). *The One Minute Manager Builds High Performing Teams*. Harper Collins.
9. © Alan Chapman 1995–2006. From the free resources website www.businessballs.com. Not to be sold or published. Alan Chapman accepts no liability for any issues arising.
10. Gaba DM, Fish SK, Howard SK (1994). *Crisis Management in Anaesthesiology*. New York: Churchill Linvingstone.
11. Kneebone R, *et al.* (2003). Learning the skills of flexible sigmoidoscopy – the wider perspective. *Medical Education* **37** (Suppl. 1).
12. Kneebone R, *et al.* (2006). Assessing procedural skills in context: exploring the feasibility of an Integrated Procedural Performance Instrument (IPPI). *Medical Education* **40:** 1105–14.

Chapter 17

Problem-based learning for simulation in healthcare

Russell W Jones

Overview

- Simulation in healthcare is replete with excellent opportunities to effectively use problem-based learning (PBL).

- The value of PBL parallels the value of simulation in that both seek to equip learners with the ability to solve problems far beyond those encountered within any specific learning experience.

- Though PBL is extremely valuable for teaching many educational objectives (or outcomes), PBL is not the optimal method for teaching all simulation sessions.

- Of the numerous definitions of PBL, most have four common elements: (i) learning objectives are translated into a problem, (ii) successful solutions require an explanation, with a possible diagnosis and treatment options, (iii) learners use small group discussions to analyse and understand the problem and potential solutions, and (iv) questions or issues that are not answered within small group discussion form the basis for further learning outside the group.

- Advantages of PBL including a focus on 'real life' core information, fostering valuable transferable skills such as leadership, team work, communication and problem-solving, encouraging a deep approach to learning, and making curriculum content relevant to healthcare problems.

- Disadvantages of PBL include a requirement for teaching faculty to facilitate rather than directly impart knowledge, a scarcity of teaching faculty with this ability, the need to provide appropriate training in PBL, the time required for health professionals to fully engage in PBL, knowledge acquired through PBL possibly being less organized than knowledge acquired through traditional learning, and potential time, cost and resource implications.

- When developing PBL scenarios, designers should specify the desired educational objectives to be achieved within a session, develop one or more trigger scenarios to achieve these objectives, and write discussion questions relevant to each trigger scenario to focus learning.

- If more than one trigger is used in a particlar session, then successive triggers should add further information to the scenario in a chronological order to gradually increase the detail of the scenario.

Overview *(continued)*

♦ One of the powerful rationales for PBL is that it provides learners who may be novices with regard to a particlar objective with seminal experiences that allow them to develop a memory of a broad range of known cases. This aids novices to approach a healthcare problem using a similar strategy to that used by experts.

♦ The best scenarios are often developed by multidisciplinary teams that allow input from a variety of different perspectives.

♦ Wherever possible PBL scenarios should be based on de-identified real patients, or composites of real patients, in order to ensure healthcare professionals appreciate that they may encounter the same or similar problems in practice.

♦ When choosing a scenario, designers should consider what content experts believe should be taught relevant to the intended learning objectives.

♦ Beyond the scenario, the single greatest factor that influences the success of PBL is the facilitatory ability of the teacher.

♦ Adequate training of facilitators is essential for any PBL session to function optimally.

17.1 **Background and definition**

By its very nature simulation in healthcare is replete with excellent opportunities for the effective use of problem-based learning (PBL). When appropriately applied PBL is an invaluable aid to teaching specific simulation related educational objectives (or outcomes). However, whereas PBL is a valuable asset for those involved in instructional design for simulation, PBL is not the optimal method for teaching all simulation sessions. Rather PBL is most suited to teach those objectives best taught when learning commences as a problem, query or question that learners need to solve[1]. PBL goes beyond merely providing an opportunity to solve problems and, instead, makes problem solving the main reason for learning. Herein lies the power of PBL because the learner is required to solve specific problems while acquiring knowledge on how to solve similar problems[2]. In this regard the value of PBL parallels the value of simulation in that both seek to equip learners with the ability to solve problems far beyond those encountered within a specific learning experience. Considering the variety and complexity of real problems that will be encountered by those involved in healthcare it may be argued that it is this ability which becomes of greatest benefit in professional life.

PBL arose out of educational initiatives in the 1960s that were primarily based on theoretical advances in behavioural psychology. Several researchers[3–5] successfully argued that learners who commenced learning by focusing on problems before attempting to understand underlying principles, had equal or greater success than learners using a traditional approach whereby underlying principles were presented first and then applied to a specific problem. PBL was initially developed and applied within a medical education context at McMaster University in Canada by Howard Barrows[6–8] and has since grown in popularity to such an extent that most courses in western medical training incorporate at least some component of PBL.

Of the numerous definitions of PBL, most have four common elements:

♦ Learning objectives are translated into a problem.

♦ Successful solutions require an explanation, with a possible diagnosis and treatment options.

- Learners use small group discussions to analyse and understand the problem and potential solutions.

- Questions or issues that are not answered within small group discussion form the basis for further learning outside the group.

Research has revealed that experts compare a novel scenario to a real scenario with which they are familiar[9]. When applied to reasoning within healthcare it is known this ability occurs naturally within experts but needs to be learned by novices. With simulation a scenario is typically used to provide an example from which a learner may extrapolate and apply in later experience. Such a scenario fosters valuable active learning and may be related to a clinical, scientific or community problem[10]. Thus PBL offers the opportunity to provide healthcare professionals with learning experiences that will be of use throughout their professional life[2].

17.2 Value of PBL to simulation

Numerous researchers argue for the benefits of PBL[11–13] and the popularity of PBL as well as its rapid widespread adoption by the healthcare community has arisen from several powerful advantages. These include[14]:

- Making curriculum content relevant by building learning around clinical, community or scientific problems.

- Focusing learning on core information relevant to real scenarios and reducing information overload.

- Fostering the development of valuable transferable skills useful throughout life-long learning. These include leadership, teamwork, and communication, as well as problem solving.

- Facilitating healthcare professionals to become responsible for their own learning. This is an essential skill for all professionals actively engaged in their own continuing development.

- Increased motivation of healthcare professionals to learn by focusing the learning on 'real-life' scenarios.

- Encouraging a deep rather than surface approach to learning by forcing learners to interact with information on multiple levels and to a greater depth than traditional teaching approaches.

- Using a constructional approach to learning whereby learners construct new learning around their existing understanding.

Many of these advantages are particularly pertinent to simulation in healthcare and should be optimally exploited by simulation course designers.

17.2.1 Potential problems of PBL for simulation

Despite the significant advantages described above, no single education strategy is perfect for all educational situations and PBL has several significant disadvantages[14]:

- Teaching faculty are required to facilitate learning rather than to directly impart their knowledge. This may be considered inefficient and, possibly, demotivating to faculty.

- Knowledge acquired through PBL is less organized than knowledge acquired through traditional learning.

- The difficulty of training facilitators and the scarcity of teaching faculty with the skills of facilitating rather than the skills of traditional teaching.

- The time required of healthcare professionals to fully engage in PBL. This can be particularly problematic for the typically crowded simulation curriculum where time-poor faculty and learners are asked to teach and learn under significant time pressures.

- The replacement of the traditional teacher role by the facilitator, which may make it difficult for learners using PBL to emulate good traditional teachers as role models. However, learners will be better able to emulate good facilitators.

- Additional disadvantages include the significant costs, resources, and time required to train effective facilitators. PBL experts also point to concerns about the costs of implementing PBL programmes, though note that other researchers argue that PBL is not necessarily more expensive than traditional educational approaches,[15,16] and raise the issue of PBL not necessarily covering all areas within a healthcare topic[14].

When considering the use of PBL for all or part of a simulation-based learning experience, simulation course designers should be aware of the above potential problems and carefully consider how to minimize or eliminate any negative impact upon learning. Those involved with simulation in healthcare who seek additional comprehensive reviews of research evidence for and against PBL are referred to excellent articles by Albanese and Mitche11[17], Berkson[18] or Vernon and Blake[19].

17.3 Structure of a PBL scenario

There are many examples of PBL scenarios and course developers are encouraged to develop their own to match the specific needs of those healthcare professionals who form the cliental of their simulation centre. When developing PBL scenarios designers should specify the desired educational objectives (or outcomes) to be achieved by the scenario. For example, the following objectives are from the *Induction of Labour Problem 514* written by Sandra Carr[20].

17.3.1 Scenario example 1

Objectives

Upon completion of this PBL, learners should be able to:

- demonstrate an understanding of the management principles related to cardiac disease in pregnancy

- discuss the management of post-term pregnancy

- know how to manage an induction of labour, including indications, conditions to be met, and available options

- appreciate the management of a high head at term (i.e. the associated risks)

- discuss analgesic options with a patient including those based on pharmacological and non-pharmacological (complimentary) therapies, associated epidemiology, and perceptions of pain of childbirth

- describe how to detect abnormal progress in labour and understand the management principles including reasons for failure to progress, clinical signs and vacuum extraction/ forceps delivery

- practise and revise resuscitation of the newborn

- understand the immediate and subsequent management of a baby with meconium-stained liquor

- discuss identification and management of jaundice in the newborn baby

- know the routine management of the postpartum period, including involution, perineum, lochia, and potential complications (e.g. sepsis)
- appreciate the processes surrounding postnatal depression, including incidence, contributing factors, signs and symptoms, and treatment options
- recognize that labour and delivery may cause stress and distress within members of the healthcare team (including themselves) and apply non-harmful methods of dealing with this.

After specifying the intended learning outcomes to be achieved from the PBL session, scenario developers should incorporate trigger scenarios designed to fulfil these objectives. One or more triggers can then be selected by course facilitators for use with a particular group of healthcare professionals. For example, the following trigger was written by Sandra Carr to fulfil some of the objectives specified above[20].

Trigger A
Marie is a 27-year-old primigravid woman who has been seeing her GP for most of her antenatal care. She has had an uncomplicated pregnancy to date.

When Marie returns to the antenatal clinic for her routine 38-week visit you, as the Resident Medical Officer (RMO), notice a medical history of rheumatic fever.

On examination you find:

- Weight: 68 kg
- U/A: NAD
- BP: 115/70
- Oedema: fingers only
- Palpation: Fundal height 43 cm, head 5/5 ↑

Marie and partner Kevin have attended parent education classes and would like to discuss analgesic options with you.

Each trigger should be associated with related discussion questions which offer the PBL session facilitator discussion tools to focus PBL learning by the healthcare professionals participating in the session. In the case of the above trigger Carr[20] wrote the following discussion questions.

Discussion questions A

- How might a history of rheumatic fever influence Marie's management in pregnancy and labour?
- What other cardiac diseases should you know about? (Note, learners should cover cardiac disease only briefly.)
- How will they influence pregnancy and labour management?
- Is the descent of the head normal?
- Should this be investigated further?
- What analgesic options does Marie have?
- What non-pharmacological options are available?
- How do these work (e.g. gate control theory of pain)?
- What are the advantages and disadvantages of these pain management options?
- What are you thoughts on the pain of birth?

Ideally a series of successive triggers should each chronologically build upon preceding triggers. Continuing with Carr's example[20] the following triggers build upon the scenario initially created by the first trigger. Each successive trigger should add further information to the scenario which gradually increases in detail (and possibly complexity) *via* successive triggers. Note also how the discussion questions are specifically designed to achieve the PBL objectives specified at the commencement of the scenario.

Trigger B

At 41 weeks, Marie returns to the clinic with Kevin. When you palpate her abdomen you note that the baby's head has moved into the pelvis (4/5↑). All other parameters are normal.

Marie and Kevin are anxious to become parents. There have been no signs of labour commencing. They want to discuss their options with you

Discussion questions B

- How do we manage the post-term pregnancy?
- What are the potential risks or complications associated with a post-term pregnancy?
- How do we induce a labour?

What are the indications?

What conditions must be met (descent)?

How can we induce?

What are the potential complications of induction?

What are your impressions of induction of labour?

Trigger C

After discussion with the consultant a decision was made to book Marie for an induction of labour 4 days later at 41^{+4}.

Marie and Kevin came to the delivery ward where you performed an ARM (artificial rupture of membranes) and inserted an IV line for a syntocinon infusion.

Twelve hours after Marie's labour is established you are called to perform a vaginal examination. You find her cervix to be 6 cm dilated and the baby's head is at −2 station, 3/5↑ with +caput and +moulding. Marie has dilated only 2cm in the past 4 hours. Marie requests an epidural to manage her labour pain.

Five hours later Marie is examined again and found to be fully dilated. You and the midwife note that there is meconium-stained liquor and moderate variable decelerations of the foetal heart on the CTG (cardiotocograph) monitor. Marie is feeling very tired.

One hour later Marie has an assisted birth, via vacuum extraction, of a little boy, James, who is pale and floppy at birth and covered in meconium. His 1-minute Apgar score is 4.

Discussion questions C

- How can you monitor the progress of labour (partogram)?
- How do we monitor maternal and foetal wellbeing?
- What would make you think Marie's progress is abnormal?
- What are some of the reasons for failure to progress?
- What criteria must be met for a safe instrumental delivery?
- Discuss vacuum extraction and forcep delivery.
- How would you resuscitate James?
- Have you had any experience with resuscitation at a delivery? (Discuss these.)

- How is meconium-stained liquor managed at birth?
- What are the potential complications and long-term implications of meconium?
- How have you felt when at a resuscitation or instrumental delivery?
- How can you manage these feelings?

Trigger D

Three days later you are asked to perform a discharge assessment of Marie on the postnatal ward. When you walk in the paediatric RMO is assessing James for jaundice. When they leave Marie starts to cry.

She says she feels like she is not coping with James and his birth is not what she was expecting.

Discussion questions D

- How can you manage these feelings?
- How do you assess for jaundice in the newborn?
- What is the management of jaundice of the newborn?
- Why does jaundice happen in the newborn?
- Is Marie's reaction normal? When would you consider it abnormal?
- What types of postnatal mood disorders exist?
- How common is postnatal depression in our community?
- What is the routine management Marie will experience during her postnatal hospital stay?
- What discharge advice would you give Marie?

Each scenario should conclude with a series of tips for PBL session facilitators that provide pertinent suggestions to aid in the planning and optimal execution of the session. The following tips are adapted from Carr[20,21].

- Consider ensuring one learner acts as a scribe to document brainstorming, facts, learning issues, etc.
- Facilitate discussion between all learners in the PBL group.
- Establish rules for PBL early in the session. These rules should include one person to speak at any time, participation is required by all learners, all suggestions to be respectfully heard.
- Facilitators should distribute triggers to learners and provide additional information when requested.
- Periodically refocus the group by providing a verbal summary of the group's progress.
- Monitor and facilitate group interaction and behaviour.
- Accept that some groups will cover more content than others.
- Use discussion questions to guide PBL focus and to stimulate learning.
- Keep to time.
- (Scenario developers may include any additional scenario specific advice to facilitators here.)

Three further examples of PBL scenarios are provided below from Dolman[22], Carr[21], and Kilroy[23].

17.3.2 **Scenario example 2**

Objectives

Upon completion of this PBL learners should be able to:

+ develop a treatment plan
+ engage within problem solving
+ implement a strategy for treatment
+ demonstrate an ability to prioritize.

Trigger A[22]

A 42-year-old man is brought to hospital by ambulance as an acute patient. The ambulance staff report that they picked the patient up at a bar called *The Last Hope* where he had fainted after vomiting blood in the toilet. The emergency doctor examines the patient. The man is unshaven, smells of alcohol and is drowsy. His limbs are cachectic in contrast with his swollen abdomen. Before consulting the internist, the emergency doctor decides upon additional examination. While making a phone call to the internist, the accident department nurse reports that the patient is vomiting large amounts of blood again and that the blood tests show many abnormal values, including haemoglobin of 4 g/decilitre, and a significantly increased ammonia level. The prothrombin time is 14 sec.

Discussion questions A

+ What are the most likely diagnoses?
+ What further information do you need?
+ How could you optimally obtain this information?
+ Outline an appropriate treatment plan.
+ Describe your prioritization.
+ Justify your prioritization.

17.3.3 **Scenario example 3**[21]

Objectives

Upon completion of this PBL learners should be able to:

+ review the normal principles of sperm production and ovulation
+ know the male and female causes of infertility and how to investigate for these
+ be aware of the treatment options available in sufficient detail to discuss these with the infertile couple
+ explore the management of potential problems with sexuality including taking a sexual history from a couple
+ explore psychosocial issues related to infertility
+ examine societal expectations surrounding fertility and infertility.

Trigger A

Peta and Michael are both 32 years old. Peta is a nurse and Michael is a sheet metal worker. They have been married for 3 years and have been trying to conceive a pregnancy for the last 12 months. They present to you as a gynaecologist for advice and guidance. Peta and Michael don't know why they are not pregnant after trying for this long.

Neither have any significant medical history. You notice on your examination that Peta weighs 85 kg, is 160 cm tall, has acne, and a menstrual history of cycles between 35 days and 12 weeks apart (oligomenorrhoea). Your examination of Michael reveals apparently normal anatomy.

Discussion questions A

◆ What do we know about Peta and Michael?

◆ What do we need to know?

◆ What do we know about infertility?

◆ What do we need to know? How do we take a history from this couple?

◆ What advice would you give at this point?

Trigger B
The results of your investigations show that Michael has normal semen analysis with a volume of 5 mL, density of 200 million/mL and normal motility.

The investigations you order for Peta reveal anovulatory cycles, raised serum androgen index and mildly increased prolactin levels.

Discussion questions B

◆ What do these results tell us?

◆ What are the possible causes of infertility?

◆ What should you do to help this couple?

Trigger C
Four months later, after receiving your advice, Peta has lost 12 kg but is still not pregnant. She confides in you that she is concerned she will never have a child. She states that her family keep asking her when she and Michael are going to start a family. She wants you to tell her what her options are now. She also confides that she and Michael have been having a lot of arguments over the past 4 months. Peta is feeling insecure in the relationship.

Discussion questions C

◆ What are the options available for Peta and Michael?

◆ What should they think about when considering these options?

17.3.4 **Scenario example 4**

Objectives
Upon completion of this PBL learners should be able to:

◆ review ethical issues associated with specific patient religious beliefs

◆ comprehend how ethical issues may complicate diagnosis and/or treatment

◆ identify the relevance of teenage children with regard to unconscious patient care

◆ explain an evolving ethical dilemma in addition to specific legal obligations for the healthcare professional

◆ identify and discuss medicolegal and ethical issues related to familiar religious beliefs for unconscious patients.

Trigger A[23]
A patient attends your emergency department complaining of haemoptysis and chest pains. He is usually fit and well but smokes heavily. He is accompanied by his two teenage children.

The family are Jehovah's witnesses. How will you deal with the issues this patient's attendance raises?

Discussion questions A

- What issues are raised by the patient's religious beliefs?
- How might these issues complicate diagnosis and treatment?
- Of what significance are the two teenage children accompanying the patient?
- What are the primary concerns from the perspective of the healthcare professional?
- Do these concerns change at any time or under any conditions?

Trigger B

One of the patient's children states that he believes his father's health is more important than any religious beliefs and asserts that the patient would concur with this belief. By this time the father has suffered violent haemoptysis and is no longer conscious.

Discussion questions B

- What, if any, influence does the teenager's assertions have on the course of treatment undertaken by the healthcare professional?
- What are the medicolegal considerations when dealing with a conscious or unconscious patient?
- What are the primary ethical and medicolegal considerations of the healthcare professional in this situation?

17.4 Developing PBL scenarios

Within healthcare, a scenario is typically used to provide an example from which a trainee may learn. Such a scenario may be related to a clinical, scientific or community problem[10]. Part of the rationale for this approach arose from a contrast of the medical reasoning skills of novices and experts. Research revealed experts compare a novel scenario to past scenarios with which they are familiar[9]. Much of an expert's diagnostic and reasoning efforts are focused on the similarities and differences of a novel case with known cases. Therefore it is reasoned that an efficient method of educating a novice is to provide them with seminal experiences that will allow them to develop a memory of a broad range of known cases, that is, will aid novices to think like experts. In this regard the choice of PBL scenario is pivotal for the focus and ultimate effectiveness of the learning experience.

The enormous range of resources available in simulation centres as well as the considerable clinical experience of instructors on a simulation team means that the number of potential scenarios approaches the infinite and is limited only by the imagination of those involved in scenario development. This highlights the value of using a team to develop scenarios. A team of developers will allow a variety of different perspectives to be brought to focus on the scenario. Ideally this should be a multidisciplinary team as the combined efforts of such a group will ensure that scenarios are optimally robust. The simulation course designer should seek to use a PBL scenario as either a 'peg' or 'growing web'[24]. The peg may be viewed as a convenient hook upon which to arrange acquired knowledge whereas the growing web uses the problem as a focus for acquired practical understanding. Carefully structured problems ensure learners comprehensively cover appropriate knowledge, skills and abilities relevant to the desired educational objectives.

Ideally a simulation course designer should use a PBL approach if the problem scenario exhibits several characteristics[22]. The problem should:

- address one or more learning outcomes relevant to the healthcare professionals to be taught in the simulation course

- facilitate healthcare learners to raise their prior learning and experience to conscious consideration and to build upon existing knowledge

- be consistent with the stage of learning at which the healthcare professionals are located

- motivate learners and, ideally, be related to the current or future practice of healthcare professionals

- provide an overall clinical context in which new knowledge is placed

- stimulate thought and discussion, provide guidance and encourage healthcare professionals to actively seek solutions

- phrase an open-ended problem to facilitate discussion and explanation (i.e. closed problems with limited scope should be avoided).

Wherever possible PBL scenarios should be based on real patients, or composites of real patients, in order to ensure healthcare professionals appreciate that they may encounter the same or similar problems in practice. Fortunately such scenarios are reasonably easy to create within the healthcare simulation environment. Furthermore, the use of actual patients allows the designers of PBL scenarios to incorporate de-identified laboratory results, X-rays, scans and pathological materials[25]. When choosing a scenario, designers should consider what topic area experts believe should be taught relevant to the intended learning objectives as well as the prevalence, severity, magnitude, treatability and intervention effectiveness[25,26]. Once a scenario has been developed it should be piloted with an audience of healthcare professionals representative of the intended simulation clients for whom the scenario was developed.

17.5 Facilitating PBL

Beyond the PBL scenario the single greatest factor that influences the success of a PBL programme is the facilitatory skill, knowledge and ability of the teacher. Such is the importance of facilitation that, within PBL, the teacher is usually referred to as the 'facilitator'. Adequate facilitator training and experience is essential for any PBL session to function optimally[2,25,27,28]. PBL is a non-traditional approach that differs significantly from traditional teaching. Of the pool of potential instructors available to a simulation centre it is likely that few will be familiar with a true PBL approach and even fewer will be able to facilitate PBL sessions without additional training and experience. If PBL is used in simulation then it is essential that those instructors who will undertake the facilitation of PBL sessions receive adequate and appropriate training in facilitation.

In true PBL the facilitator does not direct learning, dominate conversation or provide direct answers to questions (unless this is necessary for the preservation and progress of the scenario). Instead the facilitator becomes a learning guide who assists learners develop their own reasoning and hypothesizing while concomitantly allowing learners to evaluate these hypotheses and assess their own knowledge, skills and abilities[2,6]. The facilitator achieves this by continually monitoring and stimulating the PBL process and interpersonal dynamics of the group. Tools for the facilitator are the phrasing of open questions, guiding feedback, managing group dynamics, challenging learner's knowledge and understanding, and raising pertinent facts or issues in a timely manner.

Facilitator competence must include[14] the facilitation of small group learning; a comprehensive understanding of the PBL program such that the facilitator can relate immediate and future learning opportunities to the PBL scenario and guide healthcare professionals to these opportunities; and a global understanding of the overall educational curriculum so that the facilitator can place discrete problems within the global educational experiences of the learners. The abilities of facilitators to establish effective two-way communication with learners, empathy and an open and trusting atmosphere have also been shown to be important[29]. Effective use of PBL within healthcare simulation will best occur if instructors who are not experienced in any of the above are provided with the necessary instruction and experience prior to their involvement as a PBL facilitator in simulation. Once this experience has been gained each facilitator should be fully briefed about the problem and related learning[30] as well as the relationship of the problem and intended learning to the scenario.

Research has shown that content area experts may endanger PBL by exerting too great a director role and reducing the effectiveness of collaborative learning[31] as well as directly answering learners questions, devoting greater amounts of time to the development of learning issues than learners devote to solving them, and by talking 'too often and too long' [32]. However, it is likely that a content area expert, who has been correctly taught in the procedures and nature of PBL, should be able to successfully facilitate a PBL session while resisting reverting to a traditional mode of teaching. Such a facilitator would be ideally placed to be able to limit the extent to which they provide solutions to learners, consistent with a PBL approach, yet able to provide the minimal level of clinical structure necessary for learners to obtain optimal benefit from PBL[33,34]. However, whereas the extent to which a facilitator is required to be a content expert is a matter of some debate within the literature, all PBL specialists agree that adequate training in the role of facilitator is essential for the success of a PBL programme. Those designers of simulation courses who are interested in developing the PBL skills and abilities of their instructors are referred to excellent references by Barrows[27] and Irby[35].

References

1. Charlin B, Mann K, Hansen P (1998). The many faces of problem-based learning: a framework for understanding and comparison. *Medical Teacher* **20**: 323–30.

2. Jones RW (2006). Problem-based learning: description, advantages, disadvantages, scenarios and facilitation. *Anaesthesia and Intensive Care* **34**: 485–8.

3. Foord M (1964). Inductive versus deductive methods of teaching area by programmed instruction. *Educational Review* **16**: 130–6.

4. Gagne RM, Brown LT (1975). Some factors in the programming of conceptual learning. *Journal of Experimental Psychology* **66**: 325–31.

5. Markle SM (1964). *Good Frames and Bad: a Grammar of Frame Writing*. John Wiley and Sons, New York.

6. Barrows HS, Tamblyn RM (1976). An evaluation of problem-based learning in small groups utilising a simulated patient. *Journal of Medical Education* **51**: 52–4.

7. Barrows HS (1985). *How To Design a Problem-based Curriculum For Pre-clinical Years*. Springer, New York.

8. Neufeld VR, Barrows HS (1974). The "McMaster philosophy": an approach to medical education. *Journal of Medical Education* **49**: 1040–50.

9. Bordage G, Lemieux M (1991). Semantic structures and diagnostic thinking of experts and novices. *Academic Medicine* **66**:, S70–72.

10. Harden RM, Davis MH (1998). The continuum of problem-based learning. *Medical Teacher* **20**: 317–22.

11. Schmidt HG, Machiels-Bongaerts M, Hermans H, tenCate TJ, Venekamp R, Boshuizen HP (1996). The development of diagnostic competence: comparison of a problem-based, an integrated, and a conventional medical curriculum. *Academic Medicine* **71**: 658–64.

12. Shin JH, Haynes RN, Johnston ME (1993). Effect of problem-based, self-directed undergraduate education on life-long learning. *Canadian Medical Education Journal* **148**: 969–76.

13. Westberg J, Jason H (1993). *Collaborative Clinical Education: the Foundation of Effective Health Care*. Springer, New York.

14. Davis MH, Harden RM (1999). AMEE medical education guide no. 15: problem-based learning: a practical guide. *Medical Teacher* **21**: 130–40.

15. Nieuwenhuijzen-Kruseman AC, Kolle LF, Scherpbier AJ (1997). Problem-based learning at Maastricht: an assessment of cost and outcome. *Education for Health* **10**: 179–87.

16. Sefton AJ (1997). From a traditional to a problem-based curriculum: estimating staff time and resources. *Education for Health* **10**: 165–78.

17. Albanese MA, Mitchell S (1993). Problem-bases learning: a review of literature on its outcomes and implementation issues. *Academic Medicine* **68**: 52–81.

18. Berkson L (1993). Problem-based learning: have the expectations been met? *Academic Medicine* **68**: S79–88.

19. Veron DT, Blake RL (1993). Does problem-based learning work? A meta-analysis of evaluative research. *Academic Medicine* **68**: 550–63.

20. Carr S (2001). *Induction of Labour Problem Number 514*. Faculty of Medicine and Dentistry, the University of Western Australia.

21. Carr S (2001). *Infertility Problem Number 505*. Faculty of Medicine and Dentistry, the University of Western Australia.

22. Dolmans D, Snellen-Balendong H, Wolfhagen I, van der Vleuten C (1997). Seven principles of effective case design for a problem-based curriculum. *Medical Teacher* **19**: 185–9.

23. Kilroy DA (2004). Problem based learning. *Emerg Med J* **21**: 411–3.

24. Margetson D (1998). What counts as problem-based learning? *Education for Health* **11**: 193–201.

25. Barrows HS (2000). *Problem-based learning applied to medical education*. Southern Illinois University School of Medicine, Springfield Illinois.

26. MacDonald PJ (1991). Selection of health problems for a problem-based curriculum. In: Boud D and Feletti G. *The Challenge of Problem-based Learning*. Kogan Page, London.

27. Barrows HS (1988). *The tutorial process*. Southern Illinois University School of Medicine, Springfield Illinois.

28. Barrows HS, Tamblyn RM (1980). *Problem Based Learning: An Approach to Medical Education*. Springer, New York.

29. Schmidt HG, Moust JH (1995). What makes a tutor effective? A structural-equations modelling approach to learning in problem based curricula. *Academic Medicine* **70**: 708–14.

30. Eagle CJ, Harasym PH, Mandin H (1992). Effects of tutors with case expertise on problem-based learning issues. *Academic Medicine* **67**: 465–9.

31. Silver M, Wilkerson LA (1991). Effects of tutors with subject expertise on the problem-based tutorial. *Academic Medicine* **66**: 298–300.

32. Crosby J (1997). Learning in small groups. *Medical Teacher* **19**: 189–202.

33. Davis WK, Nairn R, Paine ME, Anderson RM, Oh MS (1992). Effects of expert and non-expert facilitators on the small group process and on student performance. *Academic Medicine* **67**: 470–74.

34. Schmidt HG (1994). Resolving inconsistencies in tutor expertise research: does lack of structure cause students to seek tutor guidance? *Academic Medicine* **69**: 656–62.

35. Irby DM (1996). Models of faculty development for problem-based learning. *Advances in Health Sciences Education* **1**: 69–81.

Chapter 18

Research in simulation

Alexander Garden

Overview

- Good research is based upon the application of sound research methods to a worthwhile question, after a thorough literature review.
- The choice of method should be based upon the nature of the question.
- Much simulation-based research relates to the investigation of human performance.
- The measurement of performance is often complicated by the need to ensure that the measurements are valid and reliable representations of underlying theoretical concepts referred to as constructs.
- The experimental design needs to ensure that appropriate covariates are measured, otherwise it will be impossible to exclude alternate explanations for the research findings.
- Sources of artefact, particularly subject–experimenter effects, must be adequately controlled.
- Because the research may not have any direct benefit to participants, and because of the frequent power imbalance between investigators and participants, there are potentially complex ethical issues.

18.1 Introduction

This chapter aims to provide a practical discussion about problems and concerns that are commonly encountered while engaging in research using patient simulation. Research is 'the systematic investigation into and study of materials and sources in order to establish facts and to reach new conclusions'[1], and entire textbooks of research methods are devoted to the key concepts embodied within this definition[2–4]. Medical simulation includes a range of technologies, and its breadth of use spans skills training[5], performance evaluation[6], the determination of drug dosing regimes[7] and epidemiology[8]. Irrespective of the specific domain and technology that is used, the defining feature is the absence of an actual patient[9] and the underlying rationale is based on a range of potential benefits (Table 18.1). From a research perspective these are particularly enticing, for example, in terms of the potential to enable a high degree of experimental control.

From a practical perspective, the key concepts when undertaking research using simulation are the development of worthwhile and feasible research questions, the use of appropriate research methods, and then the dissemination of the findings, typically as a conference presentation or written publication. This chapter is largely confined to problems and challenges that are encountered when undertaking research that uses high fidelity patient simulation. For the most

Table 18.1 Theoretical benefits of simulation in healthcare

- No risk to patients
- Efficient use of training time
- Scheduled clinical experience
- Reproducible clinical situations
- Economical and cost effective
- Standardized clinical situations
- Graduated complexity of clinical problems

part this research falls within the disciplines of applied behavioural research and applied education research, and the experimental methods thus draw heavily on those disciplines.

18.2 **Worthwhile and feasible research**

The origins of a research question are typically the investigator's curiosity, linked by an appropriate literature search to pre-existing knowledge. It is easy to fall into the trap of failing to undertake an adequate literature review before undertaking a research project, and this has recently been identified as a common flaw in simulation-based educational research[10]. In the era of computerized databases such as PubMed, ERIC and the Science Citation Index, the main difficulty when undertaking a literature review is limiting the results of a computerized search to a manageable number of potentially relevant publications, and the assistance of a medical librarian can be invaluable.

Although the essence of a worthwhile question is one that will generate new and important knowledge, from a practical perspective this often ends up being an economic decision based upon funding priorities. It is thus important to have a clear understanding of the funding patterns of the body from whom funding is sought. This applies to both the amount of money and nature of the project. For example there is no point in asking for $50,000 from a body that usually funds applications of less than $10,000. In competitively funded research, the project will be evaluated in terms of significance, scientific merit, research methods, and the expertise and track record of the investigators. It is thus sensible to assemble a team of investigators to provide all the needed expertise, including an established researcher.

There are many worthwhile questions that could theoretically be addressed using simulation, and the main issue often relates to narrowing the question to one that is feasible. The evaluation of a project's feasibility involves a consideration of whether it can be completed with the proposed budget (it is easy to underestimate the true cost), with the proposed participants (will people really agree to be studied in the proposed manner), and in the planned time-frame. Because simulation facilities are very expensive resources operating under tremendous financial pressure, the facilities are usually shared with other users. Typically this means that courses for fee-paying students are the primary sources of revenue, and these take priority over research. Availability of the facility for research is thus reduced, and equipment is more likely to be moved, lost or broken. These problems can be a cause of lost productivity and frustration for the research team, and they are a real threat to research feasibility.

18.3 **Methods**

The purpose of research methods is to ensure that data are collected in a systematic and ethical manner, and that they are appropriately analysed and interpreted, with conclusions that pay due diligence to competing or alternate explanations. Broadly speaking, research methods can be classified as either quantitative or qualitative. Quantitative research methods are designed to enable the logical testing of hypotheses using statistical tests to analyse data that are obtained through formal experimentation (with manipulation of the variables involved) or from observational studies. The other methodological paradigm is qualitative research and this has been widely used in the social sciences such as anthropology, sociology and education. Qualitative approaches are particularly useful when attitudes, beliefs, and socially located phenomena are under investigation. Qualitative research has been described as intrinsically exploratory[11], and it involves undertaking observations that are analysed using descriptive and interpretive approaches, with hypotheses developed to explain the data[12]. Quantitative and qualitative methods are both established research paradigms with supporting bodies of literature[2,4,11,13]. The choice of method should be driven by the question, with the two approaches viewed as complementary rather than competing[12,14]. Quantitative research has dominated mainstream biomedical research and it forms the main theme in this chapter, although a brief discussion of reliability and validity in qualitative research is included.

18.3.1 Quantitative research

Notwithstanding the importance of statistical analysis in quantitative research, it is the author's opinion that research training within medical education places excessive emphasis on statistical methods and insufficient attention upon other aspects of research methods such as measurement, experimental control and sources of artefact or bias. This opinion was supported in a recent meta-analysis of simulation-based educational research, where six consistent flaws were described, four of which did not relate to statistical problems (Table 18.2)[10].

This chapter draws upon established research methods from psychology and education[3,4,13] to place emphasis upon issues related to measurement (including reliability and validity) and experimental control (including sources of artefact).

18.3.1.1 Measurement

Scientific conclusions regarding the presence or absence of an experimental effect are based upon the interpretation of measurements made in relation to an intervention. Valid and reliable measurement is thus at the heart of experimental research, and important early decisions in any research endeavour are what to measure and how to measure it. In addition, because confidence in experimental findings hinges upon their ability to be replicated, experimental control is required, including a clear definition of the circumstances under which the experiment took place.

Research that addresses behaviour, performance or learning, frequently requires the measurement of abstract concepts (rather than physical quantities) for which appropriate measurement

Table 18.2 Consistent flaws in simulation-based educational research[10]

- Poor knowledge of literature beyond the scope of immediate specialty
- Lack of awareness of basic research design for education, behavioural science and clinical discipline
- Poor attention to the measurement properties of the educational and clinical research variables, particularly reliability
- Properties of educational intervention, such as strength and integrity, seldom described
- Inconsistent statistical reporting conventions, with failure to report indices of central tendency (e.g. mean), dispersion (e.g. standard deviation), and effect size
- No attention to statistical power

instruments may not be readily available. To give a concrete example, we might want to measure competence in crisis resource management, and so we need a tool with which to measure a theoretical concept called 'competence in crisis resource management'. One solution is to use a pre-existing tool with accepted psychometric properties, the other is to create a new measurement tool. Either way, the construct of interest or the 'latent variable'[15] is operationalized into something that can be measured or observed. Typically a scale or test is created with the assumption that it reveals the level of the underlying theoretical variable (in this case 'competence in crisis resource management'). The difficulty this poses for the researcher is the need to establish that the scale or test actually measures the construct of interest (i.e. is a valid measurement), and that this can be measured in a replicable manner (i.e. that it is a reliable measure).

Validity of measurement Validity in this context refers to the extent to which a measurement tool actually measures what it is theoretically measuring and it is thus the most basic consideration in any research activity. In the measurement of theoretical constructs it is important to ensure that the measurement adequately represents the construct of interest and that other constructs are not being measured as well as, or instead of, the construct of interest. The concept of validity can be a source of confusion because numerous definitions have been created to cover different types of validity (Table 18.3). The underlying idea is quite simple and these 'types' of validity really just reflect different dimension of a single concept. An authoritative discussion of these principles can be found in *Standards For Educational And Psychological Testing*[16]. These Standards place emphasis on the different sources of evidence for validity (Table 18.4). There is no single and encompassing test of validity, and the determination of which aspects of validity are important in any particular situation is based upon the purpose for which the test or

Table 18.3 Types of validity[3,4,13]

Type	Description
Construct validity	This is an overarching concept that is supported by the other forms of validity and requires that[17]: ◆ The construct is clearly defined and embedded in a theoretical framework that defines its relationship to other constructs. ◆ Ways to measure the hypothetical constructs are developed. ◆ Empirical testing relationships between constructs and their observable manifestations. For example, supports the discriminant validity in we would expect a high correlation between measures of theoretically related constructs (convergent validity) and low correlation between unrelated constructs (divergent validity).
Content validity	The items in the scale or test should reflect the domain of interest. Typically this is achieved through consensus among experts. Each content area that is relevant to the construct should be represented.
Criterion-related validity	This refers to the strength of association between the 'new' measurement and an accepted standard measure (a criterion) of the construct of interest. For example we might expect senior clinicians to perform better than their juniors[18]. Typically this is calculated as a correlation coefficient. Criterion validity encompasses concurrent validity and predictive validity, where correlations are made with criteria at this point in time (concurrent) or in the future (predictive).

Table 18.4 Sources of validity evidence[16]

Source	Description
Test content	Does the test content appropriately reflect the construct that it is purporting to measure? Important considerations include the potential for construct 'under-representation' when the test fails to capture important aspects of the construct, and 'construct-irrelevance', where matters that are irrelevant to the construct are measured.
Response processes	This refers to both the examinee and the judge. For example do other skills that are not directly related to the construct help with performance in a test; and in the case of the judges or raters, are they judging the same thing?
Internal structure of the test	For example, if the internal structure of a test is expected to reflect increasing difficulty, then a novice and an expert would be expected to perform differently on different test items. Internal structure is also used to assess reliability.
Relationship to other variables	This might include performance on related and unrelated constructs, and might involve experimental and correlational evidence.
Consequences of testing	For example if performance is used to determine entrance into a vocational training program, and the performance is not domain-relevant, then the validity is questionable.

evaluation is being undertaken, in conjunction with available theory, empirical evidence, and expert judgement[16]. As practical suggestions, Kazdin (page 200[3]) recommends that the number of theoretical constructs that are measured in any one experiment should be minimized and that more than one index of the construct of interest (e.g. more than one measure of 'crisis management expertise' in the above example) should be measured. Most authors are critical of the concept 'face validity', a term which basically means that 'it is reasonable and obvious that the items in a measurement scale assess what they are purported to measure'. The term is fraught because the underlying assumptions may be wrong, and the name given to a measurement tool frequently reflects the intent of its creators, rather than supporting evidence.

Reliability and measurement error Reliability in this context refers to the consistency or stability of measurement[3] (i.e. the tendency to obtain the same result with repeated measurement). As was the case with validity this is fundamentally a simple concept that can be rendered confusing because multiple dimensions have been given names that suggest different types of reliability. Any form of measurement is subject to a degree of variability, and the difference between the 'true' measurement and a single observation defines measurement error. If the measurement error is randomly distributed, then with sufficient repetitions of the measurement, the error will average to zero and we will have a 'true' measurement. The magnitude of measurement error is important because it determines the number of repetitions that are required to determine the 'true' value, and thus defines the value of a single measurement. It is also important to distinguish between random error (which averages to zero) and systematic error such as some form of offset in a measurement instrument, because the latter constitutes a form of bias that threatens validity.

When a theoretical construct is being measured, the sources of measurement error become more complicated than in the measurement of physical quantities. For example if we administer a 'crisis resource management competence' tool before and after an educational intervention and we find improved performance, what does this mean? Did the participant improve or did he or she make greater effort on the second administration? Was the participant so anxious on the pre-test that performance was impaired? Was the second rating undertaken using less stringent subjective criteria? There are clearly numerous sources of measurement error and they can be divided into contributions from the research subject, from the tool used and from the person undertaking the rating.

A range of statistical tests are typically undertaken to determine the main sources of error, the size of the error, and the degree of generalizability across alternate forms of the test or different study populations[16]. These statistical tests (Table 18.5) are based upon either correlation or analysis of variance, and the choice of test is determined by the aspect of reliability that is to be quantified. There is not one test that answers all questions, although generalizability coefficients address most. The final decision regarding the degree of reliability that is required in a particular situation is a matter of professional judgement, based upon the purpose of the measurement. For example if an individual's 'crisis management performance' score is close to a cut-score that will be used in a high-stakes decision, such as who would graduate from a vocational training programme, then reliability is critical, whereas if the score is top of the class and there is no prize, then reliability is less critical.

Table 18.5 Sources of reliability evidence[4,15,16]

Source	Description
Test–retest coefficient	The correlation between scores on an identical test administered at different times. If the test is re-administered soon after the first administration, then the result will be influenced by memory of the test, whereas with a long test–retest interval there may be real change due to uncontrolled confounding influences. The stability of the underlying construct is used to guide the inter-testing interval. Obviously if we are testing the effect of an intervention, we might expect change.
Internal consistency coefficient	The correlation among items within the test, hence also called the reliability of components. This typically produces an inflated estimate of reliability.
Alternate-form coefficients	Correlation between scores on parallel or equivalent forms of test administered in two independent testing sessions. Split-half correlation uses two halves of a single test rather than two distinct tests.
Rater-reliability	Inter-rater and intra-rater reliability are particularly important when the test score involves a high level of subjective judgement. In clinical psychology testing, a reliability coefficient of ≥ 0.85 is typically regarded as appropriate[2]. To achieve this degree of reliability, appropriate training and evaluation are required.
Generalizability coefficient	Based upon generalizability theory, analysis of variance is used to estimate the magnitude and source of variability in test results. For example, if differences between raters contribute most of the variance in performance evaluation scores, then generalizability across observers will be reduced.
Test item function	Based upon item response theory, enables the investigator to summarize how well the test discriminates among individuals with different levels of the construct being evaluated (i.e. provides a mathematical estimate of precision of measurement).

18.3.1.2 Experimental design

Statistical tests can only tell us the likelihood or probability that a given experimental finding has occurred due to chance. Statistics cannot tell us **why** an experimental effect was found, this is inferred from the experimental design including the appropriate control of confounding variables. Behavioural science is riddled with examples of covariates that must be measured to avoid erroneous conclusions. For example, in research into the effects of sleep loss upon performance, a classical error is failure to consider the improvement in performance that usually results from practise with the measurement tool. Failure to provide adequate control, with careful consideration of the influence of covariates, results in invalid research where the findings cannot be adequately explained or cannot be generalized beyond the immediate experiment.

Artefact arises when the experimental findings are caused by factors other than those intended by the experimenter[4]. The avoidance of artefact requires a clear understanding of those factors which are known to influence the measurement of interest and then the use of impeccable experimental technique to avoid errors in data handling and analysis. Artefact is particularly important in psychological research because of a range of potential subject–experimenter effects (Table 18.6). When determining the cause of an experimental finding it is always important to ensure that the experimental protocol has been a carefully administered using clear, consistent and unambiguous instructions and to then ask: What, in the delivery of this experimental protocol, is really functioning as the intervention[3]?

The double-blind, randomized controlled trial (perhaps placebo controlled) is the gold standard in the evaluation of medical therapy, and the same principles are applied in behavioural science. It may be impossible to blind the subjects regarding the purpose of the experiment or the nature of the treatment. For example, in the author's experiments into the effects of fatigue upon performance in a simulation environment, the hypothesis was obvious to anyone with a rudimentary knowledge of the determinants of human performance, and it was impossible to conceal from participants that they had been at work for 15–16 hours when they entered the fatigued condition[19]. Irrespective of the ability to blind participants, it is particularly important that those who are rating performance should be ignorant in terms of the

Table 18.6 Subject–experimenter effects as sources of artefact in behavioural science[3,4]

Effect	Description
Experimenter expectancy	Experimenter's expectations are conveyed unintentionally to the research subject and influence the results.
Experimenter characteristics	Age, gender, ethnicity, friendliness, attitudes and status of experimenter may all influence the subject's behaviour. This provides a threat to the generalizability (external validity) of the findings.
Cues from the context of the experiment	This includes aspects of the experiment such as instructions given to the subject, the room where the experiment takes place. These are also called demand characteristics of the experimental situation.
Effect due to roles taken by the subject	Subjects volunteer for research for personal reasons and frequently try to place themselves in a positive light, particularly if there is a power imbalance with the researcher or investigator. For example: ◆ Good subject (tries to please the experimenter) ◆ Negativistic subject (tries to disprove research hypothesis) ◆ Apprehensive subject (anxiety influences performance)

participants' experimental condition. The so-called Hawthorne Effect is a well known example of the placebo effect whereby participation in a study of workplace productivity resulted in performance improvement irrespective of the intervention (page 112[4]).

Randomization of participants into treatment and control groups, with matching for covariates (e.g. anxiety) or inclusion of covariates in the statistical analysis, are designs that can reduce the risk of artefact.

18.3.1.3 Statistical risk

There are two important statistical risks to address.

◆ The first is the risk of reporting a statistically significant effect that does not actually exist. This is the Type I error and a probability (known as α) of 0.05 is the traditional threshold for an acceptable level of risk. The Type I error is usually well understood and does not warrant further discussion, except to note that it has been suggested that an appropriate value for α in exploratory studies is 0.1 rather than 0.05[21].

◆ The second risk is of failing to find a statistically significant difference when an effect is really present. This is the Type II error and the probability of this (known as β) is typically expressed in terms of statistical power, the probability of finding an effect if it exists. Power is thus mathematically defined as $1-\beta$. The traditional value for acceptable power is 0.8, i.e. a 20% chance of failing to detect an experimental effect that is really present.

The importance of power rests in the interpretation of negative studies and in the planning of studies, particularly the calculation of sample sizes. Statistical power has three determinants[20]; α (the probability of making a Type I error), the effect size (the degree to which the hypothesized phenomenon exists) and the reliability of the sample results. The power of a study will increase if α is reduced, if the effect size is increased, or if the reliability of the sample results are increased (through either increasing the sample size or reducing the variability of the data)[20]. These are relatively simple concepts. For example in a paired t-test, the t statistic is calculated as the difference between group means divided by the standard error of difference scores, and a large t-value is more likely to be statistically significant for any given value of α. The standard error (i.e. the numerator in the calculation of t) is equal to the standard deviation divided by the square root of the sample size. Hence an increase in the difference in means (effect size), an increase in sample size or reduction in standard deviation will increase the likelihood of finding a statistically significant effect (i.e. will increase the power). Although the concepts are intuitive the actual calculation of power is complex and requires the use of either an appropriate statistical programme or nomograms such as those published by Cohen[20].

18.3.2 Validity and reliability in qualitative research

Thus far this chapter has focussed upon issues related to quantitative research methods. A brief divergence is now presented to introduce the application of validity and reliability within the context of qualitative research methods. A variety of approaches have been described to ensure validity (Table 18.7) and reliability (Table 18.8) in qualitative research. There is a continuum in the application of these concepts to qualitative research. At one pole is the extreme relativist view whereby all research perspectives are viewed as unique, valid in their own terms, and there are multiple perspectives[22]. However an extreme relativist view limits the extent to which finding can be generalized and so it is important to be aware of less extreme positions that are expressed as standards that are acceptable to traditional biomedical journals[23,24]. Although the research paradigm and the tools that are applied are different from quantitative research, the basic meaning of reliability and validity are unchanged.

Table 18.7 Validation techniques in qualitative research[25,26]

Method	Description
Triangulation	The use of more than one measure (data source and type, method of investigation, researcher, or theory) to corroborate the interpretation.
Theoretical sampling strategies	Theory regarding the phenomenon under investigation is used to drive sampling, rather than statistical considerations. Subjects are sampled until 'saturation' is reached (no new themes are evident) and a search is made for contradictory, outlying or negative cases, and particular attention is paid to these.
Respondent validation	The research participant's interpretation is included in the analysis.
Check for researcher effects	Personal and intellectual biases that have shaped the researcher's thinking, including the relationship between researcher and subjects and the context of the research.

18.4 Ethics, deception, and conflicts of interests

There are important ethical issues to address in research involving human participants within the simulation environment. Campbell *et al.*[27] provide a practical framework that breaks the ethical issues of research into four parts: scientific validity, risk and benefit analysis, the provision of information and obtaining consent, and the presence of procedures to ensure ethical conduct. This section focuses upon risks and benefits, and information and consent, having assumed that scrutiny by research funding agencies and ethics committees will ensure scientific validity and the presence of procedures to ensure ethical conduct.

18.4.1 Risks and benefits

In research that offers no specific advantage to the participants there must be minimal if any risk associated with participation. One of the assumptions underlying simulation is that it causes no harm. This is unproven, and in research involving the evaluation of performance, there could be unforeseen effects such as potential risks attributable to emotional response to the experience. The risks can be difficult to determine and this requires careful and unbiased peer review during the planning stages. There are a range of potential solutions. For example in studies of the effects of sleep loss upon performance, it has been the author's practice to use an anonymous third party reporting mechanism to monitor the safety of participants and others, and to provide taxis for fatigued participants.

Table 18.8 Evaluation of reliability in qualitative research[25,26]

Method	Description
Coder reliability	In studies where data are classified (coded) into different phenomenological categories, inter-coder and intra-coder reliability should be checked, and typically be in the 90% range (reliability = number of agreements / total number of agreements and disagreements)(page 64[25])
Clear audit trail	A clear description of the process of data collection and analysis, including the relationship between these processes, so that the reader can decide if the process is valid, and can potentially replicate the study.

18.4.2 **Information and consent**

The provision of sufficient information for participants to make a free choice to participate in the absence of coercion is a fundamental ethical principle. However, research involving human behaviour is fraught with a dilemma caused by potential effects that the provision of information may have upon participants' subsequent performance. A controversial solution to this problem is to undertake some form of deceptive research. Deception consists of a spectrum ranging from total misrepresentation of the purpose of the research through to failure to mention all the details and to undertake covert or unobtrusive measures. The practice is controversial because it involves a breach of participants' trust by the investigator, and because participants cannot give bona fide consent when information has been deliberately withheld. For those unfamiliar with the concepts of experiments with deception, it is worth spending time reading about the obedience experiments of Stanley Milgram. Three criteria have been suggested in the justification of deceptive studies (page 503[3]):

- ◆ The investigators are able to convince external reviewers that there is no alternative.
- ◆ The degree of deception is warranted.
- ◆ The magnitude of potential harm is low.

To minimize any potential harm, it is important to ensure that participants are appropriately debriefed after the experience. The details of what constitutes appropriate debriefing are ill defined. For example, by whom should it be done and when? From the perspective of the participant it should be done at the end of the experimental session, whereas from the perspective of the investigator, it should be after all participants have been studied. The extent of any harm and the effectiveness of the debriefing should probably be evaluated during a pilot study.

Even in the presence of full information, the process whereby consent is obtained deserves special consideration because frequently there is an unequal relationship between the investigators and the participants. For example numerous studies have been undertaken by specialist anaesthetists using anaesthesia registrars as the experimental participants. In special relationships such as these it can be difficult to ensure that consent is freely given, and for participants to be confident that they can withdraw at any time without prejudice. At the Sleep-Wake Research Centre it has been our practice to engage a third party in the recruitment process when undertaking sensitive research. This ensures that those who decline to participate remain anonymous to the investigators[28].

Another problem with research in the simulation environment is the presence of conflicts of interest. A conflict of interest is defined as any situation in which an investigator may have an interest or obligation that can bias, or be perceived to bias, a research project (page 536[3]). There are numerous examples in the anaesthesia literature where investigators have undertaken research using equipment in which they have a financial interest. Although situations of this sort present a conflict of interest, it needs to be acknowledged that much of the progress in simulation has been achieved because investigators showed enterprise and were willing to take a personal financial risk. However, when the investigator stands to gain in a material way based upon the research findings (such as an increase in sales if their product is shown to be effective) I would argue that it is better for the research to be undertaken by third parties who do not have a financial interest in the tool being studied.

18.5 **Conclusion**

The purpose of this chapter is to provide an introduction to simulation-based research and to emphasize common concerns and flaws in experimental methods. The main focus has been upon quantitative research methods, the dominant research paradigm. Qualitative research methods are touched upon and they should to be considered, particularly if the study is exploratory. Many of the problems that arise in simulation-based research relate to difficulties caused by the need to measure theoretical constructs rather than physical quantities and the need to ensure that the measurement tools are both valid and reliable. The need to use experimental methods from behavioural and educational research cannot be overemphasized, particularly the need to ensure that there is appropriate experimental control and the measurement of relevant covariates. This requires a clear understanding of the related literature. It is important to calculate statistical power, firstly to determine sample size and secondly to appropriately analyse negative finding (e.g. no difference between treatments). Although placed at the end of the chapter, the matter of ethics needs to be considered early in the planning of research endeavours. Ethical considerations are particularly critical in research where there is likely to be no direct benefit to the participants, and where there is often a power imbalance between the investigator and the participant. These are frequent considerations in simulation-based research, particularly where participant performance is under investigation, and so the ethical concerns should be addressed as part of the initial assessment of the feasibility of a research project.

References

1. Soanes C, Stevenson A, Eds. (2006). *Concise Oxford English Dictionary*. 11th ed. Oxford: Oxford University Press.
2. Denzin NK, Lincoln YS, Eds. (1994). *Handbook of Qualitative Research*. Thousand Oaks: Sage Publications.
3. Kazdin AE (2003). *Research Design in Clinical Psychology*. Fourth ed. Boston: Allyn and Bacon.
4. Rosenthal R, Rosnow RL (1991). *Essentials of Behavioral Research: Methods and Data Analysis*. 2nd ed. Boston: McGraw-Hill.
5. Martin KM, Larsen PD, Segal R, Marsland CP (2004). Effective nonanatomical endoscopy training produces clinical airway endoscopy proficiency. *Anesth Analg* **99**(3): 938–44.
6. Rosenblatt MA, Abrams KJ (2002). The use of a human patient simulator in the evaluation of and development of a remedial prescription for an anesthesiologist with lapsed medical skills. *Anesth Analg* **94**(1): 149–53.
7. Anderson BJ, Holford NH (1997). Rectal paracetamol dosing regimens: determination by computer simulation. *Paediatr Anaesth* **7**(6): 451–5.
8. Hethcote HW, Van Ark JW, Karon JM (1991). A simulation model of AIDS in San Francisco: II. Simulations, therapy, and sensitivity analysis. *Math Biosci* **106**(2): 223–47.
9. Dawson S (2006). Procedural simulation: a primer. *Radiology* **241**(1): 17–25.
10. McGaghie WC, Issenberg SB, Petrusa ER, Scalese RJ (2006). Effect of practice on standardised learning outcomes in simulation-based medical education. *Med Educ* **40**(8): 792–7.
11. Kirk J, Miller ML (1986). *Reliability and Validity in Qualitative Research*. Newbury Park: Sage Publications.
12. Jones R (1995). Why do qualitative research? *British Medical Journal* **311**: 2.
13. Kazdin AE (ed.) (2003). *Methodologic Issues and Strategies in Clinical Research*. Third ed. Washington, DC: American Psychological Association.
14. Holland R, Hains J, Roberts JG, Runciman WB (1993). Symposium–The Australian Incident Monitoring Study. *Anaesth Intensive Care* **21**(5): 501–5.
15. DeVellis RF (2003). *Scale Development Theory and Application*. Thousand Oaks Sage Publications.
16. Joint Committee on Standards for Educational and Psychological Testing of the American Educational Research Association, the American Psychological Association, and the National Council on Measurement in Education (1999). *Standards for educational and psychological testing. 1st Impression 2002*. Washington, DC: American Educational Research Association.

17. Clark L, Watson D (1995). Constructing validity: Basic issues in scale development. In: Kazdin AE (ed.). *Methodological Issues and Strategies in Clinical Research*. Third ed. Washington, DC: American Psychological Association: 207–31.

18. Devitt JH, Kurrek MM, Cohen MM, *et al.* (1998). Testing internal consistency and construct validity during evaluation of performance in a patient simulator. *Anesth Analg* **86**: 1160–4.

19. Garden AL (2006). *Fatigue, Sleep Loss and Anaesthetists' Performance: Subjective Effects and Simulation Studies*. PhD Thesis Dunedin: University of Otago.

20. Cohen J (1988). *Statistical Power Analysis for the Behavioural Sciences*. 2nd ed. Hillside, New Jersey: Lawrence Erlbaum Associates.

21. Cohen J (1992). A power primer. *Psychological Bulletin* **112**: 155–9.

22. Hammersley M (2004). Some reflections on ethnography and validity. In: Seale C, Ed. *Social Research Methods – A Reader*. London: Routledge Student Readers: 241–5.

23. Mays N, Pope C (2000). Qualitative research in health care. Assessing quality in qualitative research. *British Medical Journal* **320**(7226): 50–2.

24. http://resources.bmj.com/bmj/authors/checklists-forms/qualitative-research, accessed 10 March 2007.

25. Miles MB, Huberman AM (1994). *Qualitative Data Analysis*. 2nd ed. Thousand Oaks: Sage.

26. Pope C, Ziebland S, Mays N (2000). Analysing qualitative data. *British Medical Journal* **320**: 114–6.

27. Campbell A, Gillett G, Jones G (2001). *Medical Ethics*. 3rd ed. Oxford: Oxford University Press.

28. Gander P, Purnell H, Garden A, Woodward A (2007). Work patterns and fatigue-related risk among junior doctors. *Occupational and Environmental Medicine* **64**:733–8.

Part 4

Applied simulation

Chapter 19

Simulation in nursing education and practice

John M O'Donnell and Joseph S Goode Jr.

Overview

- Simulation in nursing education is not a new concept but until recently was a relatively obscure educational methodology.
- As technology has advanced in step with access, use of human simulators and companion curriculum has penetrated all levels of nursing education.
- There are multiple educational entry paths to nursing and it is essential to be familiar with these before identifying appropriate targets for simulation and designing curriculum.
- The current US and international nursing shortages are adversely impacting healthcare delivery, and projected future shortages argue for the leveraging of technologies such as simulation for education, retention, and credentialing.
- The history of previous simulation efforts in nursing education, such as the Simulation Gaming Movement, can offer insights into current efforts at integration of mannequin based simulation into curricula, as well as horizontal and vertical curricular development.
- A variety of educational theories, models or frameworks are available to guide the development of nursing simulation educational and research programmes.
- Examples of nursing simulation for addressing specific clinical problems include developing communication skills, part-task training, full-task training, objective structured clinical exams (OSCE), and simulation training for nursing specialty practice.

19.1 Introduction

The use of simulation is neither new nor unfamiliar for most nursing educators. As professionals we have not been crediting many common nursing educational activities as 'simulation'. Role playing and other forms of nonpatient interaction have long held a role in nursing educational approaches, with static mannequins such as 'Mrs Chase' in the 1930s foreshadowing the evolution of SimOne®, the first high fidelity simulator by three decades[1–3]. The introduction of advanced, yet affordable, patient simulators has encouraged their widespread acquisition, and pushed nursing educators to explore this educational approach. While simulation training is not a panacea or whole-cloth replacement for traditional education in either the clinical or classroom settings, thought leaders in nursing education perceive the approach as supplementing clinical training, enriching current clinical experience, and in reinforcing didactic principles.

Advantages for use of simulation education in healthcare have been described by many authors and include:

◆ Hands-on experience with rare events

◆ Hands-on experience with high-risk patient situations

◆ Guaranteed exposure to clinical experiences that are difficult to obtain

◆ Developing and establishing benchmarks for performance, which can be measured in the simulated environment and potentially transferred to patient care

◆ Flexibility in that the experiences are not contingent upon or designed around the care of real patients

◆ Similar context to actual clinical experience

◆ Opportunity for self-reflection and assessment (built into debriefing) absent in the clinical setting because of practicality

◆ Practise of both cognitive and psychomotor skills in patient care in an environment that is safer for provider and patient[4–15].

In this section we will describe simulation targets in nursing, approaches to curricular integration, education theories and models supporting approaches, important nursing simulation efforts described in the literature, and specific approaches that have been used in research and nursing educaton.

19.2 Target audience for use of simulation in nursing

19.2.1 Overview of nursing education in the USA

Nursing is a profession in evolution, with multiple levels in the nursing educational ladder that extend from Nurse Aides to Advanced Practice Nurses (Table 19.1). A key advantage in using simulation is the ability to offer nursing students across this hierarchy a consistent and reproducible experience similar to clinical practice.

Nursing education encompasses a broad spectrum of backgrounds and settings for training. Practice also varies widely between institutions and states. Standard didactic education may be efficient, but it lacks proven effectiveness in assuring skill acquisition and is weak in supporting social or contextual learning. The breadth and scope of nursing practice combined with increasingly limited access in training with some patient populations (paediatrics, obstetrics, critically ill, etc) represents an opportunity to guarantee all students at least a surrogate experience in personally managing problems that arise in specialized populations.

Nursing is at its core a hands-on profession. However, nurses entering practice are not required to demonstrate skills that would be considered essential to practice. What would be necessary to effect this change would be consensus standards constituting benchmark skills or abilities. Key challenges to such standardization are the many entry points into the profession and the resultant lack of homogeneity in degree preparation. In the USA, State Boards of Nursing (SBN) typically establish the passing level on the professional nurse (RN) and practical nurse (LPN) licensure exams (NCLEX RN and NCLEX PN) within each state – however, this is a knowledge or knowledge application to clinical scenarios-type examination that does not contain a practice component. Other professions are now considering the use of hands-on demonstration simulation for entry level and recertification exams for their members. How, when and in what manner this hands-on, competence demonstration approach might be used in the nursing profession is an important question, given the large number of nursing professionals, the diversity of educational preparation, and the variability within state regulated scopes of practice.

Table 19.1 Overview of US nursing educational preparation and licensure

Title	License or certification	CE required	Educational background and length	Clinical role
Nurse Aide (NA)[194]	Yes (by state)	Yes (12 hours/year)	State approved programmes require minimum of 75 hours including 16 hours of supervised clinical	Clinical support services including direct patient care (bathing, transfers, vital signs and clinical procedures such as bladder sonography, and simple dressings)
Licensed Practical Nurse National Federation of LPN[195, 196]	Licensure – NCLEX-PN	Varies by State	Technical, Vocational, Hospital-Based Programmes – 1 year	Clinical Care Under Supervision of RN, MD, DMD
Diploma (RN)[197]	Licensure – NCLEX-RN	Varies by State	2–3 years Hospital-based, skill-focused, minimal theory base	Full scope of RN practice as defined by SBN
Associate Degree (RN, AD)[197]	Licensure – NCLEX-RN	Varies by State	2–3 years Community college or nursing school-based, skill-focused, moderate theory base	Full scope of RN practice as defined by SBN
Bachelor of Science Degree (RN, BSN)[197]	Licensure – NCLEX-RN	Varies by State	4-year, University-based degree. Significant theory base combined with practicum.	Full scope of RN practice as defined by SBN
Advanced Practice Nurse (Certified Registered Nurse Anaesthetist (CRNA), Nurse Practitioner (NP), NurseMidwife, Clinical Nurse Specialist (CNS)[197]	Licensure – NCLEX-RN Specialty license (APRN) or specialty certification (NP) by State. CRNA credential recognized by all states	Yes (by specialty)	Masters or Doctorate Degree	Expanded scope of practice defined by SBN, clinical institution, and professional organization.

19.2.2 US nursing shortage and simulation

There are currently 2.9 million nurses in the US workforce. Despite this seemingly impressive number, the average nurse's age is 48 years, with up to 40% of practicing nurses projected to retire in the next 5 years[16–18]. As a result, the healthcare system is again facing a severe nursing shortage, with experts predicting a deficit of as many as 1 million RNs by the year 2020[16,17,19].

Factors contributing to the current US nursing shortage include nurses leaving the workforce, nursing injury, increased patient acuity, expansion of services, the aging nursing workforce and the aging of the patient population. Several authors have linked inadequate RN staffing or nurse to patient ratios with poor patient outcome and nursing burnout[20–24]. The education system charged with meeting the demand presented by this impending nursing shortage includes over 1500 schools for professional (RN) nursing education in the USA, with most holding membership in one of two collegiate associations. These organizations are the American Association of Colleges of Nursing (AACN) and the National League for Nursing (NLN). Both organizations provide educational support and access to affiliated accreditation services. Because the US Department of Education (USDE) requires that accreditation is an independent function, the two organizations are affiliated with independent accrediting arms that must adhere to USDE standards. Respectively, the AACN is associated with the Commission on Collegiate Nursing Education (CCNE) while the NLN is affiliated with the NLN Accrediting Commission (NLNAC). The AACN has published a series of *Essentials* documents for baccalaureate, masters, PhD and now doctorate of nursing practice (DNP) education. In contrast, the NLN has developed the *Excellence in Nursing Education Model* ©, which is more generic and outlines eight core elements for any successful nursing educational programmeme to achieve and sustain excellence[25]. These guidelines are valuable in the development of curriculum and mission, and ultimately are used by the accrediting bodies in assessment of the overall quality of educationalprogrammes. However, neither the *Essentials* guidelines or the NLN elements specifically prescribe the exact psychomotor, communication, attitude or critical thinking skill sets each student or nurse must possess prior to sitting for an examination such as the NCLEX (RN licensure). Each individual school is thus responsible for meeting the demands of both their accreditors and the State Board of Nursing regulators. Ultimately, individual nursing schools determine the mix of theory and specific practice skill that students must acquire through classroom and clinical experiences. Predictably, this system of individualized implementation carries the risk of preparation variability related to patient care. Annual surveys by the National Council of State Boards of Nursing (NCSBN) continue to indicate that a substantial percentage of new graduates (17.7–19.7%) from both RN and LPNprogrammes report difficulty with patient care assignments. Areas of inadequate preparation cited are:

- working effectively within the healthcare team
- analysing multiple types of data when making patient-related decisions
- delegating tasks to others
- understanding underlying pathophysiology related to a patient's condition
- difficulty caring for large groups of patients[26,27].

These activities have potential for simulation education targeting with the added advantage of addressing a valid 'real world' need.

19.2.3 International nursing shortage

Compounding the US nursing crisis is a concurrent global nursing shortage. This shortage is associated with increases in migration, both within countries and across national borders[28,29]. The scarcity of healthcare professionals such as nurses has been highlighted as one of the key obstacles in attaining the United Nations Millennium Development Goals (MDG)[29]. Campbell notes that some sub-Saharan African countries have actually regressed in areas that are significant indices of health, in no small part resulting from a migration of skilled nurses[28]. While this migration is not new, the targeted, aggressive recruitment by developed countries of nurses from developing countries is a new phenomenon[28,30]. The World Health Organization (WHO) and the International Council of Nurses (ICN) have both taken strong positions against the practice of 'nurse poaching'[31]. It is difficult to gauge the exact numbers of migrating nurses because of inconsistency in reporting, and often inferences must be made indirectly. For example, UK work permit approval data show that the primary source of migrant workers in the UK is from India, with 12% of those targeted to the healthcare sector[29]. Kline states that the primary 'donor' countries are Australia, Canada, the Philippines, South Africa and the UK, with the primary recipient countries being Australia, Canada, Ireland, the UK and the USA[32]. While this list is suggestive of some circular mobility of the available nursing pool, making it difficult to quantify, it is clear that Australia, the UK and the USA are the final destination for the largest number of migrating nurses[32]. The impact of nurse migration and the nursing shortage in the developed world is of concern, but the effect on already fragile healthcare infrastructures in the developing world has the potential for creating further increases in the healthcare equity gap[30,32,33]. Part of the reason for the disproportionate impact is that the front-line provider role of the nurse is even more critical in the developing world[29]. Some of the reasons for the nursing shortage are the same in both the developed and developing world[28,34,35]. Migration is usually attributed to low pay, job risk (i.e. infectious diseases such as HIV or TB), inadequate resource planning resulting in increased work loads, poor infrastructure, poor working conditions, and limited opportunities for advancement[28]. Combining with these problems in the developing world is the potential for unstable political climates, international conflicts, high rates of violent crime, and excessive taxation levels. Often nursing jobs are viewed as a major source of returning currency, as money is frequently sent home to support relatives left behind. Some nations actually develop nurse training programmes with the goal of exporting the nurses, much like a commodity[28,32,33]. This practice, however, is beginning to backfire under the new realities of the international nursing supply and demand equation, because even former 'export' nations are suffering from healthcare workforce deficits[31,33].

Many solutions have been suggested, including innovative programmes for expanding the nurse force supply, and attempts to share nursing resources on a regional level[28]. One problem exacerbating the shortage is that traditional nursing curricula often don't match healthcare needs in developing countries. For example, western models of nursing education focus on areas such as acute treatment of myocardial infarction because of the prevalence of coronary artery disease. However, disease distribution and mortality in developing nations typically arises from diseases like malaria, acute respiratory infections, and diarrheal illness[28]. In refocusing developing country nursing curriculum, a consideration for addressing this issue might include education of highly effective advanced practice nurses. In the USA, the expansion of the role of advanced practice nurses has resulted in positive health outcomes and demonstrated both efficacy and efficiency in patient care[36–38]. In developing countries, advanced practice nurses could be used to supervise substitute healthcare workers who are already being used. Developed nations also need to work cooperatively to stem the flow, perhaps agreeing to help facilitate the reintegration of returning nurses to their home countries. Some countries, such as the UK, have issued codes of practice for ethical recruitment[29]. Contributing to the crisis in developing countries is the concurrent loss of educators, with the global nursing shortage also being reflected in the shortage of nursing faculty[32,33,35,39]. Distance education could be used to address the need for both primary and continuing education in developing nations[28]. Rosenkoetter recommends aggressive programmes to fill faculty positions, encourage international faculty exchanges and to use technology and distance learning to facilitate nursing education[35]. While many authors call for the use of technology to help in stemming the tide of nurse migration from the developing to the developed world, there is little in the literature to suggest exactly how this would be implemented.

In areas where the infrastructure could support it, the use of distance education technology combined with simulation could be useful. For example, O'Donnell and Goode are currently investigating whether the type of intravenous catheter insertion training given to student registered nurse anaesthetists results in differences in intravenous catheter insertion skill in the real world[40]. One arm of this protocol explored the use of the Laerdal Inc. Virtual IV™ (VirIV) system with an instructor interacting with the trainee via internet videoconferencing software (Apple, Inc. iChat™). Data collection is ongoing, but if it can be shown that no significant difference exists between the videoconference group and standard training groups, this could serve as a model to expand the reach of a limited number of nursing instructors using specific simulation and communication tools.

19.2.4 Nursing target summary

Simulation education for nurses presents the opportunity for benchmarking core nursing skills ranging from simple task performance to complex interventions requiring advanced decision making ability. Acceptance of this simulation approach as an evaluation of competency is mixed, with one study indicating that only 41.9% of surveyed undergraduate and 34.9% of graduate nursing programmes agree with this concept[41]. There currently is significant variability in educational preparation of entry level nurses, with differences in accreditation standards and both a national and international nursing shortage. In our analysis, it is unlikely that the concept of 'standardized practice demonstration' as a component of licensing, practice or accreditation will arise from the 'bottom-up' at the educational programmeme level. It is more likely to be driven 'top down' by nursing professional associations and visionary leaders who recognize the value of this approach in demonstrating quality and competency among their constituents. This pathway would be analogous to initiatives within the medical community. Given the rapidly changing healthcare environment and the ongoing momentum of the national and international patient safety movements, it is likely that pressure to move toward competency-based training and education using simulation will also arise from public pressure or governmental regulation[42–44].

19.3 Integration of simulation into nursing curricula

Integration of simulation education into nursing curricula remains a challenge for nurse educators, from novice to expert nursing educators[45–50]. The concept of integration requires planning and a priore faculty time allocation in order to realize the full potential of simulation resources. Table 19.2 summarizes papers describing curricular integration of nursing simulation content categorized by student level and country of origin. In 2004, Nehring et al. published survey data from a small sample (n=34) of nursing programmes that had purchased a Medical Education Technologies Inc. Human Patient Simulator (METI-HPS®).[41] Community college-based nursing programmes reported using their simulator more frequently for advanced medical-surgical courses while university-based programmes reported more frequent use in basic skills courses. The most common applications reported across both undergraduate and graduate nursing programmes were in teaching assessment skills (90.5%) and in managing critical events (85.7%). University nursing programmes offered more content on management of rare conditions than did community college programmes (66.7% versus 8.3%)[41]. Most respondents indicated that they were using simulation as a component within their overall clinical time requirements (57.1%), supporting the use of simulation as a way to fill gaps in available clinical experiences. How simulation resources are being used within an overall curriculum is also of interest. Nehring reported that most community college and university nursing programmes were using their HPS for less than 5% of their overall curriculum. While 58.1% of programmes reported good faculty acceptance

Table 19.2 Summary of papers describing curricular integration of nursing simulation content

Author	Year	Country	Educational group targeted	Type of paper	Brief
Hoffman	2007	US	Student – UGN	Educational Research	Use of standardized knowledge tool (BKAT-6) to demonstrate effectiveness of simulation education in generating area specific knowledge improvement.
Alinier	2006	UK	Student – UGN	Educational Research	Use of high fidelity simulation exposure to demonstrate change in performance on OSCE exam.
Diefenbeck	2006	US	Student – UGN	Descriptive	Describes development of a nurse residency model incorporating simulation for improved competency, increased accountability, resource efficiency and patient safety.
Kneebone	2006	UK	Student,Professional – PN,MD	Descriptive	Use of patient focused simulation. Combines SP with HPS
O'Donnell	2006	US	Student – UGN, GN	Descriptive	Describes integration of simulation across graduate and undergraduate curriculum
Parr	2006	US	Student – UGN	Descriptive	Describes integration of simulation in an undergraduate critical care nursing course
Robertson	2006	US	Student – UGN	Descriptive	Describes integration of simulation in an undergraduate obstetric nursing course
Schoening	2006	US	Student – UGN	Educational Research	Study of the integration of simulation in an undergraduate obstetric nursing course. Focus is on the role of the educator in promoting outcome.
Wakefield	2006	UK	Student – UGN, MS	Educational Research	Describes teams of nursing and medical students using patient communication skills to break bad news
Wilford	2006	UK	Student – UGN, MS	Review Paper	Review of simulation history and integration into UK nursing curriculum.
Wisborg	2006	Norway	Professional – PN, MD	Observational study	Describes use of low fidelity simulators in training of multidisciplinary trauma teams Focus on communication, cooperation and leadership
Decker	2005	US	Student – UGN	Descriptive	Describes integration of a high fidelity simulation exercise in mass casualty responses into the undergraduate curriculum

Continued

Table 19.2 (continued) Summary of papers describing curricular integration of nursing simulation content

Author	Year	Country	Educational group targeted	Type of paper	Brief
Hravnak	2005	US	Student – GN	Descriptive	Describes integration of high fidelity simulation into the technical and cognitive preparation of ACNP and CNS students.
Jeffries	2005	US	Student, Professional – UGN, GN, PN	Descriptive	Describes elements of a framework for nursing simulation curricular development
O'Donnell	2005	US	Student – UGN	Descriptive	Describes integration of simulation in undergraduate obstetric and paediatric nursing courses
Nehring	2004	US	Student, Professional – UGN, GN, PN	Educational Research	Presents cross-sectional data on 34 Schools of Nursing using the METI human patient simulator (HPS).
Seropian	2004	US	Educators	Descriptive	Describes design of facilities, faculty training and curriculum in developing a simulation educational programme
Spunt	2004	US	Student – UGN, GN	Descriptive	Describes integration of a mock code program incorporating undergraduate and graduate students
Alinier	2003	UK	Student – UGN	Descriptive	Describes the use of part-task simulation training/skill practice incorporated within OSCE exam.
Griffiths	2003	US	Professional – PN	Descriptive	Describes a programme using human simulation as a component of the return of inactive nurses to bedside practice
Scherer	2003	US	Student – GN	Descriptive	Describes integration of high fidelity simulation into the preparation of ACNP students
Nehring	2002	US	Student – UG, GN	Review Paper	Overview of capability and use of human patient simulators in technical skills, competency based instruction and critical incident management

Content categorized by student level and country of origin. UGN = Undergraduate Nursing; GN = Graduate Level Nursing; PN = Professional Nurse; MD = Medical Doctor; MS = Medical Student.

of the technology, 93.8% of schools indicated that no more than a quarter of their faculty actually used the HPS, with 75.8% indicating that only one faculty member was primarily responsible for oversight and running of the simulator. Further, Nehring's data indicates that often there is no extra compensation, either in monetary terms or in release time, for taking on this large responsibility.[41] While limited by numbers and the selected population (only purchasers of the METI simulator), the overall picture painted by Nehring's study seemed to be that of much interest in simulation, but no consistent approach in how to prioritize use, develop faculty or gain release time for development. In addition, without succession planning, those facilities dependent on a single 'simulation expert' to run everything are at risk of having their programmes fail should the expert be lost due to death, injury or new employment.

19.3.1 Historical perspective: the simulation gaming movement and nursing education

As early as 1915, John Dewey (an early and influential 20th century humanist and educational scientist) observed that in society, learning occurs incidentally by day-to-day social interactions and formally through systems devised to teach societal newcomers. Dewey was intrigued by the role of play (or games) in the acquisition of knowledge and attempted to integrate play and games into formal educational processes[51]. Starting in 1912, Gestalt theorists including Wertheimer, Koffka, Kohler and Lewin studied the relationship of thinking and experience. These scientists identified the value of reflective thinking in the process of active learning similar to that which occurs during simulation. Reflective learning helps to develop new insights into performance and should allow generalization with transference to new situations and conse-quent long-lasting learning[52]. Adult educational theory postulates that adult learners seek out and obtain critical information and that they also lean upon previous life experience to make decisions in context. Adults also prefer to engage in active problem solving activities as opposed to receiving abstract theoretical content[52].

In 1966 Cruikshank defined simulation as "realistic games to be played by participants in order to offer them lifelike problem solving experiences related to their present or future work"[53]. Abt (1970) proposed the 'Oxymoron-Learning Strategy' that focused on teaching learners through complex simulation games. A key element of this approach is to offer learners only a portion of the complete information needed to solve a problem. Learners then attempt to solve clinical problems in the simulated game with incomplete information, which is a consistent characteristic of real world interactions[52]. Greenblat in 1971 reported the use of simulation and games by sociologists as a useful tool in healthcare provider education and defined simulation as "an operating model of central features and elements of a real or proposed system, process or environment"[54]. In later work, Greenblat demonstrated broad utility and applications of 'simulation gaming' across multiple professional domains[55].

Coleman (1973) described 150 research projects conducted at Johns Hopkins over 7 years to establish that simulation games are an effective means of teaching students and conveying knowledge[56]. Lowe in 1975 first described the use of simulation games as a nursing educational methodology[57]. In a review of simulation gaming in nursing, Clark (1976) described a variety of situations where application of gaming theory to development of realistic, case-based scenario games patterned to simulate real world events can be used within the nursing educational process. Clark noted that a 'simulation game' offers distinct advantages of engagement and the ability to interact in a complex way with fellow players. Typically a 'simulation game' provides rules, constraints, goals/objectives and some payoff or 'win' delineated by the author or instructor. Students must assume 'roles' within the game and concepts such as cooperation, collaboration, competition, power dynamics, and wealth distribution can be incorporated[58]. Some simulation games can be stand-alone if directions and learning objectives are sufficiently inclusive, while others require up-front instruction and post-game debriefing. Simulation games can be constructed for small groups (2–3 players) or large groups (20–40 players). The game itself can be played in front of a group of observers or in a more private setting with all participants engaged. In a simulation game designed to impart experience in the nurse–patient interaction, one group of students can assume the role of the 'nurse' while a second group are 'patients', with the object of the game focused on appropriate nurse–patient communication, with points awarded for correct responses[58–60].

Advantages proposed for the simulation gaming approach are that simulation games:

- are preferred to traditional lecture
- effectively convey factual information
- can result in attitude change
- allow experiential learning
- are conducted in a safe environment
- provide a wider range of possible educational experiences
- provide a responsive environment that can give learners a sense of immediacy and involvement
- allow practice in decision making in a timeless environment
- provide experience of a high-cost environment in a low-cost model
- can be standardized
- can simultaneously teach in multiple domains (i.e. cognitive, psychomotor and affective)
- avoid the pitfalls of interruptions or unplanned events that occur in the clinical setting[58].

In a follow-up study, Clark found that students who acted in the role of instructors or teachers within the game environment learned significantly more than their counterparts who were assigned to the student role during the simulation[61].

Disadvantages or problems that were identified in simulation gaming include:

- lack of full understanding of the consequences of an action to a real situation
- lack of learner preparation for their role
- poorly designed games
- more time consumption on both the front and back ends for educators
- educators may not have the expertise to design the games
- educators may be uncomfortable with a new format
- lack of prospective evidence on validity and reliability
- lack of standardized development tools
- cost in development and administration of the simulation game[52,56,58,62].

Developments in the 'simulation gaming' movement parallel the current trajectory of mannequin-based simulation within nursing education. Nursing instructors using the simulation gaming approach were urged to consider the following practices that remain relevant for computer controlled part-task or full-task training simulators. These recommendations included:

- developing clear and specific learning objectives
- curricular fit
- structure of the activity
- availability of pre-tests and post-tests

- playability (does the activity work the same way each time or is it inconsistent?)
- pragmatics or operational issues (cost, time, available tools, training requirements, and space).

Maidment and Bronstein[63] published a paradigm for construction of simulation games. This paradigm is as appropriate today for mannequin-based simulation as it was over 30 years ago for simulation gaming efforts. Maidment and Bronstein recommended the following steps in developing and deploying an effective simulation game:

- elect an approach in light of course objectives and student needs
- prepare specific objectives
- collect data
- construct a model and rules governing the activity
- design specific materials
- execute
- evaluate all aspects.

Becker reviewed these principles of gaming and simulation and pointed out that two additional steps should be added to the initial planning for a simulation game: describing the object system to be simulated, and specifically determining and describing how the object system currently works[62].

The simulation gaming movement continues to enjoy advocates but never realized its full potential as a standard component within nursing educational programmes. Many elements of development, deployment and evaluation of both mannequin and game-based simulation overlap as previously described. However, there are several factors that were absent during the rise of the simulation gaming movement that promise sustainment of mannequin-based simulation. These include the:

- example of required simulation training in the airline industry and military[64,65]
- 1999 Institute of Medicine Report that advocated for use of simulation as a safety tool[42]
- emergence of the National Patient Safety Movement[44]
- Joint Commission sentinel event reporting process and resultant annual National Patient Safety Goals[43]
- requirement for more stringent provider credentialing and competency evaluation[66–68]
- ethical benefit of preliminary skill development occurring on non-human, non-animal models[69]
- increasingly litigious healthcare environment leading risk management departments to recognize the potential value of the approach[70–75].

19.3.2 Curricular integration and nursing education

Several themes emerge from the nursing simulation literature with respect to curricular integration and course development. Curricular mapping at both the undergraduate and graduate levels cross referenced with nationally recognized healthcare accreditation standards, nursing education accreditation requirements, and standards of practice and patient care can be used to inform this process. The movement from mapping to implementation can be assisted through use of constructs or frameworks that define best practices, primary components and key variables[8,15,47,49,76–78]. One approach would be to embed simulation throughout a curriculum where appropriate, instead of viewing simulation exercises as independent set-pieces[12,47,79]. Many educators describe use of simulation activities to help attain key clinical educational benchmarks or provide students with a surrogate experiential learning opportunity for rare but critical (or crisis) events[4,8,46,79–83]. Well constructed simulation educational experiences can allow measurement of knowledge, technical skill proficiency, familiarity with and use of complex equipment in a realistic context and development of decision making or critical thinking skills[46,84–87]. The need for integration and use of simulation to 'raise the bar' across nursing educational programmes is supported by several national reports that have cited deficiencies in nursing educational preparation that contribute to lack of preparation of graduates at a time of a worsening nursing shortage[26,27,86,88,89]. Compounding the problem is a shortage of nursing educators who already are burdened with teaching, research and service responsibilities. For these professionals, the prospect of developing and implementing a new teaching approach requiring additional skill and effort is daunting. Simulation has been identified by some advocates as a means of decreasing these faculty burdens. As a result, several myths have arisen surrounding simulation education including:

- simulation is an 'easy' fix
- simulation will save time
- simulation will save money
- good clinical and didactic educators will be good simulation educators
- simulation is efficient[90].

The reality is that simulation education is a new pedagogy and requires faculty effort and planning to produce a quality outcome. Simulation activities consume significant financial and personnel resources and most nursing educators, regardless of their experience in didactic or clinical education, must develop new skill-sets to be effective simulation educators. O'Donnell[91] describes integration of a crisis management programme in a nurse anaesthesia educational programme, with the development and planning time required for a 1-day (8-hour) course reported conservatively as 345 hours. The total time commitment ultimately is determined by the simulator used, the curriculum and faculty development required, the length and frequency of the course, and the number of student participants. Faculty development is key as many nursing faculty remain unfamiliar with the methods and are unsure of how to blend the simulation experience into the traditional educational model[47]. A thoughtful, deliberate and goal directed approach is needed to maximize value while avoiding over-burdening faculty. It is important for advocates to stress these inherent challenges and clearly state that development of quality simulation curricula is time-consuming in preparation and delivery. One approach in helping faculty begin the process is to encourage them to 'wrap' existing lecture content around a relatively simple simulation event that involves application of didactic concepts to clinical care. A group of scenarios can then be built that eventually form the nucleus of a full simulation course. In this stepwise approach, a body of simulation materials can be generated with direct integration of specific didactic content to the simulation training[47].

To address the nursing shortage, Schools of Nursing have attempted to increase admissions, with a resultant increase in competition for clinical opportunities. At the same time, patients are becoming more aware of their right to receive safe, high-quality care. The conjunction of these trends has resulted in greater complexity in designing appropriate clinical placements, especially when considering access to vulnerable populations and rare experiences. Carefully designed simulations have potential to provide realistic 'hands-on clinical training' in these areas and may represent the only opportunity for students to manage patient problems independently. This independent management element highlights a true superiority of simulation over actual clinical practice as there are ethical issues inherent when novice trainees develop initial clinical skill through practice on real patients[69]. Importantly, some nursing education programmes report that they consider simulation experiences a component of overall clinical time.[41] In an ideal world, specialty simulation education activities would closely parallel the student's exposure to the same experiences in the clinical setting. For example, integrated didactic and simulation paediatric components could immediately precede or coincide with the trainee's clinical rotations in paediatrics. This integration of didactic, simulation and clinical experience would assist with assimilation of content and promote deeper understanding. However, this approach may not be possible or practical depending on available faculty, space and simulator resources. Curricular mapping can help to guide development efforts, with each successive simulation experience building upon preceding ones. In both the undergraduate and graduate settings, as didactic knowledge base and clinical experience increase with progression through the curriculum, the richness and complexity of the simulation experience should also increase [92].

One intriguing option that can help to enhance the richness of the overall simulation programme is the use of virtual patients (VP)[93–95]. Virtual patients are computer-based, video-taped standardized patients (SPs) or computer generated figures (avatars) that present real-life conditions or problems. VPs allow a standardized and interactive experience and appear to be as effective as SPs in generating comfort, confidence, screening capability, and consequent skill[93]. Open access VP cases are available at Harvard and many other US medical schools, with most involving videotaped interaction with SPs[95, 96]. One aspect of the VP approach being explored at Birmingham City University the creation of a core set of computer avatars[97]. An avatar is a screen-based representation of a human, capable of relatively complex actions including facial expressions and physical responses. Students interact with, interview and can obtain pertinent data on these avatar-based VPs. Simulation mannequins can then be moulaged to represent these screen based 'patients' so that students can interact with the corporal form of the VP during the simulation environment encounter[98]. The potential for continuity of care is clear in this approach. Avatars can also have virtual physical changes that would be difficult to replicate realistically in a videotaped SP (i.e. long-term effects of chronic liver failure or diabetes). Properly integrated, these VPs could be followed across time (which can be compressed in the virtual world to accelerate aging and chronic disease affects) and through a curriculum allowing for reinforcement of concepts related to both short-term and long-term diagnosis, planning and intervention[99–103]. In a fully integrated model, students would interact with and care for these patients in an array of structured low and high fidelity simulation training sessions. At the graduate level, students in a variety of specialty disciplines would interact with the same set of VPs for both intradisciplinary and interdisciplinary simulation exercises, allowing for focus on critical patient safety issues including communication and coordination of complex plans of care.

19.3.3 Vertical and horizontal curricular development in nursing and across disciplines

The development of both vertical and horizontal training objectives can be used to maximize efficiency of a nursing simulation programme and its resources. Vertical simulation programme development means that a single simulation course or scenario can be used across novice to expert practitioners. This model requires development of level specific objectives, an increasing degree of complexity of the scenario, and matching level of autonomy of action within the scenario to the (presumed) capability of the student. For example, a single obstetric concept such as care of the postpartum patient can be used to develop benchmarks for management of basic problems such as postpartum cramping, epidural opioid-induced urticaria, recovery from epidural anaesthesia or even spinal headache. In the vertical model, novice nursing trainees would be expected to assess, identify and report issues to their instructor and to intervene, with direct assistance and supervision available. Clinically experienced trainees would be expected to complete these tasks more rapidly and independently with smooth coordination of other members of the team. Expert level participants would be expected to autonomously manage the situation and also be able to interact expertly with other healthcare team members in management of more severe complications that could be added, including excessive bleeding, hypotension, and complex psychosocial issues. Prompting of students for completion of the simulation tasks would be more directive for the novices and potentially absent for the experts, allowing a graded continuum for both completion of course objectives and in performance evaluation[8,77,78].

Horizontal simulation programme development can reflect interdisciplinary and multidisciplinary approaches within a simulation course or scenario, with objectives modified as appropriate for each professional domain. The horizontal development approach supports the ability for contemporaneous or combined simulation courses between nurses and other healthcare professionals. In interdisciplinary training, the methods of each profession are used in development and analysis while in the multidisciplinary model the methods of a single profession or discipline are used in development and analysis of the simulations[104]. An example of horizontal course development in simulation using both multidisciplinary and interdisciplinary approaches is in rapid response or medical emergency team (RRT/MET) simulation. In this training paradigm doctors, nurses and respiratory therapists share the overall objective of improved team performance in a code as measured by simulator 'survival' post-arrest event. A flat hierarchical model based on a process improvement or 'patient safety paradigm' is used, with roles being interchangeably assumed throughout the course by individuals from different professions. Because the overall goal of treatment is medical management of arrest or near arrest, the course has a multidisciplinary element. At the same time, participants from several professional domains are engaged in evaluation of important performance elements including communication, cooperation and teamwork. This diversity of input in evaluation also reflects elements of interdisciplinary training, as each professional domain contributes expertise according to their skill and professional experience[105].

19.4 Models or frameworks used in nursing simulation education and research

There are a variety of theories, models and constructs that can be used to structure nursing simulation educational development (Table 19.3). The value of a model or construct is to provide an educator-focused tool that helps to organize development and implementation of a student-centred simulation curriculum. Because nursing simulation educational pedagogy is in the developmental phase, these constructs or models remain diverse in nature, with no model demonstrating clear superiority through prospective evaluation. However, several authors have identified 'best practices' from nursing and healthcare literature that are useful in development and organization of mannequin-based simulation educational offerings. As mentioned in our earlier discussion, these 'best practices' closely parallel guidelines in development of high quality simulation games that were proposed in the 1960s and 1970s.

19.4.1 Nursing process

The first descriptions of nursing as a 'process' occurred in the late 1950s and early 1960s, eventually evolving from a three-step to a five or six-step process as outlined in the 1973 American Nurses Association (ANA) standards[106]. State Boards of Nursing were quick to integrate these nursing

Table 19.3 Summary of educational models used in nursing simulation with examples of application

Model	Description	Potential application	Simulation literature examples
Nursing Process	Five-step or six-step descriptive conceptualization of nursing practice	◆ Multilevel and multinational nursing simulation development (universally understood) ◆ Scenario-level design, programming and evaluation ◆ Critical thinking exercise	Annett (2000) O'Donnell et al.(2003, 2005, 2007) McCausland (2004)
Benner Theory and Dreyfuss Model	Acute care Nursing practice: movement from novice to expert	◆ Overall curricular development in nursing ◆ Novice trainees to experts ◆ Benchmarking ◆ Longitudinal training ◆ Critical thinking exercise	Issenberg (2005) Larew (2006)
Chickering & Gamson	Principles for good Practice in design of undergraduate Nursing education	◆ Development of simulation learning systems and courses ◆ Development of complementary didactic material	Jeffries (2005) Issenberg (2005) Bremner (2006)
Kolb Learning Styles	Movement along information processing and perception continuums	◆ Design of individualized or cohort-based learning activities ◆ Evaluation stratified by style ◆ Critical thinking exercise	Kolb (1984) Lowdermilk (1991) Sandmire (2000, 2004) Hauer (2005) Issenberg (2005)
Situated Learning Theory	Individual learner oriented. Knowledge accumulation across all human activity. Knowledge is socially embedded.	◆ Context specific curricular development ◆ Multidisciplinary training ◆ Critical thinking exercise	Cooper (2005) Devita (2005) Kneebone (2006) Wisborg (2006)
Hierarchical Task Analysis	Ergonomic theory and methodology for description, measurement and evaluation.	◆ Development of curriculum and evaluation tools in measuring performance of individuals, tasks, processes and systems	Annett (2000) O'Donnell (2006, 2007) Goode (2007)

process steps into Practice Acts as legitimate features in the role of a registered nurse[106]. The steps of the nursing process typically include: Assessment, Diagnosis, Planning, Implementation and Evaluation (ADPIE), with Outcomes Identification a common sixth step[107]. This nursing process construct is taught in the USA as well as in many other countries around the world. It has been incorporated into training guidelines by the Canadian Nurses Association and, in some form, throughout educational programmes in the UK[106].

The use of the nursing process as a model in structuring nursing simulation course content was first reported by O'Donnell in 2003. The ADPIE structure was used to individualize simulation programing in the Laerdal SimMan operating system (Fig. 19.1) in a manner that would resonate with nurses, regardless of the type of educational programme[108,109].

Burns *et al.* describe the use of the integrated ADPIE process combined with communication assessment (ADPIE-C) in teaching freshmen undergraduate students[109]. McCausland described the use of the nursing process to create objectives for developing a heart failure simulation and in evaluation of student performance[110]. The greatest benefit of using the nursing process as a model for development, implementation and assessment in nursing simulation pedagogy derives from its broad acceptance as a description of nursing practice and integration within nursing curriculum around the world. However, one weakness that we have observed during application in simulation education is the confusion surrounding the diagnosis step. A nursing diagnosis is a standardized description of the patient state matched with both antecedent conditions and potential nursing actions. Lists of standardized nursing diagnoses are overseen and published by

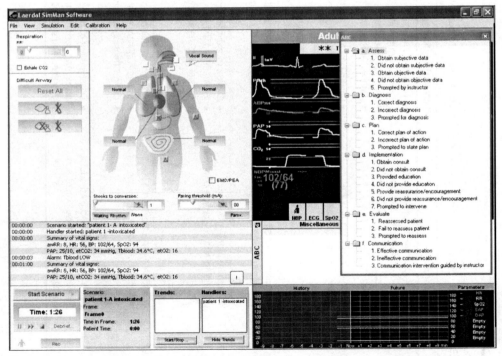

Fig. 19.1 Example of Nursing Process Programming as an 'ABC Handler' in Laerdal Inc. Simulation Software Interface. Patient is a college student who is both intoxicated and hypothermic after a motor vehicle collision. Reproduced with permission of Laerdal Medical.

an international organization (North American Nursing Diagnosis Association) dedicated to describing nursing work[111]. The concept of 'nursing diagnosis' remains prevalent in educational circles and has evolved because bedside nurses' scope of practice does not include making a medical diagnosis. Nursing diagnosis advocates purport that these statements are designed to empower nurses, standardize 'hospital languages', and provide clarity in patient care. Dorothy del Bueno, who developed the screen based PBDS evaluation system, suggests that nursing faces a 'crisis' with inadequate preparation of new nurses. del Bueno goes on to suggest that one important reason is the confusion and lack of clear communication that arises between providers because of the ongoing use of nursing diagnosis terminology[86]. Leonard describes failure in communication between providers as a lack of being 'in the same movie'. He identified this disconnect as a core component of many adverse outcomes[112]. The Joint Commission sentinel event and root cause analysis reporting programme cites failure of communication as the single most common factor in evolution of sentinel events[113].

While we are not advocating that entry-level nurses engage in independent medical diagnoses, we have found that use of the nursing diagnosis 'nomenclature' during simulation events is in fact confusing to both students and instructors. During initial attempts to use the nursing diagnosis language we also discovered that this 'language' is not shared by other members of the healthcare team. As an example, when simulating a cardiac event, the primary goal is to be able to clearly describe the patient problem and communicate with other health team members in order to implement timely and effective care. If nursing diagnosis terminology were used, the following diagnoses might all be considered acceptable when admitting this patient to an ICU setting: risk for infection, disturbed sleep pattern, deficient diversional activity, and decreased cardiac output[114]. In our use of nursing process for programing and evaluation, we encourage use of standard clinical terminology or physiological descriptors (tachycardia with hypotension, low cardiac output, cardiac problem) or if more appropriate, a simple factual description of the patient behavioural state (patient with chest pain) in place of the less direct nursing diagnosis terminology. In our model, we use common clinical terminology to promote improved student comprehension, allow direct connection to the clinical world and enhance ability to include disciplines outside of nursing as participants in the scenarios.

19.4.2 Critical thinking

An important nursing competency is to apply critical decision-making skills in routine and emergency situations. Critical thinking is typically defined as a 'thought process' that should directly correlate with expertise; as a nurse moves from the novice to expert level of practice, critical thinking skills should concurrently improve. Though its exact nature remains elusive, critical thinking is valued by both clinicians and educators as the core attribute needed for appropriate decision making[115,116]. This concept is supported by mid-range nursing theories such as those developed by Benner[116,117].

Many approaches have been advocated for development of this critical skill including computer simulations, videotaped vignettes, role playing and simple skills lab simulation. All have been inconsistent in demonstrating improvement in critical thinking[118–121]. A variety of standardized tools have been used in an attempt to measure critical thinking development in nursing and include the Watson Glaser Critical Thinking Appraisal (WGCTA), the Confidence in Critical Thinking Subscale of the California Critical Thinking Disposition Inventory (CCTDI), Performance Based Development System (PBDS), Elements of Thought Instrument (ETI) or the Nursing Performance Simulation Instrument (NPSI)[84,86,122–126]. Still, evaluation of critical thinking skill within the current learning and teaching environment remains a challenge despite the availability of these assessment tools. After more than 15 years of focus on critical thinking within the nursing educational system, some authors suggest that little or no progress has been demonstrated in improving graduate preparation and mastery of this skill, with as many as 65% of new nurses incapable of making correct clinical decisions when faced with a videotaped patient care scenario[86].

With thoughtful design, simulation sessions can be created presenting the student with a spectrum of patient problems requiring appropriate decision making and that can potentially stimulate critical thinking. Multiple authors have recommended using hands-on practice simulations to assist in the development of nurses critical thinking skills[46,79,82,127–130]. Most reports in this area are qualitative or descriptive and do not include quantitative measurement and evaluation of the critical thinking 'construct'. One challenge is to develop and deploy tools within simulations which can allow critical thinking pathways to be measured in a summative fashion. In this way, researchers can leverage the simulation environment to describe critical thinking development and skill of varying levels and types of providers. Several studies use outcome measures as surrogate markers for clinical thinking, showing improvement in clinical judgment and thus inferring improved critical thinking processes. In an exploratory study, Lasater describes the measurement of confidence, aptitude, skill, and experience as they relate to development of clinical judgment with the assumption that improved clinical judgment would reflect improved critical thinking.[76] Henrichs reports a qualitative study of nurse anaesthesia students that used a METI human patient simulator (HPS) and prescripted problem events as the baseline condition. Post intervention interviews were conducted with students reporting perceived improvement in problem solving, decision making and critical thinking[82].

19.4.3 Use of the Benner theory and the Dreyfuss model

Patricia Benner, in her landmark text *From Novice To Expert: Excellence And Power In Clinical Nursing Practice*, developed a theory of nursing practice for the acute care setting that emphasizes the progression across the spectrum of practice from the novice to the expert level[131]. This theoretical construct incorporates the use of the Dreyfuss model in acquisition of knowledge and skills crucial to the development of proficiency[131]. The five levels of proficiency include:

- Novice
- Advanced beginner
- Competent
- Proficient
- Expert.

According to Benner, these "levels reflect changes in two general aspects of skilled performance. One is a movement from reliance on abstract principles to the use of past, concrete experience as paradigms. The other is a change in the perception and understanding of a demand situation so that the situation is seen less as a compilation of equally relevant bits and more as a complete whole in which only certain parts are relevant."[117].

Benner's model depends on the acquisition of expertise through clinical experiences, but does not specifically define how a trainee might gain these experiences or how more rapid progression to higher levels of practice could be facilitated. This weakness is highlighted by Field in an analysis of the value of learning from clinical experience alone. Field asks the rhetorical question of the Benner approach "would the transition from novice to expert be obtained more efficiently with educational and in particular, mentor support?" Field speculates on several key aspects of clinical expertise development including mentor support within a robust clinical experience and the need for both rich dialogue and adequate time for student reflection[132]. Importantly, simulation has the potential to address all of these elements.

Larew *et al.* describes use of the Benner theory and the 'novice to expert' model in development of a unique nursing simulation training protocol. Recognizing the varying levels of trainees exposed to their simulation experience, the protocol incorporated a baseline patient with several cues pointing to the actual problem. A series of ascending prompts were developed to guide the trainee through the process from problem recognition to intervention. The authors note anecdotally that expert nurses required less time from recognition to resolution of the underlying problems than did novices during early testing of the protocol[78]. This study supports the underlying Dreyfuss principles of expertise development as well as the concept of using vertical integration of simulation training within a nursing curriculum.

19.4.4 Best practices in nursing simulation education

In 2003, the Laerdal Medical Corporation partnered with the National League of Nursing (NLN) and awarded a 3-year grant designed to promote development of teaching, learning and testing models for simulation within the nursing domain. A total of eight sites were chosen and a four-phase design was used. Dr Pamela Jeffries from the University of Indiana (Bloomington, IN, USA) acted as the NLN Project Coordinator. Jeffries has pointed out that simulation training done without a good supporting model results in difficulties identifying what does and does not work. The Laerdal-NLN project resulted in a nursing simulation resource text published by NLN as well as a proposed exemplar model for simulation education in nursing which was "intended to provide a context for relating a variety of likely variables" that might be incorporated into simulation course development and measurement. The studies conducted within the four phases demonstrated significant changes in self confidence, knowledge and satisfaction among participants[133].

The Laerdal-NLN 'Simulation model' draws heavily on the use of Chikering and Gamson's seven principles for good practice in undergraduate education. These practices are defined as active learning, prompt feedback, student/faculty interaction, collaborative learning, high expectations, allowing for diverse learning styles and time on task. Throughout the Laerdal-NLN model, these seven principles are used as a resource in the creation and implementation of simulation training modules[133,134]. The model also includes four major domain areas (teacher, student, educational practices, and design characteristics) each with associated variables. These domains and their associated variables interact to determine simulation course outcomes, with success being dependent on each of these primary domains. Nursing instructors, for example, must be comfortable not just with the simulation environment, but also in adjusting from an instructor-centric to a student-centric educational approach[15,109] Additionally, this model supports an expectation that students should come prepared to the simulation, requiring a significant degree of self-motivation and direction.

Bremner *et al.* also attempt to define best practices in nursing simulation education through an analysis of simulation literature and development of both qualitative and quantitative assessment tools. Their specific purpose was to develop best practices from the perspective of the end users of simulation, in this case, novice nursing students. Baccalaureate students in their first clinical nursing course were exposed to a simulation exercise, after which they answered Likert scale questions and were asked to provide feedback in written form. From the qualitative written responses, themes were identified and then categorized in the following four domain areas: teaching/learning utility, realism, limitations, and confidence/comfort. Quantitative findings indicated that students highly valued the sessions (95%), felt the experience should be mandatory (68%), were more confident in physical assessment (61%) and served to relieve stress associated with clinical (42%)[135]. Best practices advocated by these authors and based upon the student responses included:

- establishing clear learner outcomes
- clearly connecting course and clinical objectives to the simulation session
- establishing ongoing training and supervision of faculty, staff and participants
- collaborating with participants and faculty in planning, implementation and evaluation of each session
- offering a debriefing session after each simulation experience[135].

These best practices mirror those of Jeffries and many other authors and suggest that both students and educators are able to identify, at least qualitatively, some of the same strengths and weaknesses of simulation-based education. We would suggest however that training and supervision of faculty should be clearly differentiated from training and supervision of students (#3). This is also our recommendation for the planning, implementation and evaluation component (#4).

19.4.5 Other models/theories as potential frameworks in nursing simulation education

Kolb learning styles

The Kolb learning styles model has potential for development, evaluation and process mapping within nursing simulation education. In this model, two intersecting continuums are identified. The processing of information continuum stretches from 'watching to doing' and incorporates reflection as well as experimentation. The perception continuum moves from 'concrete experience (feeling) to abstract conceptualization (thinking)'. Kolb's theory describes the impact of learning styles (described as accommodating, diverging, converging and assimilating) on where individual learners fall on the intersection of these two continua. While no convincing evidence demonstrates that application of this model can effectively alter learning outcomes in the classroom environment, it holds promise in effectively describing processes which occur in the simulation arena. The Kolb model reflects disparate learning styles that are often described in simulation educational circles and may provide useful context for restructuring or conceptualizing simulation educational experiences for team training or for specific trainee domains[136–138].

Situated learning

Situated learning theory assumes that knowledge is accumulated during the course of performing various activities[139,140]. As Clancey describes, learning occurs constantly, across all human activity. Situated learning does not mean that people learn only through 'trying something out' but emphasizes that learning is a cumulative, continuous and life-embedded process that encompasses all senses, aspects and domains[141].

This theory is especially valuable in understanding issues surrounding multidisciplinary team simulation. While situated learning is an individual learner oriented model, the learner's conceptualization of what they are supposed to be doing can constrain understanding of their role within a group and attendant knowledge development. That is, knowledge is partially socially embedded and therefore learning is dependent on socially mediated collaborative processes that can be either positive or negative. Clancy explains this as 'constituting an evolving membership and capability to participate in different forms'[141]. This type of model can play an important role in the horizontal integration of simulation education exercises such as in Anaesthesia Crisis Resource Management

(ACRM) and Rapid Response Team Training (RRT) courses. As previously discussed, simulation training for Rapid Response Teams emphasizes task completion with de-emphasis of who completes the task. Optimization of this 'roles and goals' approach can be impeded when a learner arrives with a conceptualization of his or her 'place' in the healthcare hierarchy that limits their actions (i.e. task X is within a doctor's role, not a nurse's). As providers across different domains recognize that there is some interchangeability among roles, a fundamental alteration can occur in their individual construct of the team function and their role within it. Situated learning theory provides understanding of this conceptual shift by emphasizing that significant change in the 'way of thinking' can occur as "any complex system of work and learning has roots in and interdependencies across its history, technology, developing work activity, careers, and the relations between newcomers and old-timers and among workers and practitioners"[142,143].

This emphasis on system change by recognition of learners' societal and social role within the system can help to inform the construct of the 'community of practice' a definition which implies a group of people, frequently from varying backgrounds and disciplines, who coordinate their activities to achieve a goal. This concept of community of practice speaks directly to modern healthcare systems delivering complex plans of care that rely increasingly on multidisciplinary efforts to carry out those plans. Clancey identifies three key concepts that can inform nursing simulation education in the horizontal integration and team training milieu:

- knowledge is the ability to participate in a community of practice
- learning is becoming a member of a community of practice
- tools facilitate interaction within a community of practice.[141]

Simulation appears to offer unique tools to facilitate learning and perhaps retention under these conditions.

19.4.6 **Overlap with Best Evidence Medical Education (BEME)**

Issenberg et al. undertook a review of all medical simulation literature to identify which aspects of high-fidelity simulations result in the most effective learning[144,139] Because the literature demonstrates a lack of consistency in simulation approaches, true meta-analysis was not possible. Data extraction from 109 articles with outcome data yielded a list of the 'right conditions' to facilitate learning in the simulated environment. These conditions were reported as:

- Feedback is provided during the learning experience
- Learners engage in repetitive practice
- Simulation is integrated into the overall curriculum
- Learners practice with increasing levels of difficulty
- Adaptable to multiple learning strategies
- Clinical variation
- Controlled environment
- Individualized learning
- Outcomes clearly defined and measured
- Validity of the simulator.

It is clear that Issenberg et al.'s listing of these best educational conditions is, at its heart, a synthesis of multiple learning theories and educational models. For example, the need for feedback is identified in Chickering and Gamson's seven principles as well as in Benner's model and by inference in Kolb's learning styles[134,136–138]. The need for repetitive practice, clinical variation and individualized learning are also echoed in Benner, Kolb, Chickering and in Situated

Learning Theory. Effective simulations in nursing education, then, must draw upon a variety of educational models or theories to fully leverage the advantages of this emerging pedagogy. Regardless of theoretical underpinnings, the ability to measure outcomes remains a challenge but a thorough understanding of the structural framework of the educational approach may be a useful guide in designing these metrics.

19.4.7 Hierarchical task analysis

While validated models and strong educational theory foundations are crucial to designing effective nursing simulation educational tools, the ability to compare simulation and real-world outcomes as a means of determining educational efficacy remains a problematic and elusive goal. As this approach moves into the realms of competency verification, certification and licensure, metrics must be developed which are reproducible and can accurately correlate simulated and real world performance. One approach from the discipline of ergonomics that is beginning to demonstrate utility in simulation evaluation is systematic task analysis. Emerging in the early days of large-scale factory based production lines, task analysis is the process of defining either a job or the particular task or set of tasks within a job[145]. A subtype is the Hierarchical Task Analysis (HTA). As the name implies HTA not only lists each step in a particular task but analyzes the steps and attempts to place them in the order in which they should or could be performed[145–147]. HTA has been used extensively in ergonomics research and field work for over 30 years with most task analyses following HTA methodology. HTA theory is "based on goal-directed behaviour comprising a sub-goal hierarchy linked by plans"[145]. Three main principles govern the use of HTA and can be summarized as follows:

- Each task is an operation that can be defined in terms of its goal, which is the objective of the overall system in terms of production units, quality or other criteria.

- Each operation or task can be broken down into sub-operations or task steps. Each task step can then be defined by a sub-goal measured in terms of its contribution to the overall system goal, and therefore measurable (and relevant) in terms of the overall performance standards and criteria.

- The important relationship between tasks and sub-tasks is that sub-tasks are included within the overall task (a hierarchical relationship). Sub-tasks of the main tasks are typically proce-duralized, but do not necessarily have to be accomplished in a specific sequence[145].

These three guiding principles make HTA methods highly flexible so that they can be used to analyse anything from an isolated procedure to team performance to the overall function of an entire system[145]. There is a conventional nomenclature to HTA with the highest operational level being the task or operation as defined by its system-level objective or goal. The system-level goal is sometimes called the super-ordinate goal. Each super-ordinate goal is defined by its component sub-goals, which in turn can be broken down into more sub-goals. Typically when employing HTA, guidelines are developed which describe the temporal and order relationship between levels of description (e.g. x followed by y, followed by z or x and y in any order followed by z)[145].

Because HTA involves the process of description and then re-description of a system in terms of its goals and sub-goals, the process can go on for any number of iterations. This characteristic makes HTA a powerful, approach for detailed deconstruction of complex tasks[145]. One of the more difficult aspects of the HTA process is knowing the detail level at which to stop the analysis as there are no specific formulas or guidelines that indicate a definitive endpoint[145]. Task analysis methodology as applied to training in health care holds much promise in evaluating performance in both the simulated and real world settings. O'Donnell and Goode have begun exploring this approach across a range of studies. One approach was to use an intravenous catheter insertion simulator in conjunction with a ten-step IV insertion process as a means of standardizing intravenous catheter insertion training of student registered nurse anaesthetists[40]. In another study, nurses were trained to a 10-Point Patient Transfer Protocol as part of a Department of Defense funded back injury prevention project[148]. In both studies, the idealized ten-step process provided both the structure for the training intervention and the metric to evaluate performance. Notably, both 10-Point Protocols were specifically structured so that performance measurement could be done in both the simulated and clinical settings using the exact same metrics.

19.5 Simulation of specific clinical problems: an overview

19.5.1 Developing communication skills – the core of patient safety

Communication has been identified as a critical element in the delivery of patient care for all levels and domains of healthcare workers. Despite this recognition, it is clear that structured development of communication skills at both the trainee and practitioner levels has not reached a level of proficiency that offsets the potential for poor outcomes related to communication errors. This is strikingly evidenced by statistics compiled by the Joint Commission on Accreditation of Health Care Organizations (JCAHO) tabulating the root causes of sentinel events from 1995 through 2006. This report highlights communication as the most consistent variable implicated in error through root cause analysis of sentinel events across all categories with inadequate training in second place[113]. Alteration of the culture of communication promises to be a substantial challenge and it may be that communication skills are best taught in the experiential realm and not in the classroom where the primary goal is information delivery and processing, not application. Simulation training is an opportunity for improvement through practicing the language of effective communication in a realistic healthcare setting. This practice may more permanently imprint these processes with subsequent improvement in real world communication[149–153]. Additionally the simulation setting, because of its ability to replay a process or scenario over and over, can also be used to identify and avoid common communication errors within professions and across multidisciplinary teams[149–154].

Structured communications tools such SBAR (situation, background, assessment, recommendation) can easily be incorporated into a variety of simulation scenarios after a brief orientation to the rules of engagement[112]. Communication skills such as SBAR can be woven into nursing curriculum in a vertical manner by incorporating communication components into every simulation experience, even 'simple' part-task psychomotor simulations. One example would be the integration of a communication module into a simulation-training course for intravenous catheter insertion. This could take the form of an SBAR style phone call between the attending physician and the nurse with regard to confirmation of the order and the intended use of the catheter (i.e. if for blood products, selection of the appropriate gauge). More complex simulations would integrate communication skills to varying degrees, dependent on the overall course goals. Across a nursing curriculum, the continued emphasis on communication from the earliest formative phases of training will reinforce its importance as a link in the chain of patient safety[78,112,128,149,153,155–175].

19.5.2 Part-task training

Perhaps the most widely used type of simulation is that of part-task training to teach a specific psychomotor skill. There are many reports of such educational approaches and a wide variety of devices on which to train. CPR mannequins, rubber arms for intravenous or arterial line insertion, intubating/mask ventilation heads, central line insertion models and spinal/epidural models are just a few of the wide range of devices available[40,64,148,176]. Part-task trainers continue to increase in sophistication and improve in terms of fidelity. In the past there were two primary problems with these generally low fidelity training devices. First, the part-task trainers were relatively static. That is, conditions were set, usually at a normal anatomic level, and variances in anatomy and pathology were either not able to be presented or were of a limited range. Second, assessment could only be based on instructor observation with very little in the way of an objective measurement system (i.e. success with a rubber tubing IV arm was demonstrated by fluid return through the IV catheter with little evaluation of technique or associated processes). Recent technical innovations have presented the opportunity to enhance the use of part-task training. Several devices have emerged that incorporate sophisticated sensors to provide evaluation of the physical performance of the task[40,64,148,176]. Among the most interesting are developments with virtual intravenous line insertion trainers and gynaecological exam mannequins. The gynaecological exam mannequins are anatomically of high fidelity and incorporate a series of sensors to measure whether specific anatomic exam areas were assessed and what degree of pressure was exerted on these points during the exam[177]. The IV insertion trainers typically employ a haptic device that does not necessarily correspond to any particular portion of the anatomy, though the trainee can interact with it in the same way as a real patient (stretching the skin at the insertion site, adjusting the angle of the catheter insertion, etc.). The corresponding computer display allows for a wide array of choices in anatomy, insertion site, size of catheter and level of difficulty of insertion. Every mechanical movement is measured and scored, and some versions rate performance on associated tasks such as tourniquet placement and use of personal protective gear. Incorporating these types of sophisticated assessment tools into a part-task trainer moves the process from a purely psychomotor exercise to one of combined skill and critical thinking. For example, the IV insertion trainer requires that decisions be made based on patient acuity and proposed medical or surgical intervention. Clearly this is the type of thought process that goes on in the real world of patient care. However, at the earliest stages of nursing training, psychomotor skills are frequently segregated from the critical thinking component. The developments in part-task trainer technology, when combined with a well designed process and instructional plan, means that even at the earliest levels of nursing training, critical thinking components can potentially be associated with task training. Additionally, the ability to break a task into its component parts and measure performance opens up opportunities in other areas of performance measurement.

19.5.3 Objective structured clinical exams

Objective structured clinical exams (OSCE) are widely used in teaching and assessment of clinical skills in medical schools across the world. This methodology, building on the use of SPs standardizes the preparation of medical students for examination and patient interaction[178]. First described in 1975 by Harden et al., OSCE has only recently begun to gain popularity in nursing education[179,180]. The primary barriers to use of OSCE exams revolve around access and cost, with nursing use of OSCE exams more prevalent in the UK and Canada[180–182].

Rogers et al. described use of OSCE exams in preparation of medical students for critical care skills and reported significant improvement across multiple domains[183]. Alinier et al. studied second year Diploma of Higher Education in Nursing programme students in the UK. These students would be equivalent to sophomore or junior-level Bachelor of Science in Nursing (BSN) students in the USA. Using a pre-test, post-test design and an OSCE, participating students were assigned to either the control group (normal didactic and clinical content) or to the intervention group (normal didactic and clinical content, plus simulation exercises). Alinier reported statistical significance in post-test results with those students in the simulation group scoring higher on the post-simulation OSCE[184].

While OSCE exams using simulated patients show promise and have been broadly adopted in medicine, their role in the development of nursing simulation programmes is unclear. Because most US nursing schools do not have access to SPs due to cost or availability, SP based OSCE exams are unlikely to become a common component of nursing curricula. As previously described, screen or avatar-based VPs may hold promise in this area. Due to the electronic nature of the interaction, these experiences could be introduced within nursing curricula and are available from any web-based computer station with appropriate software. The primary cost of VP based systems is found in the development phase with some free-ware and commercial versions currently available[93–96,100].

19.5.4 Nursing simulation training in specialty areas

With simulation, it is possible to train large groups of providers in patient scenarios which, though common, might pose a threat to patient safety if performed incorrectly. Examples in nursing practice include:

- procedures such as endotracheal intubation, difficult airway management, central line insertion, and fibreoptic bronchoscopy
- management of acute pathophysiological conditions, such as shock, arrhythmia, hypotension, or haemorrhage
- team response during cardiac arrest, trauma resuscitation, or out-of-hospital rescue[8].

The simulation setting offers the potential to play out each of these types of scenarios consistently from individual trainee to individual trainee or from group to group allowing for comparison and evaluation. Attention to detail in the programing of simulations is critical, especially given a report of statistically significant variability in the reproducibility of programed haemodynamic trend modules[185]. Each educational scenario will have its own tolerance level for such variance, and this must be determined during the planning phase. Obviously, little variability can be tolerated when considering whether to use this type of simulation as a high-stakes evaluation tool.

19.6 Nurse anaesthesia

One particular benefit of simulation is that all trainees can experience rare or crisis events and receive immediate feedback with an opportunity for expert modeling and correction. The domain of nurse anaesthesia has demonstrated significant simulation interest. O'Donnell et al. describes the development of an Anaesthesia Crisis Resource Management (ACRM) course for nurse anaesthesia students. This paper describes the development of the course and the operational elements required. Key factors to success of the course included administrative support, faculty training, detailed scheduling, technical support and alpha testing of scenarios for validation. Scenarios were staged in five different hospital settings to replicate varying levels of support services from tertiary medical centers to rural practice. Students' ratings of the course were highly positive, scenarios were believable, the varied practice settings were useful and students felt free to participate in debriefing[48]. In a qualitative study, Henrichs et al. described nurse anaesthesia student perceptions in management of simple to complex problem events during their training programme. Students were exposed to four simulator sessions and were asked to manage both the anaesthetic and the problem event. Students reported apprehension, uneasiness and fear, but they recognized the educational value. Lack of reality, lack of knowledge in management of crisis events and anxiety were noted disadvantages. Reported improvement in confidence and clinical preparation as well as a perception of improved critical thinking were the advantages cited[82]. Hotchkiss *et al.* studied the authenticity of the simulation experience in crisis events. In this study, the authors exposed nurse anaesthesia students to a series of brief clinical crisis vignettes which were videotaped. Three raters with significant operating room environment experience rated the films using a pilot tested authenticity tool. Reliability of the rating tool was established (k = 0.75–0.90). Failure to effectively mirror actual OR culture, hypervigilance and lack of reality due to brevity of the scenarios were identified as weaknesses[11]. In a doctoral thesis, Oswaks demonstrated the use of simulation with novice nurse anaesthesia students. Core clinical skills including laryngoscopy, intubation and mask ventilation were taught within the simulation environment. Improved intubation and laryngoscopy performance was reported with no decrease in efficiency compared to standard training[6] Register *et al.* described the use of simulation to demonstrate and serve as a backdrop in detailed analysis of intrapulmonary shunt. The simulator used was a METI HPS®. A literature review was combined with a series of simulator demonstrations and data collection exercises. The outcome was a full description and analysis of shunt for students and faculty. Overall results were positive with one key weakness identified: a failure of the simulator oxygen saturation to fall as desired[186].

19.6.1 Sedation nursing

Farnsworth *et al.* conducted a study of RN conscious sedation skill development using simulation. In this quasi-experimental study, participants took a written pre-test followed by education and scenario-based skill evaluation. Upon completion of the course, participants completed a written post-test with statistically significant improvement in score. Practical exam scores were 5.5 on a 6.0 scale and satisfaction levels were high. These authors indicated that training in sedation and analgesia using simulation was both valuable and effective[187].

19.6.2 Resuscitation and critical care

Nehring and Lashley describe use of a simulator integrated in their undergraduate curriculum. The authors describe center development, equipment, potential uses and plans for additional utilization. The focal point of the course was to allow students an opportunity to independently manage critical incidents[79]. Spunt *et al.* described the use of a 'mock code' as an integrated component within an undergraduate nursing curriculum[4]. Other authors have described integration of simulation content into acute care and critical care undergraduate electives with focus placed on development of patient care skill, communication ability and patient safety behaviours[9,188]. Marsch *et al.* tested the ability of first responders to adhere to algorithms of cardiopulmonary resuscitation using a simulated cardiac arrest in an intensive care environment[189]. The physician–nurse teams functioned well in areas such as recognizing the arrest and calling for help, but there were significant delays in the initiation of basic life support and defibrillation. Observations such as this support the need for additional training in crisis team management, helping to drive the development of the Rapid Response Team concept, which draws from the concept of interactive gaming simulation[54,55,60]. Sweeney describe the integration of a core set of simulation scenarios[4] into a critical care elective. These scenarios were within the METI® programme for Nursing Curriculum Integration (PNCI). The PNCI is a set of 90 preprepared and preprogrammed scenarios. Four scenarios were chosen and were integrated into a critical care elective. Post-course evaluation data reflected high student and faculty ratings of the value and use of simulation training[46]. Hravnak *et al.* described integration of high fidelity and part-task training simulation in both Acute Care Nurse Practitioner and Acute Care Clinical Nurse Specialist graduate programmes. Students received part-task training in invasive monitoring placement combined with full context high fidelity simulation in preparation for management of critical events in the ICU setting. These authors reported positive responses from preceptors, instructors and participants[83]. Brady et al. propose an integrated online simulation curriculum as an innovation in critical care orientation. These authors describe a potential collaborative venture and describe the advantages inherent in a course shared among a conglomeration of hospitals[190]. Hoffman et al. describes the integration of human simulation educational modules within an undergraduate critical care course. Students (n=29) were exposed to simulation events across a 14-week term divided into 7 weeks of clinical and 7 weeks of simulation. Basic Critical Care Knowledge Assessment Test, Version 6 (BKAT-6) was administered in a pre-test, post-test design. Student knowledge gain was significant in 6/8 BKAT subscales. The two BKAT domains that failed to show improvement, also did not have a corresponding simulation training component[191].

19.6.3 Obstetrics

Thompson et al. reported extension of the rapid response team concept to the obstetric setting in implementation of 'preeclampsia drills'. In this study, simulation was used as a diagnostic tool to identify unit deficiencies. The primary outcome was improvement in subsequent simulated eclampsia events[72]. Cioffi et al. investigated the impact of simulation training on midwifery student performance. Simulation was compared with standard training with students in the simulation arm demonstrating increased ability to collect data, increased confidence in the data and themselves and more rapid decision making during subsequent simulation scenario testing[192]. O'Donnell and White describe the development of obstetric and paediatric scenarios in undergraduate education. These authors used a pre-test, post-test design for knowledge and attitude evaluation. Significant gains in knowledge, confidence and perceived skill were reported[77]. Robertson describes the use of human simulation scenarios in combination with a birthing simulator (Gaumard Noelle®) in offering undergraduate students a realistic obstetric experience[193]. Robertson reports a high degree of student satisfaction with the approach. Schoening et al. evaluated undergraduate nursing student perceptions of a preterm labour simulation. Participants reported that the simulation scenario improved confidence and met course objectives. Qualitative feedback emphasized the value of practice in hands-on management, teamwork, communication skills and decision-making[15].

19.7 Conclusions

Simulation education in nursing has a long history extending from static mannequins (Mrs Chase)[2,3] to the simulation gaming movement, and continuing with today's high fidelity mannequins. Despite challenges, affordable high fidelity simulation devices (Laerdal SimMan®, METI- HPS®, Gaumard NOELLE®) are becoming increasingly integrated within the educational preparation of nurses. Simulation education cannot replace all aspects of traditional clinical training; however, its value as a supplement and in some cases a surrogate for clinical experience is gaining credence. Administrative support, dedicated faculty willing to develop new skill sets, substantial financial and space resource commitments, an intent to gather data to quantify value and improve process, and willingness to abandon or alter old approaches in light of new evidence are essential elements in successful nursing simulation programmes.

Simulation educational targets include assuring experience in rare events, providing standardized training in common events, developing key cognitive and psychomotor skills, measuring or benchmarking professional competence and in specialty certification/credentialing. Simulation educators across a variety of domain areas in nursing (undergraduate, graduate, anaesthesia, critical care, paediatrics and obstetrics etc) are generating a body of literature in support of the impact and efficacy of simulation science. Nursing simulation research targets include evaluation of competency, efficiency in professional nursing education, efficacy in comparison to alternative methods, retention of skills and knowledge, improving training efficiency and in assessing translation of simulation to clinical care.

In order for the mannequin based simulation movement to avoid being relegated to the fate of the simulation gaming movement in nursing, ongoing scholarship must demonstrate more than student satisfaction and faculty recognition of effectiveness. Fit of simulation education within the overall spectrum of nursing preparation at all levels must be rigorously examined with value clearly established and communicated through ongoing publication and scholarly presentation.

References

1. Abrahamson S (1997). Sim One–a patient simulator ahead of its time. *Caduceus* **13**(2): 29–41.
2. Herrmann EK (1981). Mrs. Chase: a noble and enduring figure. *Am J Nursing* **81**(10): 1836.
3. Price AL (1939). The autobiography of Sally Chase. *Am J Nursing* **39**: 25–7.
4. Spunt D, Foster D, Adams K (2004). Mock code: a clinical simulation module. *Nurse Educator* **29**(5): 192–4.
5. Mayne W, Jootun D, Young B, Marland G, Harris M, Lyttle CP (2004). Enabling students to develop confidence in basic clinical skills. *Nursing Times* **100**(24): 36–9.
6. Oswaks JSD (2002). The use of simulated clinical experiences to improve competency in the novice anesthesia provider [DNSc], The University of Tennessee Center for the Health Sciences.
7. Fontaine DK, Norton C (2001). Beyond the essentials. Teaching critical care to undergraduate and graduate students in nursing. *Critical Care Nursing Clinics of North America* **13**(1): 13–24.
8. O'Donnell JM, Beach M, Hoffman L (2005). Human Simulation Training in the ICU: Applicability, Value, and Disadvantages. *Critical Care Alert* **13**(6): 45–8.
9. Long RE (2005). Using simulation to teach resuscitation: an important patient safety tool. *Critical Care Nursing Clinics of North America* **17**(1): 1–8.
10. Alinier G, Hunt WB, Gordon R (2004). Determining the value of simulation in nurse education: study design and initial results. *Nurse Education in Practice* **4**(3): 200–7.
11. Hotchkiss MA, Biddle C, Fallacaro M (2002). Assessing the authenticity of the human simulation experience in anesthesiology. *AANA Journal*;70(6): 470–3.
12. Rystedt H, Lindstrom B (2001). Introducing simulation technologies in nurse education: a nursing practice perspective. *Nurse Education in Practice* **1**(3): 134–41.
13. Wildman S, Reeves M (1997). The value of simulations in the management education of nurses: students' perceptions. *Journal of Nursing Management* **5**(4): 207–15.
14. Kneebone RPF, Nestel DP, Wetzel CDP, *et al.* (2006) The Human Face of Simulation: Patient-Focused Simulation Training. *Academic Medicine* **81**(10): 919–24.
15. Schoening AM, Sittner BJ, Todd MJ (2006). Simulated clinical experience: nursing students' perceptions and the educators' role. *Nurse Educator* **31**(6): 253–8.
16. Williams KA, Stotts RC, Jacob SR, Stegbauer CC, Roussel L, Carter D (2006). Inactive nurses: a source for alleviating the nursing shortage? *Journal of Nursing Administration* **36**(4): 205–10.
17. AACN (2006). Nursing Shortage Fact Sheet. *American Association of Colleges of Nursing* 1–4.
18. Unruh LY, Fottler MD (2005). Projections and trends in RN supply: what do they tell us about the nursing shortage? *Policy, Politics, & Nursing Practice* **6**(3): 171–82.
19. Murray MK (2002). The nursing shortage. Past, present, and future. *Journal of Nursing Administration* **32**(2): 79–84.

20. Buerhaus PI, Donelan K, Norman L, Dittus R (2005). Nursing students' perceptions of a career in nursing and impact of a national campaign designed to attract people into the nursing profession. *Journal of Professional Nursing* 21(2): 75–83.

21. Vahey DC, Aiken LH, Sloane DM, Clarke SP, Vargas D (2004). Nurse burnout and patient satisfaction. *Medical Care* 42(2 Suppl): II57–66.

22. Rogers AE, Hwang W-T, Scott LD, Aiken LH, Dinges DF (2004). The working hours of hospital staff nurses and patient safety. *Health Affairs* 23(4): 202–12.

23. Aiken LH, Clarke SP, Silber JH, Sloane D (2003). Hospital nurse staffing, education, and patient mortality. *LDI Issue Brief* 9(2): 1–4.

24. Aiken LH, Clarke SP, Sloane DM, *et al.* (2002) Hospital nurse staffing and patient mortality, nurse burnout, and job dissatisfaction. *JAMA* 288(16): 1987–93.

25. NLN (2006). Excellence in nursing education model. Located at: National League for Nursing, New York.

26. Li S, Kenward K (2006). *A National Survey on Elements of Nursing Education* – Fall 2004 July 2006.

27. Kenward K, Zhong EH (2006). *Report of Findings from the Practice and Professional Issues Survey* – Fall 2004 July 2006.

28. Campbell S (2006). Addressing nursing shortages in sub-Saharan Africa. *Nursing Standard* 20(51): 46–50.

29. Kirk H (2007). Towards a global nursing workforce: the 'brain circulation'. *Nursing Management (London)* 13(10): 26–30.

30. Singh JA, Nkala B, Amuah E, Mehta N, Ahmad A (2003). The ethics of nurse poaching from the developing world. *Nursing Ethics: an International Journal for Health Care Professionals* 10(6): 666–70.

31. Nelson R (2004). The nurse poachers. *Lancet* 364(9447): 1743–4.

32. Kline DS (2003). Push and pull factors in international nurse migration. *Journal of Nursing Scholarship* 35(2): 107–11.

33. McElmurry BJ, Solheim K, Kishi R, Coffia MA, Woith W, Janepanish P (2006). Ethical concerns in nurse migration. *Journal of Professional Nursing* 22(4): 226–35.

34. Oulton JA (2006). The global nursing shortage: an overview of issues and actions. *Policy, Politics, & Nursing Practice* 7(3 Suppl.) 34S–39S.

35. Rosenkoetter MM, Nardi DA (2006). White paper on global nursing and health: a brief. *Nursing Outlook* 54(2): 113–15.

36. Hoffman LA, Miller TH, Zullo TG, *et al.*(2006) Comparison of 2 models for managing tracheotomized patients in a subacute medical intensive care unit.[see comment]. *Respiratory Care* 51(11): 1230–6.

37. Hoffman LA, Tasota FJ, Zullo TG, *et al.*(2005) Outcomes of care managed by an acute care nurse practitioner/attending physician team in a subacute medical intensive care unit. *American Journal of Critical Care* 14(2): 121–30; quiz 131–22.

38. Hravnak M, Kobert SN, Risco KG, *et al.* (1995) Acute care nurse practitioner curriculum: content and development process. *American Journal of Critical Care* 4(3): 179–88.

39. Thomas P (2006). The international migration of Indian nurses. *International Nursing Review* 53(4): 277–83.

40. O'Donnell JM, Goode JA, Odonohoe O, Choe M (2007). 07 IMSH Work-In-Progress Abstracts: The Impact of Intravenous Catheter Insertion Training Modalities On Clinical Intravenous Catheter Insertion Performance in Graduate Nursing Students. *Simulation in Healthcare: The Journal of the Society for Simulation in Healthcare* 1(1): 114.

41. Nehring WM, Lashley FR, Nehring WM, Lashley FR (2004). Current use and opinions regarding human patient simulators in nursing education: an international survey. *Nursing Education Perspectives* 25(5): 244–8.

42. Kohn LT, Corrigan JM, Donaldson MS (1999). *To Err Is Human: Building a Safer Health System.* Washington, DC, National Academy Press.

43. JCAHO (2005). *2006 National Patient Safety Goals*: Joint Commission on Accreditation of Healthcare Organizations.

44. Berwick DM (2005). IHI proposes six patient safety goals to prevent 100,000 annual deaths. *Qual Lett Healthc Lead* **17**(1): 11–12, 11.

45. Wilford A, Doyle TJ (2006). Integrating simulation training into the nursing curriculum. *British Journal of Nursing* **15**(17): 926–30.

46. Parr MB, Sweeney NM (2006). Use of human patient simulation in an undergraduate critical care course. *Critical Care Nursing Quarterly* **29**(3): 188–98.

47. O'Donnell JM, Henker R, Dixon BA, *et al.*(2006) Curricular Integration Of Human Simulation Education Across programmes: SEGUE At The University Of Pittsburgh School Of Nursing. Paper presented at: International Meeting on Medical Simulation 2006; San Diego,CA.

48. O'Donnell J, Fletcher J, Dixon B, Palmer L (1998). Planning and implementing an anesthesia crisis resource management course for student nurse anesthetists. *CRNA* **9**(2): 50–8.

49. Jeffries PR (2005). A framework for designing, implementing, and evaluating simulations used as teaching strategies in nursing. *Nursing Education Perspectives* **26**(2): 96–103.

50. Haskvitz LM, Koop EC, Haskvitz LM, Koop EC (2004). Students struggling in clinical? A new role for the patient simulator. *Journal of Nursing Education* **43**(4): 181–4.

51. Dewey J (2005). Democracy and education: an introduction to the philosophy of education. New York: Cosimo Classics.

52. Hanna DR (1991). Using simulations to teach clinical nursing. *Nurse Educator* **16**(2): 28–31.

53. Cruickshank D (1966). Simulations: New Directions in Teacher Preparation. *Phi Delta Kappan* **XLVIII**(1): 23–4.

54. Greenblat CS (1971). Simulation Games and the Sociologist. *American Sociologis* **6**(2): 161–4.

55. Greenblat CS (2001). The design and redesign of gaming simulations on health care issues. *Simulation & Gaming* **32**(3): 315–30.

56. Coleman J, Livingston S, Fennessey G, Edwards K, Kidder S (1973). The Hopkins Games programme: Conclusions From Seven Years of Research. *Educational Researcher* **2**(8): 3–7.

57. Lowe J (1975). Games and simulation in nurse education. *Nursing Mirror & Midwives Journal* **141**(23): 68–9.

58. Clark CC (1976). Simulation gaming: a new teaching strategy in nursing education. *Nurse Educator* **1**(4): 4–9.

59. Greenblat CS, Uretsky M (1977). Simulation in social science. *American Behavioral Scientist* **20**(3): 411–26.

60. Greenblat CS (1977). Gaming-simulation and health education an overview. *Health Education Monographs* **5**(Suppl. 1): 5–10.

61. Clark C (1977). Learning outcomes in a simulation game for associate degree nursing students. *Health Education Monographs* **5**(Suppl. 1): 18–27.

62. Becker C (1980). An overview of simulation games and comments on their use in baccalaureate nursing education. *Nursing Papers* **12**(1–2): 32–45.

63. Maidment R, Bronstein RH (1973). *Simulation games; design and implementation*. Columbus, Ohio: Merrill.

64. Cooper JB, Taqueti VR (2004). A brief history of the development of mannequin simulators for clinical education and training. *Quality and Safety in Health Care* **13** (Suppl. 1): i11–i18.

65. Grenvik A, Schaefer J (2004). From Resusci-Anne to Sim-Man: the evolution of simulators in medicine. *Critical Care Medicine* **32**(2 Suppl.): S56–57.

66. O'Neale M, Kurtz S (2001). Certification: perspectives on competency assurance. *Seminars in Perioperative Nursing* **10**(2): 88–92.

67. Weddle DO, Himburg SP, Collins N, Lewis R (2002). The professional development portfolio process: setting goals for credentialing. *Journal of the American Dietetic Association* **102**(10): 1439–44, 1577–1438, 1588.

68. Underwood P, Dahlen-Hartfield R, Mogle B, Underwood P, Dahlen-Hartfield R, Mogle B (2004). Continuing professional education: does it make a difference in perceived nursing practice? *Journal for Nurses in Staff Development – JNSD* **20**(2): 90–8.

69. Ziv A, Wolpe PR, Small SD, Glick S (2003). Simulation-based medical education: an ethical imperative. *Academic Medicine* **78**(8): 783–8.

70. Skupski DW, Lowenwirt IP, Weinbaum FI, Brodsky D, Danek M, Eglinton GS (2006). Improving hospital systems for the care of women with major obstetric hemorrhage. *Obstetrics & Gynecology* **107**(5): 977–83.

71. Gordon DL, Issenberg SB, Gordon MS, *et al.* (2005). Stroke training of prehospital providers: an example of simulation-enhanced blended learning and evaluation. *Medical Teacher* **27**(2): 114–21.

72. Thompson S, Neal S, Clark V (2004). Clinical risk management in obstetrics: eclampsia drills. *Quality and Safety in Health Care* **13**(2): 127–9.

73. Rosenstock C, Ostergaard D, Kristensen MS, Lippert A, Ruhnau B, Rasmussen LS (2004). Residents lack knowledge and practical skills in handling the difficult airway. *Acta Anaesthesiologica Scandinavica* **48**(8): 1014–18.

74. Mayo PH, Hackney JE, Mueck JT, Ribaudo V, Schneider RF (2004). Achieving house staff competence in emergency airway management: results of a teaching programme using a computerized patient simulator.[see comment]. *Critical Care Medicine* **32**(12): 2422–7.

75. Grenvik A, Schaefer JJ, 3rd, DeVita MA, Rogers P (2004). New aspects on critical care medicine training. *Current Opinion in Critical Care* **10**(4): 233–7.

76. Lasater K (2005). The impact of high fidelity simulation on the development of clinical judgment in nursing students: an exploratory study, Ed. Portland State University.

77. O'Donnell JM, White D (2005). Simulation Training in Obstetrics and Pediatrics for Nurses. *Hospital News* (April 2005).

78. Larew C, Lessans S, Spunt D, Foster D, Covington BG (2006). Innovations in clinical simulation: Application of Benner's theory in an interactive patient care simulation. *Nursing Education Perspectives* **27**(1): 16–21.

79. Nehring W, Lashley, F, Ellis, W (2002).Critical incident nursing management using human patient simulators. *Nursing Education Perspectives* **23**(2): 128132.

80. Fletcher JL, Fletcher JL (1995). AANA journal course: update for nurse anesthetists–anesthesia simulation: a tool for learning and research. *AANA Journa* **63**(1): 61–7.

81. Hotchkiss MA, Mendoza SN (2001). Update for nurse anesthetists. Part 6. Full-body patient simulation technology: gaining experience using a malignant hyperthermia model. *AANA Journa* **69**(1): 59–65.

82. Henrichs B, Rule A, Grady M, Ellis W (2002). Nurse anesthesia students' perceptions of the anesthesia patient simulator: a qualitative study. *AANA Journal* **70**(3): 219–25.

83. Hravnak M, Tuite P, Baldisseri M (2005). Expanding acute care nurse practitioner and clinical nurse specialist education: invasive procedure training and human simulation in critical care. *AACN Clinical Issues* **16**(1): 89–104.

84. Brooks KL (1990). Relationships among professionalism, critical thinking, decision-making and self-concept for senior nursing students in four types of nursing curricula [Ed.d.], Temple University.

85. Daly WM, Daly WM (2001). The development of an alternative method in the assessment of critical thinking as an outcome of nursing education. *Journal of Advanced Nursing* **36**(1): 120–30.

86. del Bueno D (2005). A crisis in critical thinking. *Nursing Education Perspectives* **26**(5): 278–82.

87. del Bueno DJ (1990). Experience, education, and nurses' ability to make clinical judgments. *Nursing & Health Care* **11**(6): 290–4.

88. AACN (2007). The Essential Clinical Resources for Nursing's Academic Mission. http://www.aacn.nche.edu/Education/clnesswb.htm. Accessed May 9, 2007.

89. JCAHO (2002). *Healthcare At The Crossroads: Strategies For Addressing The Evolving Nursing Crisis.* Joint Commission on Accreditation of Healthcare Organizations.

90. O'Donnell JM (2006). Technology in Teaching: PowerPoint, SimMan, and the Land of Oz: Is that a yellow-brick or megabyte road we are following? Paper presented at: American Association of Nurse Anesthetists Assembly of School Faculty; Feb 2006; San Diego, CA.

91. O'Donnell JM, Fletcher J, Dixon B, Palmer L (1998). Planning and implementing an anesthesia crisis resource management course for student nurse anesthetists. *CRNA: The Clinical Forum for Nurse Anesthetist* **9**(2): 50–8.

92. Diefenbeck CA, Plowfield LA, Herrman JW (2006). Clinical immersion: a residency model for nursing education. *Nursing Education Perspectives* **27**(2): 72–9.

93. Triola M, Feldman H, Kalet AL, *et al.* (2006). A randomized trial of teaching clinical skills using virtual and live standardized patients. *Journal of General Internal Medicine* **21**(5): 424–9.

94. Huang GC, Caughey TD (2004). Virtual Patient Reference Library The Carl J. Shapiro Institute for Education and Research at Harvard Medical School and Beth Israel Deaconess Medical Center.

95. Huang GMD, Reynolds RMPA, Candler CMD (2007). Virtual Patient Simulation at U.S. and Canadian Medical Schools. *Academic Medicine* **82**(5): 446–51.

96. Zary N, Johnson G, Boberg J, *et al.* (2006). Development, implementation and pilot evaluation of a Web-based Virtual Patient Case Simulation environment–Web-SP. *BMC Medical Education* **6**: 10.

97. Wynne N (2007). Use of Screen Based Avatars as a Component of a Fully Integrated Pre-Registration Curriculum. In: O'Donnell JM, Goode J, Eds. Orlando, Florida.

98. Wynne N (2007). Use of Computer Based Avatars as a Component of an Integrated Simulation Curriculum. In: O'Donnell JM, Ed. Description of UCE programme of avatars combined with mannekin based programme across a pre-registration curriculum ed. Birmingham.

99. Rusdorf S, Brunnett G, Lorenz M, Winkler T (2007). Real-time interaction with a humanoid avatar in an immersive table tennis simulation. *IEEE Transactions on Visualization & Computer Graphics* **13**(1): 15–25.

100. Simo A, Cavazza M, Kijima R (2004). Virtual patients in clinical medicine. *Studies in Health Technology & Informatics* **98**: 353–9.

101. Schmidt TA, Abbott JT, Geiderman JM, *et al.*(2004) Ethics seminars: the ethical debate on practicing procedures on the newly dead. *Academic Emergency Medicine* **11**(9): 962–6.

102. Alverson DC, Saiki SM, Jr., Jacobs J, *et al.* (2004) Distributed interactive virtual environments for collaborative experiential learning and training independent of distance over Internet2. *Studies in Health Technology & Informatics* **98**: 7–12.

103. Gaggioli A, Mantovani F, Castelnuovo G, Wiederhold B, Riva G (2003). Avatars in clinical psychology: a framework for the clinical use of virtual humans. *Cyberpsychology & Behavior* **6**(2): 117–25.

104. Merriam-Webster (2007). Webster's Third New International Dictionary. *Merriam-Webster Unabridged* [Electronic data base] Online dictionary. Available at: http://unabridged.merriam-webster.com. Accessed April 5, 2007.

105. DeVita MA, Schaefer J, Lutz J, Wang H, Dongilli T (2005). Improving medical emergency team (MET) performance using a novel curriculum and a computerized human patient simulator. *Quality and Safety in Health Care* **14**(5): 326–31.

106. Wilkinson JM (2007). *Nursing process and critical thinking.* 4th ed. Upper Saddle River, NJ: Pearson/Prentice Hall.

107. ANA (2004). *Nursing: Scope and Standards of Practice.* 3rd ed. Washington, DC: American Nurses Publishing, American Nurses Association.

108. O'Donnell JM, Hoffman R (2003). Enhancing Professional Competence Through High Fidelity Human Simulation. Paper presented at: University of Pittsburgh Innovations in Education Teaching Excellence Fair; November, 2003; Pittsburgh, PA.

109. Burns H, Hoffman R, O'Donnell JM (2005). Enhancing Nursing Knowledge Acquisition through an Innovative Curricular Approach Using High Fidelity Human Simulation. Paper presented at: 23rd Quadrennial International Council of Nurses (ICN) Congress, 2005; Taipei, Taiwan.

110. McCausland LL, Curran CC, Cataldi P (2004). Use of a human simulator for undergraduate nurse education. *International Journal of Nursing Education Scholarship* **1**(1): 1–17.

111. NANDA (2007). NANDA International. http://www.nanda.org/. Accessed June 9, 2007.

112. Leonard M, Graham S, Bonacum D (2004). The human factor: the critical importance of effective teamwork and communication in providing safe care. *Quality & Safety in Health Care* **13**(Suppl. 1): i85–90.

113. Joint Commission T (2006). Sentinel Event Statistics.

114. Martins DL, Garcia TR (2004). Nursing diagnostic profile of patients with myocardial infarction. *Online Brazilian Journal of Nursing* **3**(2): 6p.

115. Turner P (2005). Critical thinking in nursing education and practice as defined in the literature. *Nursing Education Perspectives* **26**(5): 272–7.

116. Paul RW, Ed. (1993). *Critical Thinking*. Santa Rosa, CA: Foundation for Critical Thinking.

117. Benner P (1982). From novice to expert ... the Dreyfus Model of Skill Acquisition. *American Journal of Nursing* **82**: 402–7.

118. Chau JP, Chang AM, Lee IF, Ip WY, Lee DT, Wootton Y (2001). Effects of using videotaped vignettes on enhancing students' critical thinking ability in a baccalaureate nursing programmeme. *Journal of Advanced Nursing* **36**(1): 112–19.

119. Peterson MJ, Bechtel GA (2000). Combining the arts: an applied critical thinking approach in the skills laboratory. *Nursing Connections* **13**(2): 43–9.

120. Jenkins P, Turick-Gibson T, Jenkins P, Turick-Gibson T (1999). An exercise in critical thinking using role playing. *Nurse Educator* **24**(6): 11–14.

121. Weis PA, Guyton-Simmons J (1998). A computer simulation for teaching critical thinking skills. *Nurse Educator* **23**(2): 30–3.

122. Brooks KL, Shepherd JM (1990). The relationship between clinical decision-making skills in nursing and general critical thinking abilities of senior nursing students in four types of nursing programmes. *Journal of Nursing Education* **29**(9): 391–9.

123. Keller R (1993). Effects of an instructional programme on critical thinking and clinical decision-making skills of associate degree nursing students [PhD], University of South Florida.

124. Saucier BL (1995). Critical thinking skills of baccalaureate nursing students. *Journal of Professional Nursing* **11**(6): 351–7.

125. Johannsson SL, Wertenberger DH (1996). Using simulation to test critical thinking skills of nursing students. *Nurse Education Today* **16**(5): 323–7.

126. Seldomridge EA (1996). The influence of confidence, factual, and experiential knowledge on speed and accuracy of clinical judgment among novice and expert nurses [PhD]. Baltimore, University of Maryland.

127. Seldomridge LA, Walsh CM (2006). Measuring critical thinking in graduate education: what do we know? *Nurse Educato* **31**(3): 132–7.

128. Medley CF, Horne C (2005). Using simulation technology for undergraduate nursing education. *Journal of Nursing Education* **44**(1): 31–4.

129. Sorenson JL (2002). *The use of simulated clinical experiences to improve competency in the novice anesthesia provider* [DNSc], The University of Tennessee Center for the Health Sciences.

130. Rauen CA (2001). Using simulation to teach critical thinking skills. You can't just throw the book at them. *Critical Care Nursing Clinics of North America* **13**(1): 93–103.

131. Benner PE (1984). *From novice to expert: excellence and power in clinical nursing practice*. Menlo Park, California: Addison-Wesley Pub. Co., Nursing Division.

132. Field DE (2004). Moving from novice to expert – the value of learning in clinical practice: a literature review. *Nurse Education Today* **24**(7): 560–5.

133. Jeffries PR (2005). Technology trends in nursing education: next steps. *Journal of Nursing Education* **44**(1): 3–4.

134. Chickering A, Gamson Z (1987). Seven Principles for Good Practice in Undergraduate Education. *The Wingspread Journal* **9**(2).

135. Bremner MN, Aduddell K, Bennett DN, VanGeest JB (2006). The use of human patient simulators: best practices with novice nursing students. *Nurse Educator* **31**(4): 170–4.

136. Sandmire DA, Boyce PF (2004). Pairing of opposite learning styles among allied health students: effects on collaborative performance. *Journal of Allied Health* **33**(2): 156–63.

137. Sandmire DA, Vroman KG, Sanders R (2000). The influence of learning styles on collaborative performances of allied health students in a clinical exercise. *Journal of Allied Healt* **29**(3): 143–9.

138. Hauer P, Straub C, Wolf S (2005). Learning styles of allied health students using Kolb's LSI-IIa. *Journal of Allied Health* **34**(3): 177–82.

139. Kneebone R (2005). Evaluating clinical simulations for learning procedural skills: a theory-based approach. *Academic Medicine* **80**(6): 549–53.

140. Yuan Y, McKelvey B, Yuan Y, McKelvey B (2004). Situated learning theory: adding rate and complexity effects via Kauffman's NK model. *Nonlinear Dynamics, Psychology, & Life Sciences* **8**(1): 65–101.

141. Clancey WJ (1995). A Tutorial On Situated Learning. Paper presented at: International Conference on Cumputers and Education; Taiwan.

142. Clancy J, McVicar A, Bird D (2000). Getting it right? An exploration of issues relating to the biological sciences in nurse education and nursing practice. *Journal of Advanced Nursing* **32**(6): 1522–32.

143. Lave J (1988). Cognition in practice: Mind, mathematics and culture in everyday life: 1988.

144. Issenberg SB, McGaghie WC, Petrusa ER, Lee Gordon D, Scalese RJ (2005). Features and uses of high-fidelity medical simulations that lead to effective learning: a BEME systematic review. *Medical Teacher* **27**(1): 10–28.

145. Stanton NA (2006). Hierarchical task analysis: developments, applications, and extensions. *Applied Ergonomics* **37**(1): 55–79.

146. Annett J, Cunningham D, Mathias-Jones P (2000). A method for measuring team skills. *Ergonomics* **43**(8): 1076–94.

147. Shepherd A (1998). HTA as a framework for task analysis. *Ergonomics* **41**(11): 1537–52.

148. O'Donnell JM, Bradle J, Goode JA (2007). 07 IMSH Peer-Reviewed Research Abstracts: Development of a Simulation and Internet Based Pilot Intervention to Evaluate Adherence to a Patient Transfer Protocol in the Real World Environment. *Simulation in Healthcare: The Journal of the Society for Simulation in Healthcare* **1**(1): 62.

149. Wakefield A, Cooke S, Boggis C (2003). Learning together: use of simulated patients with nursing and medical students for breaking bad news. *International Journal of Palliative Nursing* **9**(1): 32–8.

150. Kneebone R, Kidd J, Nestel D, Asvall S, Paraskeva P, Darzi A (2002). An innovative model for teaching and learning clinical procedures. *Medical Education* **36**(7)628–34.

151. Flanagan B, Nestel D, Joseph M et al. (2004) Making patient safety the focus: Crisis Resource Management in the undergraduate curriculum. *Medical Education* **38**(1): 56–66.

152. Blum RH, Raemer DB, Carroll JS, Dufresne RL, Cooper JB (2005). A method for measuring the effectiveness of simulation-based team training for improving communication skills. *Anesthesia & Analgesia* **100**(5): 1375–80.

153. Donovan T, Hutchison T, Kelly A (2003). Using simulated patients in a multiprofessional communications skills programmeme: reflections from the programmeme facilitators. *European Journal of Cancer Care* **12**(2): 123–8.

154. Choi J-I, Hannafin M (1995). Situated cognition and learning environments: Roles, structures, and implications for design. *Educational Technology Research & Development* **43**(2): 53–69.

155. Becker KL, Rose LE, Berg JB, Park H, Shatzer JH (2006). The teaching effectiveness of standardized patients. *Journal of Nursing Education* **45**(4): 103–11.

156. Rutledge CM, Garzon L, Scott M, Karlowicz K (2004). Using standardized patients to teach and evaluate nurse practitioner students on cultural competency. *International Journal of Nursing Education Scholarship* **1**(1): 18p.

157. Gilbert DA (2004). Coordination in nurses' listening activities and communication about patient-nurse relationships. *Research in Nursing & Health* **27**(6): 447–57.

158. Yoo MS, Yoo IY (2003). The effectiveness of standardized patients as a teaching method for nursing fundamentals. *Journal of Nursing Education* **42**(10): 444–8.

159. Nestel D, Kneebone R, Kidd J (2003). Teaching and learning about skills in minor surgery. *Journal of Clinical Nursing* **12**(2): 291–6.

160. Nestel D, Kidd J (2003). Peer tutoring in patient-centred interviewing skills: experience of a project for first-year students. *Medical Teacher* **25**(4): 398–403.

161. Mar CM, Chabal C, Anderson RA, Vore AE (2003). An interactive computer tutorial to teach pain assessment. *Journal of Health Psychology* **8**(1): 161–73.

162. Kneebone RL, Nestel D, Moorthy K, *et al.* (2003). Learning the skills of flexible sigmoidoscopy – the wider perspective. *Medical Education* **37**(Suppl.1): 50–8.

163. Kneebone R, Nestel D, Ratnasothy J, Kidd J, Darzi A (2003). The use of handheld computers in scenario-based procedural assessments. *Medical Teacher* **25**(6): 632–42.

164. Ker JS (2003). Developing professional clinical skills for practice – the results of a feasibility study using a reflective approach to intimate examination. *Medical Education* **37**(Suppl.1): 34–41.

165. Konkle-Parker DJ, Cramer CK, Hamill C (2002). Standardized patient training: a modality for teaching interviewing skills. *Journal of Continuing Education in Nursing* **33**(5): 225–30.

166. Conway J, Sharkey R (2002). Integrating on campus problem based learning and practice based learning: issues and challenges in using computer mediated communication. *Nurse Education Today* **22**(7): 552–62.

167. Kruijver IP, Kerkstra A, Bensing JM, van de Wiel HB (2001). Communication skills of nurses during interactions with simulated cancer patients. *Journal of Advanced Nursing* **34**(6): 772–9.

168. AHRQ (2001). Making Health Care Safer: A Critical Analysis of Patient Safety Practices *Evidence Report: Technology Assessment (Summary)* **43**: i-x, 1–668.

169. Takahashi M, Muranaka Y, Negishi M, Maruoka A, Koganezawa T (2000). How to create nursing CAI in the specialised course/nursing seminar in the baccalaureate programmeme. In: Saba V, *et al.*, Eds. *Nursing Informatics 2000 One Step Beyond: the Evolution of Technology and Nursing Proceedings of the 7th IMIA International Conference on Nursing use of Computers and Information Science, Auckland, New Zealand, 28 April–-3 May, 2000*: Adis International Limited: Auckland, New Zealand.

170. Ambrosiadou V, Compton T, Panchal T, Polovina S (2000). Web-based multimedia courseware for emergency cardiac patient management simulations. *Studies in Health Technology & Informatic* **77**: 578–82.

171. Brown G (1999). Technology in nurse education: a communication teaching strategy. *ABNF Journal* **10**(1): 9–13.

172. Arthur D (1999). Assessing nursing students' basic communication and interviewing skills: the development and testing of a rating scale. *Journal of Advanced Nursing* **29**(3): 658–65.

173. Foley ME, Nespoli G, Conde E (1997). Using standardized patients and standardized physicians to improve patient-care quality: results of a pilot study. *Journal of Continuing Education in Nursing* **28**(5): 198–204.

174. Baker K, Garrett E, Kirkham M (1997). The use of actresses in midwifery education. *Modern Midwife* **7**(7): 28–31.

175. Rizzolo MA (1990). Factors influencing the development and use of interactive video in nursing education. A Delphi study. *Computers in Nursing* **8**(4): 151–9.

176. Goode JA, Schumann T, Klain M, O'Donnell JM (2007). 07 IMSH Work-In-Progress Abstracts: Evaluation of a Novel System for Quantitative Assessment of Bag Valve Mask Ventilation (BVMV). *Simulation in Healthcare: The Journal of the Society for Simulation in Healthcare* **1**(1): 96.

177. Pugh CM, Youngblood P (2002). Development and validation of assessment measures for a newly developed physical examination simulator. *Journal of the American Medical Informatics Association* **9**(5): 448–60.

178. Adamo G (2003). Simulated and standardized patients in OSCEs: achievements and challenges 1992–2003. *Medical Teacher* **25**(3): 262–70.

179. Nicol M, Freeth D (1998). Assessment of clinical skills: a new approach to an old problem. *Nurse Education Today* **18**(8): 601–9.

180. Major DA (2005). OSCEs–seven years on the bandwagon: the progress of an objective structured clinical evaluation programmeme. *Nurse Education Today* **25**(6): 442–54.

181. Bartfay WJ, Rombough R, Howse E, Leblanc R (2004). Evaluation. The OSCE approach in nursing education. *Canadian Nurse* **100**(3): 18–23.

182. Alinier G (2003). Nursing students' and lecturers' perspectives of objective structured clinical examination incorporating simulation. *Nurse Education Today* **23**(6): 419–26.

183. Rogers PL, Jacob H, Thomas EA, Harwell M, Willenkin RL, Pinsky MR (2000). Medical students can learn the basic application, analytic, evaluative, and psychomotor skills of critical care medicine. *Critical Care Medicine* **28**(2): 550–4.

184. Alinier G, Hunt B, Gordon R, *et al.* (2006). Effectiveness of intermediate-fidelity simulation training technology in undergraduate nursing education. *Journal of Advanced Nursing* **54**(3): 359–69.

185. Mudumbai S, Lighthall G, Sun C, Harrison K, Davies F, Howard S (2007). 07 IMSH Peer-Reviewed Research Abstracts: Reproducibility of A Model Driven Simulator and Sensitivity to Initial Conditions. *Simulation in Healthcare: The Journal of the Society for Simulation in Healthcare* **1**(1): 45.

186. Register M, Graham-Garcia J, Haas R (2003). The use of simulation to demonstrate hemodynamic response to varying degrees of intrapulmonary shunt. *AANA Journal* **71**(4): 277–84.

187. Farnsworth ST, Egan TD, Johnson SE, Westenskow D (2000). Teaching sedation and analgesia with simulation. *Journal of Clinical Monitoring & Computing* **16**(4): 273–85.

188. Henneman EA, Cunningham H (2005). Using clinical simulation to teach patient safety in an acute/critical care nursing course. *Nurse Educator* **30**(4): 172–7.

189. Marsch SC, Tschan F, Semmer N, Spychiger M, Breuer M, Hunziker PR (2005). Performance of first responders in simulated cardiac arrests. *Critical Care Medicine* **33**(5): 963–7.

190. Brady D, Molzen S, Graham S, O'Neill V (2006). Using the synergy of online education and simulation to inspire a new model for a community critical care course. *Critical Care Nursing Quarterly* **29**(3): 231–6.

191. Hoffmann R, O'Donnell JM, Kim Y (2007). The Effects of Human Patient Simulators on Basic Knowledge in Critical Care Nursing with Undergraduate Senior Baccalaureate Nursing Students. *Simulation in Healthcare: The Journal of the Society for Simulation in Healthcare* **2**(2): 110–14.

192. Cioffi J, Purcal N, Arundell F, Cioffi J, Purcal N, Arundell F (2005). A pilot study to investigate the effect of a simulation strategy on the clinical decision making of midwifery students. *Journal of Nursing Education* **44**(3): 131–4.

193. Robertson B (2006). An obstetric simulation experience in an undergraduate nursing curriculum. *Nurse Educator* **31**(2): 74–8.

194. Traczyk J, Tharp D, Fields T, *et al.* (2002). State Nurse Aide Training: programme Information and Data. In: Services HaH, ed: United States Department of Health and Human Services: Office of Evaluation and Inspection: 1–29.

195. NFLPN (2007). LPN Education Web Page. *National Federation of Licensed Practical Nurses* [http://www.nflpn.org/. Accessed March 3, 2007.

196. USDOL (2007). Occupational Outlook Handbook: Licensed Practical and Vocational Nurses. http://www.bls.gov/oco/ocos102.htm. Accessed March 3, 2007.

197. USDOL (2007). Occupational Outlook Handbook: Registered Nurses. http://www.bls.gov/oco/ocos102.htm. Accessed March 3, 2007.

Chapter 20

Crisis resource management in healthcare

Geoffrey K Lighthall

Overview

- The outcome of many natural and manmade disasters is dictated by the interaction between underlying hazards and the human response to such conditions.

- Aviation and other high-risk industries have recognized that deficiencies in interpersonal communication and team management skills can contribute to significant loss of life.

- Teaching teamwork and behavioural skills became more successful in aviation after their incorporation into existing technical skills training programs that used high fidelity flight simulators.

- Realistic patient simulation systems were created in anaesthesiology as a vehicle for introducing crisis management principles into resident training. Anaesthesia crisis resource management (ACRM) was a prototype curriculum that resulted from these efforts.

- ACRM exposed trainees to common and uncommon anaesthesia crises, and helped develop an understanding of specific cognitive and teamwork skills that could augment responses to a variety of crises. Crisis resource management (CRM) has come to represent the latter set of skills.

- Anaesthesia's success has been replicated in a number of different healthcare fields such as intensive care and emergency medicine, where CRM skills are equally applicable.

20.1 Introduction

Crisis resource management (CRM) has come to define the cognitive and teamwork skills that facilitate management of medical events bearing a high risk to patient well being. There are various definitions for crisis, but for purposes of this discussion, the definition below will be used.

A crisis is an unplanned life-threatening event in which there is a mismatch between the ambient level of resources and those that a patient needs to regain stability.

Resources should be thought of in the broadest sense to include a wide range of personal, psychological, and material components that can be mobilized to improve a patient's course. For example, a patient with significant bleeding can be managed without too much difficulty in an operating room, since the expertise, materials and reserves for fluid and blood administration are widely available. Encountering the same patient on a medical ward is likely to be a crisis due to the novelty of the situation, a lack of personnel trained to handle the problem, and lack of key materials. The requisite skills for managing such a crisis include understanding the situation, its evolution and various solutions, and how to engage others in order to arrive at a solution. These, as well as the acquisition of additional information and help, communicating with coworkers, and making back-up plans are examples of CRM skills that can influence the overall outcome of the situation. For illustrative purposes, the key points of CRM taught in our residency training programs are listed in Table 20.1. Behavioural skills such as these have been labeled 'non-technical', in contrast to medical knowledge and procedural proficiency, which represent technical skills. Training in CRM or behavioural skills is most applicable to fields of medicine that commonly encounter crises or high-risk unplanned events, high stress, diagnostic or therapeutic ambiguity, or time pressures. CRM training is based on the premise that both technical and non-technical skills are essential to critical event management and should be developed in parallel. However, this realization has come only recently, lagging a century and a half behind the traditional paradigm of care that emphasizes knowledge and skill of the individual as the basic target of training and evaluation. Implicit to the traditional model is that those that excel will have the best outcomes. However, under stress, there is no guarantee that even the best plan will be implemented without some additional abilities in managing a diverse set of personnel, understanding one's own limitations under stress, and without deliberate attention to communication, contingency planning, and effective leadership[1]. Interest in such behavioural skills has come not from prospective evaluation of these components, but from the realization that a significant number of medical mishaps are traceable to the absence of these skills[2–4].

The role of non-technical skills and their relationship to patient outcomes had a striking resemblance to findings from research into aviation disasters of the prior decade. Inquiry into accidents revealed that in most crashes implicating pilot error, it wasn't manual skills that were lacking, but deficiencies in leadership, teamwork, communication, and planning[5]. For aviation, the tragedy of lost life is generally front-page news and subject to open investigation. The public outcry for full analysis and prevention is overwhelmingly greater than is the case of medicine, where the public's awareness of mishaps has been historically low. In both medicine and aviation, simulation of critical events is closely tied to analysis of cognition and teamwork dynamics and their role in propagating or minimizing risk to human life. Consideration of the evolution of

Table 20.1 Skill sets applicable to critical event management

Technical skills	Non-technical skills	
Medical knowledge and its application	Decision-making and cognition	Team and resource management
Physical examination	Knowledge of the team and environment	Taking a leadership role
Data evaluation	Anticipation and planning	Calling for help early
Differential diagnosis	Wise allocation of attention	Communicating effectively
Knowledge of therapeutic plans and pathways	Use of all available information and confirmation of key data streams	Distributing the workload
Hands-on skills	Use of cognitive aids (e.g. checklists, reference materials)	Mobilization and utilization of all available resources

CRM in commercial aviation and its entry into medicine provides an informative perspective on the use of patient simulation systems, and to what may turn out to be their 'higher calling'.

20.2 Origins of CRM in aviation

CRM owes its origins to a series of teamwork and behavioural training interventions originating in commercial aviation in the late 1970s (see Chapter 4). The impetus to offer such training came from a systematic study of plane crashes showing that breakdowns in communication, information sharing, and contingency planning underlie the majority of such events[6]. In one classic case, a three-member crew of a full passenger jet became occupied with a faulty landing gear indicator light while on final approach to Miami airport[7]. While distracted, the crew failed to notice that the autopilot was disengaged, or notice the low altitude warnings that would have prevented the loss of all life on board. Ideally, one would have been flying the plane, while the remaining crew sought additional verification of a landing gear problem and prepared for an emergency landing if necessary. A similar 'possible landing gear problem' led another crew to lengthen a flight in order to consume extra fuel; however, execution of this plan was flawed, and the plane ran out of fuel 12 miles short of the airport[8]. Investigators from the US National Transportation Safety Board implicated "failure of the captain to monitor properly the aircraft's fuel state and to properly respond to the low fuel state and the crewmembers' advisories regarding the fuel state" as the probable cause of the crash[8].

A series of interventions were subsequently aimed at preventing such errors through more effective use of the human resources in the cockpit. Its first iteration, cockpit resource management (CRM), consisted of discussion groups where various qualities of leadership and interpersonal behaviour were explored; this general model of leadership training was largely modeled on concepts and programmes used by corporations to improve managerial effectiveness. Early acceptance faced challenges associated with changing the *status quo*, as well as the uphill battle of winning over the individualistic culture of aircraft pilots with programmes perceived by some as 'charm school'.[9,10]

Subsequent generations of CRM took on a more holistic view of team coordination, and began to include the cabin crew and ground personnel as well. The name changed from 'cockpit ...' to 'crew resource management', in accordance with this new mindset. A major difference was a shift in focus from the abstract concepts of interpersonal dynamics, to courses that identified more specific behaviours and skills that pilots could use to function more effectively[10]. The later generations of CRM are notable for establishing firmer connections between the realities of flight command and non-technical skills, and significantly, for their greater acceptance by pilots. The improved reception was undoubtedly facilitated by the recent change of flight simulation activities from skill training sessions to full mission simulations containing scenarios that tested teamwork, communication, and decision making skills of intact crews. With this type of training, behaviours could be learned and practised by in-flight scenarios, and further explored by subsequent review of recordings[5]. This latter paradigm of crew training received considerable support by US government agencies such as the US Federal Aviation Administration (FAA), which in 1990 began requiring integration of CRM into regular flight training[10], and the National Transportation Safety Board, whose investigations of airline crashes began noting the presence of such programmes in their investigations and recommendations. CRM is not a single shot training experience, rather, it has been incorporated into the periodic simulation training and certification process that pilots undergo throughout their careers. Some evidence exists to the effectiveness of CRM training. Responses on surveys describing attitudes toward communication, crew coordination, and command responsibility are associated with higher degrees of performance when rated by trained observers during real flight and in simulated flight[11,12]. Both pilots and regulatory agencies have attributed some positive outcomes to existence of CRM programmes, the most notable being a 1989 flight of a DC-10 in which the crew needed to devise a means of controlling the plane after losing all hydraulic controls from a central engine explosion. Despite crashing in the end, the plane reached a runway and spared the lives of half on board. During this crisis the crew recruited a passenger who was a pilot to assist with controlling the plane; the cockpit voice recordings indicate a crew that was constantly updating data sources, communicating clearly, prioritizing tasks, and planning ahead. The final report issued by the National Transportation Safety Board viewed "the interaction of the pilots…during the emergency as indicative of the value of cockpit resource management training, which has been in existence at United Airlines for a decade[13]."

20.3 CRM enters the world of medicine

The evolution of CRM is notable for introducing a philosophical shift in the training of crews and in how excellence in aviation is defined, more than leaving a firm set of rules. A great deal of latitude was allowed for organizations to develop crew coordination concepts applicable to their particular set of operating conditions. The incorporation of crew resource management into the everyday activities of commercial aviation was helped by its provision of solutions to publicly visible problems, its recommendation by investigative and regulatory agencies, and an overall desire of the military and civilian corporations to preserve material assets and life. The transfer of CRM concepts to medicine occurred in contrast, largely in the absence of the public's awareness of errors and mishaps and their contribution to mortality, with little scrutiny of regulatory agencies calling for solutions, and with no organized front of patients, hospitals, or insurers clamouring for ways to minimize patient risks. Rather, CRM made its way into healthcare through a fortuitous combination of individual, temporal, and technological forces.

20.3.1 The man

CRM was introduced to healthcare through the efforts of David Gaba, an anaesthetist, patient safety advocate, capable engineer, and ardent follower of space and aviation programmes. With these interests, he was keenly aware of the development and rationale for CRM in commercial airlines and equally cognisant of the parallels between accidents in anaesthesia and those in aviation – two fields in which poor outcomes were attributable to deficiencies in non-technical skills as noted above. Shortly after a few airlines merged newly formed programmes of full-mission simulation with CRM training, Gaba was at work creating a similar experience for anaesthesia resident trainees with the construction of an operating room simulator featuring a computer-controlled mannequin 'patient'.

20.3.2 The moment

The late 1980s and early 1990s was a watershed moment for patient safety and especially in the field of anaesthesiology. At this time, investigators in this field began to explore the nature of mishaps, deaths, and cases resulting in lawsuits. Institutional developments marking this period were the establishment of the Anaesthesia Patient Safety Foundation in the USA, the Australian Patient Safety Foundation[14–16], initiation of the anaesthesia closed claims project[17] and the Australian Incident Monitoring Study. Unlike the fruits of other medical fields, administration of an anaesthetic *per se*, offers no direct benefit to a patient – only additional risk[18]. From this humble position of risk aversion, the field of anaesthesiology became a model for nearly all of the patient safety and medical error research occurring in medicine today [19,20]. The early wave patient safety interest within the field of anaesthesia brought with it some funds, which in part allowed Gaba's project to come to fruition.

Development of a realistic mannequin simulator was undoubtedly facilitated by the prior development of waveform generators, individual task trainers and electronic displays that were increasingly available at the time. Integrating these various training devices into a single high performance organism became a reasonable option for the first time due to the explosive developments in personal computers and software, and their greater affordability.

20.3.3 The machine

Through the efforts noted above, both human and material components of the operating room were assembled in an evolving set of simulators systems called CASE® (Comprehensive Anaesthesia Simulation Environment). While interactive software-based simulators were available[21], the hands on simulator was able to 'recreate the anaesthesiologists physical, as well as mental, task environment[22]'. This was considered an important adjunct to the computer trainers that assessed only *knowing what to do*. With the entire environment at hand, participants had to balance manual as well as cognitive tasks, and manage such at the same time as communicating with surgeons and managing distractions. While the philosophical drive behind this training environment changed little, dramatic improvements were made in the actual patient simulator. CASE® version 1.2 featured operator control of a computer that drove multiple perceptible clinical signs such as breathing, pulses, heart sounds and rhythm, and the ability to display such on real monitors in the operating room; a head–torso combination covered by surgical drapes served as a patient[22]. Later models featured complete mannequins and fully integrated patient responses driven by pharmacological and physiological models. Initially the simulator was placed in a real operating room, but the timing, logistics, and workload created a need for a separate facility for conducting this training; hence the concept of a dedicated simulation centre was born.

20.3.4 The philosophy

The curriculum resulting from these efforts eventually became known anaesthesia crisis resource management (ACRM). In ACRM, the anaesthesia trainee is exposed to a patient care scenario that typically unfolds into a full-blown crisis requiring additional help, material resources, and leadership from the anesthesiologist, while faculty and staff play the roles of surgeons and nurses. The scenarios therefore provide valuable experience in managing high-yield patient care problems, as well as serving as a basis for practising and learning the non-technical aspects of event management. The actual simulations are only part of ACRM; the course considered a number of additional components essential to crisis management training[23]:

- A catalogue of incidents with guidelines for avoidance, recognition and management (analogous to the pilot's emergency procedure manual)
- A theoretical framework for understanding human performance and human error
- A case study to further clarify key issues of performance and some of the vocabulary used in its analysis
- Familiarization with the environment
- Realistic hands-on simulation
- Structured debriefings of simulation performance (using audio and video recordings) that clarify both technical and CRM aspects of event management.

Unlike its component parts that were designed for training of isolated tasks, the high fidelity simulator provided an essential source of credibility to an environment designed to introduce a 'systematic approach to managing crises'[23]. CRM introduced new ideas regarding patient care, and the simulator was the messenger for these concepts. Certainly, the absence of a human patient posed no theoretical barrier to CRM training; however, the ability to introduce these concepts to the anaesthesia community in a highly recognizable manner led to almost instant approval of both patient simulation and related CRM training. Of equal importance, critical event simulations created opportunities for the conduct of research into human performance during medical crises. Prior to critical event simulation of *known problems*, the actions and behaviours of participants were largely inaccessible, because of the sporadic occurrence and sometimes unknown aetiology of such events in real life[24,25].

The CASE simulator was not the first patient simulator constructed. Abrahamson and colleagues developed a full-scale simulator in the late 1960s that was developed to train anaesthesia residents in airway management[26,27]. While the creators of this prototype simulator (called SimOne®) noted that learning on the mannequin could allow instruction to occur without compromise to patient safety, the latter idea probably had little resonance at that time. Also, the supporting computer was too large and too expensive for commercialization[28]. Overall, SimOne® was an idea that arrived before its time.

In addition to Gaba's Stanford/ Veterans'Administration programme, the modern renaissance of simulation also includes an effort led by Michael Good at the University of Florida[29]. This effort also resulted in the development of a full-scale mannequin, but with a focus on training residents to recognize various forms of machine failure and other discrete intraoperative events. The early years of simulation highlighted the fact that some aspects of anaesthesia patient care training may be best accomplished in settings outside of the operating room, or at least in the absence of real patients. It further highlighted the value of simulation as an entry point into understanding the non-technical or behavioural aspects of patient care.

Whether the behavioural concepts introduced by ACRM could be appreciated by a wider slice of the academic and anaesthesia community remained unclear. To address this, the ACRM curriculum was exported to the Harvard Department of Anaesthesiology where the curriculum was presented in a series of sessions to nurse anaesthetists, attending, and resident level anaesthesiologists. The courses were met with a high degree of approval, demonstrating both the general acceptance and exportability of the educational model and technology[28,30]. Similar degrees of success were replicated in the latter part of the 1990s as CRM courses based on the anaesthesia model were developed in emergency medicine[31], neonatology[32], critical care[33], and surgery[34].

20.4 **Crisis resource management: core concepts**

CRM offers a framework for understanding and improving upon human performance in medical crises; as such, it is intended to complement pre-learned 'technical' skills of diagnosis and disease management. Despite the intangible nature of an *approach* rather than a *set method*, a set of recurring concepts can be identified in the published reports from programmes that have implemented CRM-based curricula (Table 20.2). The set of topics presented below appears for illustrative purposes and to stimulate further thought. There is no dogmatic list of CRM principles in either aviation or medicine. Rather, individual training programmes, hospitals and disciplines may chose to emphasize certain concepts over others and develop their own set of rules or principles applicable to that practice environment. Understanding the antecedents and contributing factors to critical events and near misses within an institution is an important starting point for understanding the workplace, its inhabitants, and the training content that is likely to carry the greatest impact.

Table 20.2 Core concepts of crisis resource management

- Maintain situational awareness
- Prevent fixation errors
- Know the environment and know your teammates
- Distribute the workload
- Call for help early enough
- Practice effective leadership
- Communicate effectively
- Allocate attention wisely
- Anticipate and plan
- Use all sources of information and cross-check data streams
- Use cognitive aids to assure completeness

20.4.1 Maintain situational awareness

Situational awareness (SA) is the ability to understand the content and significance of important elements within the environment. The concept comes from military aircraft operations, but is equally applicable to any healthcare domain that deals with acutely ill individuals[35,36]. Endsley has developed a construct of SA that involves three levels[37].

- Level I is a perception of the elements in the environment, for example an understanding of patient comorbidities and current complaints, vital signs and the frequency of their acquisition, and pertinent laboratory and imaging studies.

- Level II is a comprehension of the patient's current status based on a synthesis of level I variables and an understanding of their relationship to known events. Crises are often recognized by a patient's status being different from preconceived ideas of what should be occurring.

- Level III awareness describes the ability to predict how a current set of events will lead to subsequent events. This latter level of awareness is necessary to prepare for future events and to have greater control over them – in other words, moving from a reactive to a proactive mode and creating appropriate back-up plans.

Factors that allow one to establish and maintain SA include experience, ability to solicit information from a variety of sources, and a constant refocusing on overarching priorities. Factors that impair SA are task overloading, fright or distress, psychomotor impairment (lack of sleep, drugs), and preoccupation with inconsequential tasks (fixation errors, see below). Interpersonal factors such as leadership style (specifically one that tends to squelch valuable input), pressure to conform, and lack of objectivity can also impair forming accurate and objective perceptions of a situation. SA is a more familiar term in military flight training than in healthcare. Nonetheless a number of key points of ACRM and its offspring have been derived from this concept[23,31–33].

20.4.2 Know the environment and know your teammates

Defining of a crisis as a mismatch between resources required to stabilize a patient and what is actually available, it is easy to see where knowledge of the immediate environment is important for formulating an impression of the current situation, and understanding how ambient resources may influence outcome. Some patients may be better served by bringing one or two additional elements into an environment (fluoroscopy machine or extra anaesthesiologist) instead of moving the patient to a different area. Knowing what other individuals are present and what they are qualified to do, assists greatly with team coordination and efficiency.

Further, understanding whether any other capabilities exist within a hospital (cardiac catheterization facilities, MRI) is essential for prioritization and planning during an emergency.

20.4.3 Distribute the workload

Deliberate attention to what tasks need to be done, when they are begun and completed, and what level skill is necessary to perform the task is an important part of personnel management in a crisis. Medical emergencies can create an overdependence on key personnel (bottlenecks); however these can be avoided by proper spreading of work over time and personnel. Understanding what type of tasks can be attended to by a single profession, and which can be dispensed to others is an important part of conserving key people resources for crucial times. In some of our critical care simulations, we have taken the position that *the best leaders of multiple professions are those that understand something about the workload and struggles of each profession.* Thus, having medicine residents cross-filling the roles of anaesthesiologist, nurse and pharmacist has provided these trainees with some insight into what each profession can handle at a given time, and how to redistribute some of their requests in a crisis.

20.4.4 Call for help early enough

Especially at night, some of the most skilled and experienced people are at home where they are of little use to an unstable patient. Even during the day, many are occupied with patients in the operating room or clinic. Key assets such as endoscopes, bronchoscopes, catheterization labs, operating room or ICU beds all have some lag that occurs prior to full engagement. Thus, even at the expense of bringing others into a situation where they are not eventually needed, the best care of some patients requires an early engagement of other personnel and resources. A key factor to effective use of help is knowing that certain types of help are only effective at certain times. For example, a surgeon can help with a cricothyroidotomy in a 'can't intubate/can't ventilate' scenario only if they are in the same room. Barriers to effective mobilization of others range from personal factors ("I don't want to appear weak….") to the interpersonal ("the GI people always give me a hard time when I call at night"), and cultural ("I am a senior fellow, it is *my* job to handle this type of problem.") Simulations in a controlled environment where the patient problems are known can be used to create situations where external help is needed, and the expectation that help be called can be reinforced. Unlike real life, errors can be left uncorrected to help trainees appreciate the consequences of certain actions or inactions.

20.4.5 Practice effective leadership

> The wise leader does not intervene unnecessarily. The leader's presence is felt, but often the group runs itself.
>
> J Heider, *Tao of Leadership*[38]

The leader is in charge of coordinating the activities of team members according to the needs and priorities of a given situation. Implicit in the apprenticeship model of medical training is that leadership skill derives from experience in the field. While knowledge and experience are certainly indispensable, the highest level of performance will likely result from leaders that demonstrate additional traits, such as:

- the ability to promote clear and open communication (see below)
- the ability to identify and communicate priorities

- an ability to inspire confidence
- comfort in acknowledging limitations and asking for help
- understanding personal limitations, and accepting the fact that performance may be influenced by situational and personal factors
- openness to suggestions.

From studies on group dynamics and task completion in simulated and real emergencies, it is apparent that some form of leadership structure improves team dynamics and task performance and completion[25,39,40]. Further, the leader's engagement in hands-on tasks has been suggested to impair group function and task completion[39]. While we may currently struggle to find data on what constitutes 'proper leadership' in general, crisis simulation provides an excellent means for exploring aspects of leadership and group action in specific situations. With a simulated scenario and debriefing one can quite accurately explore a number of significant questions.

- What did the team leader think was going on, and what was actually communicated to the team?
- What did the leader seek to accomplish, and what was actually accomplished?
- Were requests made but never heard or acted upon?
- How well were key tasks distributed?
- Were key personnel underused or overused?
- How well did the leader handle input and other suggestions?

Usually, discovery and discussion of failed group processes in debriefings point to specific behaviours that can be practised in subsequent encounters. In simulation training that involves multiple scenarios, we routinely see progressive improvement in leadership behaviours throughout the course, suggesting that trainees possess the ability and motivation to improve non-technical and technical skills[33].

20.4.6 Communicate effectively

Communication is the clear sending and receiving of information, directions, and assessments. It is the responsibility of every team member to understand what is said and to be understood. Clarification should be sought over making assumptions or incorrectly recalling a request. Closed loop communication, in which the responder repeats back what is requested, is an effective tool for assuring that both the content and the direction of a request were understood. Barriers to effective communication are group distractions, hierarchies, or lack of a shared model for a situation or problem. Noise, interpersonal problems, and leader behaviour can interfere with communication or the respondents' willingness to clarify a request. Crowd control, pairing requests with names, eye contact, asking if the content is understood, and avoidance of jargon can all improve the ease and fidelity of communication.

20.4.7 Allocate attention wisely

A leader's attention in a crisis is perhaps his or her most valuable asset. Of utmost importance is the maintenance of attention on information that allows an understanding of a patient's problem and the ability to monitor team activities as 'solutions' are applied. Many problems and tasks arise in dynamic environments; thus, leadership that can understand the crisis well enough to establish priorities and communicate these to team members is necessary. Unfortunately, most high risk medical professions also involve a high degree of procedural expertise, and in this way, the person who is the most qualified to be the leader may also be the person with the best manual skills. Once a leader becomes occupied with a given task, his or her effectiveness as a leader diminishes appreciably[39]. Conversely, competent execution of manual tasks loses its effectiveness when other distractions (such as the need to process information or lead a team) compete for attention. We see examples of the latter on a weekly basis on house staff cardiopulmonary resuscitation drills when the person performing chest compressions often slows down or stops compressing when distracted with conversation or rhythm interpretation. One value of CRM training with videotape debriefing (see Chapter 13) is its ability have participants see and experience the ubiquitous nature of attentional derailing.

Maintaining a degree of attentional reserve may allow a skilled leader to understand that an individual patient problem may be part of a larger issue. For example a previously healthy patient admitted with respiratory distress may be an index event to a toxic exposure or pandemic. Likewise a disruption in oxygen supply that causes unexpected hypoxaemia in an operative patient may be related to a problem of the entire building that needs immediate attention to prevent morbidity to hundreds of other patients.

20.4.8 Prevent fixation errors

Managing crises requires a flexible mindset that accepts the possibility of making incorrect assumptions or errors, but mitigates damage through constant re-evaluation of the situation and team interventions. Fixation errors result from the persistent inability to revise or employ plans in accordance to readily available data[1]. Engagement in tasks that have little relationship to the primary problem or task at hand is a common manifestation of this type of error (remember the landing gear lamp above). The risk to patients is therefore two fold.

◆ Attendance to less significant tasks reflects a poor understanding of the overall situation.

◆ The attention devoted to such tasks further distracts one's ability to step back and more fully understand the problem.

The definition of fixation errors, their source and mitigation figures prominently in nearly all healthcare CRM programmes that the author is aware of; many use some of the examples from aviation as an entry point to this discussion[7]. The value of such understanding is to be aware that crises are loaded with these traps and to be able to recognize their presence and to avoid them. Gaba and colleagues describe three main types of fixation errors[1].

◆ *This and only this...* The persistent fixation on a single problem and failing to revise a diagnosis or plan despite contradictory evidence. In some cases, the available evidence is interpreted out of context, and in others, secondary problems receive more attention than the primary problem (i.e. treating tachycardia rather than significant haemorrhage).

◆ *Everything but this...* The persistent inability to act upon a major problem. Valuable time is wasted searching for other problems, sometimes to the exclusion of treating the main problem.

◆ *Everything is OK...* The persistent belief that there is not any major problem. Commonly, reassuring signs are used to override worrisome evidence (despite anuria and the lactate of 8 mMol/L, the patient was mentally intact, so there was no real urgency to treat the patient...). Likewise, worrisome data is written off as artifactual while other data streams indicate imminent deterioration. Equipment failures, alarms and abnormal data can pose interesting challenges; in these instances sometimes the patient is actually fine, and deserves less attention than another problem. Nonetheless, declaring the patient to be 'OK' without a reasonable reassessment is problematic.

An awareness of fixation errors from CRM training may lead to specific workplace rules where applicable. Treatment protocols, mandatory help calls for specific problems, and an atmosphere where all team members feel their input is valuable are possible means to avoid fixation errors. In cardiac anaesthesia, I have a rule that when an infusion pump alarms, either the resident or attending is assigned to watch the patient and monitors *before* any attention is diverted to the pump. Emergency medicine and critical care environments may likewise wish to develop training procedures or rules for attending to a set of shifting or competing priorities that may exist within a multi-patient environment.

20.4.9 Anticipate and plan

This is a more tangible and teachable rule extracted from the goal of maintaining situational awareness. Knowing where a problem or crisis is headed, and communicating this understanding can do much to facilitate group function by helping others focus on what they need to be doing and how to prioritize work. If presented in the right manner, statements of plans act as an invitation for others to contribute their ideas to the overall process. Further, discussion of plans builds purpose and camaraderie within a group, and helps others maintain a proper state of arousal. In the process of training, it important for participants to know that there is rarely a single perfect solution to a patient emergency; rather, there is a huge array of imperfect choices that require constant reassessment and simultaneous institution of backup plans. In anaesthesia, airway management and haemodynamic instability are examples of crises requiring the practitioner to always stay one problem ahead of oneself.

20.4.10 Use all sources of information and cross-check data streams

Proper orientation in a medical crisis depends upon an accurate assessment of the patient's status. The potential for inaccurate, incomplete, or artifactual data arises in many emergencies, and requires that reactions to the data be made in response to the true reality of the situation. Data from pulse oximeters, electrocardiographic traces and arterial blood pressure monitors can elicit behavioural responses that range from no action, 'must be an artifact, the pulse ox is always falling off…' to the other extreme of administering chest compressions to a stable patient. Factors contributing to this type of problem include inexperience, lack of familiarity with the environment, and the presence of stress, distractions or personal factors that prevent a proper intake of pertinent elements (Level I situation awareness in Endsley's formulation[37]). The reader will recognize incomplete information use or aberrant interpretation of a data stream as a common type of fixation error. Potential countermeasures include use of well-practised behaviours (ABCs) or work procedures (checklists) that help establish orientation. CRM training in a simulated setting assures that behaviours and responses can be compared to *a known problem*. The latter is an improvement upon reconstruction of real-life events, because the data set and perceptions that prompted a given action can *never be compared to what was really going on*. With realistic scenarios presented in a controlled setting, factors underlying improper actions can be explored and hopefully corrected.

20.4.11 Use cognitive aids to assure completeness

Pocket cards, handbooks, and electronic assistants are almost part of the uniform worn by medical trainees, but in our experience, it is rare to see this information used in real emergencies. Why is this so? Perhaps looking things up in public projects an image of uncertainty or lack of knowledge. Or perhaps the presence of such information is simply not considered during the fright of an emergency. Following the ABCs when encountering an unsure situation is one type of cognitive scaffold that we are all trained to follow, but beyond that, medical practice – referring to medical education and the workplace – has done little to educate and implement the use of decisional support tools. Interestingly, cardiac arrest emergencies derive from a handful of patterns for which treatment algorithms have been developed and extensively published[41]. Despite this achievement, nowhere in the American Heart Association manuals is it noted that memory of algorithms may be impaired, and that it might be a good idea to designate an individual to extract the proper algorithm and assure that it is followed. Since its origin in healthcare, CRM training has consistently advocated that cognitive aids be used to provide decisional support whenever applicable. In fact, many of our trainees are a bit surprised when we ask them to carry their cards and handbooks during simulator training. Importantly, trainees should be given opportunities to experience the usefulness of different cognitive aids, and have this reinforced during the course of training. Interestingly, emergency simulations may provide some insight into the actual design of cognitive aids, and serve as a proving ground for their usefulness[42].

Types of cognitive aids:

◆ Reference manuals of critical events[1,43]

◆ Hand-held computers and databases (Palm pilot, PDAs)

◆ Internet searches at point of care

◆ Telephone consultations

◆ Poison control centres and other regional 'hotlines'

◆ Manufacturer support for medical devices (pacemakers).

20.5 Using simulation systems to provide CRM training

Critical event simulations can accommodate a diversity of training goals; however, the impact of each course is likely to be greater if one does not attempt to 'do it all at once'. The applicability of simulation systems to clinical education can be described by a spectrum of activities listed according to increased complexity.

◆ Simple skill acquisition (central line placement).

◆ Dynamic skill acquisition (airway management – dynamic because it involves decisions, integrating pharmacology, anatomy, patient state and monitor data).

◆ Pattern recognition and diagnosis.

◆ Management of a disease process – as single discipline trainees or as a team.

◆ Team management of a disease process – forming a team and initial stabilization.

◆ Team management of an evolving or complex disease process.

CRM skills are certainly most applicable to the last three items on the list, although one might argue that at every juncture of training, one should be reminded that the practice of medicine is a team endeavour. Nonetheless, it is quite likely that many of the educational objectives for the earlier listed items can be achieved quite well without the use of a simulator and at a lesser expense, and that the true value of a simulated environment is that it raises the level of the event to one where team coordination can actually make a difference in outcome.

CRM training is typically coupled to scenarios where the medical management can be challenging, but not is mysterious. If the diagnosis is too puzzling, valuable course time will be spent debating what really was going on, rather than concentrating on how a group can organize itself to deal with such a situation. Scenario design and length should be consistent with the goals of the exercise. Short scenarios are ideal for challenging diagnostic capabilities and are well suited

Table 20.3 Use of patient crisis simulation to address CRM concepts

CRM point	Scenario or condition	Rationale
Situational awareness	◆ Sepsis, obstetric disaster, bleeder, MI. Have arriving participant ask what's going on ◆ Diseases with secondary findings (i.e. tachycardia in haemorrhage)	◆ Assesses ability to understand and verbalize nature of situation ◆ Assesses whether team maintains focus on primary abnormality
Leadership	◆ High complexity cases with shifting needs (mechanical ventilation, procedures, CPR etc.) ◆ Send in senior physician when junior physician (current leader) is doing an adequate job	◆ Assesses ability to focus on priorities while maintaining view of larger problems ◆ Set up for power struggle – does leader support or take over? What is best for patient?
Use of cognitive aids	◆ Malignant hyperthermia ◆ Pulseless Electrical Activity	◆ Forces use of MHAUS* direction sheet ◆ Forces one to find list of 'five Ts and five Hs'**
Anticipation /acquiring help	◆ Haemorrhage, myocardial infarction, increased intracranial pressure ◆ Any rapidly deteriorating patient	◆ Requires engagement of others for definitive control – time sensitive disease processes ◆ Is patient receiving more attention or monitoring? ◆ Are junior-level trainees over their heads?
Check all data streams	◆ Pulseless arrest; equipment disruptions ◆ Pneumothorax, hypopnoea, bronchospasm, heart murmur	◆ Requires examination of all sources confirming pulsatile blood flow ◆ Is a team member actually examining the patient?
Distribute the workload	◆ Sepsis or haemorrhage with several tasks to attend to – send in someone asking if they can help ◆ Send in ECG tech or X-ray tech (=radiographer) who asks trainees to move away; patient has ventricular ectopic beats	◆ Assesses leader's monitoring of workload and task pairing ◆ Assesses if anyone is watching patient

Continued

Table 20.3 (continued) Use of patient crisis simulation to address CRM concepts

CRM point	Scenario or condition	Rationale
Prevent fixation errors	◆ Equipment malfunctions, pulseless patient ◆ Novel, rare, or other problems with poor outcomes (malignant hyperthermia, machine malfunction, tamponade)	◆ Whether finding is related to overall situation, whether new information changes plans or are there overriding beliefs that all is fine ◆ Can the team accept compelling information establishing a diagnosis?
Communication	◆ Data probes (information passed on to a single group member) ◆ Send in extra people, create noise	◆ Assesses presence of healthy two-way communication, willingness of junior members to contribute information ◆ Forces use of techniques such as read back that assure requests are properly received
Allocate attention wisely	◆ Pneumothorax, shock, tamponade, haemorrhage	◆ Cases requiring high level of technical skill that may force senior leader to perform procedure (assesses whether leader gets other to do the procedure, watch patient, lead team)

* Malignant Hyperthermia Association of the United States

** American Heart Association Advanced Life Support algorithm for summative evaluations of performance[44]. Longer scenarios require sustaining group attention on key problems and prevention of fixation on secondary problems.

Specific scenarios can be designed to address specific CRM points. By keeping the message of a scenario simple, the participant should leave with a vivid experience that can serve as a model for managing similar situations in real life. Some specific suggestions are made in Table 20.3.

20.6 **Summary**

Simulation systems and team level training programmes owe their origin to data demonstrating a connection between medical errors, and failings in cognition and event management. CRM represents an analytical approach based on cognitive and social psychology that has been used in aviation and medical simulation training to understand and improve upon human performance. Careful design of patient crisis scenarios can facilitate the understanding and application of CRM concepts. Unlike retrospective studies that assess medical management error well after the fact, crisis simulations with debriefings can identify and correct errors in close to real time.

References

1. Gaba DM, Fish KJ, Howard SK (1994). *Crisis Management in Anaesthesiology*. New York: Churchill Livingstone.
2. Cooper JB, Newbower RS, Long CD, McPeek B (1978). Preventable anaesthesia mishaps: a study of human factors. *Anaesthesiology* **49**(6): 399–406.
3. Graber ML, Franklin N, Gordon R (2005). Diagnostic error in internal medicine. *Arch Intern Med* **165**(13): 1493–9.
4. McQuillan P, Pilkington S, Allan A, *et al.* (1998). Confidential inquiry into quality of care before admission to intensive care. *BMJ* **316**(7148): 1853–8.
5. Helmreich RL (1997). Managing human error in aviation. *Sci Am* **276**(5): 62–7.
6. Cooper G, White M, Lauber J (1980). Resource management on the flight deck: Proceedings of a NASA/ Industry workshop (NASA CP-2120). Moffet Field, CA: NASA Ames Research Center.
7. US National Transportation Safety Board (1972). Aircraft Incident Report: #NTSB-AAR-73–14. Pertaining to Eastern Airlines Flight 401. Obtained at http://aviation-safety.net/investigation/cvr/transcripts/ (Accessed Oct 5, 2006). *Note: a currently out of print film from the US Public Broadcast System production NOVA (produced by station, WGBH, Boston MA, USA), presents a re-enactment of the final minutes of this flight.*
8. US National Transportation Safety Board (1978). Aircraft Incident Report: #NTSB-AAR-79–7; Pertaining to United Airlines Flight 173. Obtained at http://aviation-safety.net/investigation/cvr/transcripts/ (Accessed Oct 5, 2006).
9. Helmreich R (1986). Theory underlying CRM training: psychological issues in flight crew performance and crew coordination. In: Orlady HW, Foushee HC, Eds. *Cockpit Resource Management Training (NASA Conference Publication 2455)*. Washington DC: National Aeronautics and Space Administration: 15–22.
10. Helmreich RL, Merritt AC, Wilhelm JA (1999). The evolution of Crew Resource Management training in commercial aviation. *Int J Aviat Psychol* **9**(1): 19–32.
11. Helmreich RL, Foushee HC, Benson R, Russini W (1986). Cockpit resource management: exploring the attitude-performance linkage. *Aviat Space Environ Med* **57**(12 Pt 1): 1198–200.
12. Helmreich RL, Wilhelm JA (1991). Outcomes of crew resource management training. *Int J Aviat Psychol* **1**(4): 287–300.
13. US National Transportation Safety Board (1989). Aircraft Incident Report #NTSB-AAR-90–06. Pertaining to United Airlines Flight 232. Obtained at http://aviation-safety.net/database/record.php?id=19890719–1. (Accessed Oct 6, 2006).

14. Cooper JB (1997). APSF grants support key safety research. *J Clin Monit* **13**(1): 59–65.

15. http://www.apsf.org.au

16. http://www.apsf.com

17. Keats AS (1990). The Closed Claims Study. *Anaesthesiology* **73**(2): 199–201.

18. Cooper JB (1994). Towards patient safety in anaesthesia. *Ann Acad Med Singapore* **23**(4): 552–7.

19. Stoelting RK, Khuri SF (2006). Past accomplishments and future directions: risk prevention in anaesthesia and surgery. *Anesthesiol Clin* **24**(2): 235–53v.

20. Gaba DM (2000). Anaesthesiology as a model for patient safety in healthcare. *BMJ* **320**(7237): 785–8.

21. Schwid HA (1987). A flight simulator for general anaesthesia training. *Comput Biomed Res* **20**(1): 64–75.

22. Gaba DM, DeAnda A (1988). A comprehensive anaesthesia simulation environment: re-creating the operating room for research and training. *Anaesthesiology* **69**(3): 387–94.

23. Howard SK, Gaba DM, Fish KJ, Yang G, Sarnquist FH (1992). Anaesthesia crisis resource management training: teaching anesthesiologists to handle critical incidents. *Aviat Space Environ Med* **63**(9): 763–70.

24. Gaba DM, DeAnda A (1989). The response of anaesthesia trainees to simulated critical incidents. *Anesth Analg* **68**(4): 444–51.

25. Marsch SC, Tschan F, Semmer N, Spychiger M, Breuer M, Hunziker PR (2005). Performance of first responders in simulated cardiac arrests. *Crit Care Med* **33**(5): 963–7.

26. Abrahamson S, Denson JS, Wolf RM (1969). Effectiveness of a simulator in training anaesthesiology residents. *J Med Educ* **44**(6): 515–9.

27. Denson JS, Abrahamson S (1969). A computer-controlled patient simulator. *JAMA* **208**(3): 504–8.

28. Cooper JB, Taqueti VR (2004). A brief history of the development of mannequin simulators for clinical education and training. *Qual Saf Healthcare* **13**(Suppl.1): i11–8.

29. Good M, Lampotang S, Gibby G, *et al.* (1988). Critical events simulation for training in anaesthesiology. *J Clinical Monitoring Computing* **4**: 140.

30. Holzman RS, Cooper JB, Gaba DM, Philip JH, Small SD, Feinstein D (1995). Anaesthesia crisis resource management: real-life simulation training in operating room crises. *J Clin Anesth* **7**(8): 675–87.

31. Reznek M, Smith-Coggins R, Howard S, *et al.* (2003). Emergency medicine crisis resource management (EMCRM): pilot study of a simulation-based crisis management course for emergency medicine. *Acad Emerg Med* **10**(4): 386–9.

32. Halamek LP, Kaegi DM, Gaba DM, *et al.* (2000). Time for a new paradigm in pediatric medical education: teaching neonatal resuscitation in a simulated delivery room environment. *Pediatrics* **106**(4): E45.

33. Lighthall GK, Barr J, Howard SK, *et al.* (2003). Use of a fully simulated intensive care unit environment for critical event management training for internal medicine residents. *Crit Care Med* **31**(10): 2437–43.

34. Moorthy K MY, Forrest D, Pandey V, Undre S, Vincent C, Darzi A. Surgical crisis management skills training and assessment: a simulation-based approach to enhancing operating room performance. *Ann Surg* **244**(1): 139–47.

35. Wright MC, Taekman JM, Endsley MR (2004). Objective measures of situation awareness in a simulated medical environment. *Qual Saf Healthcare* **13**(Suppl.1): i65–71.

36. Gaba DM, Howard SK, Small SD (1995). Situation awareness in anaesthesiology. *Hum Factors* **37**(1): 20–31.

37. Endsley MC (1995). Toward a Theory of Situation Awareness in Dynamic Systems. *Hum Factors* **37**(1): 32–64.

38. Heider J (1988). *The Tao of Leadership: Lao Tzu's Tao Te Ching Adapted for a New Age.* New York: Bantam Books.

39. Cooper S, Wakelam A (1999). Leadership of resuscitation teams: "Lighthouse Leadership". *Resuscitation* **42**(1): 27–45.

40. Marsch SC, Muller C, Marquardt K, Conrad G, Tschan F, Hunziker PR (2004). Human factors affect the quality of cardiopulmonary resuscitation in simulated cardiac arrests. *Resuscitation* **60**(1): 51–6.

41. Cummings RO, Ed. (2003). *ACLS Provider Manual*. Dallas, TX: American Heart Association.

42. Harrison TK, Manser T, Howard SK, Gaba DM (2006). Use of cognitive aids in a simulated anesthetic crisis. *Anesth Analg* **103**(3): 551–6.

43. Runciman WB, Merry AF (2005). Crises in clinical care: an approach to management. *Qual Saf Healthcare* **14**(3): 156–63. *Note: this is the introductory article to a large collection of articles on critical events and their management.*

44. Boulet JR, Murray D, Kras J, Woodhouse J, McAllister J, Ziv A (2003). Reliability and validity of a simulation-based acute care skills assessment for medical students and residents. *Anaesthesiology* **99**(6): 1270–80.

Chapter 21

Intern training
A national simulation-based training programme to enhance readiness for medical practice

Orit Rubin, Haim Berkenstadt, and Amitai Ziv

Overview

- Medical school graduates are commonly required to participate in an internship programme, which serves as the bridging transition from the students' status to a physicians' (resident) status.

- The combination of interns' lack of experience and common low confidence level creates a threat to patient safety, and challenges the medical education system to explore thoroughly ways to smooth the transition and ensure a safe shift from medical school into actual medical practice.

- This chapter reviews the Israeli experience in developing and implementing a mandatory national simulatio n-based training programme aimed at improving interns' preparedness to practice.

- The interns' workshop programme was to be related to tasks interns are expected to encounter, to focus mainly on hands-on training and to emphasize issues related to patient safety.

- A 5-day workshop, including eight different simulation-based modules (basic life support, basic clinical procedure, mechanical ventilation, advance life support, transport, and communication and medicolegal skills) was designed, and it has been implemented since 2003 at MSR, The Israel Center for Medical Simulation.

- The workshop is complemented by a web-based self-learning system, which provides to the interns a structured and interactive learning process for each module.

- The instructors in the workshop are physicians, paramedics and nurses recruited from different hospitals in Israel, and they are all obligated to participate in a half-day 'train the trainer' workshop that is conducted by MSR's professional staff.

- In the period from 2003 to 2006, 1287 interns participated in 25 workshops (50–60 participants per workshop).

- In feedback questionnaires, participants indicated that the workshop contributed to the acquisition of essential practical experience that was not acquired in medical school and that it improved awareness to safety issues in extreme situations.

21.1 **Introduction**

The transition from the students' status at medical schools to the physicians' status at the residency programmes is commonly bridged by an internship period during which graduates of medical schools are working under close supervision. Although the internship programme is built upon the knowledge, skills and competencies acquired during medical school, the overnight change in status and level of clinical responsibilities is well recognized to be accompanied by a sense of un-readiness and anxiety on behalf of the beginning interns[1,2,3]. Thus, the combination of lack of experience and low confidence level creates a threat to patient safety, and challenges the medical education system to explore thoroughly ways to smooth the transition and ensure a safe shift from medical school into actual medical practice.

Simulation-based hands-on training, with its embedded safety and experiential qualities has been shown to be an effective educational tool to enhance readiness for medical practice. This chapter will review the Israeli experience in developing and implementing a national simulation-based training programme aimed at improving interns' preparedness to practice.

21.2 **The initiative**

In Israel, an annual cohort of approximately 450 medical school graduates is required to participate in a 1-year rotating internship. Approximately 300 of them are graduates of the four Israeli medical schools that run a 6-year programme, while the rest are graduates of foreign medical schools. The internship programme includes 8 months of statutory rotations in internal medicine, emergency medicine, surgery and paediatrics, and 4 months of elective training in two other medical domains. Interns can start their internship at any time of their choice as long as it is coordinated with the individual hospital where they are designated to be positioned. The programme is regulated and supervised by a national internship committee that include representatives from the deans' offices of the four medical schools, as well as representatives of the ministry of health and the major general hospitals in Israel.

Recognizing the need to improve the interns' readiness to practice, the internship committee initiated in 2003 the development and implementation of a mandatory simulation-based training programme (interns' workshop). The initiative stated that the interns should participate in the workshop prior to the start of their official internship period. Four guiding principles for the workshop were defined:

- Training should be driven by an internship 'job analysis', and related to tasks interns are expected to encounter.
- The workshop should focus mainly on hands-on training.
- The programme should emphasize issues related to patient safety.
- The programme should enhance interns' readiness to practice in a supervised environment.

Based on these principles, a sub-committee of clinical and simulation-based experts defined the desired goals for the training programme. These included:

- Improving participants' competency and knowledge required in emergency situations.
- Honing participants' skills in performing basic clinical procedures such as intravenous line insertion and urinary catheterization.
- Enhancing competency in interpersonal communication with patients, families, and staff.
- Improving interns' awareness of medicolegal aspects of medical practice in general and during internship in particular.

◆ Providing experiences in conditions that reflect daily interns' tasks to increase self-confidence and improve competency in dealing with extreme scenarios.

The interns' committee also decided that the workshop will be developed in cooperation with the Israel Centre for Medical Simulation (MSR), which will also be the host institution as well as responsible for the implementation and execution of the workshop[4]. MSR is a national multi-disciplinary and multimodality simulation centre, offering a wide spectrum of medical simulation experiences and technologies. These include simple task trainers, advanced task trainers for complex manual skills, computer-driven, full-body physiological mannequins, and live simulated/standardized patients (SPs) – role-playing actors – for communication and clinical skills training. MSR's setting contains a variety of training environments, one-way mirrors and sophisticated audiovisual capabilities for debriefing needs, making it ideal for educational and constructive/formative purposes.

21.3 The workshop's structure

The original workshop was designed to include eight different simulation-based modules that were conducted over a period of five consecutive training days. Over the past 3 years the workshop was slightly modified, mainly following feedback gained from trainees and instructors who participated in over 20 workshops that were conducted thus far.

While in the first few workshops the first day was dedicated to lectures aiming to refresh knowledge necessary for training, in later workshops it was replaced by a web-based self-learning platform. One reason for this change was the recognition of the participants' heterogenicity in knowledge and experience that required a more flexible, self-paced educational approach to ensure the prerequisite knowledge prior to the workshop. Another, more important reason was the understanding that more time should be used for hands-on training and not on frontal lectures.

At present, the web-based learning system serves as an integral part of the interns' training. All the prerequisite cognitive educational materials for the different modules are accessible through the system, which provides a structured and interactive learning and evaluation process. Participants are obligated to use the system to refresh their knowledge so that during the workshop they can gain the utmost from the hands-on simulation training. The system also serves for evaluation of the interns' basic cognitive knowledge by means of a mandatory pretest that all participants need to complete prior to the workshop. It also provides a platform where evaluation of the workshop takes place through feedback questionnaires completed at the end of each workshop by trainees and instructors.

21.4 The training modules

The present training programme includes 8 modules that vary in duration from a few hours to a full day (Table 21.1).

21.4.1 Basic life support

Basic life support (BLS) module (module 1) is conducted on the first day of the workshop. Given the wide variability in training and background experience of graduates of different medical schools and the importance of mastering BLS skills as an essential element in handling more complex medical tasks, this module was positioned as the first hands-on module of the workshop. This enabled a gradual increase in difficulty and complexity of the modules conducted thereafter. Experienced paramedics from the Israeli Emergency Medical Services (EMS) were chosen to be the instructors of this module and simple BLS simulators serve as the training platforms.

Table 21.1 The eight training modules

Module	Module title
1	Basic life support (BLS)
2	Basic clinical procedures
3	Basic surgical skills
4	Mechanical ventilation
5 + 6	Advance life support
7	Transport
8	Communication and medicolegal skills

21.4.2 Basic clinical procedures

Basic clinical procedures (module 2), is the module where participants are trained in basic procedures such as intravenous line insertion, urinary catheter and nasogastric tube insertion, and in the use of basic medical devices like syringe pumps and defibrillator. Training in this module is provided mostly by nurses following a web-based self learning that includes explanations of the different procedures and video clips demonstrating the actual performance. Interns then practice under supervision the various procedures on simple task trainers specially designed for each procedure.

21.4.3 Basic surgical skills

Basic surgical skills (module 3) is instructed by surgeons and focuses mostly on basic suturing skills, as applied and practiced on simple synthetic skin models.

21.4.4 Mechanical ventilation

Mechanical ventilation (module 4) is a module where interns learn the basic handling of invasive and noninvasive mechanical ventilation. This module was initiated because of the scarcity of intensive care beds in Israel. Many ventilated patients are treated in step down units located in regular medical departments, thus creating a reality where interns often face the task of handling invasive and noninvasive mechanical ventilation medical devices. This module is mostly instructed by anaesthesiologists who supervise the interns as they perform tasks on mechanical ventilation devices connected to advanced simulated platforms including artificial lung models.

21.4.5 Advance life support

Advance life support (modules 5 and 6) are two modules with increased clinical complexity that include scenario-based training on advanced cardiac life support, advanced paediatric life support, and advanced emergency room scenarios. These modules are conducted on advanced computerized full-body simulators and are instructed by emergency and intensive care physicians who debrief the interns through the audiovisual recording of each scenario. Beyond feedback on clinical aspects of the management of the acutely ill patients, interns are also debriefed on aspects related to team-work and team communication during emergency situations.

21.4.6 Transport

Transport (module 7) is considered the highlight of the acute care modules as it focuses on transport scenarios where interns are required to transport adult and paediatric 'patients' (advanced mannequins) through the different floors of the simulation centre while facing equipment failure and acute medical challenges. These scenarios are instructed by physicians from the relevant professions (paediatricians, anaesthesiologists, internists), who also make use of audiovisual recording of the transport scenarios to enhance the quality of the debriefing and better convey the important educational messages.

21.4.7 Communication and medicolegal skills

Communication and medicolegal skills (module 8) is a full-day module where participants encounter 10 different archetypical communication challenging scenarios focusing on everyday hospital milieu and common medical vignettes. Training is based on simulated/standardized patients (SPs) – highly trained actors who have been trained to respond in a 'rewarding' way when facing efficient communication skills (i.e. if the trainee is empathic, resilient or assertive when needed, the SP will cooperate to permit the trainee experience success, whereas if the trainee is not patient-oriented, the SP will exhibit resistance as in real life situations). During this training the interns' tasks include, for example, dealing with aggressive patients, calming down an agitated mother whose baby has suffered from fever-related convulsions, admitting to a self-performed medical mistake, and dealing with a mentally traumatized person who has just survived a terror attack. In this module each intern participates in two scenarios, and observes, via one-sided mirrors, four other scenarios performed by peers. All encounters are documented by the audiovisual equipment, and observed by two experts in medical communication and in medicolegal/risk management. The videotape and comments written by the experts are used for debriefing and discussion performed in groups of 12 trainees. During this session the experts are dissecting emotional and cognitive levels of the learned material to the interns as individuals and as a group. The communication module lasts for a full day and is considered extremely important by the interns' committee to emphasize the high priority given to communication skills as an important competence in healthcare delivery and patient safety.

21.5 Logistics

Each workshop includes 50–60 participants divided into eight groups of six to seven participants each. Groups perform as an integral unit throughout all the workshop modules and stations, and interns have the opportunity to experience all modules both as observers of their peers as well as carrying out and leading the various tasks/scenarios. The workshop occupies most rooms of the simulation centre (10–15 rooms each day), an average of eight instructors each day, 24 different simulators and six SPs (each playing two different roles). Three of the simulation centre staff members are fully occupied for logistic and administrative support and three more for operating the simulators.

21.6 Instructors

Initially, most of the instructors who were recruited for the workshop were physicians. However, mainly due to availability problems and training standardization issues, two thirds of the modules are currently instructed by experienced paramedics and nurses. All instructors are obliged to participate in a half-day 'train the trainer' workshop that is conducted by MSR's professional staff. This workshop is designed to brief the instructors on the workshop and its goals, to thoroughly expose them to the specific training station or scenarios they are expected to participate in, to guide them on the principles of simulation-based training and audiovisual based debriefing, and to provide them with feedback on their hands-on training skills. Each year, a refresher 'train the trainer' workshop is held for experienced and for new instructors. Over the past 4 years, over 200 instructors were trained, and served alternately in the successive workshops: 15 physicians, 14 nurses and 13 paramedics for each workshop.

21.7 Descriptive data

Over the years 2003–2006, 25 workshops have been run for 1287 interns who filled in demographic questionnaires at the beginning of the workshop and an evaluation (feedback) questionnaire at the end of the workshop. The interns' feedback was analysed and provided the basis for the gradual modification of the structure and content of future workshops that took place over the 3 years since its inception.

The workshop structure and the feedback forms were modified in 2004, and the programme and evaluation tools were a year later.

In 2005, 331 participants filled in the questionnaire (46% male, 54% female, mean age 28.5 years). Thirty four percent of the participants had obtained advanced cardiac life support training during their medical school years (two-thirds of them within the past year before the workshop), and 27% reported they had had training in emergency medicine (of these, one-third as part of hospital work as physicians assistants, one-third as part of working as medics in the Israeli EMS, and one-third as part of their army service as medics).

21.7.1 Trainee feedback

On a scale of 1–4 (where 1 stands for not at all, 2 for slightly, 3 for much and 4 for very much), 63% participants marked 3 – that they have mastered the theoretical knowledge (mean 2.7), 51% marked 3 that they have mastered the clinical competencies (mean 2.6) needed from an intern, 57% marked 3 they that they have mastered their ability to work well with other members of the medical staff (mean 3.2), and 58% (mean 3.2) marked 3 that they have mastered their ability to deal with communication problems. The mean score for the time management of the workshop was 3.6 (58% marked 4) and scores evaluating the quality of the different modules were 8–9 on a scale of 1–10 across all modules. To the question "If participation in the workshop would not have been mandatory, would you have chosen to participate in such workshop anyway?" 100% of respondents responded positively. Moreover, in the section of free text comments, many wrote comments such as "How could we have done without the workshop..." or that the workshop reflects the "most effective 5 training days I have ever received thus far" etc., indicating the high importance that the participants attribute to the workshop. Other comments and feedback information indicated that according to the participants:

- the workshop contributed to refreshing the theoretical knowledge and to the acquisition of essential practical experience that was not acquired in medical school
- the workshop improved awareness to safety issues in extreme situations
- all the topics covered in the workshop were considered to be highly important
- the e-learning component of the workshop provided a good preparation for the hands-on experiences
- the workshop should be longer to allow thorough personal training and repetition.

An interesting finding was that while most participants indicate that the workshop reduced the level of anxiety in anticipation of the internship, some of the interns reported a decrease in their self-confidence to act in extreme situations. This might be the result of the fact that for some of the participants, the experiences in the workshop were a first 'vivid prediction' of their new role and responsibilities as physicians. Another interesting finding was that throughout the year, the degree of satisfaction from the workshop remained stable even though the ratio of physicians to other health professionals in the training staff has been reduced.

21.8 Summary

The need and importance of preparing medical graduates for their encounter, as interns, with clinical situations is described. Simulation-based training in a comprehensive multidisciplinary, multimodular simulation centre is shown to be the preferred platform for such instruction and maximizes patient safety. In addition to hands-on procedures and management, the significance of communication skills is emphasized. Debriefing by instructors, including constructive feedback of peers, is a vital element in the learning process.

Simulation-based training is a valuable adjunct in enhancing readiness to medical practice and should be employed increasingly in medical schools and in crucial milestones over the course of medical training

References

1. Hannon FB (2000). A national medical education needs' assessment of interns and the development of an intern education and training programme. *Med Educ* **34**(4): 275–84.
2. Roche AM, Sanson-Fisher RW, Cockburn J (1997). Training experiences immediately after medical school. *Med Educ* **31**(1): 9–16.
3. Goldacre M, *et al.* (2003). Pre-registration house officers' views on whether their experience at medical school prepared them well for their jobs: national questionnaire survey. *BMJ* **326**: 1011–12.
4. Ziv A, Erez D, Munz Y (2006). The Israel Center for Medical Simulation: A Paradigm for Cultural Change in Medical Education. *Acad Med* **81**(12): 1091–7.

Chapter 22

Non-technical skills: identifying, training, and assessing safe behaviours

Rhona Flin and Nicola Maran

Overview

- Non-technical skills such as decision making, situation awareness, team working and leadership are the skills used to underpin the technical skills required for safe and effective practice.
- Many major incidents in a range of industries including air accidents, Chernobyl and the Piper Alpha disaster are examples of non-technical failures causing massive loss of life.
- The aviation industry recognizes that many adverse incidents have non-technical failures at their core and have responded by providing mandatory non-technical skills (CRM) training for all staff.
- Despite high numbers of adverse events in healthcare, non-technical skills are not currently explicitly taught in the medical curriculum.
- Observations and rating of non-technical skills can be carried out using behavioural rating or marker systems. Similar behaviour rating tools based on defined sets of key skills have been used in healthcare although many are adaptations of those used in the airline industry.
- Some speciality-specific behavioural marker systems for anaesthetists (ANTS) and surgeons (NOTSS) have been developed for use in both clinical and simulation environments to give feedback for training.
- Despite their apparent simplicity, in order to use behavioural rating systems accurately and reliably, raters need considerable training.
- Simulation provides the ideal setting in which to examine individual or team skills under stress. Debriefing using video allows individuals to gain insight into their own non-technical skills in such conditions. Repeated exposure to such situations allows individuals to develop their skills.

22.1 Introduction

22.1.1 What are non-technical skills?

In aviation, it has been realized for 30 years that aircraft crashes are usually not only due to mechanical failures or pilots' inadequate technical competence. Many of the errors that

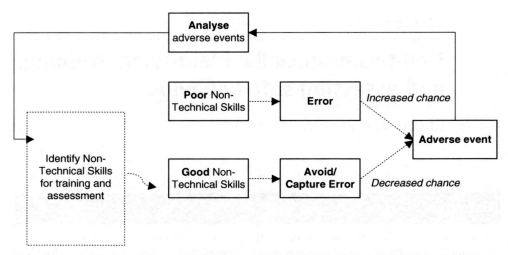

Fig. 22.1 Non-technical skills and safety. (Reprinted from Flin *et al.* (2008). *Safety at the Sharp End: A Guide to Non-Technical Skills.* Reproduced with permission of Ashgate.)

contribute to accidents across industries could have been avoided if better non-technical skills had been demonstrated by the personnel operating or maintaining the system. The term non-technical skills (NTS) is used by a range of technical professions[1], to describe what they previously referred to as 'soft' skills. In aviation, the term was first used by the European regulator and was defined as 'the cognitive and social skills of flight crew members in the cockpit, not directly related to aircraft control, system management, and standard operating procedures'[2]. These skills include situation awareness, decision making, leadership and teamwork. They complement workers' technical skills and should reduce errors, increase the capture of errors and help to mitigate when an operational problem occurs as illustrated in Fig. 22.1. NTS are also called crew resource management (CRM) skills and the civil aviation industry has pioneered the development of CRM training.

In this chapter, the terms non-technical and CRM skills can be regarded as synonymous. Following a description of the initial interest in NTS shown by the aviation industry almost 30 years ago, there is an overview of the identification, training and assessment of NTS in aviation and the more recent adoption of this approach in healthcare, using simulated as well as real environments. The focus is on individual skills within a team setting rather than on skills at the group level. For more detailed information, Flin *et al.*[3] review the principal categories of NTS for maintaining safe and efficient operations across a range of work settings, as well as how to identify, train and assess them.

22.1.2 **Individual or team skills?**

The issue of whether NTS should be trained and assessed at an individual or a team level is a topic of ongoing debate in industry. In most safety-critical settings, work is carried out by teams of technical specialists and so the work group provides the context for the individual's behaviour. The main reason for focussing on the individual is because the individual is the basic 'building block' from which teams and larger organizational groupings are formed. Moreover in many workplaces (e.g. civil aviation, the energy industry, hospital medicine), the staff do not work in the same team every day. In the larger airlines, the same pilots seldom fly together and for that reason, the focus in European aviation has been on the individual pilot's technical and non-technical competence, rather than on a crew[4]. The introduction of working time restrictions and the streamlining of medical training have forced changes to shift and rotation patterns such that team composition in hospitals is seldom fixed. Although doctors increasingly practise in interdisciplinary teams, they remain individually accountable for their professional conduct and the care they provide[5].

The counter argument is that the unit of operation is the crew and that how the team members interact to accomplish their tasks is most important. Crew members have shared responsibility for the operation and one person's behaviour will be influenced by another's. There are a number of crew rating systems used in aviation, but it should be noted that a flightdeck crew normally consists of only two pilots, both fixed in their seats, operating the same equipment, with one main external communication channel. This is very different from many healthcare teams – an operating theatre can have six to ten individuals from different professions moving around and engaged in a whole set of interacting tasks, communicating with a range of external sources. It takes considerable skill to observe all these individuals, track their communications and rate what is happening at a group level of analysis.

It is proposed, therefore, that the initial focus for training and evaluation of NTS should be on the individual. This is especially applicable in healthcare where currently many professionals are unfamiliar with the basic concepts (e.g. situation awareness) and do not have a shared vocabulary for discussing these within their own profession, never mind across professional boundaries. Single discipline training of NTS (as is now being developed for surgeons[6]) can then be complemented by training and evaluation of multidiscipline teams.

22.2 Background

22.2.1 Non-technical skills in aviation and other industries

Thirty years ago, a series of major aviation accidents without primary technical causes forced investigators to turn their attention to the behaviour of the humans operating the aircraft. In 1977, two Boeing 747 jets operated by KLM and Pan Am collided on the runway of Los Rodeos airport, causing 583 deaths. Analysis of the accident revealed problems relating to communication with air traffic control, teamwork, decision making, fatigue, and leadership behaviour[7]. United Airlines suffered a sequence of crashes in the late 1970s, also not due to technical failures. The aviation psychologists and airline captains began to scrutinize the behaviours associated with errors and accidents, reporting early findings at a NASA workshop in 1979. The emerging culprits were failures in leadership, poor team coordination, communication breakdowns, lack of assertiveness, lack of attention, inadequate problem solving, often exacerbated by stress and fatigue.

The aviation industry then realized that the maintenance of high standards of safety was going to require more than efficient technology and proficient technical skills in the system operators (e.g. pilots, engineers, air traffic controllers). It began to take a serious interest in NTS. These were not mysterious or rare behaviours, they were actually normal practices that pilots had always regarded as an essential part of good airmanship. However, these NTS had often been tacitly rather than explicitly addressed and were taught in an informal and inconsistent manner from one generation of pilots to the next[8]. Studies were commissioned by the airlines and in the USA by the Federal Aviation Authority (FAA) at the leading aviation psychology centres, such as the Crew Factors Group at NASA, Ames, and the Human Factors Research Group at the University of Texas at Austin. Working with experienced pilots, the aviation psychologists began to run experiments in the flight deck simulators, to interview pilots, to analyse accident reports, to discover which skill components either contributed to, or were effective in preventing adverse events.

Once the core NTS had been identified, then the airlines began to develop special training courses to raise awareness of the importance of these skills, to provide the necessary underpinning knowledge and practice for skill development. These were initially called cockpit resource management (CRM) courses, later amended to crew resource management as other flight crew members, such as cabin attendants, began to be involved[9].

Accidents involving inadequacies in NTS are certainly not unique to the aviation industry. In two of the world's most serious nuclear power plant incidents, Chernobyl and Three Mile Island, operator error relating to poor situation awareness and flawed decision making played a major role. The loss of the Piper Alpha oil platform with 167 deaths was caused by inadequate team coordination at shift handover, compounded by leadership failures in emergency response[10]. Shipping accidents frequently reveal examples of poor bridge team leadership, failures in crew communication and flawed decision making[11]. Consequently, many other high risk industries have introduced CRM training, such as nuclear power generation, Merchant Navy, prison service, emergency services[12,13,14]. Some organizations, for instance the UK nuclear power companies, also assess NTS of staff in safety-critical positions, such as control room operators[15].

22.2.2 Non-technical skills in healthcare

Concern about the rates of adverse events to patients caused by medical error grew in the late 1990s[16]. As many of these could be attributed to failures in NTS[17,18], medical professionals began to look at safety management techniques used in the high risk industries. Drawing on the behaviour-based approach adopted by the aviation sector to enhance safety, the acute medical specialities began to identify the NTS contributing to safe and efficient performance, so that these could be trained and evaluated. Increasing availability of simulated medical environments, such as operating theatres, ICUs, and trauma centres also offer ideal facilities for practising and debriefing healthcare professionals' NTS. The rest of this chapter discusses the identification, training and assessment of NTS in healthcare, with particular reference to the use of simulation facilities.

22.3 Identifying non-technical skills

22.3.1 Introduction

The specific NTS required for a particular occupation need to be determined by a systematic process of identification based on task analysis[19]. While the main skill categories (e.g. decision making or leadership), are similar across professions, the component elements and examples of good and poor behaviours need to be carefully specified for a given profession and task set. These can be distinctive and clearly vary from one technical setting to another. This is why it is inadvisable to use a NTS taxonomy or behavioural marker system devised for one domain (e.g. aviation) in a different work setting (e.g. healthcare).

In essence, a two-stage process is used:

- First, identify the skills and related behaviours deemed to influence safe and efficient performance.

- Second, refine the resulting list and organize it into a concise, hierarchical structure or taxonomy.

This tool then needs to be tested to ascertain usability, reliability and validity. See Fig. 22.2 for an example of the stages in the development of the NOTSS tool to rate surgeons' behaviour in the operating theatre[20].

The level of detail and scope required will depend on the purpose for which the taxonomy is being developed. A set of behaviours identified for a research tool could be more complex and

Phase 1: Task analysis

1. Literature review (*Surgery*, 2006)
2. Adverse event analyses
3. Cognitive Interviews (27 surgeons, 12 nurses)
4. Observation in theatre
5. Attitude survey (*The Surgeon*, 2006)

Phase 2: Design and development (*Medical Education*, 2006)

- Develop skills taxonomy
- Refine categories and elements (4 panels of surgeons)
- Write behavioural markers (16 surgeons)
- Prototyping and usability testing

Phase 3: System evaluation

- Establish evaluation criteria – reliability and usability
- Experimental evaluation (44 surgeons) (*World Journal of Surgery*, 2008)
- Usability trial in theatre (11 surgeons + trainees) (*Cognition, Technology and Work*, (in press))
- Make modifications to system

Fig. 22.2 Stages for development of NOTSS behaviour rating tool. (Based on: Flin R, Yule S, Maran N, Paterson-Brown S, Rowley D (2005). NOTSS: Non-Technical Skills for Surgeons. Paper presented at the European Association of Work Psychology Conference, Istanbul.)

comprehensive than one being developed for practitioners to use as the basis for training or assessment. The methods that are typically used to develop NTS taxonomies are briefly outlined below.

22.3.2 Identifying domain specific non-technical skills

The first place to look for information is the published literature for the job in question. There are hundreds of research studies published by industrial psychologists examining behaviour in the workplace, including risky environments[21] and a suitable skills set may already exist. For many occupations, a wealth of information exists on which behaviours contribute to safe or unsafe performance[22]. Organizations can also hold documentary analyses that cover NTS for a particular occupation including job assessments, task analyses, competence frameworks, training programmes, assessment and appraisal systems. If sufficient information cannot be found in these sources then, the data collection methods described below can be used.

22.3.3 Data collection techniques

If there is not a suitable taxonomy available, there are a number of techniques that can be adopted and, to enhance validity, these diagnostic tools are normally used in combination. These can be grouped into three main types.

- Questioning techniques, which involve soliciting information directly from role holders from the job under investigation using for example, an interview, a focus group or a questionnaire survey[23,24].

- Observational techniques, in which individuals are observed carrying out one or more tasks[25] can be used but this usually requires some kind of coding scheme to organize the information. These first two methods tend to be used with experienced personnel – often referred to as subject matter experts (SME).

◆ Event-based analyses, in which accident or near miss reports are examined to identify patterns of behaviours and related errors[17,26]. This includes the use of confidential reporting systems, which encourage reports of safety concerns, as well as actual events. A problem with this method in healthcare, until recently, was that these reports were seldom coded for human and organizational causal factors, being mainly concerned with clinical or technical matters.

22.3.4 Developing a skills taxonomy

The second stage of refining the skill list into a workable taxonomy with skills grouped into categories is normally carried out using panels of subject matter experts[27]. This is the methodology which has been applied to the development of the ANTS (Anaesthetists' Non-Technical Skills) and NOTSS (Non-Technical Skills in Surgery) taxonomies. For more detail, see Flin et al.[3] and there are accounts of the development of particular taxonomies and associated behaviours for individuals, see below. For whole teams, there are also descriptions of skill sets and behavioural rating methods (e.g. for neonatal resuscitation teams[24] or operating theatre teams[28]). There is also a body of research examining the behaviours of medical trauma and emergency room teams, some of which has used behavioural ratings[29,30]. To date, most of this work has been for research purposes rather than to develop NTS sets to be used by practitioners.

22.4 Training non-technical skills

22.4.1 Non-technical skills (CRM) training in aviation

As mentioned above, NTS have been trained in aviation and other industries using crew resource management (CRM) courses. The international aviation regulators have generally mandated and monitored CRM courses[31,32] and they are run by almost all air operators, as both introductory (2–3 days) and refresher courses (e.g. one day annually). Commenting on the widespread introduction of CRM training in aviation, a former 747 captain commented, *"Even error management strategies are properly trained, much to the chagrin of some old-school instructors, who still hold the conviction that we should teach pilots to be infallible (just like them)"*[8]. Regulators offer guidance on syllabi[4] but airlines design their own courses to suit their operational requirements. A typical syllabus will include the following topics; human error and accidents; situation awareness, decision making, communication, leadership, team working, stress and fatigue management. In UK aviation, the CRM instructors must be specially trained and formally qualified[32]. Reviews of studies attempting to evaluate the effectiveness of CRM training studies[14,33,34] generally report positive changes in attitudes, knowledge and sometimes also behaviour[35], but improvements in safety (e.g. reduced accident rate) have usually only been shown in military. Accident rates in commercial airlines are so low that it is difficult to use this as a sensitive outcome measure. Wiener et al.[9] give a comprehensive account of the development of the early CRM courses and there are other books available on CRM training in aviation[36,37,38,39].

22.4.2 ACRM and non-technical skills training in anaesthesia and surgery

Anaesthesia has been at the forefront of developments to train NTS in medicine with Gaba and colleagues designing anesthesia crisis resource management (ACRM) courses based on aviation CRM[40]. There is considerable interest in adapting CRM training for healthcare[41], and there are now a range of NTS courses available. Although historically focussed on the development of technical expertise, surgeons are now introducing CRM and similar NTS courses[6,42,43]. This is recognized as an important component of patient safety education for surgeons[44]. Many of the courses in healthcare are being developed in collaboration with former airline pilots with experience of CRM training. It is evident that courses are sometimes imported from aviation or other industries without adequate training needs analysis or customization[45]. Baker et al.[46] reviewing medical team training courses, including CRM, found that, *"not one of the programs was based on a comprehensive pretraining needs analysis and participants had limited opportunities to receive practice and feedback on critical teamwork skills"* (pv).

22.4.3 Principles of course design

Whichever training programme is adopted or designed, the basic principles of training design should be followed[47]. That is, there should be a systematic process of identifying the skills required for the particular profession or team, deciding how best to deliver the instruction and a method of evaluating whether the training was successful.

Typically CRM courses are staged in a classroom setting for 2 days with about 12 participants and one or two trainers. Ideally the trainers should be experienced professionals from the relevant domain who have a sufficient understanding of psychology to deliver the material. For those designing their own courses, the methods of training NTS have been outlined in a number of sources on CRM training[4,32,48]. Many of these are related to aviation but there are now descriptions and guidance for other work places, including healthcare[45,46,49]. General material on cognitive and social skills can be found in psychology textbooks. Those written for industrial psychology are most useful[21], as they show how basic psychological theory and experimental findings relating to NTS can be applied in the workplace. Flin et al.[3] outline the basic psychological background, with a range of industrial examples, for seven generic NTS. There is also a CRM Developers Forum which has a website providing resources and a discussion group, http://www.crm-devel.org. In our experience, most experienced CRM trainers are willing to allow professionals from other disciplines to sit in and observe their courses. They can also be generous with training materials.

22.4.4 Course content and delivery

Basic CRM or NTS courses provide an introduction to the concept of human error and are designed to raise awareness and convey knowledge of the main NTS, as well as influencing factors such as stress and fatigue and how these influence task performance. However in order to develop these skills, participants must be given an opportunity to put them into practice and to receive feedback and coaching. This can be done to a certain degree in a classroom setting using role play and observed group exercises but scenario based training using simulators gives trainees the ideal opportunity to take part in real task-based exercises. Video feedback is a particularly powerful way of allowing participants to gain insight into aspects of their own performance. Structured debriefing, using a skills framework or taxonomy allows identification of specific skills with illustration of positive and negative impacts of these actions. The trainers for these sessions must be skilled not only at observing and evaluating NTS but also know how to debrief them in a constructive manner. Good facilitation by an instructor should help the candidate to identify ways in which skills can be improved.

In aviation, these sessions are regarded as an important element of pilot training and they are usually referred to as LOFT (Line Oriented Flight Training). Dismukes and Smith[50] neatly describe the skills required to facilitate and debrief training and assessment sessions, designed to provide feedback on pilots' non-technical, as well as technical skills. They emphasize the need to make this an individual or team-centred experience in order to maximize learning (see also CAA[4], Appendix 9 on CRM facilitation skills). Rudolph *et al.*[51] describe a debriefing technique for medical instructors to disclose their evaluations of behaviour while eliciting trainees' assumptions about the situation and their reasons for acting as they did. Thereafter further simulator practice allows development of these skills with further feedback.

Simulator practice, with the opportunity for video feedback, is the optimal way to encourage individuals to reflect on their own NTS and to identify individual strengths and weaknesses. However, most scenarios experienced on the simulator use these skills in emergency situations and are less likely to look at use of NTS in 'everyday' or 'routine' practice. Therefore, it is vital that feedback is given, preferably using the same feedback tools, in the clinical environment on a routine basis. One of the greatest assets of the ANTS system is that it can be used in this manner giving a consistency of feedback in both the simulator (emergency) and routine clinical environments. This approach also emphasizes the importance of NTS in the prevention of critical incidents, as well as their use in crisis management.

22.5 Assessing non-technical skills

22.5.1 Assessment of CRM skills in aviation

In UK, it is now mandated[4,32] that an assessment of non-technical (CRM) skills is included into all levels of training and checking of flight crew members' performance. This builds on earlier regulations and research developments instigated across Europe by the joint aviation regulator (JAA). For example, '*the flight crew must be assessed on their CRM skills in accordance with a methodology acceptable to the Authority and published in the Operations Manual. The purpose of such an assessment is to: provide feedback to the crew collectively and individually and serve to identify retraining; and be used to improve the CRM training system.*'[52]. Where formal assessment of pilots' NTS is required, as in the UK, then specific guidelines are provided (e.g. '*CRM assessment should only be tied to the assessment of technical issues, and not carried out as a stand alone assessment. Suitable methods of assessment should be established, together with selection criteria and training requirements of the assessors, and their relevant qualifications, knowledge and skills*')(e.g. CAA 2006, Chapter 7, page 2[4]). Moreover, the examination of a pilot's CRM skills must be undertaken by a qualified CRM Instructor/ Examiner (CRMIE) who has been formally assessed as competent for this role[32]. In other countries such as the USA, there are some similar requirements for pilots' CRM skills to be evaluated[31] and there are various expert sources on this topic[19,53,54,55,56].

While a number of the larger airlines had already developed their own systems for evaluation of pilots' NTS[57], the European regulator required a generic method of evaluation of pilots' NTS that could be used across all the countries, in large and small operators. This was intended to minimize cultural and corporate differences, and to maximize practicability and effectiveness for airline instructors and examiners. In 1996, a multinational research team of pilots and psychologists developed a set of NTS (NOTECHS) that could be rated by observing an individual pilot's behaviour on the flight deck[2, 33 or 34, 58]. The NOTECHS behavioural rating system has been recommended by some regulators in Europe as one method of assessing a pilot's NTS. It is used by a number of airlines in Europe and beyond. A number of operators have customised the basic system to meet their own fleet requirements.

The NOTECHS system is designed for the assessment of an individual pilot's NTS by observing his/her behaviour in a crew setting. There are also group level assessment systems, for rating observed aspects of a crew's performance. The best known of these is LOSA (Line Oriented Safety Audit)[59,60], which is widely used in aviation to record ratings of a flightdeck crew, as well as errors and situational factors (threats). The LOSA system is a descendent of the first behaviour rating system (called a behavioural marker system) that was devised for evaluating a flightdeck crew's NTS. This system originated in the University of Texas Human Factors Research Project (then called the NASA/UT Behavioural Markers) in the late 1980s. There were two goals: the first was to evaluate the effectiveness of CRM training as measured by observable behaviours while the second was to aid in defining the scope of CRM programmes. Their research resulted in the first manual to assist check airmen and evaluators in assessing the interpersonal component of flying[61]. Originally, ratings of crew performance were made by observers assessing a complete flight from initial briefing to landing, taxi-in, and shut-down of engines.

The first set of crew behavioural markers was included by the Federal Aviation Administration as an appendix to its Advisory Circular on CRM (AC-150A). Systematic use of the markers grew as airlines enhanced assessment of crew performance and as the project began collecting systematic data on all aspects of an airline's operations in LOSA. The markers themselves were incorporated in a form for systematic observations known as the Line/LOS Checklist (LOS refers to line operational or full mission simulation). As experience and the database of observations increased, it became apparent that there was significant variability in crew behaviour during flights that needed to be captured. Accordingly, the form was modified to assess the markers for each phase of flight[62].

A validation of these markers was undertaken by classifying their impact (positive and negative) in analyses of aviation accidents and incidents[63]. The results provided strong support for the use of the markers as indicators of crew performance and their value as components of CRM training. Comparisons of the LOSA and NOTECHS markers in aviation studies have generally produced similar results[64,65]. See Flin et al.[3] for details of the NOTECHS and LOSA systems.

22.5.2 Behaviour rating systems in medicine

Behaviour rating systems for medical professionals' NTS have been developed using methods derived from the aviation studies, most typically from LOSA and NOTECHS. Examples from anaesthesia and surgery are described below.

22.5.2.1 Behaviour rating systems in anaesthesia

One of the first behavioural rating systems for assessing anaesthetists' behaviours during critical incidents was developed by Gaba and his team in Stanford for use in the simulator setting[66]. The tool was adapted from the instrument used to rate flight deck crew behaviours, which was developed at the University of Texas as described above. It covered ten crisis management behaviours including communication, feedback, leadership, group climate, anticipation/planning, workload distribution, vigilance, and re-evaluation and also included overall ratings for the individual anaesthetist and the anaesthesia team.

In Scotland, a taxonomy of NTS, the ANTS (Anaesthetists' Non-Technical Skills) system was developed using a similar design and evaluation process to that used in the development of NOTECHS. The content was derived from the research literature on anaesthetists' behaviour, as well as data from observations, interviews, questionnaires and incident analysis[23,67,68]. The system was developed as a tool for giving anaesthesia trainees feedback on NTS, primarily in the clinical environment but also for use in the simulator setting. As can be seen from Fig. 22.3, there are four main categories of skill, each subdivided into component elements and for each element a number of positive and negative examples (markers) of behaviour are provided for illustration. Each element and category is rated on a four-point scale: Good, Acceptable, Marginal, Poor.

ANTS has undergone some preliminary trials in clinical practice in the UK through the Royal College of Anaesthetists, and the Australian and New Zealand College of Anaesthetists have

Categories	Elements
Task management	• Planning and preparation • Prioritizing • Providing and maintaining standards • Identifying and using resources
Team working	• Coordinating activities with team members • Exchanging information • Using authority and assertiveness • Assessing capabilities • Supporting others
Situation awareness	• Gathering information • Recognizing and understanding • Anticipating
Decision making	• Identifying options • Balancing risks and selecting options • Re-evaluating

Examples of behavioural markers for good practice

- Confirms roles and responsibilities of team members
- Discusses case with surgeons or colleagues
- Considers requirements of others before acting
- Cooperates with others to achieve goals

Examples of behavioural markers for poor practice

- Reduces level of monitoring because of distraction
- Responds to individual cues without confirmation
- Does not alter physical layout of workspace to improve data visibility
- Does not ask questions to orient self to situation during hand-over

Fig. 22.3 The structure of ANTS (Anaesthetists' Non-Technical Skills).

recently sponsored an evaluation study. The system has been translated into German and Hebrew, and has been used to evaluate simulator training for anaesthetists in Canada[69] and in Denmark[70]. Patey[71] describes use of ANTS for training and debriefing. For further details see http://www.abdn.ac.uk/iprc/ants.

22.5.2.2 Behaviour rating systems in surgery

One of the first studies observing and recording the behaviour of surgeons and other operating theatre team members was carried out in Switzerland. Helmreich and Schaefer[25] observed operations using a set of nine categories of 'specific behaviours that can be evaluated in terms of their presence or absence and quality' 'that are essential for safe and efficient function'. Their goal was 'to develop a rating methodology that can be employed reliably by trained observers' (page 242). Using this behaviour categorization for the observations, they identified a number of instances of error relating to inadequate teamwork, failures in preparation, briefings, communication, and workload distribution. Subsequently, Helmreich *et al.*[72] designed the Operating Room Checklist (ORCL), which consisted of a similar list of behaviour categories with rating scales that could be used to assess the non-technical performance of operating teams. This was adapted from the UT marker system used in aviation and was designed to measure team behaviours rather than to rate the NTS of individual surgeons.

In a UK research study observing and rating the behaviour of paediatric cardiac surgeons, Carthey *et al.*[73] developed a 'framework of the individual, team and organizational factors that underpin excellence in paediatric surgery'. They rated seven NTS at the individual (surgeon) level, in addition to 'technical' skill. Leadership, communication and coordination were listed as team level behavioural markers. This scale does not appear to have been developed further but the authors concluded that 'behavioural markers developed to explain aviation crew performance can be applied to cardiac surgery to explain differences in process excellence between surgical teams' (page 422).

Two observational studies in operating theatres have adapted the NOTECHS method for rating airline pilots' NTS to examine surgeons' behaviour in the operating theatre[74,75]. More recently a taxonomy and behavioural rating system has been designed for rating individual surgeons' NTS, the NOTSS system[76]. This used a method similar to that employed in the development of NOTECHS and ANTS, as shown in Fig. 22.2. An example of a NOTSS rating form representing an assessment of a general surgeon's NTS is shown in Fig. 22.4. The NOTSS system has recently been tested in experimental and usability trials[77]. For details see http://www.abdn.ac.uk/iprc/notss.

A new project at Aberdeen University in Scotland is now identifying behavioural markers for theatre nursing staff. On completion of this work, behavioural marker systems, grounded in individual disciplines (http://www.abdn.ac.uk/iprc/nurses/), will offer tools for observing behaviours of the core members of the operating theatre team.

22.5.3 Implementation of non-technical skills assessment

The process of introducing the ANTS and NOTSS systems has revealed some of the difficulties of bringing a novel type of assessment system into workplace-based assessment. The basic psychological language (e.g. situation awareness) is still unfamiliar to most clinicians and therefore, there is actually a need for basic awareness training courses in NTS for both ratees and raters before trying to implement the system in training. In aviation, pilots are taught about psychological and physiological factors that influence their performance from the start of their training (Performance Limitations courses). As qualified pilots they then undertake CRM training provided by their employing airline on a regular basis. Consequently they are very familiar with

Hospital: Date:		Trainer name: Trainee name:		Operation: Right inguinal hernia repair
Category	Category rating*	Element	Element rating*	Feedback on performance and debriefing notes
Situation Awareness	3	Gathering information	2	Didn't mark side/ arrived in theatre late
		Understanding information	4	Aware of INR importance and checked
		Projecting and anticipating future state	3	Take more of a lead in op – i.e. requesting retractions
Decision Making	3	Considering options	3	Be more explicit about relative merits of options
		Selecting and communicating option	2	Not sure about sutures/ mesh sizes etc...
		Implementing and reviewing decisions	4	Readily vocalised concerns
Communication and Teamwork	2	Exchanging information	2	Did not relate well to anaesthetist
		Establishing a shared understanding	3	Waited for trainer to take the lead
		Co-ordinating team activities	3	Did not enquire about pt condition from anaesthetist
Leadership	3	Setting and maintaining standards	4	Followed theatre protocol but didn't mark side
		Supporting others	4	Good rapport with trainee OPD and scrub nurse
		Coping with pressure	3	At times seemed to carry on regardless - oblivious to important anatomy – too focused on other things

Fig. 22.4 Completed NOTSS rating form for a trainee general surgeon's performance on a hernia repair. (Adapted from: Yule S, Flin R, Paterson-Brown S, Maran N, Rowley D, Youngson G (2008, in press). See one, do one, debrief one. *Cognition, Technology and Work*)

the cognitive and social skills influencing performance. Basic knowledge of the factors influencing human performance should be introduced to the medical curriculum at undergraduate level to allow NTS to be properly developed in postgraduate training. The introduction of patient safety to the undergraduate medical curriculum[78] is beginning to address this deficiency.

The evaluation of NTS may be undertaken for both training purposes as described above or for a more formal assessment. More formal assessment can be a contentious issue, especially if it becomes part of a competence assessment or licensing procedure. For either purpose, the general principles of performance assessment apply[79], although there are particular considerations to be taken into account when using a behavioural rating system to assess NTS for licensing. In this case, such as in civil aviation in the UK, then specific guidelines need to be developed (see CAA[32] Chapter 7, page 2). In the UK, concern about licensing and revalidation of doctors[80] is starting to raise the prospect of competence assurance being introduced across the medical career. Klampfer et al.[81] offer guidance for those considering using behavioural marker systems for summative assessment.

◆ Raters require extensive training (initial and recurrent). They also need to be 'calibrated' – that is, their ratings need to be anchored onto the rating scale in a consistent manner.

◆ The rating systems do not transfer across domains and cultures without adaptation (e.g. western behaviours in eastern cultures, or from aviation to medicine).

◆ The rating systems need proper implementation into an organization, and need management and workforce support. It is recommended that a phased introduction is required to build confidence and expertise in raters and ratees. Consideration needs to be given to how rating information will be stored and accessed (as with any other performance data held on file).

◆ Application of the rating system must be sensitive to the stage of professional development of the individual, and to the maturity of the organizational and professional culture (e.g. whether used as a diagnostic, training and/or assessment tool).

◆ Any use of the system must consider contextual factors when rating behaviour (e.g. crew experience, workload, operating environment, operational complexity).

When using a behaviour rating system for competence assessment, there are additional considerations because the formal assessment of non-technical aspects of performance presents significant challenges. The rating system must capture the context in which that assessment is made (e.g. crew dynamics and experience, operating environment, operational complexity, current conditions). For example, in a team, the behaviour of one crew member can be adversely or positively impacted by another, which could result in a substandard or inflated performance rating. Marker systems should be designed to detect and record such effects.

Most behaviour rating systems consist of a set of observable skills and rating scales on which to record the evaluations. The identification of skill sets was described above and these usually include examples of behaviours that signify whether the skill is being demonstrated. Rating scales come in a range of formats and need to be carefully designed.

The behavioural rating method that is used needs to meet a number of psychometric conditions, such as reliability and validity. Flin *et al.*[3] discuss these in more detail along with the design and use of behavioural rating skills for NTS assessment. In order to achieve the optimum quality of ratings, the raters must be properly trained. The training requirements for raters should not be underestimated. The danger is that behaviour rating systems look deceptively simple. Considerable skill is required to make accurate observations and ratings, and to give constructive feedback to those being rated. The following are recommended for a training course in behaviour rating and feedback:

◆ minimum 2–5 consecutive days training (depending on prior experience)

◆ ideal group size, 8–12 people

◆ half-day training follow-up (e.g. meeting, feedback *via* telephone) after rating practice.

The training for raters should deliver the following:

◆ Make explicit the goals for use of the rating system (e.g. formal assessment, developmental feedback, organisational audit).

◆ Explain the design of the rating system, as well as content and guidelines for its use.

◆ Review main sources of rater biases (e.g. hindsight, halo, recency, primacy) with techniques to be used for minimization of these influences.

◆ Present the concept of inter-rater reliability and the methods that will be used to maximize it.

◆ Illustrate and define each point of the rating scale and different levels of situational complexity with video examples, discussions and hands-on exercises.

◆ Provide practical training with multiple examples.

◆ Include calibration with iterative feedback on inter-rater reliability score.

◆ Teach debriefing skills as appropriate.

◆ Conclude with a formal assessment of rater competence.

22.6 **Conclusion**

In healthcare, as in other workplaces, human errors are common and it is clear that they are not only caused by technical malfunctions or lack of clinical skill. Workers' social and cognitive skills also play an important role in causing or protecting against adverse events. As simulation facilities have developed in medicine, there has been an increased recognition that that these offer an ideal opportunity for the development and evaluation of practitioners' NTS. Recent advances in the identification of skill sets, the design of training courses and the availability of behaviour rating systems are beginning to provide the necessary tools for enhancing the practice of NTS in medicine.

References

1. Heath C (2000). Technical and non-technical skills needed by oil companies. *Journal of Geoscience Education* **48**: 605–12.
2. Flin R, Martin L, Goeters K-M, Hoermann J, Amalberti R, Valot C, Nijhuis H (2003). Development of the NOTECHS (Non-Technical Skills) system for assessing pilots' CRM skills. *Human Factors and Aerospace Safety* **3**: 95–117.
3. Flin R, O'Connor P, Crichton M (2008). *Safety at the Sharp End. A Guide to Non-Technical Skills.* Aldershot: Ashgate.
4. CAA (2006). *Crew Resource Management (CRM) Training. Guidance for Flight Crew, CRM Instructors (CRMIs) and CRM Instructor-Examiners (CRMIEs).* CAP 737. Gatwick: Safety Regulation Group, Civil Aviation Authority. http://www.caa.co.uk.
5. General Medical Council (2006.) *Good Medical Practice. Working with Colleagues / Working in Teams.* Paragraphs 41–42. London: GMC.
6. Flin R, Yule S, Maran N, Paterson-Brown S, Rowley D, Youngson G (2007). Teaching surgeons about non-technical skills. *The Surgeon* **5**: 86–9.
7. Wieck K (1990). The vulnerable system: An analysis of the Tenerife air disaster. *Journal of Management* **16**: 571–93.
8. Lodge, M. (2002) Airline captain. In R. Flin & K. Arbuthnot (Eds.) *Incident Command. Tales from the Hot Seat.* Aldershot: Ashgate.
9. Wiener E, Kanki B, Helmreich R, Eds. (1993). *Cockpit Resource Management.* San Diego: Academic Press.
10. Flin R (2001). Piper Alpha: Decision making and crisis management. In: A Boin, U Rosenthal, L Comfort, Eds. *Managing Crises: Threats Dilemmas and Opportunities.* Illinios: CC Thomas.
11. Hetherington C, Flin R, Mearns K (2006). Safety at sea. Human factors in shipping. *Journal of Safety Research* **37**: 401–11.
12. Flin R, O'Connor P, Mearns K (2002). Crew Resource Management: improving safety in high reliability industries. *Team Performance Management* **8**: 68–78.
13. Okray R, Lubnau T (2004). *Crew Resource Management for the Fire Service.* Tulsa: PennWell.
14. Salas E, Wilson K, Burke S, Wightman D (2006). Does Crew Resource Management training work? An update, an extension and some critical needs. *Human Factors* **48**: 392–412.
15. Flin R (2006). *Safe in their Hands? Licensing and Competence Assurance of Safety Critical Roles in High Risk Industries.* University of Aberdeen. Report to the Department of Health, London. Available at http://www.abdn.ac.uk/iprc.
16. Vincent C (2006). *Patient Safety.* London: Churchill Livingstone.
17. Reader T, Flin R, Lauche K, Cuthbertson B (2006). Non-technical skills in the intensive care unit. *British Journal of Anaesthesia* **96**: 551–9.
18. Yule S, Flin R, Maran N, Paterson-Brown S (2006). Non-technical skills for surgeons: a review of the literature. *Surgery* 139: 140–49.
19. Seamster T, Keampf G (2001). Identifying resource management skills for pilots. In: E. Salas, C. Bowers and E. Edens (Eds.) *Improving Teamwork in Organizations. Applications of Resource Management Training.* Mahwah, NJ: LEA.
20. Flin R, Yule S, Maran N, Paterson-Brown S, Rowley D (2005.) *NOTSS. Non-Technical Skills for Surgeons.* Paper presented at European Association of Work Psychology Conference, Istanbul, July.
21. Landy F, Conte J (2007). *Work in the 21st Century. An Introduction to Industrial and Organizational Psychology.* (2nd ed.) Oxford: Blackwell.
22. Barling J, Frone M, Eds. (2004). *The Psychology of Workplace Safety.* Washington: American Psychological Association.

23. Fletcher G, Flin R, McGeorge P, Glavin R, Maran N, Patey R (2004). Development of a prototype behavioural marker system for anaesthetists' non-technical skills. *Cognition, Technology and Work* **6**: 165–71.

24. Thomas E, Sexton J, Helmreich R (2004). Translating teamwork behaviours from aviation to healthcare: development of behavioural markers for neonatal resuscitation. *Quality and Safety in Health Care* **13**(Suppl. 1): i57–i64.

25. Helmreich R, Schaefer H (1994). Team performance in the operating room. In M. Bogner (Ed) *Human Error in Medicine*. New Jersey: Lawrence Erlbaun.

26. Thomadsen B (2007). Medical failure taxonomies. In: P. Carayon (Ed.) *Handbook of Human Factors and Ergonomics in Health Care and Patient Safety*. Mahwah, NJ: LEA.

27. Yule S, Flin R, Paterson-Brown S, Maran N, Rowley D (2006). Development of a rating system for surgeons' non-technical skills. *Medical Education* **40**: 1098–104.

28. Undre S, Healey A, Darzi A, Vincent C (2006). Observational teamwork assessment in surgery: A feasibility study. *World Journal of Surgery* **30**: 1774–83.

29. Mackenzie C, Craig G, Parr M, Horst R, the LOTAS Group (1994). Video analysis of two emergency tracheal intubations identifies flawed decision making. *Anesthesiology* **81**: 911–19.

30. Marsch S, Muller C, Marquardt K, Conrad G, Tscan F, Hunziker P (2004). Human factors affect the quality of cardiopulmonary resuscitation in simulated cardiac arrests. *Resuscitation* **60**: 51–6.

31. FAA (2006). Advanced Qualification Program. Advisory Circular 120–54-A. Washington: Federal Aviation Administration.

32. CAA (2006) *Guidance Notes for Accreditation Standards for CRM Instructors and CRM Instructor Examiners*. Standards Doc. 29 Version 2. Gatwick: Civil Aviation Authority.

33. O'Connor P, Hormann H-J, Flin R, Lodge M, Goeters K-M, the JARTEL group (2002). Developing a method for evaluating crew resource management skills: A European perspective. *International Journal of Aviation Psychology* **12**: 265–88.

34. O'Connor P, Flin R, Fletcher G (2002). Evaluating CRM. *Human Factors and Aerospace Safety*, 2,217–255.

35. Goeters K-M (2002). Evaluation of the effects of CRM training by the assessment of non-technical skills under LOFT. *Human Factors and Aerospace Safety* **2**: 71–86.

36. Jensen R (1995). *Pilot Judgment and Crew Resource Management*. Aldershot: Ashgate.

37. Macleod N (2005). *Building Safe Systems in Aviation. A CRM Developer's Handbook*. Aldershot: Ashgate.

38. Salas E, Bowers C, Edens E, Eds. (2001). *Improving teamwork in organizations: applications of resource management training*. Mahwah, NJ: LEA.

39. Walters A (2002). *Crew Resource Management is No Accident*. Wallingford, UK: Aries.

40. Howard S, Gaba D, Fish K, Yang G, Sarnquist F (1992). Anaesthesia Crisis Resource Management training: teaching anesthesiologists to handle critical incidents. *Aviation, Space and Environmental Medicine* **63**: 763–70.

41. Pizzi L, Godfarb N, Nash D (2001). Crew Resource Management and its applications in medicine. In: K. Shojana, B. Duncan, K. McDonald & R. Wachter. *Making health Care Safer. A Critical Analysis of Patient Safety Practices*. Rockville: MD: AHRQ: 501–10.

42. Bleakley A, Hobbs A, Boyden J, Walsh L (2004). Safety in operating theatres. Improving teamwork through team resource management. *Journal of Workplace Learning* **16**: 83–91.

43. Brennan S (2006). NOTSS course (non-technical skills for surgeons). *BMJ Careers* **9** (sept): 98.

44. Sachdeva A, Philibert I, *et al.* (2007.) Patient safety curriculum for surgical residency programs: Results of a national consensus conference. *Surgery* **141**: 428–41.

45. Flin R, Maran N (2004). Identifying and training non-technical skills for teams in acute medicine. *Quality and Safety in Health Care* **13** (Suppl. 1): i80–i84.

46. Baker D, Beaubien M, Holtzman A (2006). *DoD medical team training programs: An independent case study analysis*. Publication 06–0001.Washington: AHRQ.

47. Goldstein I, Ford K (2002). *Training in Organizations*. Belmont, CA: Wadsworth.

48. Salas E, Wilson K, Burke S, Wightman D, Howse W (2006). A checklist for Crew Resource Management training. *Ergonomics in Design* **14**: 6–15.

49. Baker D, Salas E, Barach P, Battles J, King H (2007.) The relation between teamwork and patient safety. In: P. Carayon, Ed. *Handbook of Human Factors and Ergonomics in Health Care and Patient Safety.* Mahwah, NJ: LEA.

50. Dismukes K, Smith G, Eds. (2000). *Facilitation and Debriefing in Aviation Training and Operations.* Aldershot: Ashgate.

51. Rudolph J, Simon R, Dufresne R, Raemer D (2006). There's no such thing as 'nonjudgmental' debriefing: A theory and method for good judgment. *Simulation in Healthcare* **1**: 49–55.

52. JAA (2001). JAR OPS Regulations 1.940, 1.945, 1.955, 1.965. Hoofdorp: JAA.

53. Baker D, Mulqueen C, Dismukes K (2001). Training raters to assess resource management skills. In: E Salas, C Bowers, E Edens, Eds. *Improving Teamwork in Organizations. Applications of Resource Management Training.* Mahwah, NJ: LEA.

54. Baker D, Dismukes K (2002). Special issue on training instructors to evaluate aircrew performance. *International Journal of Aviation Psychology* **12**: 203–22.

55. Beaubien M, Baker D, Salvaggio A (2004). Improving the construct validity of line operational simulation ratings: Lessons learned from the assessment center. *International Journal of Aviation Psychology* **14**: 1–17.

56. Holt R, Boehm-Davis D, Beaubien M (2001). Evaluating resource management training. In: E Salas, C Bowers, E Edens, Eds. *Improving Teamwork in Organizations. Applications of Resource Management Training.* Mahwah, NJ: LEA.

57. Flin R, Martin L (2001). Behavioural markers for Crew Resource Management: A review of current practice. *International Journal of Aviation Psychology* 11: 95–118.

58. Avermaete, van J, Kruijsen E, Eds. (1998). *NOTECHS. The Evaluation of Non-Technical Skills of Multi-Pilot Aircrew in Relation to the JAR-FCL Requirements.* Final Report NLR-CR-98443. Amsterdam: National Aerospace Laboratory (NLR).

59. Helmreich R (1999). CRM training, primary line of defence against threats to flight safety, including human error. *ICAO Journal* **54**: 6–10.

60. Helmreich R, Klinect J, Wilhelm J (2003). Managing threat and error: Data from line operations. In: G Edkins, P Pfister, Eds) *Innovation and Consolidation in Aviation.* Aldershot: Ashgate.

61. Helmreich R, Wilhelm J (1987). Reinforcing and measuring flightcrew resource management: Training Captain/Check Airman/Instructor Reference Manual. *NASA/ University of Texas at Austin Technical Manual 87–1.* Austin, TX: The University of Texas, Human Factors Research Project.

62. Helmreich R, Butler R, Taggart W, Wilhelm J (1995). The NASA/ University of Texas/ FAA Line/ LOS checklist: A behavioural marker-based checklist for CRM skills assessment. Version 4. Technical Paper 94–02 (Revised 12/8/95). Austin, Texas: University of Texas Aerospace Research Project.

63. Helmreich R, Butler R, Taggart W, Wilhelm J (1995). Behavioral markers in accidents and incidents: Reference list. NASA/UT/FAA Technical Report 95–1. Austin, TX: The University of Texas, Human Factors Research Project.

64. Hausler R, Klampfer B, Amacher A, Naef W (2004). Behavioral markers in analysing team performance of cockpit crews. In R. Dietrich & T. Childress (Eds). *Group Interaction in High Risk Environments.* Aldershot: Ashgate.

65. Thomas M (2004). Predictors of threat and error management: Identification of core nontechnical skills and implications for training systems design. *International Journal of Aviation Psychology* **14**: 207–31.

66. Gaba D, Howard S, Flanagan B, Smith B, Fish K, Botney R (1998). Assessment of clinical performance during simulated crises using both technical and behavioural ratings. *Anesthesiology* 89: 8–18.

67. Fletcher G, McGeorge P, Flin R, Glavin R, Maran N (2003). Anaesthetists' non-technical skills (ANTS). Evaluation of a behavioural marker system. *British Journal of Anaesthesia* **90**: 580–8.

68. Patey R, Flin R, Fletcher G, Maran N, Glavin R (2005). Developing a taxonomy of anaesthetists' non-technical skills (ANTS). In: Hendriks K, Ed. *Advances in Patient Safety: From Research to Implementation.* Rockville, MD: Agency for Healthcare Research and Quality.

69. Yee B, Naik V, Joo H, *et al.* (2005). Non-technical skills in anesthesia crisis management with repeated exposure to simulation-based education. *Anesthesiology* **103**: 214–8.

70. Rosenstock E, Kristensen M, Rasmussen L, Skak C, Ostergaard D (2006). Qualitative analysis of difficult airway management. *Acta Anaesthesiology, Scandinavia* **50**: 290–7.

71. Patey R (2007). Non-technical skills and anaesthesia. In: J Cashman, R Grounds, Eds. *Recent Advances in Anaesthesia and Intensive Care 24.* Cambridge: Cambridge University Press.

72. Helmreich R, Schaefer H, Sexton J (1995). The operating room checklist. Technical Report 95–10, NASA/University of Texas/FAA, Austin Texas.

73. Carthey J, de Leval M, Wright D, *et al.* (2003). Behavioural markers of surgical excellence. *Safety Science* **41**: 409–25.

74. Catchpole K, Giddings A, Wilkinson M, Hirst G, Dale T, de Leval M (2007). Improving patient safety by identifying latent failures in successful operations. *Surgery* **142**: 102–110.

75. Moorthy K, Munz Y, Forrest D, *et al.* (2006). Surgical crisis management skills. Training and assessment. *Annals of Surgery* **244**: 139–47.

76. Yule S, Flin R, Paterson-Brown S, Maran N, Rowley D, Youngson G (2008). Surgeon's Non-technical skills in the Operating Room: Reliability Testing of the NOTSS Behavior Rating System. *World Journal of Surgery* **32**: 548–556.

77. Yule S, Flin R, Paterson-Brown S, Maran N, Rowley D, Youngson G (in press). See one, do one, debrief one. *Cognition, Technology and Work.*

78. Patey R, Flin R, *et al.* (2007). Patient safety: helping medical students understand medical error. *Quality and Safety in Health Care* **16**: 256–259.

79. Fletcher C (2004). *Appraisal and Feedback. Making Performance Review Work. (3rd ed.)* London: Chartered Institute of Personnel and Development.

80. Donaldson L (2006). *Good Doctors, Safer Patients.* London: Department of Health.

81. Klampfer B, Flin R, Helmreich R, *et al.* (2001). *Enhancing performance in high risk environments: Recommendations for the use of Behavioural Markers.* Daimler Benz Foundation. Available from: http://www.abdn.ac.uk/iprc.

Chapter 23

Simulation training programmes for rapid response or medical emergency teams

Elizabeth A Hunt, Nicolette C Mininni, and Michael A DeVita

Overview

- Simulation was initially used in the aviation industry to train pilots how to fly a plane. The programme developed into cockpit and later crew resource management (CRM) training, which focused on team training as an equally important part of simulation training to optimize flight safety.
- Rapid response systems (RRS) use medical emergency teams (METs), within hospitals to respond to patients who are clinically deteriorating on the wards *before* they suffer a respiratory or cardiopulmonary arrest, to improve patient safety.
- Simulation training is effectively being used to train MET team members.
- Important concepts learned from CRM training used in MET training:
  1. 'Flattening the hierarchy' within teams is an important way to improve communication between team members.
  2. Practising ways to improve 'situational awareness' keeps all members of a team 'on the same page' and allows them to identify and deal with problems more quickly.
  3. 'Closed loop communication', 'assertive communication', use of SBAR and AMPLE are all methods to improve communication between team members.
- A key component of effective simulation training is thoughtful feedback and debriefing.
- Simulation training is being used to train ward staff how to take care of a patient during the 'first 5 minutes' of a medical emergency, while waiting for a MET response.

23.1 Introduction

Simulation has been used to analyse teamwork, find areas of deficiency, and to improve team performance in several different industries. Recently, simulation has been used to assess the skills of medical emergency teams (MET) and rapid response teams (RRT), as well as a tool to improve team performance. In this chapter we will describe a few examples of industries that have successfully used simulation as a key component for team training as a template for medical professionals to follow and expand upon, and then discuss how lessons learned have been and may be applied to MET and RRT.

23.2 Simulation for aviation team training

Simulation has been used to improve team function and safety in the aviation industry successfully for many years. Interestingly, while simulation has been used to train pilots since 1911 (individual skills training: 'how to fly'), it was not used for team training *per se* until recently[1,2]. Then, in 1979, the aviation industry studied the causes of airline crashes and identified that most disasters had a series of errors preceding them (both technical and human). The most common human cause of these tragedies was a failure in communication[3]. By analysing cockpit communications stored on flight recorders, they were able to identify patterns of communication and behaviour that failed and directly contributed to the outcomes.

In order to prevent future events, team courses were developed to avoid the most common errors. A new type of simulation training was developed that was originally called cockpit resource management. This training exercise was required training for all pilots; however, the pilots were still only required to *pass* the technical skills and not the cockpit resource management course. While communication within the cockpit may have improved, it was recognized that important communication-related errors were still occurring, among all important members of the team, such as the flight attendants, the air traffic control tower, and of course, pilots. Therefore, training was altered to emphasize the importance of effective communication between all members of the team; the course was renamed crew resource management (CRM). In the late 1980s, the system for assessing competency of pilots was changed such that they had to demonstrate proficiency of technical skills as well as communication and team functioning during simulation exercises[2,3].

This brief history of the development of the CRM programme in aviation highlights several lessons for the medical community. The fact that simulation training was most effective in preventing disasters only after communication (team) skills were perceived to be as important as technical (flying) skills instructs heathcare providers, to emphasize both as well. Improved team functioning requires team training. If healthcare is a set of team activities, then focus on team training may improve teamwork in healthcare as it helped it in aviation (Table 23.1).

The second concept to glean from aviation's CRM is the importance of 'flattening the hierarchy'. This phrase refers to giving team members autonomy and responsibility, as well as diminishing communication barriers between team members. In particular, improving communication both to and from the leader is considered essential to success. A third basic concept is 'situational awareness', which refers to members of the team understanding their role in the team as well as the importance of communicating changes in the state of the patient and/or situation to others so that everyone is making decisions based on current information. A fourth concept that is being promoted in healthcare is the practice of 'closed loop communication' to improve accuracy of communication. In closed-loop communication, the receiver repeats back to the speaker the information s/he heard for confirmation by the speaker. For example, the leader may say, "Linda, please place an IV". Linda should reply, "You want me to place an IV". Later, Linda might update, "the IV is in," and the leader reply, "the IV is in." This method helps to increase situational awareness

Table 23.1 Important concepts learned from aviation industry crew resource management courses

- ◆ Team skills are as important as technical skills in error prevention
- ◆ Flat hierarchies improve communication
- ◆ Situational awareness impacts data transfer and team behaviours
- ◆ Closed loop communication decreases communication errors
- ◆ Assertive communication may help avoid errors

because key information is both accurate and repeated. A fifth concept is 'assertive communication', which refers to the practice of team members recognizing important new information and making sure it is transmitted effectively. It is essential to train team members to speak up especially when they believe an error in management is taking place. This concept is closely related to the principle of flat hierarchy. For example, should the team leader respond to a question incorrectly, team members recognizing the error should raise the issue. While this may create a 'battle' for leadership, if the commentary is patient centred rather than focusing on the error, it is usually well accepted. An example is, "Leader, the patient received Dilaudid (hydromorphone). Nalaxone may allow him to protect his airway and perhaps he will not need endotracheal intubation," as opposed to stating "Leader, you are wrong". The latter provokes a defense response whereas the former tends to focus on the issue.

Below, we will describe how various medical simulation groups have applied these concepts to their Rapid Response Team (RRT) simulation training sessions in order to optimize the effectiveness of the training. We will now discuss lessons learned from another industry that has high performing teams who have used simulation to improve team performance.

23.3 Lessons learned from high performance teams

Highly functional teams exhibit coordinated behaviour directed towards a single goal, or a coordinated set of goals. Two models for coordination are hierarchical and non-hierarchical. In hierarchical models, a team leader assigns responsibilities, coordinates activities, and makes decisions; it is based largely on the CRM aviation model. In non-hierarchical models, exemplified by a NASCAR pit crew, each member of the team has pre-assigned (or self-assigned) roles and duties, and reports along predetermined lines in a non-hierarchical manner. In the latter model, when applied to medicine, there is no 'team' leader *per se* because the team members have preassigned duties, but there would be a 'treatment' leader, a person focused on what diagnostics and treatments are required. The distinction is that the 'team' leader has duties both to team process as well as data analysis and treatment decision making, while the 'treatment' leader would only have responsibility for prioritizing data acquisition, performing data analysis and decision making regarding therapeutics. In the non-hierarchical model, the team members must know their individual duties before the event for success to be achieved routinely. When designed well, these duties are coordinated, or choreographed, with others' duties to address prioritization and efficiency. Once designed, they can be taught and then practised to perfection. Benefits of this model include more rapid task completion, especially early in the response, planned coordination of activities, ease of teaching and assessing team performance because of objective, prioritized task load, and an equitable distribution of duties (avoiding duty overload).

The more common hierarchical approach is somewhat more typical of crisis resource management (CRM), based on civil aviation, and espoused by a number of authors, most notably Gaba and Raemer[4–8]. The non-hierarchical is based more on a NASCAR pit crew or Advanced Trauma Life Support (ATLS), with its pre-assigned roles and responsibilities. In the setting of RRT responding to a medical crisis, DeVita *et al.* has used the term Crisis Team Training (CTT) to distinguish it from traditional CRM methodology[9]. Professionals trained using the CTT method have delineated roles and responsibilities, and a choreographed response. In this model, responders self-assign to predetermined roles based upon their skills, and then perform the duties ascribed to those roles. This pattern unloads the treatment leader of the responsibility for team management and allows the leader to focus on patient needs instead.

The bottom line is that teams function better if the roles and responsibilities are clear and have been practised repeatedly. The NASCAR pit crew is a prime example of the type of teams that use simulation to streamline the design of the response, master role clarity, and to optimize communication in order to create a unit that functions synergistically so that the team is more than the sum of its parts. This brief discussion of how various industries have used simulation training to optimize team functioning leads us to our primary discussion, of how hospitals can use simulation in order to improve the manner in which RRTs function and ultimately to save more lives.

23.4 Brief history of medical emergency teams and rapid response systems

Medical Emergency Teams (MET) were first described in Australia by Lee and then in the USA by DeVita[10,11]. The MET is a pre-organized group of professionals and equipment that are dispatched to a patient's bedside anywhere within a hospital. All reports of successful MET processes used a standardized and objective set of MET criteria that are vital sign limits, which if exceeded, require a MET activation or other triggers such as specific patient symptoms (excluding acute change in mental status or chest pain) or concerns that staff have about the patient. The hope is to be able to swiftly identify suddenly critically ill patients outside the intensive care unit, and then to immediately provide critical care resources to correct the 'needs-resources' mismatch. Studies which have demonstrated benefit are summarized in a recent consensus conference report, but a large cluster randomized trial of MET demonstrated no benefit[12,13].

While the actual effect of METs on the incidence of in-hospital cardiopulmonary arrest is still not clear, what is clear is that the large majority of patients who suffer an in-hospital cardiopulmonary arrest while on the wards have preceding signs and/or symptoms that are harbingers of what is to come. The goal of MET systems is to make sure that:

- these patients are identified as early as possible
- experts in critical care evaluate these patients as quickly as possible in order to optimize patient outcomes.

A group of international experts met during the first consensus conference on medical emergency teams in 2005 and described the four key components of a successful RRS. This included the:

- event identification/ response trigger (afferent arm)
- responder/treatment team (efferent arm)
- quality improvement and feedback
- administrative oversight.

Theoretically, simulation can be used to address each of these arms, but it has already been used by some hospitals to train healthcare teams on the efferent and afferent arms of the MET and finally as a quality improvement tool to modify the response design (DeVita, unreported)[14,15]. There are several forms of efferent teams that the consensus conference defined. While the names of these efferent arm teams have been inconsistently used in the literature, the following is a summary of the terms as defined by members of the consensus conference. The first is a nurse-led response, which is termed a RRT, the second is a MET, which is a physician led team. Both these teams act in response to a crisis situation. The third team has been termed critical care outreach (CCO). These teams may be physician or nurse led, but differ from RRT and MET in that they are proactive. They routinely round on high-risk patients like those recently discharged from intensive care, or those receiving high-risk treatments in an effort to prevent crises as well as cardiac arrest. All three team forms are trainable using simulation, though the CCO is a lower acuity intervention that may be less error prone.

23.5 Examples of simulation training for rapid response systems

Simulation training programmes for RRT and MET are still in their infancy. The first reference to simulation training for MET appears in 2004 and other authors have shown some of the potential of this type of training[14,16–18]. While most RRS training programmes have some medical content as part of the training (such as a review of medical guidelines for resuscitation or algorithms for goal directed therapy in shock), simulation training has predominantly focused on improving team performance. The courses point out that teamwork is the structural underpinning of successfully delivering appropriate medical care. Techniques differ between programmes, but primary intervention focused on effective communication, division and coordination of labour, and teamwork to achieve common goals is universal. Johns Hopkins, Harvard, Penn State and the University of Pittsburgh are a few of the medical schools that use simulation for training RRT and MET (Table 23.2). In this case, the goal of a simulation training programme is to develop a group that can organize and coordinate behaviors to become an effective team. This requires that teammates assume roles and carry out the responsibilities to assess, treat, stabilize, and triage the patient. Training is also effective for the afferent (crisis detection) arm as well. University of Pittsburgh has a "First Five Minutes" simulation training programme intended to teach nursing staff how to recognize a crisis, call for help, and what to do until the team arrives.

At the University of Pittsburgh a simulation programme, titled Crisis Team Training, (CTT), is used to train the MET and RRT responders[19]. One of the challenges of training is that members of a MET or RRT vary from institution to institution and even among different hospitals within a healthcare system. The problem of training team members to a choreographed plan is compounded by the *ad hoc* nature of the team. When a MET or RRT is called, staff members assigned to respond for a specific area of the hospital or for a shift may never have worked with other team responders. Teaching participants to respond to a crisis situation by assuming a role, performing the associated responsibilities and using effective communication skills is the focus. While a 'huddle' at the beginning of a work shift may serve as an opportunity to coordinate or plan duties (especially for institutions with a single defined team), many institutions may find this impractical due to staffing imperatives. Therefore, one goal of CTT is to teach the team a specific organizational plan, including roles, duties associated with each role, how to assume roles, to perform responsibilities or tasks (Fig. 23.1), and finally to communicate effectively.

Many team courses require participants to pre-register for class. Some maintain a multidisciplinary student mix to reflect a similar composition to the hospital's MET. University of Pittsburgh trains nurses (ICU and non-ICU), physicians (critical care, specialty care and primary care), respiratory therapists, nursing assistants, pharmacists, and physician's assistants in the same class. Each class must have at least three disciplines represented in order to foster an interdisciplinary approach and enable best cross training. Online pre-course materials, demographics and simulator experience surveys are required to be completed prior to class. The beginning of the class day consists of brief didactic lecture presented by a course facilitator, or a team exercise using networked videogaming technology. However, most of the programme uses simulation

Table 23.2 Principles of crisis resource management

- Roles – leaders and followers
- Communication – closing the loop
- Support – calling for help
- Resources – getting what you need
- Global assessment – an open mind

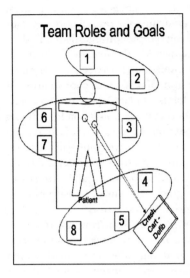

Role	Responsibility
1. Airway Manager	Assess, count respiratory rate, assist ventilation, intubate, check pupils
2. Airway Assistant	Assist airway manager, oxygen and suction setup, suction as needed.
3. Bedside Assistant (RN &/ ICU RN Backup)	Provide SBAR, psychologically support patient, check pulse, obtain vital signs, pulse oximeter placement, assess patent IVs, push meds.
4. Crash Cart Managerr (ICU RN &/ Pharmacist)	Deploy equipment, (AmbuBag-Board-Pads-Paper record), prepare meds, run defibrillator.
5. Treatment Leader	Assess team responsibilities, data, direct treatment, set priorities, triage patient.
6. Circulation	Check pulse, place defib pads, perform chest compressions.
7. Procedure	Perform procedures, IVs, chest tubes, CBS, ABG and provide additional patient history.
8. Data Manager (Usually an ICU RN)	Role tags, AMPLE, lab results, chart, record interventions.
Aide	Bring CBS machine, patient chart and requested equipment to bedside.

Fig. 23.1 Rapid response team roles, responsibilities and bedside position.

crisis scenarios, including a high fidelity full body simulator. Nine scenarios have been developed based on common crisis events. The simulation includes patient charts that include short patient history, allergies, medications and current vital signs, lab values and diagnostics. These human and non-human factors increase the realism of the simulation.

Each scenario begins by one participant being given some patient information, after which s/he needs to assess the patient. The initial participant is expected to identify whether there is a crisis (2 of 9 scenarios are null or non-crisis events), activate the team, and communicate the relevant information essential to proper treatment of the patient. Each scenario is videorecorded, enabling playback, analysis and debriefing by the facilitator and participants. Comprehensive debriefing tools have been created to score participants on behaviours that fall into three categories:

♦ communication

♦ organizational tasks

♦ therapeutic tasks[20].

The programme does not focus on diagnosis and treatment of the crisis as much as to focus on to the impact of and how to organize quickly and communicate effectively. Trainees learn that

Table 23.3 Data probes for each of the nine scenarios used in the University of Pittsburgh's crisis team training course. The scenarios are acute myocardial infarction, ventricular tachycardia, opioid overdose, subarachnoid haemorrhage, ventricular fibrillation, null, acute postoperative haemorrhage, tension pneumothorax, and null (DNR)

Data probe 1	Data probe 2
EKG	Complaint of chest pain
Complaint of racing heart	Monitor showing ventricular tachycardia
History of opioid administration	Pulse oximetry
History of subarachnoid haemorrhage and unclipped cerebral aneurysm	Unequal pupils
Absent circulation	Ventricular fibrillation on monitor
Diphenhydramine administration	Normal vital signs
Low blood pressure	Low hct
History of IJ line insertion	Absent breath sounds on right
Chart order for DNR	Absent respiration

teamwork leads to more rapid and accurate diagnosis and treatment. Imbedded in the scenario are so-called 'data probes', which are essential pieces of information that must be communicated to the team to treat the patient correctly. Examples include an ECG showing ST elevation, a patient complaint of palpitations, a chest X-ray showing a tension pneumothorax, or a history of bleeding (Table 23.3) Effectiveness at assessing and communicating these pieces of data are tracked and graded. The course directors believe that while this method does not record or evaluate all communication, it does provide a window into the team's ability to share key information. Additional communication assessments are built into the debriefing tool and are as simple as verification that vital signs were documented on a crisis event sheet or therapeutic intervention orders were given, received and carried out (i.e. closed-loop communication).

23.5.1 Debriefing review and feedback

Immediate review of behaviour and debriefing are the core of simulation education. Participants have the opportunity to discuss actions and team performance, particularly as they relate to the designed response. Through debriefing and the use of a debriefing tool (which supports facilitators in emphasizing key learning objectives), performance can be analysed to demonstrate improvement in communication and task completion between scenarios[19]. Perceptions of performance can be compared to actual performance, enabling trainees to learn how to gauge their own performances in the future. In self-evaluation, 91% of CTT participants rated themselves as able to communicate with others more effectively and able to coordinate actions with other team members after completing the course. Over a 20-month period, April 2005 through November 2006, a cumulative graph representation serves as the benchmark for current students participating in CTT programmes. Participant feedback *via* graphics compares current participants to the cumulative benchmark of all other programmes in areas of communication, organization and therapeutic tasks (Fig. 23.2). Performance assessment also includes patient survival of the simulated crisis. Together, participants and facilitator determine if the patient survived (based on maintenance of basal physiological needs), experienced a critical incident

Assessing Role Performance

60 seconds Session 1 ORGANIZATION TASKS THERAPEUTIC TASKS					
Station	Team Member	Items	CT	Save	TCT
Airway Manager		Identify self	N		N
		Name tag	N		N
		Move Bed from wall	N/A		
		Stand in appropriate position	Y		Y
		Count respiratory rate	N		N
		Assess: is airway open	N		N
		Open airway	N/A		
		Assist ventilation (Mouth to mask, or Bag-Mask)	N		N
Airway Assistant		Identify self	N		N
		Name tag	N		N
		Obtain Airway Bag	N		N
		Stand in appropriate position	Y		Y
		Give mask/bag to airway manager	N		N
		Set up oxygen	N		N

Fig. 23.2 Part of the scoring sheet used in the University of Pittsburgh CTT course. Two roles are exhibited, along with duties that need to be accomplished within 60 seconds of scenario start. Note: some tasks are organizational while others are therapeutic in focus.

(some error that may have caused harm), or died. Simulation training for RRT brings together individuals with a variety of healthcare provider backgrounds and minimal experience working together as a team, breaks down the essential skills necessary to organize quickly in order to assess patient, examine essential data, communicate effectively, and deliver appropriate care.

The Johns Hopkins Children's Centre uses simulation training as part of their quality improvement effort for both the efferent and the afferent arms of the RRS. The afferent arm of a RRS involves the ward staff who must identify that there is a problem and then trigger the MET to the patient's bedside. Each month, simulated medical emergencies known as 'mock codes' are held on one of the paediatric wards in an actual patient bed space. These mock codes are organized by the chairman of the paediatric CPR committee, the paediatric chief residents, the children's centre head nurse educator, and the nurse manager for the floor where the mock code will occur. This multidisciplinary committee (part of the administrative arm of the RRS) sets the learning objectives prior to each mock code. A high fidelity mannequin is taken to the room and is hooked up to any equipment that an actual patient in that setting would be on, and then the call button in the room is triggered, asking for help. This methodology keeps the staff unaware that an event is to occur. Most scenarios involve a patient who is medically unstable, but not yet in cardiopulmonary arrest. During debriefing the educational team emphasizes specific triggers for the MET (e.g. seizures with apnoea, acute mental status changes, and desaturation unresponsive to initial manoeuvres.) The mock codes helped us to recognize that the ward staff was given too many tasks and perhaps as a result were not prioritizing initial assessment and treatment of airway, breathing and circulation[21]. This led to the development of a curriculum entitled *The First Five Minutes*. This curriculum is focused on when to call for help, how to call for help and what to do during the first 5 minutes. Of interest, both the Johns Hopkins Children's Centre and the University of

Pittsburgh independently created a curriculum entitled *The First Five Minutes*, highlighting that both institutions have noted a need to improve the quality of the first responder's actions when caring for patients who become critically ill on the wards. Tasks include the ward nursing staff functioning as 'first responders', and not merely preparing the room for the MET or code team. The new process enabled us to empower the nursing staff to act by calling for help when they (or the parents) sense that a child is not doing well, even if there is no objective vital sign abnormality. Any time our quality assurance process identifies a real patient in whom the MET was not called or was called later than we would have liked, that case is incorporated into the next mock code.

We also use simulation training to improve the efferent arm of the RRS. The mock codes described above start with the afferent arm component, but then move on to include the efferent arm (the actual MET). During these mock codes, we address specific medical crises (e.g. severe asthmatic exacerbation, and supraventricular tachycardia). Nevertheless, the primary focus of the simulation exercise remains how the team functions (even as we assess medical knowledge). We concentrate our teaching on:

- diagnosing environmental barriers (i.e. any issues related to staff being able to find or use the equipment)
- assessing information transfer from the ward staff to the MET
- cooperation between the MET and the ward team.

During the debriefing, we discuss communication among the ward staff and the MET. In our training, we emphasize the importance of quickly establishing leadership and roles, as well as other issues that are integral to good team functioning (e.g. closed-loop communication, situational awareness, flattening of the hierarchy and assertive communication). Each of these is addressed during the debriefing with specific examples from the mock code that just occurred. We emphasize that these mock codes include the actual team members that would be responding to a real emergency on that particular day. This exercise allows the individuals to practice organizing to make a well functioning *ad hoc* team. Participants include the physician trainees, the paediatric intensive care unit (PICU) nurses, PICU respiratory therapists, pharmacists, a chaplain and a security guard. Pharmacy, for example, considers these exercises an integral component for training their staff on how to listen and speak up during the chaotic atmosphere of a medical emergency, thus optimizing their efficacy. For example, when conducting a mock code about a severe asthmatic in respiratory failure who requires intubation, the most experienced airway person was attending a simultaneous emergency, thus leaving the paediatric residents in charge. We noted that the paediatric residents were struggling with what pharmacological agents to use for the intubation, while the experienced pharmacist had already prepared ketamine, lidocaine and succinylcholine, based on his experience. Unfortunately, he had not communicated his knowledge to the team. The mock code helped him realize how valuable his input is to the team and may make him more likely to speak up during the next emergency.

Johns Hopkins has recently recognized the importance of the concept of 'training to success'. For their large, multidisciplinary team, this means that problems observed during a mock code or real code response that they wanted to prevent in the future, they would re-enact in a simulated setting to allow the team to practice until they perfected the response. Examples include ineffective handoffs and failure to communicate. Another common sociological problem was encountered after Johns Hopkins converted from a traditional cardiac arrest Team to a MET. Some response team members questioned being summoned especially if the patient was not in cardiac arrest. They made remarks such as "This wasn't a real code," or "I left the unit for *this?*" These types of remarks may cause the ward team to feel guilty or ashamed, and may create a barrier to future calls that may result in patient harm. Therefore, the training sessions include simulations where the patient has recovered by the time the team has arrived. For this scenario, learning objectives include performing an adequate patient assessment, maintaining appropriate interactions with ward staff, and understanding the potential impact that negative commentary may have on future events.

Simulation may be used to enhance training for most health professional disciplines. For example, the Children's Centre nursing educators use simulation while training their ward nurses on the role they should play during the 'first five minutes' of a medical emergency, on when and how to call the team, and their role once the whole team arrives. Pharmacy uses simulation to train their pharmacists on their role in a MET call, including practising finding the appropriate drugs rapidly in the emergency drug box, anticipating what drugs will be needed and rapidly drawing up emergency medications in a safe manner. Finally, the residents who will be carrying the MET beeper that month participate in a monthly 'teaching mock code training session'. This involves a 2-hour session in which the residents run through ten 'mini mock codes' that focus on the following issues:

- establishing a leader
- clarifying the pre-established MET team member roles
- specifically assessing and frequently reassessing airway, breathing, and circulation
- practising performance of important skills such as bag–valve–mask ventilation, chest compressions, intraosseous needle placement, and defibrillation
- practising effective communication patterns mentioned above, such as closed-loop communication, situational awareness and assertive communication.

In our system, the residents participate in a 'teaching mock code' early in their ward month and again during the multidisciplinary surprise mock code described already. The institution performs competency testing annually for all nursing staff and paediatric resident staff using simulation[22]. This annual testing allows us to remediate any obvious deficiencies in skills and/or knowledge and identifies gaps in our training that can then be addressed in future exercises.

The examples above describe how two different hospitals have used simulation to enhance their physician led RRS. In Canada, simulation has been used to train nurses who staff their nursing led teams, called critical care outreach teams. These programmes teach and examine adherence to protocols related to assessment and treatment of common problems, such as hypoglycaemia.

Simulation has also been used to train MET members on individual skills, such as airway management, central venous line insertion, intraosseous line insertion, defibrillation, transcutaneous pacing, and decompression of a tension pneumothorax.

23.6 **Simulation training to improve team communication in crisis**

Medical simulation can be used to teach communication skills as well as technical skills. Communication in a crisis should occur between nurses, physicians (both trainee and staff), respiratory therapists, and pharmacists. Typically, when a nurse recognizes a patient in crisis, the communication skills used are based on the traditional nursing paradigm of 'assess, plan, implement and evaluate'. Often, the nurse reports the crisis to the physician (or team) beginning with the assessment and moves through history *before* describing the current situation. Some nurses are trained to avoid attaching a medical diagnosis to the situation. As a result, nurses can be said to 'feed the facts' and expect the team or physician to come up with the diagnosis. In this hierarchical model, even if an experienced nurse believes that a tension pneumothorax is the problem, they are not empowered to start off an interaction with their perception of what the problem or diagnosis might be. Rather, they are taught to share what they have observed during their assessment so that the physician has the information needed to make the diagnosis. In a crisis, this is inefficient and may delay intervention. The CRM principles, calling for help, using closed-loop communication, maintaining an open mind and getting the resources you need, help improve efficiency and effectiveness (Table 23.2). This is a change to traditional nursing communication that can and should be incorporated into RRS training using simulation.

Several acronym tools exist to facilitate rapid team communication.

SBAR is the acronym for: Situation, Background, Assessment, and Recommendation[23]. When the team arrives after a call is made, the ward staff must in a few sentences summarize the problem and the urgency of the situation. SBAR establishes a standardized format for communication that has a positive effect on the team[23]. The assessment comes after the situation and a description of the urgency is included early in the communication.

The principles of CRM, support (calling for help), communication (closing the loop) and global assessment (an open mind) are outlined in the following SBAR scenario.

- **Situation** – call made for RRT. Caller has seconds to construct 3–5 sentences that describe the urgency of the situation and the problem.

    "Mr. Collin's respiratory situation has been deteriorating rapidly the last 5 minutes. His oxygen saturation is not responding to the increase in oxygen and his level of alertness is deteriorating."

- **Background** – focus on what is the clinical background to the current situation and relevant information.

    "Mr. Collins is a 24-year-old patient with cystic fibrosis, awaiting lung transplant. He has a history of several spontaneous pneumothorax episodes."

- **Assessment** – statement of what the problem is and current vital signs.

    "I am unable to hear breath sounds on his right side at this time and I think he has a pneumothorax. Blood pressure is dropping from earlier, it is now 80/40 and the heart rate is up from 88 to 136. I have reviewed his chart and he has no known allergies, I also think it is important that you are aware he just finished lunch."

- **Recommendation or request** – what would I do to correct it?

    "I think he needs a stat portable chest X-ray and I need you to see him now."

In many SBAR scenarios, responders arrive at different times to a crisis call. Keeping the situation part of the communication succinct decreases chatter that interferes with effective communication. Responders can promote communication by arriving and asking "What's the situation" *versus* using other words that may sound challenging. By including the word 'situation' the nurse may be reminded to think of SBAR and be prompted to use this more effective communication pattern. The process of using the same, standardized phrase in a particular clinical situation in order to enhance communication is referred to as using critical language. A similar phraseology has been used at the University of Pittsburgh: when the team arrives, they ask, "How can we help?" rather than, "Why did you call?" The suggested communication promotes the caller to express the critical needs.

When team members arrive, either individually or as a group, they should each assume their role and begin organizational and therapeutic tasks to help the patient in crisis. Critical data can be collected rapidly if the team members each follow the AMPLE mnemonic as it pertains to their responsibility: Allergies, Medications, Past medical history, Last meal/Latest Labs, and Event (what is the crisis).

AMPLE is a second acronym that is useful in crisis management, and perhaps better when responders do not know the patient. AMPLE not only serves as a background assessment tool but also a safety assessment because it assess for allergies and medications that are often part of the cause of the crisis situation.

In simulation, whether training the use of SBAR or AMPLE, patient scenarios can be developed with an allergy and medication history that must be communicated effectively for safe and effective treatment. For example, a scenario might be created with an oncology patient who has developed septic shock, requiring rapid fluid resuscitation as well as delivery of antibiotics. The scenario may be designed with a patient history of anaphylaxis to cephalosporins. Whether or not the team delivers a cephalosporin to the simulated patient, a 'teaching moment' has been created. During the debriefing, the facilitator may probe the potential for error, and assess using standardized methods like SBAR or AMPLE for sharing information. Allowing the team to discover this information during the debriefing can promote both learning and retention in a safe setting. (It is safe because a patient does not experience a critical error, and consequently there is less psychological burden on the person who makes the error.) It also allows the team to practice the use of these effective communication tools. Debriefing of simulation exercises should highlight both examples of effective and ineffective communication and allow participants an opportunity to re-enact a piece of the scenario and practice effective communication.

23.7 Feedback and debriefing

Feedback is an essential component of effective simulation training. The most common format of simulation exercises is for a medical scenario to progress uninterrupted, and then for feedback to be given to the participants on their performance during the debriefing. However, for some simulation exercises, it may be beneficial to interrupt and give feedback as soon as an error is observed, so that the error can be replayed and corrected, and then the simulation exercise continues. Debriefing tools can be used as a scoring mechanism (Table 23.3) or as a tool to ensure consistency between programmes and serve as prompts to cover important points (Fig. 23.3). Some advocate that the debriefing should take twice as long as the simulation exercise (e.g. simulation 5 minutes, debriefing 10 minutes). University of Pittsburgh uses only 3 minutes of simulation (to force focus on early organization) and then programmed debriefing of 15 or more minutes.

A key component of a debriefing is for the participants to become aware of the quality of their performance. An interesting phenomenon that has been described is when an individual is unaware that they are not doing their job effectively. This has been labeled 'unconscious incompetence'[24].The University of Pittsburgh noted that when the participants of MET simulation exercises grade their own performance after the first team exercise of the day at their simulation centre, participants consistently grade themselves well above their actual performance. However, after viewing videos of their performance and debriefing based on objective performance criteria, they become much more capable of assessing their performance accurately in subsequent scenarios. In spite of continued inadequate teamwork, the group is aware of the quality. They achieve what is called 'conscious incompetence': they are aware of poor performance[24]. As they improve their performance they may achieve 'conscious competence': they perform competently and are aware that they have done so[24].

A recent study by Savoldelli explicitly revealed the importance of debriefing[25]. Anaesthesia residents participated in a simulation exercise and were graded on their non-technical skills. Each resident was randomized to receive either no debriefing, debriefing with oral feedback assisted by video or debriefing with oral feedback but no video assistance. Afterwards, all

Debrief 1: Roles
Section 2 Focus: Perception of Organizational Performance

Teaching Points

- To avoid chaos, devote time and effort to organization
- Choosing roles aids in organization
- Best team performance requires not just ABC (Airway, Breathing, Circulation), but OABC (Organization, Airway, Breathing, Circulation)

TASKS: Complete all of the tasks prior to continuing to the need debriefing section
☐ Display results of Perception of Team Work from Auto Debrief Tool
☐ Review Questions with participants
☐ Teaching Points were made

Questions for Participants

- ☐ Was the team' response chaotic or organized?
  - Elicit opinions and rationale
- ☐ What would improve your organization?
  - Elicit "Leadership, "knowing your own role, "Planning, "Practice, "Communication
- ☐ What rules would you make to improve team organization?
  - Elicit some roles, list tasks and priorities, sense of division of labor
- ☐ What tasks should be accomplished within the first 60 seconds of a crisis response?
  - Elicit as many tasks as possible
- ☐ Which of those tasks are organizational tasks and which are patient care tasks?
  - Analyse priority trainees have placed on organization
  - often participants omit organization Explore what organizational tasks should be done
- ☐ Which is a higher priority during the first 60 seconds
  - Explore rationale for prioritizing organizational tasks over treatment tasks
  - Discuss OABC

Lecture   R & G   Video   ScoreSheet   Graphs   Continue

Fig. 23.3 Page two of the four-section debriefing tool. The facilitator uses the tool to direct debriefing. Note: hyperlinks to other training tools: lectures, Roles and Goals poster, video playback, score sheet and performance graphics.

residents participated in a second simulation exercise. Those with no debriefing showed no improvement in their performance, while those who were debriefed showed significant improvement in their performance. The debriefings with and without video assistance were equally effective[25]. This study is consistent with the vast experience of those who use simulation as a training tool. Debriefing is indeed an integral component of effective simulation training.

23.8 Summary

RRS have been introduced to a large number of medical facilities across the world. The goal of the system, whether the efferent arm is a MET or RRT, is to identify patients whose clinical status is deteriorating and to rapidly deploy the necessary human and material resources to meet the patient's needs. These systems may represent a huge change in culture, as well as require new team skills especially if the response teams are *ad hoc* in nature. Both issues, culture and skills, lend themselves to simulation training. Simulation training methodology has been successfully used to improve team performance, including individual and team skills involving knowledge, communication skills, and efficient distribution of resources that are integral to effective team operations.

References

1. Mohler SR (2004). Human factors of powered flight: The Wright brothers' contributions. *Aviat Space Environ Med* **75**: 184–8.
2. Helmreich RL, Merritt AC, Wilhelm JA (1999). The evolution of Crew Resource Management in training in commercial aviation. *Int J of Aviat Psychol* **9**: 19–32.

3. Hamman WR (2004). The complexity of team training: what we have learned from aviation and its applications to medicine. *Qual Saf Health Care* **13** (Suppl.): 72–9.

4. Gaba DM, Fish KJ, Howard SK (1994). *Crisis Management in Anesthesiology.* Churchill Livingstone, Inc. Philadelphia, Pennsylvania.

5. Holzman RS, Cooper JB, Gaba DM, Philip JH, Small SD, Feinstein D (1995). Anesthesia crisis resource management: real-life simulation training in operating room crises. *Journal of Clinical Anesthesia* **7**: 675–87.

6. Howard SK, Gaba DM, Fish KJ, Yang G, Sarnquist FH (1992). Anesthesia crisis resource management training: teaching anesthesiologists to handle critical incidents. *Aviation Space & Environmental Medicine* **63**: 763–70.

7. Blum RH, Raemer DB, Carroll JS, Sunder N, Felstein DM, Cooper JB (2004). Crisis Resource Management training for an anaesthesia faculty: a new approach to continuing education. *Medical Education* **38**: 45–55.

8. Sica GT, Barron DM, Blum R, Frenna TH, Raemer DB (1999). Computerized realistic simulation: a teaching module for crisis management in radiology. *American Journal of Roentgenology* **172**: 301–4.

9. DeVita MA, Schaefer JS, Wang H, *et al.* (2005). Improving medical emergency team (MET) performance using a novel curriculum and a full-scale human simulator. *Qual Safety Healthcare* **14**: 326–31.

10. Lee A, Bishop G, Hillman K, *et al.* (1995). The medical emergency team. *Anaesth Intensive Care* **23**: 183–86.

11. DeVita MA, Braithwaite RS, Mahidhara R, *et al.* (2004). Use of Medical emergency team response to reduce hospital cardiopulmonary arrests. *Qual Safety Health Care* **13**: 251–54.

12. DeVita MA, Bellomo R, Hillman K, *et al.* (2006). Findings of the first consensus conference on medical emergency teams. *Crit Care Med* **34**: 2463–78.

13. MERIT study investigators (2005). Introduction of the medical emergency team (MET) system: a cluster-randomised trial. *Lancet* **365**: 2091–97.

14. DeVita MA, Schaefer J, Lutz J, Dongili T, Wang H (2004). Improving medical crisis team performance – A Celebration of the Life of Peter J. Safar, MD and Proceedings of the Second Annual Safar Symposium. *Critical Care Medicine* **32** (Suppl.) S61–S65.

15. Smith GB, Osgood VM, Crane S (2002). ALERT – a multiprofessional training course in the care of the acutely ill adult patient. *Resuscitation* **52**: 281–6.

16. Kim J, Neilipovitz D, Cardinal P, Chiu M, Clinch J (2006). A pilot study using high-fidelity simulation to formally evaluate performance in the resuscitation of critically ill patients: The University of Ottawa Critical Care Medicine, High-Fidelity Simulation and the Crisis Resource Management I Study. *Critical Care Medicine* **34**: 2167–74.

17. Burke CS, Salas E, Wilson-Donnelly K, Priest H (2004). How to turn a team of experts into an expert medical team: guidance from the aviation and military communities. *Quality & Safety in Health Care* **13** (Suppl.): i96–i104.

18. Lighthall GK, Barr J, Howard SK, *et al.* (2003). Use of a fully simulated intensive care unit environment for critical event management training for internal medicine residents. *Critical Care Medicine* **31**: 2437–43.

19. DeVita MA, Schaefer J, Lutz J, Wang H, Dongili T (2005). Improving medical emergency team (MET) performance using a novel curriculum and a computerized human patient simulator. *Quality & Safety in Health Care* **14**: 326–31.

20. DeVita M, Lutz J, Mininni N, Grbach W (2006). A novel debriefing tool: Online facilitator guidance package for debriefing team training using simulation. *Simulation in Healthcare* **1**: abstract.

21. Hunt EA, Walker AR, Shaffner DH, Miller MR, Pronovost PH (2008). Simulation of in-hospital pediatric medical emergencies and cardiopulmonary arrests: highlighting the importance of the first 5 minutes. *Pediatrics.* **121**: e34–43.

22. Hunt EA, Nelson KL, Shilkofski NA, Haggerty J (2006). Performance of Crucial Resuscitation Maneuvers during Simulated Pediatric Cardiopulmonary Arrests: The Effect of an Educational Intervention. *Simulation in Healthcare* **1**: abstract.

23. Leonard M, Graham S, Bonacum D (2004). The human factor: the critical importance of effective teamwork and communication in providing safe care. *Quality & Safety in Health Care* **13** (Suppl.): i85–i90.

24. Flower J (1999). In the Mush. *The Physician Executive* **25**: 64–6.

25. Savoldelli GL, Naik VN, Park J, Joo HS, Chow R, Hamstra SJ (2006). Value of debriefing during simulated crisis management: oral versus video-assisted oral feedback. *Anesthesiology* **105**: 279–85.

Chapter 24

Simulation in paediatrics

Louis Patrick Halamek and Kimberly Allison Yaeger

Overview

- Paediatric healthcare differs from adult healthcare in significant ways and these differences must be considered when building paediatric simulation programs.
- Identifying the learners and learning objectives are mandatory first steps in creating a successful simulation program.
- It is helpful to think in terms of discrete cognitive, technical and behavioural skills when writing learning objectives.
- The metrics used to evaluate trainees and programs must be aligned with the skill sets underlying the learning objectives.
- Close collaboration between paediatric healthcare professionals and industry will be required to address the serious deficiencies in paediatric human patient simulators.

24.1 Introduction

Before discussing paediatric simulation-based training, it is important first to define what is meant by the term 'paediatric'. The adjective paediatric applies to the period of human development from birth (0 days) to young adulthood (21 years) of both male and female patients. Paediatric patients range from those born at a gestational age of 22–23 weeks (a little more than halfway through a full-term, 40-week pregnancy) and a birth weight of approximately 500 g, to young adults standing 2 m in height and weighing more than 100 kg. The anatomical, physiological, developmental, and psychological differences found across this spectrum of patients are wide ranging, and present tremendous challenges for those healthcare professionals charged with their care. These differences also present great challenges for those involved in paediatric simulation-based training. Realistically, simulating the wide range of body sizes, anatomial features, vital signs, physiological responses etc, present in this group of very diverse patients is a daunting challenge. Because of the complexity of paediatric healthcare, a large number of subspecialties have evolved over the past century. Just as in adult healthcare the field of paediatrics includes physicians, nurses and allied healthcare professionals with expertise in areas such as newborn intensive care (neonatology), paediatric critical care, cardiology, pulmonology, gastroenterology, nephrology, anaesthesiology, general surgery, cardiothoracic surgery, and multiple other medical and surgical domains.

Healthcare professionals caring for children are faced with a myriad of challenges. In addition to treating complex diseases careful consideration of the child's developmental stage and the necessary involvement of family in the decision-making process must be included. Training professionals to provide competent, compassionate, and developmentally appropriate care has been a difficult process secondary, in part, to the limitations of the traditional training paradigm that does not provide sufficient opportunity for hands-on practice in interacting with children and their families. David Kolb, a renowned educational theorist, identified the importance of experience in adult education[1]. His theory, known as the experiential learning theory (ELT), has become widely accepted as an important contribution to the body of literature describing adult education. Kolb described a cycle of learning in which students are able to process new information from their own frame of reference, create new concepts, and test them through active experimentation. This cycle closely parallels the methodology of simulation-based training.

Kolb's cycle is comprised of four major steps that are along a continuum of learning[2]. The cycle is comprised of:

- concrete experience
- observation and reflection
- forming abstract concepts and generalizations
- testing implications of concepts in new situations.

It is possible to capture each step of this cycle in a paediatric simulation-based training programme.

24.2 Rationale for paediatric simulation

Why devote an entire chapter to paediatric simulation-based training? Children are not small adults and paediatric simulation is not adult simulation on a smaller scale. As one can see from the preceding section, there is no standard paediatric patent akin to the '70 kg adult white male', so often described in the adult literature. Thus the focus of this chapter is to highlight those unique aspects of paediatric simulation-based training rather than repeat information found elsewhere in the text.

One question that must be answered early on is this: Given that most children are healthy and rarely present healthcare professionals with serious management issues, why develop a programme in paediatric simulation-based training in the first place? Most children ARE healthy – and that is a major reason why paediatric simulation makes sense. In many ways serious paediatric pathology is the classic low frequency, high-risk event that lends itself well to simulation-based training. Many paediatric healthcare professionals seldom get the opportunity to manage a serious disease process let alone a true life-threatening emergency. Even for those for whom a sufficient number of opportunities do exist, one must question whether it is acceptable to essentially practice on real living patients who are not capable of providing informed consent on their own. While parents do act as surrogate decision makers for children below the age of consent, few want to contemplate that their child is to be someone's first spinal tap, first intubation, first thoracostomy tube placement, or first intestinal resection. Thus one may argue that the ethical imperative for simulation is stronger in paediatrics than in any other field of healthcare[3].

Paediatric healthcare professionals work in environments just as complex, dynamic, and highly technical as any found in adult medicine. This can be confirmed by walking into a neonatal or paediatric intensive care unit and standing at the bedside of a patient with persistent pulmonary hypertension of the newborn on extracorporeal membrane oxygenation (ECMO) or a paediatric patient with multisystem organ dysfunction receiving high frequency oscillatory ventilation (HFOV), inhaled nitric oxide (INO), dialysis, and inotropic support. Demands for succinct and accurate transfer of information while under intense time pressure and the need to interact with young overwhelmed parents acting as surrogate decision makers for patients who are too ill to speak for themselves are also inherent in these environments. Thus the professionals working in these environments must possess not only the content knowledge and technical skills required to understand and treat the disease process but also behavioural skills to allow them to respond appropriately while under intense pressure.

One subspecialty of paediatrics, neonatal–perinatal medicine, is unique in that the soon-to-be paediatric patient (the fetus) exists inside of an adult patient; in addition there may be one, two, three or more paediatric patients awaiting birth inside of that pregnant adult female patient. In this instance, the possibility of a sick mother delivering a sick newborn creates a situation where optimal training occurs only when the paediatric and adult teams train together[4]. The multitude of events (from both the maternal and neonatal perspectives) that can complicate human birth make this an especially appealing target for simulation-based training[5].

23.3 Building a successful paediatric simulation programme

The specialty of paediatrics is not a newcomer to simulation as defined in its broadest sense. Low fidelity examples of simulation are common in the field, ranging from role-playing exercises used in communication training to skills stations and 'megacodes' found in programmes such as the neonatal resuscitation programme (NRP) of the American Academy of Pediatrics (AAP) and the paediatric advanced life support programme (PALS) of the America Heart Association (AHA). However, higher fidelity training is just now finding its niche within paediatrics and its various subspecialties. Higher fidelity refers to training that uses real human actors or realistic patient simulators conducted in an authentic healthcare environment using working medical equipment where trainees are able to achieve a 'suspension of disbelief' and behave as they do when caring for real human patients in the clinic or hospital. An example of this type of simulation is found in the Centre for Advanced Paediatric and Perinatal Education (CAPE) located at Packard Children's Hospital on the campus of Stanford University[6]. Some of the simulation-based training programmes currently conducted at CAPE have been in existence since 1997[7–12]. A partial listing of the paediatric and obstetric programmes that are conducted at CAPE is listed in Table 1.

So what does it take to build a successful paediatric simulation programme and in what ways does that process differ from similar endeavours in adult simulation? Note that this discussion is focused on building a simulation *programme*, not a simulation *centre*. Although usable space in a location convenient to trainees is at a premium in most medical centres, creating a simulation

Table 24.1 Simulation-based training programmes at the Center for Advanced Pediatric and Perinatal Education (CAPE)

- NeoSim (neonatal resuscitation)
- SimTrans Neonatal (neonatal critical care transport)
- ECMO Sim Neonatal (neonatal ECMO)
- PediSim (paediatric resuscitation)
- SimTrans Paediatric (paediatric critical care transport)
- ECMO Sim Paediatric (paediatric ECMO)
- OBSim (obstetric rsuscitation)
- SimTrans OB (obstetric transport)
- Sim DR – The Simulated Delivery Room (perinatal team training)
- Disclosure of Unanticipated Consequences
- Perinatal Counseling
- End-of-life Counseling

ECMO, extracorporeal membrane oxygenation

Table 24.2 Steps in building a successful paediatric simulation programme

- Determine the relative balance of service (training and education) and investigation (research)
- Identify the learners
- Establish learning objectives
- Determine the optimal learning methodology
- Train instructors
- Write the curriculum
- Secure the necessary physical resources (space, equipment, patient simulators)
- Continuously evaluate both the programme and the instructors

centre is, in many ways, easier than building a simulation programme. A simulation centre requires space and equipment. A successful simulation programme requires a number of components:

- dedicated, talented personnel with an understanding of adult learning and a vision for training and education that goes beyond passive exercises such as lectures
- solutions to the logistical problems that arise when undertaking training, especially training of multidisciplinary teams
- a sustainable budget.

Whereas a simulation centre, in its strictest sense, requires dedicated space, a simulation programme can be conducted in space that has flexible use and not devoted solely to simulation-based training.

Based on the experience gained at CAPE in the past decade, building a successful simulation programme requires a number of steps. These steps are listed in Table 24.2 and described in detail in the paragraphs that follow.

One of the first steps in developing a successful paediatric simulation-based training programme is to determine the relative balance of service (training and education) and investigation (research in areas such as adult learning, human performance and patient safety) that will be undertaken. There is no right or wrong mix of effort; the answer will depend on the interests and talents among those running the programme and the resources available to them.

Identifying the learners is another important early step. Who will be the primary target audience? Will there be more than one target audience? How large is each target audience? Does the target audience consist primarily of novices (students/professionals with little clinical experience) or experts (seasoned clinicians)? Without answers to these questions one risks expending a great deal of time and effort in developing a curriculum and putting resources in place to implement that curriculum only to find that it fails to meet the needs of the learners. This is especially important in paediatrics where resources may not be as abundant as in other specialties where reimbursement rates are higher and more resources are available for training and education.

Once the learners are identified appropriate learning objectives must be established. This is another key step that cannot be left out or delayed until later in programme development. Why? Learning objectives drive everything in simulation-based training: scenario design, equipment used, content of debriefing, evaluation tools, etc. Poorly defined learning objectives are likely to lead to substandard learning experiences and ill-prepared trainees. Identifying learning objectives makes it possible to identify measures of assessment that will demonstrate that new knowledge has been gained[13]. It is helpful when determining learning objectives to consider the types of skills that learners must acquire in order to achieve those objectives. In general, these skills fall into three major categories: cognitive ('what we think' or content knowledge), technical ('what

Table 24.3 A partial list of skills necessary for successful intubation of the newborn

Cognitive skills

- Know the indications for intubation of the newborn
- Know how to recognize these indications when present
- Know what equipment (size of endotracheal tube, laryngoscope blade) to use in order to accomplish intubation
- Know the indicators of a successful intubation

Technical skills

- Know how to assemble the laryngoscope
- Know how to hold the laryngoscope
- Know how to use the equipment to expose the airway to view
- Know how to insert the endotracheal tube into the airway
- Know how to assess for proper placement of the endotracheal tube in the airway
- Know how to secure the endotracheal tube to the airway

Behavioural skills

- Communicate effectively with team members regarding the need for intubation, specific pieces of equipment, etc
- Distribute the workload so that specific tasks are assigned to the team members most likely to carry them out successfully
- Delegate responsibility and supervise appropriately
- Call for help when necessary

we do' or hands-on, manual interventions), and behavioural ('how we think and do') when working under time pressure[14]. Here is an example: An important learning objective in neonatal–perinatal medicine is effective, safe intubation of the newborn. In order to achieve this learning objective one must master the abbreviated list of skills found in Table 24.3. As can be seen from this list, effective and safe intubation of a neonate is a learning objective that is achieved only by integrating multiple elements of the three major skill sets.

The process of developing pertinent learning objectives includes determining whether the learners' needs are best met by training as a single discipline or as part of a multidisciplinary team and deciding whether novices can/should be integrated with experts during training. Consideration also should be given to an estimation of the length of time required for acquisition of particular skills, their half-lives, and the timing of retraining. Many recommendations for the length and frequency of training experiences are not evidence based and are arbitrary at best. While certainly there are learning objectives that are common to all fields of paediatric healthcare even these require some modification based on the specific attributes of the patient population being simulated. While not unique to paediatric simulation-based training these issues are especially relevant to paediatric simulation because of the wide spectrum of patient sizes, varying physiologies, and distinct disease states that are seen in the paediatric population.

Once learning objectives are specified one can then determine the optimal learning methodology for achieving those objectives. A word of caution here: Simulation may not be the optimal learning methodology for all of the learning objectives that are identified. For example, learning objectives that consist primarily of cognitive skills or content knowledge may be best acquired by reading self-study manuals and textbooks or interacting within online learning environments. Similarly technical skills that require many repetitions in order to achieve mastery may be optimally acquired and refined by working with task trainers at skills stations (as opposed to practice within comprehensive high fidelity environments). However, for learning objectives that are primarily behavioural in nature or that encompass components of all three skill sets, simulation is an ideal learning methodology; it is reasonable to hypothesize that most learning objectives in healthcare belong in this category.

After establishing that simulation-based training is the optimal methodology for achieving the learning objectives that have been identified, appropriate human resources must be put in place. While it is relatively easy for a single instructor to deliver a lecture to an audience numbering in the hundreds, the instructor:trainee ratio is much higher for simulation-based training because of the hands-on, experiential nature of the methodology. Another important aspect of simulation-based training to consider is the intimate relationship that tends to develop between instructors and trainees (and among the trainees themselves) as they work through highly realistic scenarios and detailed debriefings capable of evoking both visceral and emotional responses. Thus simulation instructors must display a skill set different from that of their colleagues functioning in more traditional training environments.

This is yet another area where paediatric simulation-based training involves unique considerations. Because of the long history of low fidelity simulation in paediatrics one might think that recruiting experienced instructors would be easier than in other healthcare domains where that is not the case. However it is also possible (even probable) that a percentage of those instructors have become so enamored of the traditional, didactic, instructor-focused methodologies that it is difficult or impossible for them to embrace a new methodology that:

♦ focuses on learning rather than teaching
♦ gives more control over the learning environment to the trainees
♦ places much of the responsibility for learning on the trainees
♦ integrates cognitive, technical and behavioural skills
♦ does not lend itself necessarily to tightly scripted deliveries of content knowledge defined by time (i.e. the 45 minute lecture)
♦ de-emphasizes written tests in favour of performance-based assessments of skills that are carried out while under realistic time pressure generated by changes in patient physiological state.

Simulation-based training transfers the locus of learning from the instructor to the learners, meeting them at their baseline. The learning process is driven by the trainees as they problem solve during scenarios and then reflect on their actions during facilitated debriefings. Constructivism is an adult learning theory that describes learning as an active process where the trainee constructs, generates and assimilates new information into an existing knowledge base. Instructors are therefore expected to provide students the building blocks of knowledge in a logical, sequential fashion[15].

In addition to those considerations, anecdotal experience hints that different personality types populate different healthcare domains. For example professionals working in paediatrics may in general have different personality traits than those in surgery or psychiatry. The impact of this perceived difference on how trainees learn, handle criticism, and respond to stressors such as time pressure is an area ripe for research.

Simulation programmes that involve research require the contributions of professionals with special skills, including but not limited to framing well-defined hypotheses, fulfilling the requirements of institutional review boards, obtaining informed consent, gathering data, maintaining the confidentiality of subjects, abstract presentation and manuscript preparation. Once again this is a component of paediatric simulation that presents its own special challenges, especially when dealing with patients who are too young to provide consent themselves.

Table 24.4 Sample paediatric scenario template

- Name of scenario (event)
- List of trainees: name, job description, years of clinical experience
- Learning objectives
- Room setup
- Mannequin preparation
- Medical equipment needed
- Other props
- Simulator instructors: name, role
- Initial conditions
- Brief history of event
- Mannequin vital signs, physical exam findings
- Laboratory, radiological and other diagnostic studies
- Confederates and role in scenario
- Anticipated interventions and outcomes
- Debriefing points

Once the learners and the learning objectives are identified and colleagues are recruited to assist in developing the programme, it is time to write the curriculum. The learning objectives and the cognitive, technical and behavioral skills implicit in each learning objective should be explicitly listed and referred to whenever questions arise as to how to proceed with curricular development. It is helpful to use a scenario template such as the one in Table 24.4 to insure that a uniform and comprehensive approach is maintained. Scenarios should be based on learning objectives and only secondarily on the type of patient simulator used; unfortunately the opposite is often true. Current paediatric patient simulator technology has many limitations, some of which are due to the inappropriate extrapolation of adult simulator features to their paediatric counterparts. In view of this those designing paediatric scenarios need to identify the visual, auditory and tactile cues that are important in allowing trainees to suspend their disbelief that they are working with simulated rather than real patients and appreciate the fact that a number of these cues will need to come from components of the training environment other than the patient simulator. Debriefing is an important curricular component of paediatric simulation-based training and videotape is a highly useful tool for providing an objective time-coded record of the events of the scenario; as such, videotape serves as the basis for the debriefing. The experience at CAPE over the past decade indicates that trainees highly value the opportunity to critically reflect on their performance with feedback coming from instructors trained in debriefing as well their peers[16]. Debriefing is another topic covered elsewhere in this text in more detail. The length of the curriculum may vary from relatively brief (less than 1 hour) to day-long programmes encompassing a number of realistic scenarios followed by constructive debriefings. Ultimately the length of the training depends on how long it takes the trainees to master the learning objectives.

Physical resources (space, equipment etc) are important components of any programme but large expenditures of capital should not be undertaken until extensive progress has been made with the previous steps. A commonly made mistake is to purchase an expensive human patient simulator as a first step, then end up wondering:

- how it can be used to facilitate learning in your target audience
- how it actually works (where's the ON switch?)
- why you spent all that money on it in the first place!

Until it is clear who the learners will be and what they will be learning it is difficult to know what tools will be needed to facilitate that learning.

The current state of the art in paediatric human patient simulators is inadequate to meet the needs of the diverse group of professionals that might benefit from widespread implementation of simulation-based training. The full range of patient sizes represented in the paediatric patient population is underrepresented by the paediatric simulators that are commercially available. Most of these simulators are not capable of indicating their state of relative health or disease. Of those that do harbour some type of internal physiological modeling, the models are often based on adult physiology and adapted in some way for the paediatric patient. This type of engineering ignores the unique anatomy and physiology of paediatric patients and results in a substandard learning experience for all. Areas where extrapolation of adult physiology to paediatric patients may result in significant inaccuracies include:

- Cyanotic congenital heart disease with persistent low haemoglobin oxygen saturation (SaO_2): The low SaO_2 (70–85%) commonly seen in these patients is compensated for by unusually high haematocrits that insure adequate oxygen content and delivery and are completely compatible with survival. When SaO_2 in this range is seen in adults it usually presages ventricular fibrillation and death.

- Right-to-left shunting of un-oxygenated blood through a patent ductus arteriosus: The ductus arteriosus normally closes off in the days following birth at full term; thus there is no anatomical equivalent in the adult.

- Congenital malformations such as diaphragmatic hernia (CDH): CDH, with its concomitant pulmonary parenchymal and vascular hypoplasia, may be associated with persistent pulmonary hypertension of the newborn, significant right-to-left shunting of un-oxygenated blood, and severe cyanosis and acidosis. Again, there is no anatomical equivalent in the adult population.

- Cardiac death: In the neonatal and paediatric populations death is usually preceded by bradycardia followed by asystole. In adults dysrhythmias such as ventricular fibrillation usually constitute the terminal event.

- Events preceding death: In the paediatric population respiratory failure is a far more common cause of cardiac arrest than intrinsic cardiac disease. In the adult, cardiac disease is the usual underlying cause of cardiac arrest.

- Drug metabolism: Drug metabolism is developmentally regulated and thus can differ not only from that of the adult but also from that of older or younger peers in the paediatric population.

Until there is better collaboration between industry and paediatric healthcare professionals with knowledge of both paediatric medicine and simulation-based training significant inadequacies will continue to plague efforts to achieve higher fidelity and improved training experiences.

Access to space is often a challenging issue in a healthcare facility or health professions school. It is important to understand that proximity to trainees and instructors is likely to be more important than other characteristics (size, appearance, etc.) in selecting space. Proximity to trainees provides them with the easy access that will allow them to benefit from the opportunities present within the space. Proximity to instructors is a key in fostering the development of multidisciplinary training programmes. This is another key to building a successful paediatric simulation programme. Without the involvement of multiple paediatric domains and disciplines it will be extremely difficult to maintain financial viability unless the programme is supported by an extensive endowment. Most importantly the benefits of simulation-based training will not reach the widest audience possible and the paediatric patient population will not be adequately served.

Once space is made available (either a permanent training space or temporary space that is used for other purposes when not used for training) it should be furnished with working medical equipment. Equipment needs are also a special consideration in paediatric simulation as a variety of equipment size and type is necessary to care for the wide range of patient size encountered in the paediatric population. In addition, a multidisciplinary paediatric simulation programme will need to accommodate the needs of professionals from multiple paediatric domains and disciplines, all of whom require specific pieces of equipment in order to deliver care. Finally, do not forget that storage space will also be necessary (the bigger the programme, the bigger the storage needs). Once again, even though paediatric patients may be smaller in size than their adult counterparts, higher fidelity paediatric patient simulators require just as much or more in the way of supporting equipment (air compressors, range of laryngoscope blades sizes, etc.).

Once a programme is underway, ongoing evaluation is a necessary component if the programme is to evolve and be successful. Training programmes should be evaluated every time that they are conducted and this information reviewed prior to the next programme. This is especially true when a programme is in the early phase or rollout period; it can be very helpful to recruit expert clinicians as trainees and request that they cast a very critical eye when completing the programme evaluation. This is a great way to find out what works and what does not work prior to opening the programme to general audiences. Another vital component of the evaluation process is critique of instructors by trainees and by their fellow instructors. Immediately upon the close of a training programme all instructors should be debriefed during which all aspects of their performance are reviewed.

24.4 **Challenges in paediatric simulation**

Certainly there are many challenges in building a successful paediatric simulation programme. This section will discuss some of those that are more commonly encountered

High fidelity simulation-based training represents a paradigm shift in paediatric healthcare education and training[17–20]. As such it usually takes some period of time for instructors to recognize its value, become willing to change their own (old) patterns of behaviour, and acquire the skills necessary to become proficient at it. In general instructors fall into one of three groups:

- Early adopters who see it, get it, and immediately want to become a part of it.
- The 'wait'n'see-ers' who find the concept interesting but are not yet convinced they can/should become involved.
- The 'naysayers' who are highly resistant to change and either cannot or will not contemplate it.

In order to be successful in implementing change one must embrace and reward members of the first group, work with those in the second group, and readily identify those in the third group so as to avoid investing time and energy in attempts at converting them (unless, of course, they control important resources). So as not to seem unfairly critical, the same three groups may be encountered within the simulation community itself. For example, one may find that a unique approach to some aspect of simulation-based training that works well in the paediatric domain but is foreign to non-paediatric domains is rejected as not being 'true simulation'. Any innovator must expect such questions and criticisms and be able to provide thoughtful responses to them.

Resistance to change may also occur on an institutional level. Officials responsible for managing education and training budgets may question why traditional lecture settings involving relatively large numbers of trainees and smaller numbers of instructors should be replaced by experiences demanding a much higher instructor:trainee ratio. And they would be correct in their skepticism

Table 24.5 Some benefits of paediatric simulation-based training

- Permits training in environments (intensive care) that are usually inaccessible to less experienced trainees
- Creates training opportunities for rarely encountered but highly challenging/risky situations (resuscitation, delivery of difficult news)
- Allows for training opportunities in paediatric domains ranging from general paediatrics to intensive care, counseling to highly technical areas such as extracorporeal membrane oxygenation
- Permits formal objective performance assessment

if the learning objectives involve only cognitive skills (content knowledge). Once again, here is where the long history of widely accepted paediatric training programmes complicates efforts to embrace simulation as a methodology. Proponents of paediatric simulation-based training must be able to explain the unique benefits their programmes offer; some of these are listed in Table 24.5.

Sustainability is a particularly important issue for paediatric simulation programmes. Unless one is fortunate enough to work at a children's hospital, paediatrics is often a small (<10%) component of the care delivered at community and university hospitals. As mentioned previously it is extremely difficult for any single paediatric subspecialty to generate enough revenue or provide enough service to maintain a viable programme. The key to avoiding this situation is to actively recruit paediatric colleagues to form multidisciplinary teams who take ownership of and pride in their simulation programmes. Sharing resources with the adult programmes will also help to defray overall costs and create potentially powerful collaborations and interesting programmes (such as combined neonatal–obstetric team training). On an institutional level, a paediatric simulation programme should be one component of a comprehensive programme to enhance human performance and improve patient safety[21]. Indeed organizations such as the Joint Commission on Accreditation of Healthcare Organizations (JCAHO) has already made recommendations for simulation-based training in the perinatal domain[22].

A simulation programme should not just be maintained; rather it must grow and evolve to meet the changing educational needs of trainees. This growth and evolution requires active management of the programme and this includes anticipation of problems, facilitation of solutions and proactive identification of opportunities. In order to understand what it will take to achieve fiscal sustainability one must have a clear understanding of the sources of expense and revenue; one can then develop a realistic business model. Business models will vary based on a number of factors including but not limited to:

- the size of the programme and potential user base
- the ratio of time spent providing training (service) to that involved in research or other academic activities.

Multiple sources of support – tuition, contracts, grants and philanthropy – should be sought.

24.5 **Future directions**

High fidelity simulation-based training has the potential to revolutionize paediatric healthcare education and training but this potential will be reached only if it is developed and implemented in a logical manner. The process outlined previously is one that can serve as a model not only on a local level for an individual simulation programme but also on a national level for institutions, professional societies and other large groups involved in simulation-based training.

The relative paucity of realistic paediatric patient simulators, while in some ways an impediment, also provides an opportunity – an opportunity to 'do it right' from the start.

An ongoing dialogue needs to be established between the healthcare professionals who care for children and the engineers and others who design and build paediatric patient simulators. This dialogue can be established only if those involved speak the same language. Healthcare professionals need to become more familiar with adult learning theory and focus on determining the right methodologies to meet whatever learning objectives are set. They must appreciate the limitations of hardware and software in modeling paediatric physiology and understand the fact that patient simulators do not need to have 100% fidelity to real humans in order to be useful as training tools. Those in industry must develop a better understanding of the visual, auditory and tactile cues that are important to clinicians in determining the state of relative health or illness in their patients and find cost-effective ways to incorporate those cues into the simulators they produce. Long-term relationships must be built so that product development and improvement can continue uninterrupted until useful, cost-effective, upgradeable simulators are commonplace. An early example of this type of interaction is the request for proposals (RFP) developed by the NRP of the AAP for the development of a true neonatal patient simulator; it is available as a PDF document titled *Desired Features for Industry for the Development of a Realistic Neonatal Human Patient Simulator*[23]. The simulator characteristics listed in this RFP were based on the learning objectives of the NRP and driven by its vision to move training in neonatal resuscitation toward a more immersive experience based on the tenets of adult learning theory.

Development of hybrid technologies that combine materials like the plastics used for physical patient simulators with visual displays and haptic interfaces capable of generating the images and tactile sensations associated with patient care will create learning opportunities that are currently impossible to achieve in the absence of a real patient. This combination of physical and virtual reality is sorely needed in paediatrics and obstetrics for the following reasons:

◆ Paediatric patients come in many different sizes and while it is not necessary to simulate every conceivable stage of human development it is nevertheless important to simulate those stages where significant differences in anatomy and physiology dictate different approaches to care. An obvious example of this is the neonate – there are many anatomical and physiological differences between preterm and term neonates and these mandate careful consideration when selecting pharmaceuticals, determining the size of catheter for insertion into the umbilical artery, etc.

◆ Purely mechanical devices are unlikely ever to be able to simulate vaginal birth, with enough fidelity to generate sufficient suspension of disbelief by trainees, in a cost-effective manner. The same is true of highly invasive procedures such as cesarean section.

Thus combinations of physical whole body simulators with virtual reality interfaces designed to compensate for the physical simulators' limitations will play a major role in paediatric and obstetric high fidelity simulation.

Collaboration with professionals with a variety of backgrounds is needed to move the field forward. Involvement of those with experience in human factors, psychometrics and other related fields will be helpful in sorting out the important methodological issues facing healthcare educators. Those in quality improvement and risk management can serve as useful resources in determining priorities for training and in providing objective data to assess the outcomes of any training programme. Finally working with colleagues with expertise in healthcare finance will provide guidance in analysing the cost–benefit ratio of simulation-based training. Given the financial constraints in paediatric healthcare these relationships are arguably more important in paediatric than adult simulation.

Multidisciplinary team training will eventually become the norm in healthcare. To accomplish this the artificial barriers among physicians, nurses, allied healthcare professionals and administrators must be first recognized and then actively dismantled. This may occur within the next decade as those who are heavily invested in the more traditional methodologies retire and are replaced by a generation that is more comfortable with a collaborative approach to training. The term 'disruptive technology' describes the rapid evolution that occurs when a technological breakthrough allows business to capitalize on its potential; this term was coined by Clayton Christensen in 1997[24]. Christensen later changed his terminology to 'disruptive innovation' in 2003; this may be a reasonable description of the potential of the simulation-based training methodology to change education and training in healthcare[25]. If not self-motivated and self-regulated by professional and hospital associations within healthcare itself such change will likely be driven by outside forces such as industrial regulatory bodies and the government. Just as in the delivery of healthcare to patients, a movement to evidence-based practice (of training and education) will be undertaken requiring that methodologies and technologies be validated *via* single centre and multicentre trials.

24.6 Conclusions

Despite the fact that simulation-based training in paediatrics and obstetrics is in its early stage we can draw some conclusions from the work that has been done thus far in healthcare and other related fields:

◆ Not all that is taught is learned.

Intense focus must be placed on facilitation of learning rather than teaching and on the needs of the learners rather than the teachers.

◆ Simulation is a methodology, not a technology.

While technology can be a useful tool for the acquisition of cognitive, technical and behavioural skills, it cannot, in and of itself, overcome poorly designed learning objectives and curriculum.

◆ Simulation is a useful learning methodology for healthcare professionals ranging in experience from novice to expert and can be employed in multiple areas of paediatric healthcare training.

In paediatrics the intended result of any endeavour must be to improve the care of children. When expending paediatric healthcare resources one must be assured that any investment will yield results that benefit children, either directly or indirectly. Supporting paediatric simulation-based training as a way to help healthcare professionals deliver better care to children is an investment that will likely return a high yield.

References

1. Kelly C (1997). David Kolb, the theory of experiential learning and ESL. *The Internet TESL Journal* 3(9) 1–5E.
2. Miettinen R (2000). The concept of experiential learning and John Dewey's theory of reflective thought and action. *International Journal of Lifelong Learning Education* 19(1): 54–72.
3. Ziv A, Wolpe PR, Small Sd, Glick S (2006). Simulation-based medical education: an ethical imperative. *Simulation in Healthcare* 1(4): 252–6.
4. Halamek LP. Agency for Healthcare Research and Quality Web M&M. Mortality and Morbidity Rounds on the Web. Spotlight Case. Obstetrics. A slippery slide into life. URL: http://webmm.ahrq.gov/case.aspx?caseID=112
5. Murphy AM, Halamek LP (2005). Simulation-based training in neonatal resuscitation. *NeoReviews* 6(11): e489–92.
6. http://www.cape.lpch.org

7. Halamek LP, Kaegi DM, Gaba DM, *et al.* (2000). Time for a new paradigm in paediatric medical education: Teaching neonatal resuscitation in a simulated delivery room environment. *Paediatrics* **106**(4): e45. URL: http://www.paediatrics.org/cgi/content/full/106/4/e45

8. Murphy AM, Halamek LP (2005). Simulation-based training in neonatal resuscitation. *NeoReviews* **6**(11): e489–92.

9. Anderson JM, Murphy AA, Boyle BB, Yaeger KA, Halamek LP (2006). Simulating extracorporeal membrane oxygenation (ECMO) emergencies to improve human performance, Part I: Methodologic and technologic innovations. *Simulation in Healthcare* **1**: 220–7.

10. Anderson JM, Murphy AA, Boyle BB, Yaeger KA, Halamek LP (2006). Simulating extracorporeal membrane oxygenation (ECMO) emergencies, Part II: Qualitative and quantitative assessment and validation. *Simulation in Healthcare* **1**: 228–32.

11. Wayman K, Yaeger KA, Sharek PJ, *et al.* (2006). Simulation-based medical error disclosure training for paediatric healthcare professionals. Accepted for publication: *Journal of Healthcare Quality.*

12. Eppich WJ, Adler MD, McGaghie WC (2006). Emergency and critical care paediatrics: use of medical simulation for training in acute paediatric emergencies. *Curr Opin Pediatr* **18**(3): 266–71.

13. http://www.park.edu/cetl/quicktips/writinglearningobj.html

14. Halamek LP (2006). Simulation-based training: Opportunities for the acquisition of unique skills. *Virtual Mentor* 2006;8:84–7. URL: http://www.amaassn.org/ama/pub/category/15877.html

15. http://portal.acm.org/citation.cfm?id=238386.238476&coll=portal&dl=ACM&CFD= 1285945& CFTOKEN=81748579.

16. Yaeger KA, Murphy AA, Coyle MW, *et al.* (2004). Perceptions of high fidelity simulation-based neonatal and paediatric training. In: Patankar MS, ed. *Proceedings of the First Safety Across High-Consequences Industries Conference* [book on CD-ROM]. St. Louis, MO: Saint Louis University: 205–8.

17. Halamek LP, Kaegi DM, Gaba DM, *et al.* (2000). Time for a new paradigm in paediatric medical education: Teaching neonatal resuscitation in a simulated delivery room environment. *Paediatrics* **106**(4): e45. URL: http://www.paediatrics.org/cgi/content/full/106/4/e45

18. Yaeger K, Braccia K, Coyle MW, *et al.* (2004). High fidelity simulation-based training in neonatal nursing. *Adv Neonatal Care* **4**: 326–31.

19. Weinstock PH, Kappus LJ, Kleinman ME, Grenier B, Hickey P, Burns JP (2005). Toward a new paradigm in hospital-based paediatric education: the development of an onsite simulator programme. *Pediatr Crit Care Med* **6**(6): 635–41.

20. Ziv A, Erez D, Munz Yet al. (2006). The Israel Centre for Medical Simulation: A paradigm for cultural change in medical education. *Acad Med* **81**(12): 1091–7.

21. Halamek LP (2003). Improving performance, reducing error, and minimizing risk in the delivery room. In: *Fetal and Neonatal Brain Injury: Mechanisms, Management, and the Risks of Practice.* Sunshine P, Stevenson DK, Eds. St. Louis, MO: Mosby Year Book. 3E.

22. http://www.jointcommission.org/SentinelEvents/SentinelEventAlert/sea_30.htm

23. http://www.aap.org/nrp/about/about_sitemap.html

24. Christensen CM (1997). *The Innovator's Dilemma.* Harvard Business School Press. Boston, MA.

25. Christensen CM (2003). *The Innovator's Solution.* Harvard Business School Press. Boston, MA.

Chapter 25

Obstetric simulation

Shad H Deering

Overview

- Emergencies in obstetrics are not uncommon and may result in significant morbidity and mortality for the mother and the fetus.

- Obstetric simulators are relatively inexpensive and easier to use than those required for other specialties.

- New task trainers and birthing simulators will continue to improve and become available.

- A well thought out curriculum and evaluation forms are essential to provide realistic and beneficial training.

- Practising for obstetric emergencies with simulation training has the potential to significantly decrease maternal and fetal/infant morbidity and mortality, and is now recommended and recognized by major regulatory bodies.

- Obstetric simulation may also lead to decreases in malpractice claims, and several insurance carriers now offer discounts in malpractice premiums when their providers attend simulation training for obstetric emergencies.

- Both teamwork and technical performance are important components to evaluate during training.

- Training done on the actual delivery unit may be more beneficial than in a labouratory setting, as it allows for the assessment of technical skills and the opportunity to evaluate for systems issues that can be corrected.

- Research and validation of obstetric simulation has been published, and more and more data are demonstrating the benefits of this approach.

25.1 Brief history and background

There are few areas of medicine where simulation training is more necessary and potentially beneficial than obstetrics.

Given the current medicolegal climate in developed countries, where there is the expectation of a perfect outcome with every delivery regardless of complications, the inability to predict when many common emergencies will occur on the labour and delivery ward, and the difficulties presented by resident work hour restrictions of 80 hours per week in the USA, obstetrics is the ideal field in which to apply simulation training.

While cost is always a consideration with regards to simulation, obstetrics is fortunate in the sense that, for a relatively small investment, a wide range of simulations can be run, and a large number of providers trained with minimal yearly upkeep costs. For example, a full-size birthing mannequin can be purchased for between $US2,500 and $US20,000 and all the basic emergencies discussed in this chapter can be run with it. When compared with the average payment for an obstetrics malpractice claim in the USA over the past several years, which the Institute for Healthcare Improvement reports was 2.5 million dollars between 1997 and 2003, it is obvious that the simulator will pay for itself if even a single bad outcome is prevented.

The objectives of this chapter are to provide the reader with a good understanding of the current state of obstetric simulation, how to construct and run scenarios, and provide evidence that can be used to convey the importance of the training and the benefits it provides.

25.2 Available obstetric simulators

There are several companies that supply a wide range of obstetric simulators, with more being made available every year. What follows is a reasonable representation of some of those used most often and those the author is most familiar with, but there are some different models, and new models are always becoming available.

25.2.1 Birthing mannequins

Birthing mannequins range from the lower portion of the female torso without legs to a complete adult female with arms and legs. Determining exactly which one is best for your needs is a balance of cost and the anticipated use. The good news about obstetric simulation is that even the most expensive birthing mannequins only cost about half as much as those used for other specialties, and the upkeep and yearly expenses to maintain them and continue the training are also minimal. For example, the most expensive birthing mannequin from Gaumard Scientific is around US$30,000, while a basic laparoscopic surgical trainer may be more than US$100,000.

Two of the more common birthing mannequins in use are the NOELLE® mannequin made by Gaumard Scientific and the PROMPT® birthing trainer, which is produced by the company Limbs and Things.

25.2.1.1 NOELLE® birthing mannequin

The NOELLE® mannequins are generally full-size females complete with arms and legs, though there are more simple birthing mannequins that only include the lower torso without the legs. (Fig. 25.1) There are several different models of this mannequin available, and some of them include dual monitors that allow the trainer to show both the fetal heart rate tracing and maternal vital signs. The full size mannequins by Gaumard allow for most all of the obstetric simulations included in this chapter to be run. The fetus may be delivered either by a motor that is contained within the abdomen, or pushed out by hand. Specific features of the mannequin with regards to the individual simulations are discussed in detail in the following sections.

25.2.1.2 PROMPT® birthing simulator

The PROMPT® birthing simulator consists of the lower torso of an adult female, and includes only the top portions of the thighs (Fig. 25.2) The birthing fetus that is included on some models contains a force-feedback mechanism that allows the trainer to monitor the amount of force applied during delivery. In order to control the fetus during delivery with this model, it requires someone playing the part of the patient to sit on the bed and push the fetus out.

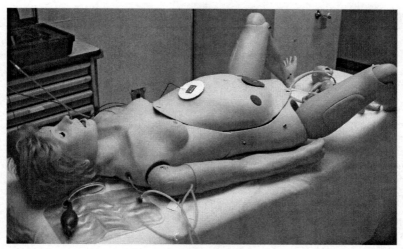

Fig. 25.1 NOELLE® mannequin (Gaumard Scientific, Florida).

A list of the simulations that the NOELLE® and PROMPT® birthing trainers can support can be found in Table 1 and internet links for these manufacturers can be found at the end of this chapter.

25.2.2 **Specific task trainers**

There are a number of specific task trainers that are available for obstetrics at this time, though most all of the simulations discussed in this chapter can be accomplished on standard birthing mannequins. The most common procedures that can be taught with task trainers are episiotomy, perineal laceration repair and amniocentesis.

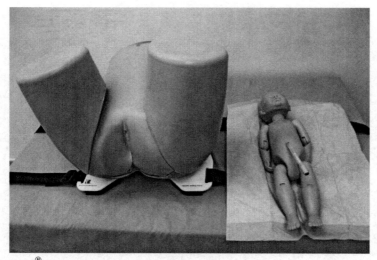

Fig. 25.2 PROMPT® birthing trainer (Limbs and Things, Bristol, UK).

Table 25.1 Simulations that can be run with specific birthing simulators.

NOELLE®

- ◆ Spontaneous vaginal delivery
- ◆ Forceps delivery
- ◆ Vacuum delivery
- ◆ Breech vaginal delivery
- ◆ Umbilical cord prolapse
- ◆ Shoulder dystocia
- ◆ Postpartum haemorrhage
- ◆ May monitor maternal vital signs with specific models
- ◆ Fetal heart rate tracing interpretation (with specific models)
- ◆ Internal monitor placement/AROM

PROMPT® birthing simulator

- ◆ Spontaneous vaginal delivery
- ◆ Forceps delivery
- ◆ Vacuum delivery
- ◆ Breech vaginal delivery
- ◆ Umbilical cord prolapse
- ◆ Internal monitor placement
- ◆ Shoulder dystocia
  - • Ability to monitor actual force applied to fetus during delivery

25.2.2.1 Episiotomy

There are several models available and described in the literature for training and practising episiotomy and third/fourth-degree laceration repairs. These range from homemade simulators, such as using a thawed beef tongue or a carwash sponge, to more advanced anatomical models[1]. The Limbs and Things models are probably the most realistic at this time, and have been used at different centres in validation studies[2]. A picture of an episiotomy model is seen in Fig. 25.3, and the different models are discussed in more detail later in the chapter.

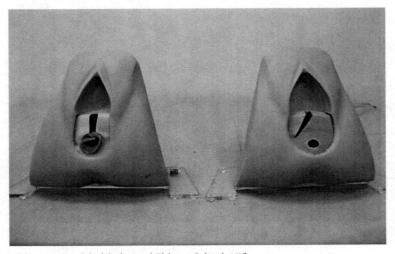

Fig. 25.3 Episiotomy models (Limbs and Things, Bristol, UK).

25.2.2.2 Amniocentesis/cordocentesis

A commercially available amniocentesis/cordocentesis trainer is available from Limbs and Things (Bristol, UK). The model contains two separate placentas and simulated umbilical cords that can be refilled with mock blood to practice both amniocentesis and cordocentesis. The model is relatively simple to use, and the only issue we have found in working with it is that there is no representation of subcutaneous tissue, so the procedure is significantly easier than real life.

25.3 Essential components for obstetric simulations

The most important components of obstetric simulation are actually very simple. First, you must have a dedicated champion in the department who will schedule and run the desired simulations. There are many places that have purchased expensive mannequins only to have them sit in a room because, while they have good intentions, they do not have a person to implement the training. The second critical component is a standard obstetric simulation curriculum, which this chapter is meant to assist with developing. While it is definitely beneficial to have the ability to practice on simulators, it is just as important to have a defined instructional curriculum on the different procedures/emergencies and standards of performance for your institution.

Didactics In order to ensure that you are teaching each trainee the appropriate material, it is best to write out a short didactic handout about the simulation procedure/emergency. This will help to prevent confusion because all staff tend to have slightly different approaches/information about the various conditions. While you can and should use standard textbooks and journals to create these short handouts, it is also important to include your institutional protocols or standards as well. An example of our didactic handout for a shoulder dystocia can be seen in Addendum A.

Instructions for simulations For each simulation, create an instruction packet for the staff who will run the simulation. This should include a brief overview of the simulation as well as a simple flow diagram of how to run the drill. This flow diagram should explain how the simulation begins, and define a clear point at which the simulation will end. For example, with a shoulder dystocia scenario, it begins as they enter the room and the fetal head is made to deliver. At our institution, the simulation continues until the trainee delivers the posterior arm, performs a Zavenelli manoeuvre, or states that they do not know any other manoeuvres that they can do.

Another area that should be covered in the instructions is the role of any additional personnel other than the staff running the scenario. For instance, if you are going to have someone play a nurse or family member, make sure to include their role and basic responses in the instructions so they are standardized for all the participants. We have found that if you can add a concerned and vocal 'family member' to the simulations that it adds a lot to the reality of the situation and we highly recommend doing this if you are able.

In addition, we usually include a basic troubleshooting list and common questions that the trainee may ask and what the standard response will be during the scenario for each question. An example of these instructions can be seen in Addendum B.

Clinical scenarios It is important to write a brief clinical scenario for the trainee to read prior to beginning the simulation. Ideally, the scenario should have some basic background information about the patient and their medical history and at least one risk factor for the complication they are going to encounter, but not every risk factor known so that the person can easily guess exactly what they will encounter. As you run drills again at later times, amend the clinical scenarios as you see fit (see Addendum C).

Evaluation forms When making a grading form for your simulation, it is usually easiest to include both objective and subjective sections. For example, the objective section should have simple yes or no questions regarding the actions taken by the trainee during the simulation. (See Addendum D for an example of the grading form for shoulder dystocia.) The subjective section may include a standard Likert scale and is meant to assess more global issues such as, how well did the person perform overall or how prepared was the person doing the simulation?

I always encourage people creating these data forms to discuss the important performance measures with their staff and local experts, because these may vary between sites at times and local standards of practice should be used. After you have designed your grading form, the best way to determine if it works well is to record someone, even yourself, going through the simulation and then having two or three people watch and grade you and comment on the evaluation forms themselves. This will allow you to see if the form is simple enough for them to understand how to fill it out, if they are relatively consistent in their assessments, and if there is anything you might want to add or delete from the forms as well.

Feedback session There is a definite skill to giving feedback after simulation, and entire courses have been developed to assist with this process. I usually go through a brief didactic about the procedure/emergency and then talk about specific areas where people tend to make mistakes. After this, allow the trainees to practice on the actual mannequin with supervision and assist them in anything they have difficulty with.

25.3.1 How to conduct simulation training sessions

Exactly how you run the training sessions will depend on how many staff you have to run the simulations, how many people you have to train, and time constraints. For example, you will set things up very differently if you are trying to train 20 residents in a 4-hour session *versus* only 4. If there are larger numbers of trainees, then group teaching afterwards may be more efficient than the individual debriefing that can be accomplished with smaller numbers. It is important, however, that you allow trainees to practice physically on the mannequin after/during the debrief, and to practice the skills you are trying to teach.

One of the most significant challenges is what to do with trainees between simulations as others run through the simulation, because having them just sit around is a waste of valuable time. Some ways to decrease any down time are to either have two or three stations that they rotate between and then do additional teaching/training after they have completed all stations or have the trainee write a procedure or delivery/event note after they go through the simulation. These notes can then be used as part of the debriefing process and provide a good opportunity for instruction on documentation after emergencies/procedures.

For many of the obstetric scenarios the actual simulation part only requires about 5 minutes, so you can realistically have multiple people run through them and then bring them together afterwards for feedback, instruction, and additional practice on the simulator.

In general, here is how we run our simulation training exercise for shoulder dystocia:

Step 1: The birthing mannequin is set up in a room on a delivery table with legs in stirrups. The staff controlling the fetus places the fetus and harness in the abdomen.

Step 2: The trainee is given the clinical scenario just outside the room. They take a few minutes to read it and then enter the room and the scenario begins.

Step 3: After the simulation ends, the trainee is told not to discuss the simulation with others and goes outside the room and writes a delivery note while the simulation staff grade their performance with the grading forms. If there are other people in the group, they run through the simulation one at a time and follow the same procedure.

Step 4: The trainees are brought back in and given a copy of their grading form. They are given a brief didactic lecture on shoulder dystocia and the manoeuvres are then practised on the birthing mannequin and fetus, and additional feedback is given during this time.

*NOTE: For emergency simulations, such as shoulder dystocia or a postpartum haemorrhage, we do not have the staff interact with regards to teaching or instruction during the simulation. This allows the trainee to experience some of the real stress that they will encounter during the real event. Debriefing and teaching is done afterwards. For specific tasks and non-emergent procedures, such as cervical examinations or internal monitor placement, we generally provide more instruction during the training rather then making them wait until the end.

25.4 Location of obstetric simulation training

There is currently a significant amount of debate about where obstetric simulation training should occur, with reasonable arguments for several different approaches. For the most part, the decision must be made between conducting training on the labour and delivery unit or at a separate dedicated location.

The benefit to conducting training at a location away from labour and delivery is that the staff involved are less likely to be pulled into other clinical duties during the simulation training time. In addition, if you can procure a permanent space, then you do not have to set up and then put away the equipment and you have a better ability to consider installing videorecording devices, which are helpful in training and debriefing. It is, though, often difficult to find space, but fortunately you generally do not need much more than a single small room for all of the obstetric simulations discussed in this chapter.

On the other hand, training on the actual labour and delivery ward adds a degree of realism that you cannot achieve in the lab. By making people practice where they perform, you can not only ensure that they do the appropriate procedures correctly, but also evaluate teamwork better and see what unique systems problems they may encounter. For example, if you simulate a shoulder dystocia and the staff asks the nurse to call for help, if you are on your labour and delivery unit, that nurse has to find the phone, use the correct phone number, or physically go and find the appropriate person in the exact same manner as they will during a real dystocia. If the simulation is done in a lab, then the act of finding someone to help can be simulated, but it does not translate as well. The down side to training on the actual labour and delivery unit is that scheduling may be difficult as the acuity at any given time cannot be predicted with certainty, and patient safety will always trump training. Another logistical issue is that you will have to transport the mannequin to the unit for training if it is not normally stored in that area.

Where you decide to conduct your training will depend on multiple factors, as discussed above. If you are training students, residents, and staff on procedures, this can be accomplished well away from the labour and delivery ward. If you have the ability and desire to provide a more realistic team approach, then simulation training on labour and delivery may be a better choice.

25.5 Specific obstetric procedures and simulations

25.5.1 Procedures

25.5.1.1 Episiotomy/laceration repair

A model produced by Limbs and Things is available that can simulate cutting an episiotomy and repairing a simple episiotomy. There are also models for repair of third and fourth-degree

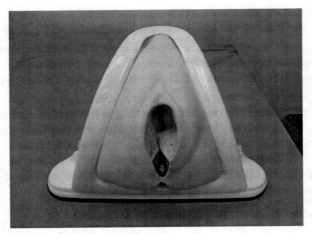

Fig. 25.4 Episiotomy models (Limbs and Things, Bristol, UK).

lacerations (see Figs.25.3 and 25.4) These models simulate the deep tissues relatively well and they have replaceable tissue blocks so that after they are used (we get about 30–40 repairs per block) they can simply be replaced without purchasing an entire new model. This is the model used by Nielsen *et al.* in their study where they developed an OSATS (Objective Structured Assessment of Technical Skills)[2].

Both a car wash sponge and beef tongue can be used to simulate an episiotomy, and there are some publications that describe exactly how to do this[1]. It is also important to remember to thaw the tongues before starting the simulation!

Gaumard Scientific has vulvar inserts that can be placed on their standard birthing mannequin that allow for suture of episiotomy. These inserts, however, are made of a basic plastic that does not simulate the deeper tissue well, sutures tend to rip through easily, and the material does not last through many repairs.

The simulations can be set up either as a pure instruction station, where you teach the trainee how to perform the episiotomy and then repair the laceration, or with a clinical scenario that forces them to choose the correct sutures and then perform the repair. We usually begin our academic year with an instructional station and then later in the year repeat the simulation training with a graded exercise complete with the clinical scenario and same type of evaluation tools described previously.

25.5.1.2 Cervical examinations

The NOELLE® mannequin has a cervix that the fetus can deliver through. It does a reasonable job when the fetal head is well-applied to the cervix, but it is very pliable to allow the fetal head to deliver, so it feels like a multiparous cervix and can easily be stretched, which makes standardizing the dilation difficult. The easiest way to teach cervical dilation with this model is to check the cervix yourself and then have the trainee check and then explain to them if they are correct or what their error is. The newer models have a stretchable plastic that is significantly more realistic than the previous cloth models.

25.5.1.3 Internal monitor placement and artificial rupture of membranes

These skills can be practised on any of the standard birthing mannequins. In general, we give the trainees a brief didactic on the indications and contraindications for these procedures, demonstrate them on the mannequins, and then allow the trainees to practice while asking them questions.

Artificial rupture of membranes (AROM) At this time, we teach this skill using a standard NOELLE® birthing mannequin with the cervix in place, and ensure that the head is well-applied to the cervix. I then demonstrate the proper way to insert the amniohook, with the hook down and protected by the finger, and then how to rotate it around, rupture the membranes, and then rotate it back down and remove, taking care not to injure the vaginal tissue. While other birthing mannequins may be used, the presence of a cervix is helpful, which the PROMPT® trainer does not have at this time.

Fetal scalp electrode (FSE) placement After the didactics, you should use the same FSE that is used on your labour and delivery unit. We teach the trainee how to identify the bony part of the skull, and then the mechanics of twisting the electrode and removing the sheath. The main limitation with teaching this procedure is the fetal head on the mannequin. With the NOELLE® mannequin, the regular delivery fetus has a hard plastic head and will not work, however, the vacuum delivery fetus works well. The PROMPT® trainer has a smooth head that can also be used for FSE placement.

25.5.1.4 Leopold manoeuvres

In order to perform Leopold manoeuvres, the fetus is placed into the abdomen in a known position and the different manoeuvres are performed. This is somewhat difficult to do with most of the available models, but some things can be done to make it slightly easier.

With the NOELLE® mannequins, there is an inflatable insert that goes into the abdomen that pushes the fetus closer to the abdominal wall. If you then use the thinnest abdominal wall cover (not the one with the inflatable air cells) then this will give you the best tactile sensation. Some of the models have foam inserts and these can be easily removed to improve your ability to palpate the fetus. Because the birthing mannequins are all hard plastic, even when you can feel the fetus, it is difficult to determine the vertex from the breech, but you can usually teach the trainee how to feel the fetal back at least.

With the PROMPT® birthing mannequin, there is only the lower part of the abdomen present, so it is not possible to palpate the superior pole in a realistic manner. The way the fetus sits in the pelvis also makes it difficult to palpate the presenting part from the abdominal route as well.

25.5.1.5 Spontaneous vaginal delivery

For this type of exercise, you are generally working with people either at the beginning of their training, or those who you feel may be called on to perform a delivery in an emergency. You can run this scenario with the same format as discussed previously, but in general, we tend to provide more instruction during the actual simulation with regards to hand placement and traction.

This skill can be taught on a number of different birthing trainers. On some mannequins, such as the upper level NOELLE® products, there is a mechanical device that pushes the fetus through the birth canal. Others generally require the staff to push the fetus through the canal and the head onto the perineum. In our institution, because of the time involved in using the motor (usually at least 5 minutes for a delivery), we simply stand by the side of the mannequin and push the fetus out with one hand under the gown and abdominal cover.

With any of the simulations that require delivery of the fetus, lubrication is the most important part of the simulation. Most birthing mannequins come with silicone lubricant, but when you run out of this, ultrasound gel works just as well, and is easy to procure from the labour unit.

25.5.1.6 Counseling for obstetric procedures

Both the forceps and vacuum scenarios described later in the chapter offer a great opportunity to provide instruction in how to counsel patients appropriately for an operative vaginal delivery. Because the counseling that is done tends to be different for an emergency operative delivery for fetal distress than it would be for the indication of maternal exhaustion, we include different scenarios during our training.

In order to make sure the trainee has the opportunity to counsel the patient during their simulation, if they begin to apply either forceps or a vacuum without first counseling the mannequin patient, we have the staff who plays the part of the 'spouse' or 'family friend' say something like "that looks dangerous", which usually prompts them to stop and counsel the patient.

After the simulation is over, you can review the counseling that was done, or in many cases what was not done, with the trainee and go over exactly what is expected in the situation.

25.5.1.7 Documentation

After the actual simulation is completed, many scenarios, such as shoulder dystocia and operative vaginal deliveries, lend themselves well to having the trainee write a delivery note summarizing their care. This is a good exercise because it can not only give them something to do if they are waiting for another station, but also provides a good opportunity to review their documentation to ensure that all key elements are included.

This technique has been described in the literature with regards to shoulder dystocia notes. In a descriptive study of delivery notes after a simulated shoulder dystocia, the authors found that only 18% of the providers mentioned which shoulder was anterior during the delivery, which is important as the anterior shoulder is the one where you would anticipate an injury if one occurred, and that 67% recorded fewer than 10 of the 15 key components that were graded[3].

25.5.2 Obsetric emergencies

25.5.2.1 Shoulder dystocia

Shoulder dystocia is, unfortunately, a very common obstetric emergency and occurs in 1–3% of all deliveries, depending on how exactly it is defined. Of all obstetric simulations, there is the most information and data on this simulated complication. It is also important to note that there is a published abstract that reported a significant decrease in neonatal injuries (12.8% to 3.6%, $P < 0.0001$) after implementation of shoulder dystocia simulation drills[4].

In 2004 we published a study where residents were randomized by training-year level to simulation training with a NOELLE® mannequin in shoulder dystocia management *versus* standard didactic training[3]. Several weeks later, all the residents, without prior notice, went through a shoulder dystocia simulation and their performance was evaluated by staff physicians blinded to their training status. We found that simulation-trained residents performed significantly better than their untrained counterparts in all aspects of their management and accomplished delivery of the fetus is less than half the time as untrained residents. Similar findings were recently reported by a group using the PROMPT® birthing trainer as well[5].

The NOELLE® and PROMPT® birthing trainers are the two main models that are available to simulate a shoulder dystocia at the present time.

NOELLE®: This is a full-size birthing mannequin. This simulator does not have a mechanism to actually keep the fetus in the abdomen, and simulates a shoulder dystocia by having the internal motor push the head of the fetus out and then have it retract slightly. In order to conduct this simulation in a realistic manner, you must fashion a harness for the delivery, because other-

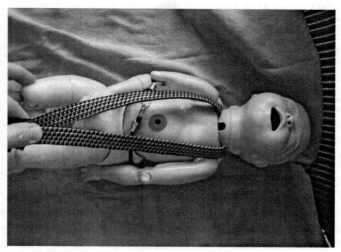

Fig. 25.5 Dystocia harness.

wise, when the delivering provider pulls on the fetal head after delivery, the baby will just deliver. Pictures of this can be seen in Figs. 25.5 and 25.6.

In addition, when we do this simulation, we do not use the internal motor, but rather just have the training staff play the role of the 'father' or 'mother' and they stand on the side of the patient and simply push the fetus out until the head delivers and then restitutes. It is important to remove the cervix when doing this drill as well as ensure that the fetus is well lubricated with either the silicone-based gel that it comes with or sonogram gel. After delivery of the fetal head the staff holds onto the harness as the trainee attempts to deliver. The fetus is allowed to deliver at whatever endpoint you have set. (We have generally used posterior arm delivery or Zavenelli manoeuvre as our endpoints.)

PROMPT®: The major difference with the PROMPT® trainer (Fig. 25.2) is that you have the staff person physically sit on the delivery table/bed and act like the patient, because it only includes the

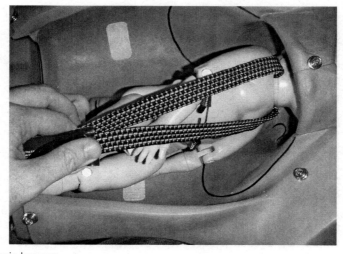

Fig. 25.6 Dystocia harness.

lower part of the abdomen. In addition, when McRoberts position is done, this only involves rotating the upper thighs upwards as there are not full legs on the model. The major benefit of this model as compared to the NOELLE® mannequin is that the fetus has a force-feedback mechanism in the neck. During the simulated dystocia, the staff sitting on the bed must grasp the inferior portion of the fetal torso as the trainee attempts to deliver the fetus. The fetus attaches to a laptop through the umbilical cord and real-time feedback can be seen on the screen with regards to how much force the person is applying.

The other thing that is different with this trainer is that the perineum is more realistic in appearance and from a tactile sense than the NOELLE® model, but it is significantly more difficult for the operator to push the fetal head through the canal.

25.5.2.2 Postpartum haemorrhage

Even with advances in obstetric care, postpartum haemorrhage (PPH) is a significant cause of maternal morbidity and mortality, resulting in approximately 140,000 deaths worldwide[6]. To address this issue, clinical drills to improve the management of this emergency have been recommended by the US Joint Commission on Accreditation of Healthcare Organizations (JCAHO).

Currently, there is a commercially available simulation module available from Gaumard Scientific that consists of an inflatable uterus which is attached to a perineum and has tubing that will carry simulated blood from an external IV bag through the uterus and out of the cervix. The external IV bag is inflated with the included pump and it pushes a good amount of blood through in a continuous manner that will provide the 'audible bleeding' and dripping onto the floor that often accompanies a PPH. The uterus can be made to be atonic and soft, or firm by using the hand pump that is attached and comes out of the abdomen (Fig. 25.7). While there is a separate line that goes to the lateral edge of the cervix to simulate a cervical laceration, there is not currently a way to make this act like arterial bleeding (i.e. pulsating), but this may come in the near future.

This PPH module has recently been used in a multicentre trial. The investigators found that, when the standard for stopping a PPH included performing fundal massage and administering

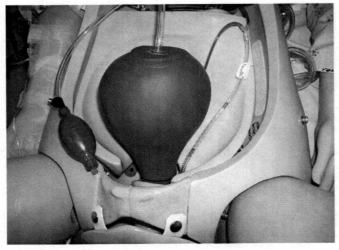

Fig. 25.6 Postpartum haemorrhage model (Gaumard Scientific, Florida).

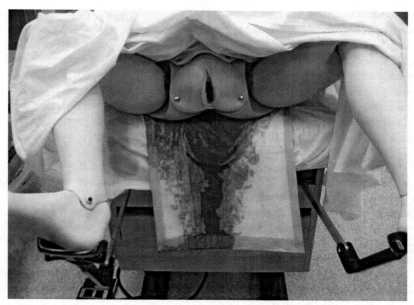

Fig. 25.7 Postpartum haemorrhage model (Gaumard Scientific, Florida).

two medications correctly (correct dose and route of administration), only 55% of the residents were able to correct a PPH within 5 minutes[7]. In addition, the same number of residents made at least one error during the simulation in the medications they requested.

Running a postpartum haemorrhage scenario When setting up the PPH scenario, it is important to not only have the simulator bleed, but to also give additional feedback about the patient's vital signs as this will move the simulation along and provide added emphasis/stress for the trainee. This can be accomplished either by having the staff verbally provide worsening vitals at designated intervals (i.e. at 30 seconds, 60 seconds, 120 seconds, etc) or with the assistance of the maternal vital sign software that comes with the more sophisticated NOELLE® mannequins.

The staff generally stands to the side of the mannequin and the blood reservoir is hidden by the patient's head under a sheet/towel. It is important to have the head/upper torso of the NOELLE® mannequin at about a 45° angle because this allows the blood that comes out of the cervix to drain out of the vagina. If you do not elevate the mannequin, then the simulated blood may pool and come out of the lower back. Another design issue with the haemorrhage module is that, while there is a rectum where you can place Misoprostol if desired, the perineum is not sealed between the posterior vaginal opening and the rectum and the blood sometimes runs directly down to the rectum rather than out of the vagina. We have used things like duct tape and even sutures to approximate this area to keep it closed so that the blood comes out of the vagina.

At the beginning of the simulation, the clamp from the pressure bag with the simulated blood reservoir is unclamped and the uterus is made to be 'boggy'. There are generally two staff required for this model, one to grade/observe, and one to manage the scenario as the nurse. The nurse stands at the head of the bed and starts the bleeding by releasing the clamp before the trainee enters the room so that there is some already on the perineum when they enter the room. (The blood reservoir provides 5–8 minutes of bleeding before running out.) In our scenario, we have the nurse tell them the initial vital signs when they enter the room, which includes slight tachycardia and a borderline low blood pressure. At specific time intervals, such as 30 seconds, 60 seconds, and 120 seconds, the trainee is given additional vital signs which become progressively worse if they have not corrected the haemorrhage. While you can simply do this verbally, if you have the NOELLE® model with the vital signs monitors, then you can simulate these changes with that software as well.

For this PPH simulation, we generally allow the bleeding to occur until the trainee evaluates for vaginal lacerations, performs fundal massage, and administers two different medications correctly, but you can decide on your own endpoints based on your institutional protocols and desires.

25.5.2.3 Eclampsia

Because of the rarity of eclamptic seizures with current obstetric care, and magnesium sulphate seizure prophylaxis, eclampsia is an important emergency to simulate.

Simulation of eclamptic seizures has been reported in one study and the results published in the literature. In the only published study by Thompson *et al.*, they described using 'eclampsia drills', which were conducted in various places in the hospital without warning with a human playing the 'simulated patient'[8]. After they simulated an eclamptic seizure the team of providers that responded was evaluated and briefed on how well they had performed. In this study, they identified multiple system deficiencies that led to the hospital placing specific 'eclampsia packets' in multiple locations in the hospital.

At this time, there is not an obstetric mannequin available that will simulate an eclamptic seizure by actually convulsing, but there may be some value in performing these drills with either a human patient actor or with one of the available birthing mannequins and simply calling people to the emergency and stating that she is pregnant and just had a witnessed seizure. In order to do this, we would recommend using the same essential components discussed earlier in the chapter, and evaluating those who respond to the emergency based on your institution's protocols for this emergency.

25.5.2.4 Breech vaginal delivery

Although current recommendations for delivery of a singleton breech are now for a primary Caesarean section in order to decrease the risk of fetal injury, patients still present either preterm or in advanced labour at the point where a vaginal breech delivery is inevitable[9]. Because of this, it is important that all residents are trained how to deliver the breech fetus, and currently simulation is the only viable method with which to teach this skill[10].

In a recent article, residents from two separate institutions were evaluated on their performance of a simulated breech vaginal delivery both before and after training with a standard NOELLE® mannequin[11]. In this study, residents scored significantly better after training with regards to their overall performance and safety in performing the breech delivery.

This simulation can be accomplished easily with either a full-size or basic pelvic model as long as you have an articulating fetus. While the full-size NOELL® mannequin has a motor that can push the fetus through the vaginal opening in a breech position, it is easier and more realistic to have an assistant with a hand under the patient's gown and abdominal cover push the fetus out. One important thing to remember in this simulation is to remove the internal cervix as this tends to make the birthing fetus get stuck during the delivery. On the other hand, if you want to simulate head entrapment, the new cervix available with the NOELLE® mannequin, which is a soft and stretchable plastic, is a significant improvement over the previous cloth cervix included on earlier models. The PROMPT® birthing model can also simulate a breech vaginal delivery and does not have a cervix that needs to be removed.

During the simulation, the trainee should not only call for appropriate assistance, but also perform the correct manoeuvres to affect a safe delivery. This can include the placement of Piper forceps and the reduction of a nuchal arm if desired as well. Performance is graded with evaluation forms that are similar to those described earlier in this chapter.

25.5.2.5 Operative vaginal delivery

The ability to perform an operative vaginal delivery is an important skill that all providers who deliver babies should have. While there is a notion that vacuum deliveries are safer than using forceps, both have risks and the current medical legal climate is such that they are done less and less, which makes simulation training for these all the more important.

Another benefit to the simulators is that, after the trainee goes through the simulation, you will have the opportunity to review their performance by actually opening up the abdominal cover and showing how to place the instruments.

These scenarios are generally run according to the protocols listed earlier. Some helpful hints are as follow:

- **Decide on the urgency of the simulation** Operative deliveries may occur in an emergent or non-emergent situation. For example, using a vacuum for delivery when a patient has maternal exhaustion is very different than if there is a fetal bradycardia to the 60s. The scenario you decide to use will affect both your set-up and expectations for how the trainee should react (i.e. in a non-emergent scenario, expect a much more lengthy discussion of risks and benefits of the procedure with the simulated patient than in the emergent one, and grade accordingly).

- **Use of fetal heart rate (FHR) tracings is helpful if available** For operative vaginal deliveries, we often use the FHR software with the NOELLE® model to simulate a concerning fetal heart rate tracing or prolonged bradycardia. This adds an element of stress and realism that is very helpful in recreating an actual situation as best possible. In the absence of this, you can remind the trainee of the fetal heart rate every 15–30 seconds during the scenario. Other ways to reproduce a fetal bradycardia is with an EKG rhythm simulator or the abdominal speaker which comes with some of the NOELLE® models and can be monitored with your regular fetal doppler equipment, or by taking FHR tracing paper and simply drawing a concerning tracing on it.

- **Set-up of the delivery table** Have a normal delivery table set up and keep all operative devices out of sight. This will force the trainee to ask for the correct device. It also allows you to test their knowledge of instruments. For example, if they ask for forceps, you should ask what kind they would like, or you can have a separate covered table you can uncover and allow them to choose. (If you do this, you can have the correct type for the clinical situation and then others to see if they can pick the correct ones.) You can also throw in some additional challenges to see if they catch them, such as mismatched forceps or the incorrect tubing for the vacuum device!

- **Selection of birthing fetus** For the PROMPT® birthing trainer, you can use the same birthing fetus for both a vacuum and forceps delivery. For the NOELLE® mannequin, the hard plastic birthing fetus has a rubber face that goes on over the hard plastic head that provides good traction with the forceps. There is a separate vacuum delivery fetus for the NOELLE® model as well that is usually ordered separately, but is very inexpensive. This fetus has a much more pliable head, but the arms and legs do not articulate so it is not really useful for other types of deliveries.

Forceps delivery For our forceps simulations, we set up the scenario for either an emergent delivery or for maternal exhaustion. The scenario is also written to direct the trainee to choose a specific type of forceps and the fetus is placed in the pelvis to do this as well (i.e. if you want to teach rotational forceps, then the fetus would be in an occiput transverse or occiput posterior position). When the trainee asks for forceps, we have several pairs to choose from. This forces them to not only know what to ask for, but also to be able to recognize them. The specific instruments you use will depend on what you normally use at your institution.

During the actual application of the forceps, most birthing mannequins do not have good enough soft tissue to hold the first blade in place, so you will need an assistant to do this or they often fall to the floor. Another issue with all of the birthing fetuses is that they are generally not as large as a term fetus, so the forceps placement on the fetus will not be exactly the same as real life.

The birthing fetus with the PROMPT® model is made of softer plastic and traction is generally not a problem, but because the fetal head does not turn to the side very easily, when the trainee applies traction, the staff holding the birthing fetus needs to help push from above and rotate the fetal shoulders to allow for delivery.

Vacuum delivery The scenarios for the vacuum delivery simulations are almost identical to the forceps scenarios, as the indications are often similar. You should always try and use the vacuum devices that your institution uses and test them on the birthing fetus prior to running the simulation real time.

Lubrication for the fetal head is essential in order to obtain a good seal with the vacuum for delivery. With the NOELLE® mannequin, a specific vacuum delivery fetus is required to perform this type of delivery, while the basic birthing fetus that comes with the PROMPT® model is suitable for both forceps and vacuum deliveries.

25.5.2.6 Emergency Caesarean section

The author is not aware of any good models currently available that simulate the ability to perform an actual Caesarean section at this time, however, at least one company is in the process of producing an abdominal cover that will allow this.

For the present time, simulations that would require an urgent or emergent Caesarean section are still valuable with regards to both determining when it is appropriate to move to the operating room (such as a prolapsed cord or a non-reassuring fetal heart rate tracing) and evaluating the labour and delivery team's teamwork, such as the ability to contact the scrub technician and anaesthesiologist, and response time in getting to the operating room to effect delivery. An example of this type of scenario that can be run is that of a prolapsed umbilical cord.

In order to perform this scenario, the birthing mannequin is placed in a regular hospital bed on the labour and delivery unit and the fetus is placed in the pelvis, but the umbilical cord is made to preceed the fetal vertex. Fetal heart rate decelerations may be simulated as discussed previously and the trainee is called in to evaluate the patient for sudden onset decelerations. On examination, they should recognize the complication and call for help and initiate plans to move to the operating room in an expeditious manner.

Important areas to focus on with this training are recognition of the complication, communication with other members of the team, and time from recognition to arrival in the operating room.

25.5.3 **Teamwork training**

Any simulation training that uses the birthing mannequins is an opportunity for teamwork training and evaluation. The challenge involved in doing this usually stems from being able to have the ancillary staff available to participate and finding a time that is not too busy on labour and delivery if that is where the training will take place.

Teamwork training also brings up another very strong argument to conduct simulation training on the actual labour and delivery unit itself rather than in a separate location or lab. By running simulations on the floor, it will be the actual environment where the emergencies will take place in real life, and you will have the opportunity to identify any systems issues that may be a problem as well that you cannot in a lab or remote location.

Key things to remember when performing Teamwork training include:

- Inform ancillary staff of plans for simulation training: When planning on evaluating the entire team's performance on a simulation exercise, you must discuss the plans for training with all services who make up the team. This includes nursing personnel, paediatrics, anaesthesia, and the administrative staff on the unit. While you do not have to tell them when the 'emergencies' will occur, they should all be aware that they will at some point. As an example, the first time that we conducted a simulated shoulder dystocia drill at our institution, we did it during the night shift and decided not to call the paediatricians because we had not yet warned them about our plans. We even went as far as to specifically instruct the ward secretary not to call them. However, in the excitement of the simulation, the nurse who emerged from the room and asked her to call paediatrics was stressed enough that the secretary did call the paediatricians, who came running down the hall!

- Inform any patients on the floor of the planned training: If you are conducting training on your labour and delivery unit, it is wise to have a provider go to any rooms in proximity to the one you will be using and inform the families and patients that if they hear a commotion in the hallway that you are conducting a drill and not to be alarmed.

- Coordinate simulations with the head nurse: If training is occurring on the labour unit, then you should coordinate with the head nurse on the day of the simulation to ensure that the acuity of the floor is such that they can accommodate the training.

- Debriefing is key, but must be done correctly: Because it is difficult for any provider to hear that they made mistakes in front of others, we recommend that the debriefing is conducted in two parts, or a 'dual debrief'.

The first part of the debriefing should include all providers and personnel who responded to the emergency. Questions should be asked in a non-threatening manner and initially be general.

Each group (i.e. the obstetric care provider, anaesthesia, paediatrics, nursing, and support staff) should be asked what they thought was done well, and what could be done better or differently from their perspective the next time this emergency is encountered. These suggestions should be recorded and passed on to other staff as lessons learned and the next time a simulation is run, you will be able to see if your team did better.

Another area to focus on during the debriefing is the communication between team members. Make sure and ask if everyone felt that they were in the loop with what was going on during the simulated emergency and address ways to make this better for the next time.

If there are specific interventions that people did not know how to do, such as McRobert's position during a shoulder dystocia, or where to go and obtain forceps, then you can demonstrate these on the mannequin or show them how to find the appropriate instruments or supplies.

The second part of the 'dual debrief' will involve only the providers who actually performed procedures. For this part, excuse the ancillary staff and everyone except usually the few who did things to the mannequin during the simulation. At this time, go over their actions during the procedure. For example, if the simulation was a shoulder dystocia, review the actions they took and their technical performance of the manoeuvres used. By doing this without everyone else present, they are less likely to feel threatened or singled out for any mistakes, and you also have the opportunity to let them practice on the mannequin and teach at that time.

25.6 **Conclusions**

Simulation training in obstetrics has the potential to prevent a significant number of poor outcomes. It is an essential part of training today and can be accomplished with a small investment of both time and funding.

References

1. Sparks RA, Beesley AD, Jones AD (2006). The "sponge perineum:" an innovative method of teaching fourth-degree obstetric perineal laceration repair to family medicine residents. *Fam Med* **38**(8): 542–4.

2. Nielsen PE, Foglia LM, Mandel LS, Chow GE (2003). Objective structured assessment of technical skills for episiotomy repair. *Am J Obstet Gynecol* **189**: 1257–60.

3. Deering SH, Poggi S, Hodor J, Macedonia C, Satin AJ (2004). Evaluation of residents' delivery notes following a simulated shoulder dystocia. *Obstet Gynecol* **104**: 667–70.

4. Wilson L, Ash J, Crofts J, Sibanda T, Draycott T (2006). Does training reduce the incidence of fetal injury in cases of shoulder dystocia? *Simulation in Healthcare* **1**(3): 185.

5. Crofts JF, Benedetti TJ (2006). Shoulder dystocia training: Comparison of existing training and a new mannequin with force feedback. Oral presentation, APGO/CREOG meeting, Mar 2006, Orlando, FL.

6. American College of Obstetrics and Gynecology (ACOG) (2006). Practice Bulletin, Postpartum Hemorrhage #76, October 2006.

7. Deering, SH Chinn M, Hodor J, Benedetti T, Mandel L, Goff B (2006). Validation and testing of a postpartum hemorrhage simulator for instruction and evaluation of resident. APGO/CREOG Annual Meeting, Orlando, FL, Mar 2006.

8. Thompson S, Neal S, Clark V (2004). Clinical risk management in obstetrics: eclampsia drills. *BMJ* **328**: 269–71.

9. Hannah ME, Hannah WJ, Hewson SA, Hodnett ED, Sagai S, William AR (2000). Planned caesarean section versus planned vaginal birth for breech presentation at term: a randomised multicentre trial. *Lancet* **356**: 1375–83.

10. Queenan JT (2004). Teaching infrequently used skills: vaginal breech delivery. *Obstet Gynecol* **103**(3): 405–6.

11. Deering SH, Brown J, Hodor J, Satin AJ (2006). Simulation training improves resident performance of singleton vaginal breech delivery. *Obstet Gynecol* **107**: 86–9.

Useful websites for obstetric simulation

Supplies/models:

http://www.Gaumard.com

  NOELLE® birthing mannequin (full-size patient)

http://www.limbsandthings.com

  PROMPT® birthing simulator (pelvis and upper legs)

  Episiotomy and anal sphincter trainers

  Amniocentesis model

http://www.clinicalinnovationseurope.com

  Sophie's Mum birthing simulator (Pelvis and upper legs)

  Cervical examination model

Curriculum and simulations:

http://www.acog.org/creogskills

  Compilation of teaching models by CREOG

Addendum A: Shoulder dystocia didactic

Shoulder dystocia

Definition: This complication occurs when the shoulders fail to deliver either spontaneously or with gentle downwards traction after the fetal head has delivered. It is usually a result of the anterior shoulder being wedged behind the pubic symphysis. Because a lengthy delay in delivery can cause significant injury to the fetus, it is imperative to have a well-rehearsed plan of action so that delivery can occur in an expedient and safe manner. It is also important that your assistants and/or nurses are well prepared for this drill.

Incidence: This complication occurs in 0.6–1.4% of vaginal deliveries of vertex fetuses. The recurrence risk is reported as 1–16%[1]. When a shoulder dystocia does occur, a brachial plexus injury may occur 4–40% of the time, but only 10% of these will be permanent[1].

Risk factors: Although there are well-known risk factors for a shoulder dystocia, most cases cannot be predicted. Some risk factors include:

- Previous shoulder dystocia
- Diabetes
- Fetal macrosomia (> 4000gms)
- Maternal obesity
- Multiparity
- Postterm gestation (42+ weeks)
- Previous history of a macrosomic fetus
- Epidural anaesthesia
- Induction of labour
- Operative vaginal delivery

Prevention: Because this complication is generally unpredictable, prevention is not usually possible and, if risk factors are present, the physician must be ready to take action should the complication occur.

In certain cases, however, such as when the estimated fetal weight is >5000 g in a nondiabetic patient, > 4500 g in a diabetic patient, a prophylactic Caesarean section may be performed[2].

Elective induction of a patient with presumed macrosomia in an effort to avoid shoulder dystocia is not supported by the literature or ACOG[3].

Treatment: There are many standard manoeuvres that are undertaken when a shoulder dystocia occurs. While there is disagreement about exactly what order to do them in, there are some simple manoeuvres that should be initially attempted. What follows is an ordered list of possible manoeuvres that can be attempted and a detailed description of each. It is important to note that most shoulder dystocias will resolve with only a few manoeuvres and that the more extreme interventions are, fortunately, not often required.

- **McRobert's manoeuvre:** Almost universally, the initial manoeuvre is McRobert's maoeuvre, which involves hyperflexion and abduction of the patients' legs back to flatten the lumbar lordosis and potentially free the impacted shoulder. After this manoeuvre is done, attempt again to deliver the anterior shoulder with gentle downward traction on the fetal head.

Adapted from Deering SH. *Labour and Delivery Essentials*, 2002 and published with permission.

- **Suprapubic pressure:** This is often performed at the same time as McRobert's manoeuvre. An assistant stands up on a stool or high enough to provide downward pressure just above the pubic symphysis in an attempt to dislodge the anterior shoulder. It is important to remember NOT to apply fundal pressure as this has been associated with worse fetal outcomes.

- **Modified Woods screw manoeuvre:** This manoeuvre is meant to turn the shoulders to an oblique position in order to deliver the child. It is performed by placing two fingers behind the posterior shoulder and rotating the child's anterior shoulder to release to release it from behind the symphysis.

- **Rubins manoeuvres:** This is actually two manoeuvres, with the first being an attempt to disimpact the anterior shoulder by transabdominal manipulation and the second using a hand vaginally behind the anterior shoulder to move it into an oblique angle for delivery by abducting the shoulder which will decrease the fetal diameter that must be delivered.

- **Delivery of the posterior shoulder:** A hand is placed into the posterior portion of the vagina and the posterior elbow grasped and swept across the body to deliver the posterior arm. When this occurs, the anterior shoulder will almost always deliver easily. If this is too difficult because there is minimal room posteriorly, a generous episiotomy may be cut to create additional room. (*This manoeuvre is often used before a Woods screw or Rubins manoeuvre.)

- **Generous episiotomy:** If it is very difficult to perform the rotational manoeuvres listed previously, then an episiotomy, and even a proctoepisiotomy (which intentionally extends into the rectum) may be made, although there is debate as to whether or not this is helpful as the limiting factor is seldom the posterior soft tissue.

- **Fracture of the clavicle:** The fetal clavicle can be fractured by placing two fingers underneath it and pulling outwards. It should not be pushed towards the fetus as the sharp ends could result in a fetal pneumothorax if the fracture occurs towards the lung. This manoeuvre is actually more difficult than it sounds, but may allow for compression of the fetal shoulder towards the thorax if successful.

- **All-fours manoeuvre:** This manoeuvre involves having the patient move from her back to a position on her hands and knees. It may free the anterior shoulder by rotation of the patient's pelvis. In patients with an epidural, however, this may be a very difficult position to move into.

- **Symphysiotomy:** To perform this manoeuvre, the patient is placed in lithotomy position and a local anaesthetic is injected into the skin and ligament of the symphysis pubis. Some form of urinary catheter inserted into the urethra and it is then deviated to the side with a vaginal hand. The ligament of the symphysis is then incised inferiorly with the initial incision starting at the junction of the upper and middle third of the ligament. The scalpel is then rotated 180 degrees and the remaining upper third of the ligament is incised pushing superiorly. The symphysis can then be opened approximately 2.5 cm to allow for delivery of the anterior shoulder[4].

- **Replacement of the fetal head (Zavanelli manoeuvre):** This is a last-ditch effort if all reasonable efforts have failed to deliver the fetal shoulder. In doing this, the cardinal movements of labour are reversed and the fetal head is flexed and replaced into the vagina and upwards while the patient is quickly moved to the OR for an emergent Caesarean section. The risk of significant fetal morbidity and mortality is increased greatly when this manoeuvre is required.

After delivery of the fetal shoulders, regardless of how long the delivery took, you should collect a section of the umbilical cord for cord gases.

It is imperative to sit down with the parents to explain exactly what occurred and what measures you took to deliver their child after the delivery is over. When things have calmed down, make sure you counsel them regarding the risk of recurrence should they decide to have another child. It is also extremely important to meet with everyone involved in the delivery or present in the delivery room and write a detailed note in the chart noting the time of delivery of the head, what manoeuvres were performed, what the time of delivery of the impacted shoulder occurred, which shoulder was stuck (left or right), Apgar scores, umbilical cord gases, and whether or not the child was moving its extremities after delivery. (Make sure you include the paediatrician's names in your note as well.) In addition, you should always dictate a delivery note as a supplement to your written note as soon as you have all of the pertinent information.

References

1. American College of Obstetricians and Gynecologists: Shoulder Dystocia. *Practice Bulletin* 40, November 2002.
2. Rouse DJ, Owen J, Goldenberg RL, Cliver SP (1996). The effectiveness and costs of elective Cesarean delivery for fetal macrosomia diagnosed by ultrasound. *JAMA* **276**: 1480–6.
3. Sanchez-Ramos L, Bernstein S, Kaunitz AM (2002). Expectant management versus labour induction for suspected fetal macrosomia: A systematic review. *Obstet Gynecol* **100**: 997–1002.
4. Wykes CB, Johnston TA, Paterson-Brown S, Johanson RB (2003). Symphysiotomy: a lifesaving procedure. *BJOG* **110**(2): 219–21.

Addendum B: Instructions for shoulder dystocia simulation

Shoulder dystocia scenario

Personnel required

- Staff to control fetus and maternal mannequin (1)
- Assistants to provide assistance with manoeuvres (1–2)
- Staff to film procedure (1 – or may use tripod)

Equipment required

- NOELLE® birthing simulator
- Fetus with dystocia harness
- Standard delivery table (bulb suction, Kelly clamps, scissors, etc)
- Digital videocamera
- Chronograph (may use watch with timer or even a second hand)

Scenario set-up

- Wrap the nylon strap around the birthing fetus such that the strap is hidden between the neck and body, then wrap it around so that the anterior arm (which will be the right one for this scenario) is held in by the strap as well, then tie the strap. Make sure to leave the posterior arm free so that they can deliver it during the simulation.
- Place the NOELLE® model in low lithotomy position and place the fetus with the harness on in the OA position.
- Close the abdominal cover over the fetus and pull the gown over the abdomen, making sure you can grasp the harness with your hand. (I suggest grabbing the harness with

your dominant hand as some residents will pull VERY hard during the delivery, which is something you should give them feedback on afterwards!)

Basic hints

- ◆ Use plenty of lubrication for the fetus. The mannequin comes with some silicone lubricant and works well, but sonogram gel works well when you run out of this.
- ◆ Remove the cervix that comes with the model as it generally will hold up the fetus and it is not needed for this simulation.
- ◆ Make sure and tell the resident to only simulate an episiotomy if they feel that one is necessary and NOT to actually cut the mannequin!

Answers to common questions

- ◆ If they ask for paediatrics or other help, have the assistant tell them that they are on their way.
- ◆ You do not have any more history than what the resident received before they walked into the room.
- ◆ You can have the 'OR' opened up but cannot move back there either before or after the delivery because it is being cleaned.
- ◆ You do not know any manoeuvres or how to help them, but can help provide McRoberts position or suprapubic pressure if they ask and show you how.
- ◆ Feel free to ask the resident why the fetus is turning blue as they are trying to deliver the baby!

Flow diagram of simulation

Give trainee clinical situation prior to entering the room

Trainee enters room

Primary staff plays the role of the husband and informs the resident that she is having a contraction and she has to push.

Push the fetal head until it delivers and then have the fetus restitute such that the right fetal shoulder is anterior and then apply traction on the harness and do not allow the shoulders to deliver.
*(At this time, begin the timer to measure the head-to-body delivery interval)

Trainee should recognize shoulder dystocia and begin manoeuvres.

Respond to manoeuvres with feedback if they ask if the shoulder is delivering.

If/when the resident attempts to deliver the posterior arm, allow the fetus to deliver. (If they do not attempt to deliver the posterior arm, then proceed until they do a Zavenelli or they say that they do not know anything else to do.)

Ask the trainee how long they think the head-to-body delivery interval was and record both this and the actual time on the data sheet.

$\downarrow$

Inform trainee of the following information:
APGARS 6/8
Birthweight = 4100 g
Baby is moving both extremities

After delivery
Have the trainee sit down and write a delivery note. When they are done with this, review their note and performance with the provided grading sheets, give them feedback, and demonstrate any mistakes and the appropriate techniques.

Addendum C: Clinical scenario for shoulder dystocia simulation

Clinical scenario

Mrs B.J. is a 35-year-old G2P1001 at 41+1 weeks gestation. Her prenatal course has been complicated by advanced maternal age (AMA),with a normal amniocentesis and a positive 1-hour glucola, with a negative 3-hour glucose tolerance test (GTT). She presented in active labour and was given an epidural for pain relief, and progressed well. She was C/C/+1 at her last check, and has been pushing for approximately 90 minutes with a reassuring foetal heart rate tracing (FHRT).

Please remember

- Treat the simulation as real as possible.

- If you need to cut an episiotomy, please simulate this and do not actually cut the mannequin.

Addendum D: Evaluation form for shoulder dystocia simulation

Shoulder dystocia evaluation form

Trainee # / Name _____ Date _____
Training Site _____ Grader _____

Training Level: (Circle One) PGY-1 PGY-2 PGY-3 PGY-4 Staff Midwife Fellow

1. Assess actual performance during shoulder dystocia drill:

CRITICAL TASKS:

Recognizes situation as a shoulder dystocia	Yes	No
Calls for additional help	Yes	No
Calls for paediatrics	Yes	No
Applies gentle traction to attempt delivery	Yes	No
Uses McRobert's manoeuvre	Yes	No
Uses Suprapubic pressure	Yes	No

IMPORTANT TASKS:

Attempts oblique maneuver (Woodscrew or Rubin)	Yes	No
Episiotomy	Yes	No

Attempts to deliver posterior arm	Yes	No
Drains the bladder	Yes	No
Fracture of the clavicle	Yes	No
Symphisiotomy	Yes	No
Zavenelli	Yes	No
Collects cord blood for gases	Yes	No

Noted head-to-body time: _____   Actual head-to-body time: _____

1. They performed manoeuvres in timely fashion

Strongly disagree					Neither agree or disagree					Strongly agree
0	1	2	3	4	5	6	7	8	9	10

2. They performed most manoeuvres correctly

Strongly disagree					Neither agree or disagree					Strongly agree
0	1	2	3	4	5	6	7	8	9	10

3. Overall, how well did they perform during the shoulder dystocia scenario?

Extremely poor					Average					Outstanding
0	1	2	3	4	5	6	7	8	9	10

4. How prepared do you feel they were for this complication (shoulder dystocia)?

Not prepared at all					Reasonably prepared					Very prepared
0	1	2	3	4	5	6	7	8	9	10

Chapter 26

Simulation in emergency medicine

John A Vozenilek and Mary D Patterson

Overview

- Emergency medicine simulations reflect the fast paced and chaotic nature of the emergency department.
- As such, these simulations may include multiple 'patients' and reflect the importance of surge and prioritization in emergency practice.
- Simple task trainers are valuable procedural training tools for medical students and junior graduate physicians.
- More sophisticated simulators present opportunities to develop and practice complicated decision making and management skills as well as the management of multiple simultaneous patients.
- Simulation integrated curricula are being used for emergency medicine postgraduate programmes.
- Simulation provides a method of ensuring exposure to a standard set of critical and seasonal conditions as opposed to relying on chance or random patient presentations to the emergency department.
- The use of simulation for teamwork and communication training for emergency teams is a developing area of focus.
- The evaluation of competencies for emergency medicine trainees and the development of simulation-based certification processes for emergency medicine practitioners is a relatively new use for emergency medicine based simulation.
- Simulation is a valuable means of assessing professionalism and communication skills – particularly around the delivery of 'bad news'.
- Simulation is becoming recognized as a valid tool for the evaluation of new systems and equipment before their actual use in the clinical environment.

26.1 Introduction

Simulation-based exercises in emergency medicine tend to be brief and fast paced. This emulates the practice of emergency medicine (EM), where the focus is on making diagnoses and initial stabilizing interventions. This is not to say that EM simulations are simple. Those attempting to capture the essence of the practice of EM in the simulated environment quickly conclude that there are a remarkable variety of cases and training events that fall within the purview of the emergency specialist. Since improved patient care and patient safety are generally the goals of EM simulations, the recognition of internal and external factors that can optimize or degrade patient care are key. Simulations will often focus on required skills in multiple simultaneous patient management (including mass casualty exercises). For this reason, EM-based simulation centres are more likely to use a number of devices, rather than the classic model of the single simulation unit.

A common misconception is that EM simulation training is primarily focused on the application of algorithms like those provided by the American Heart Association for advanced cardiac life support or paediatric advanced life support, etc. While these standardized courses emphasize knowledge and a structured approach to a particular set of clinical problems, they do not incorporate any skills related to teamwork and communication, which are critical to the practice of EM. EM-based simulations are rich in diversity and complexity, drawing heavily upon the benefits of experiential learning and cycles of training and focused debriefing.

As in the practice of EM itself, simulations designed to meet the needs of the emergency care provider may range from the patient with a sore throat or sprain to the critical patient suffering a myocardial infarction. These and many other patients must be triaged, evaluated, and managed simultaneously. The 'open' format of the typical emergency department often leads to situations in which doctors and nurses must simultaneously manage patient care and interact with patient family members. Using standardized patients concurrently with mechanical simulators therefore carries obvious educational advantages.

Another important aspect of emergency care is the concept of prioritization and 'flow' in times of crisis. Current modes for simulating these events include exercises on paper, computer-based exercises, so called 'smart' patients, high fidelity patient simulators, or any or all modes used in combination. These efforts can be effective not only for emergency practitioners, but also for the hospitals and systems in which they operate. The simulation of 'surge' (the influx of more patients than the system is equipped to handle) and the development of 'surge capacity', the solutions to an overwhelming influx of patients, are critically important in light of the concerns for pandemic disease and viral threats.

26.2 Curricula

As a relatively young specialty, much of the guidance related to curriculum and practice of EM in general originates in the USA, Europe, Australia, and New Zealand. Several documents may serve as useful starting points for developing a curriculum of educational simulation events for EM applications. The first document is a product of the American College of Emergency Physicians (ACEP). The most recent *Model of the Clinical Practice of Emergency Medicine* is jointly approved by the American Board of Emergency Medicine, ACEP, Council of Residency Directors, Emergency Medicine Residents Association (EMRA), Residency Review Committee for Emergency Medicine (RRC-EM), and the Society for Academic Emergency Medicine (SAEM), and approved by the ACEP Board of Directors in 2005[1]. Its original purpose, as defined in the document, is 'a listing of common conditions, symptoms, and diseases seen and evaluated in emergency departments'. As such this document provides a framework for the types of cases or training that would be suitable for trainees in EM.

For resident physicians, a second document, created by members of the Society for Academic Emergency Medicine and called the *Model Curriculum for Emergency Medicine Residency Training*, provides learning objectives that are helpful in crafting simulation-based exercises[2].

The Medical Student Educators interest groups within SAEM have at the time of this writing also created a model curriculum for use within a clinical rotation in EM. Though none of these documents is specific to simulation within EM, they are helpful in creating goals for learners. In 2002, Steven McLaughlin *et al.* published *Human Simulation in Emergency Medicine Training: A Model Curriculum*, which more specifically sets goals[3].

EM residents in the Harvard University programme and others at the time of this writing use a simulation-integrated modular curriculum[4]. The traditional lecture-based curriculum is surveyed for simulation compatibility, and simulation cases are crafted to provide experiential learning. The use of high fidelity simulation expands the teaching tools available to educators, but integrated curricula of this type are labour and time intensive. Educators interested in this model must keep in mind the learning objectives for a given training event, and if lower fidelity models or training methods are a better fit, use these alternatives.

26.3 Medical student education

The use of electromechanical simulator devices for educational training is not limited to the clinical rotations in medical school. Medical students from a variety of institutions are currently using these devices for practical correlation to pharmacology, physiology, and other core curricula. The presence of physical findings as well as dynamic vital signs as exhibited by these devices allows for a demonstration of the physical effects of medications, toxidromes (a constellation of signs and symptoms associated with ingestion of or exposure to specfic toxic substances), and medical conditions such as shock. However, it is also clear that the novice in EM can benefit from simpler and less expensive simulation tools[5–7].

For any trainee, it is essential that the prerequisite educational 'building blocks' be in place before entering simulation training. For medical students who have not yet encountered the concepts of fluid overload or Starling's curve, a training session with a high fidelity simulator that demonstrates all of the cardinal signs of congestive heart failure may tend to be over detailed. These student's peers, however, who already have some familiarity with these concepts, will gain more from the simulator session. To better prepare the first group of students for the simulation experience on congestive heart failure, they might be 'prepped' with a variety of screen-based simulations that reinforce the relevant basics of human physiology and anatomy. These programmes are available from a variety of commercial sources. Preparation of students (providing detailed didactic information and expectations) prior to the immersive learning experience helps them extract and retain the greatest amount of educational value from simulation.

Particularly with respect to technical and procedural skills, a static model or task trainer is entirely sufficient during initial exposure and practice of various procedures. A learner who has never held a laryngoscope and does not know which hand to use does not require a computerized mannequin whose tongue swells or that simulates laryngospasm. A static task-trainer is adequate for the initial introduction and practice of endotracheal intubation. Likewise, chicken legs suffice for the practice of intraosseous line insertion, and other static task-trainers provide an initial introduction to urinary catheter insertion or lumbar puncture. The progression from simple procedural skill practice on static models to the incorporation of critical thinking and teamwork skill practice with an interactive and more sophisticated dynamic simulator is entirely consistent with the principles of graduated challenges in simulation education.

For learners in the clinical rotations of training, the electromechanical simulator devices have considerably more utility. Despite the variable fidelity present in the current state-of-the-art manikins, the ability to convey a clinical scenario to a novice learner is invaluable. Medical student rotations in EM are typically brief and heavily emphasize the clinical exposure. Many disease entities within the scope of EM practice are seasonal, however. Medical students may therefore graduate without ever encountering a case of croup, bronchiolitis, or the presentation of a patient with heat prostration. Since the 'best cases' in EM are typically those involving the most critically ill patients, medical students' exposure is often limited.

The simulation environment allows a clerkship director the opportunity to plan the cases to which the medical student will be exposed. This ability provides even distribution of the presentations irrespective of season or the influence of chance presentation. In a 4-hour training sequence, a medical student could manage four presentations of shock, ranging from septic, hemorrhagic, neurological, and cardiovascular, and receive a debriefing based on the specific learning objectives on each topic.

It is important to study the effect of simulation training on the medical student educational process. However, such studies are highly labour-intensive and difficult to perform in a blinded fashion, and thus far findings have been inconclusive. Despite such challenges, there is a significant ethical drive to provide educational experiences for medical students in the safe and controlled simulation environment. One study on patient attitudes towards medical student procedures indicates that if the skill has been mastered on a simulator, patients are generally more accepting of medical students performing procedures on them[8].

For medical students the goal may not be exposure to a particular disease entity, but how to utilize the system for diagnostic decision making. One benefit of an immersive simulation environment is the opportunity to educate students on resource utilization (e.g. laboratory, radiology, and other support services), and then to evaluate their abilities in this domain. Medical students faced with a diagnostic puzzle and offered all of the diagnostic tools available to them in the emergency environment can test their own internal diagnostic algorithms. This is particularly effective in an immersive simulation environment, where there is a focus on creating a suspension of disbelief. Provision of laboratory data mock-ups, radiographs, ECGs and even video clips of patient findings allow the educator to portray a clinical scenario and provide an opportunity to evaluate the medical student's understanding of the diagnostic workup.

26.3.1 Procedural trainers for medical students

Currently, medical schools in the USA do not subscribe to a common list of procedures that are required for training prior to graduation. The escalating demands on medical education to remain current with advances in medicine and technologies result in the shunting of procedural competencies to postgraduate training. There is, however, a clear need for procedural practice and basic competence. A medical student rotating in the emergency department will be exposed to a variety of basic procedures, such as intravenous access, central venous access, arterial blood gas, lumbar puncture, urinary catheterization, suturing, and splinting. A variety of task trainers, available from multiple commercial sources, exist to provide opportunities to 'see one and do one' on a simulator rather than on a patient. Typically these devices are designed with adequate fidelity in order to present the anatomic landmarks and cues required to carry out a particular procedure.

There is evidence that task trainers for procedures such as intravenous insertion adequately reproduce the procedure for novices, are well accepted, and can discriminate between novices and experts[9]. In Germany, simulation has been used to reinforce, train, and evaluate medical students' responses to various cardiac arrhythmias. As compared with those taught traditionally, the medical students using simulation believed the simulation was more effective in linking theory to actual practice[10]. Roger Kneebone has developed simulations that combine standardized patients and task-trainers. Typically the task-trainer is adjacent to or draped in a suitable location attached to the standardized patient. This allows the student to interact with the standardized patient while performing the procedure. This type of simulation recreates the technical aspects of a procedure, but also the non-technical, interpersonal aspects of treatment, including explanation of the procedure to the patient and assent of the patient[5].

There are recognized ethical imperatives for medical students and residents to develop procedural competence 'as far away from the patient as possible'. Historically, physicians in training mastered procedures on the poor or disadvantaged. This practice is no longer considered acceptable[11]. The old adage of 'see one, do one, teach one' should become: 'see one, practice till competency in a simulated setting, and then do one on a patient'.

26.4 Postgraduate education in emergency medicine

In the USA, the Healthcare Finance Administration enacted regulations mandating strict faculty supervision of residents and residents' procedures approximately 10 years ago. This resulted in less independence and fewer opportunities for autonomous case management for graduate physicians. In the last three years, restrictions of resident work hours have been implemented with the goal of improving patient safety and decreasing medical errors related to fatigue. This restriction in work hours was not accompanied by a lengthening of postgraduate specialty training. Paradoxically, the decrease in clinical exposure increases the likelihood that an individual resident will finish training having cared for fewer patients, having less experience in managing critical conditions, and having performed fewer procedures for which technical competencies are mandated. These two regulatory requirements, though well intentioned, have diluted the practical clinical experience and retarded the development of the critical thinking and decision making skills of graduate physicians. The critical question is whether the widespread use of simulation training can in effect 'concentrate' the learning experience and promote an equivalent degree of competence with an overall decrease in clinical exposure.

There is a growing body of information in the medical literature regarding the use of simulation for resident education. Reznek has written, "Superior patient care and optimal physician training are often mutually exclusive in the clinical setting, and consequently live-patient training has several significant shortcomings"[12]. These limitations include the increased risk of complications for the patient, the inability to guarantee procedural opportunities (the presentation of a particular type of case or procedure is random), the inability to provide repeated or graduated opportunities for practice of a particular procedure, and the ethical obligation to intervene if one sees an error in progress. There is no opportunity for a resident to learn from a mistake under controlled conditions without harm to a patient[12]. In EM, the development of competence is complicated by the sheer number of procedures and varied types of diagnostic and management challenges in which mastery must be attained prior to completion of training.

In addition to the need to develop knowledge and procedural skill expertise in EM, there is also a critical need to develop decision making skills. Satish states that: treating patients often requires more than factual knowledge... The physician or medical team is thus often challenged by VUCAD (volatility, uncertainty, complexity, ambiguity and delayed feedback)....the medical decision maker may not possess the information processing skills that provide the needed mental model to perceive, understand, and respond optimally to such highly complex challenges[13].

Satish has suggested that strategic management simulations may provide a way to assess strengths and weaknesses as well as train for these kinds of situations. Strategic management simulations are complicated simulations designed to assess the individual's response to stress and ability to process information and make decisions appropriately. These do not typically involve medical crises but complicated disasters like a dam break, which residents have described as 'just like dealing with multiple serious problems in the emergency department'[14]. While these types of simulations have been used widely in non-healthcare industries, their use in healthcare is limited. Surgical residents have been evaluated for their ability to gather, process, prioritize, and act on information in a simulated dam break. A strong correlation was found between performance in this simulation and faculty evaluations of abilities. While these types of simulations do not evaluate content knowledge, targeted training in these types of information processing and decision making skills has resulted in significant improvements in these skills[14].

The Accreditation Council for Graduate Medical Education (ACGME) is responsible for the accreditation of postdoctoral medical training programmes within the USA. The goal of ACGME's Outcomes Project is to document an individual's growth toward competency as a physician. This organization aims to improve patient care through the growth of physician competency. The core competencies as defined by ACGME require residents to demonstrate particular behaviours. The core competencies of medical knowledge (defined as current knowledge and application of same during care) and patient care (appropriate and compassionate care) are particularly well suited to the simulation environment for assessment and critique. This organization has identified simulation as an acceptable means to document a trainee's growth to full professional status[11].

As in the case of medical student education, the role of chance plays heavily in a programme director's desire to document direct observations in the clinical arena. The simulation environment allows for the assessment of a particular skill set, whether it is knowledge-based, systems-based, or procedural. For EM there is particular emphasis on the resident's achievement of the 'skills necessary to prioritize and manage the emergency care of multiple patients'[15]. As such, immersive simulation centres which are used for emergency specialist training should present opportunities to engage the trainee with multiple patients sequentially or simultaneously.

In 2005, when the ACGME added procedural competencies and chief complaint-based competencies, residency programme directors again looked to simulation as a necessary and useful tool. The Residency Review Committee (RRC) in EM specifically indicates at the time of this writing that simulation is an acceptable mode for the documentation of procedural competency. Within their guidelines for procedures and resuscitations the specific numbers of procedures required for a resident to complete are presented (Table 26.1).

Table 26.1 Emergency medicine postgraduate procedural requirements (US)

Adult medical resuscitation	45
Adult trauma resuscitation	35
Bedside ultrasound	40
Cardiac pacing	06
Cardioversion/defibrillation	10
Central venous access	20
Chest tubes	10
Conscious sedation	15
Cricothyrotomy	03
Disclocation reduction	10
Intubations	35
Lumbar puncture	15
Paediatric medical resuscitation	15
Paediatric trauma resuscitation	10
Pericardiocentesis	03
Peritoneal lavage	03
Vaginal delivery	10

From ACGME Emergency Medicine Guidelines: http://www.acgme.org/acWebsite/RRC_110/110_guidelines.asp#res

Interestingly, similar postgraduate training programmes in the USA, such as the Pediatric Emergency Medicine fellowship, do not require programme directors or their trainees to document a specific number of procedures. Programmes are required to track procedures but not achieve minimum numbers of procedures. In these instances individual programme directors may dictate how their trainees accomplish internally set goals for procedural competency. Neither the American Board of Emergency Medicine nor the Pediatric Emergency Medicine sub-board of the American Board of Pediatrics has specified the number of procedures that may be performed in a simulated environment as opposed to a clinical environment in order to satisfy their requirements. This ambiguity has placed residency and fellowship directors in the difficult position of attempting to accurately 'guess' how these requirements may best be fulfilled. As programme directors set forth to respond to their review committees, simulation can be a powerful tool to help answer the following questions: What competencies are expected for each year of training? What are the measurable competency objectives for each year of training? How are these objectives measured? How are deficiencies remedied? Clear and specific guidance from these boards and the residency review committees is necessary if simulation is to be used extensively for this purpose.

Advances in patient care have led to additional focus areas for training. In the case of the increased attention to early goal-directed sepsis management, increased numbers of internal jugular cannulations were being performed in the emergency department. This need occurred concurrently with the increased use of ultrasound for the guidance of central line placement. This need created a training gap, one to which a variety of simulation manufacturers have responded. The original task trainers for central venous cannulation were helpful for the training the psychomotor skills for a 'blind' technique. Newer task trainers allow for the use of real ultrasound as well. Currently many programmes use a variety of ultrasound training devices, such as phantoms or other integrated devices. New protocols will require this flexibility of design, and as medicine evolves, of necessity so will the tools used to train clinicians.

In the USA the RRC 'expects that programmes will assess the competency of residents to handle key chief complaints in EM'. Specifically stating that 'At the time of programme review, the programme will demonstrate how it assesses resident competency for three chief complaints over the course of the training programme. The programme can use a variety of tools including direct observation, check-lists, simulations, etc.' Members of the SAEM Committee for Technology in Medical Education, in partnership with the Association of American Medical Colleges have created a peer-reviewed online case library which may have a role in assisting programmes in their approach to fulfilling this requirement[16].

In addition to technical competencies as described by the ACGME and the various specialty medical boards, it has been recommended that communication and teamwork training be incorporated as an integral part of postgraduate medical training. The ACGME states that 'Residents must demonstrate interpersonal and communication skills that result in effective information exchange and teaming with patients and professional associates'. In addition they must have the ability to 'work effectively with others as a member or leader of a healthcare team'[17].

Simulation is recognized as one method of evaluating the professionalism of EM residents – another component of the ACGME requirements. Gisondi and colleagues included a 'professionalism performance assessment tool' as part of an Emergency Medicine Crisis Resource Management Course offered to EM residents. The authors incorporate ethical dilemmas into the simulated medical crises and evaluated the performance of the residents for medical management and ethical competency. Specifically residents were asked to deal with the issues of patient confidentiality, informed consent, withdrawal of care, procedural practice on the recently deceased, and the use of 'Do Not Resuscitate' orders. A checklist was used to rate critical actions for each simulation. The authors demonstrated that their assessment of resident competency in this domain directly correlated with the number of years of training[18]. The improvement in skills in this area of simulation training lends face validity to the use of simulation for both education and assessment of this particular competency.

26.5 Ultrasound simulation

EM has relied upon diagnostic bedside ultrasound for decades and has taken an increasingly active role in the preparation of residents and attending physician staff for the proper use of this powerful tool. Typical training includes didactic training coupled with direct observations of examinations by experts and/or recordings of ultrasound exams. Ultrasound simulator devices are currently in use for EM training and may become more frequently found in training programmes in EM.

The currently available ultrasound simulator devices were initially intended to train registered ultrasound technicians. These devices create a facsimile of the ultrasonographic findings on a display as the trainee passes the 'ultrasound probe' across a mannequin instrumented with sensors. The simulator typically is housed within a unit which simulates the controls presented to the user on a real ultrasound device. In this way trainees may operate controls and fine tune their skills interfacing with the device as well as practice the manoeuvres and hand-to-eye coordination required for successful ultrasonography.

The major advantages of these devices are that trainees may swiftly engage a number of normal, normal variants, and abnormal findings, depending on the 'case' presented. Some simulators have an instructor mode, which allows the trainee to track and emulate the proper location of the ultrasound probe on the mannequin for a given exam. These devices may be used independently or in conjunction with other training and allow flexibility for scheduling. Patient models are not required and serious pathologies may be repeatedly simulated in a controlled training environment.

In 2001 ACEP created a policy statement entitled *Emergency Ultrasound Guidelines*[19]. This document, in combination with the previously published ultrasound curriculum by Mateer *et al.*, may serve as a guideline for simulation-based ultrasound curricula[20]. To date these devices produce fair to good fidelity, but still require augmentation with live patients or patient models to produce more realistic assessments of competency. The ACEP document predates the increased use of ultrasound simulators in EM training, and mentions that 'computer simulations of sonography can be useful additions in teaching and assessing the psychomotor component'. More explicitly, the document advocates the use of patient models, such as those who are on peritoneal dialysis, to simulate abnormal findings. Clearly the computer-based ultrasound simulator will eventually find its way more formally into training.

26.6 Continuing medical education opportunities

Continuing medical education (CME) opportunities in EM are numerous and diverse. As in other educational venues, high fidelity simulation devices and task-trainers may be used to augment standard didactic presentations or to create an immersive training experience for CME. The demand for this type of training is relatively high and as content becomes more interactive this is increasingly attractive to adult learners. The downside of training of this type remains its labour-intensive nature for the instructor. It is our experience that training for this cohort requires even more preparation.

Simulation is highly used for continuing procedural skills practice for high-acuity, low-frequency events. Difficult airway skills education, such as fibreoptic intubation, laryngeal mask airways, and other novel equipment are easily and safely performed using airway task-trainers or high fidelity simulation devices. There are currently several commercial providers of CME that use high fidelity simulation.

One successful offering for practising physicians fills the need for participants to refresh their approach to emergencies in the office setting. One study of unannounced paediatric mock code scenarios and focused debriefing indicated that following the event, offices were more likely to establish written protocols and engage in life support certifications[21]. Emergency physicians are viewed as proficient in acute care management by colleagues in office-based practices. Emergency physicians serve as expert faculty and may assist by reinforcing lessons learned during residency or introduce new concepts, such as the use of automated external defibrillators. Hospitals may also look to emergency physicians to train staff on rapid response teams, dedicated to the early recognition of declining patient status and providing therapeutic interventions before a patient suffers cardiac or respiratory failure.

Following the terrorist events of 2001, increased funding for training resulted in the greater use of simulation for disaster preparedness and mass casualty training in the USA. The Advanced Bioterrorism Triage Course, Advanced Disaster Life Support, and other offerings are examples of courses that integrate high fidelity simulation fully into a curriculum designed for physicians out of training[22–24].

26.7 Delivery of bad news and disclosure of error

The delivery of bad news is inherent to the practice of EM, though few practitioners receive formal training or practise these skills. The advent of simulation training has encouraged the rehearsal and practice of these behaviours in a simulated setting, most often using simulated family members. In fact, the simulation may begin with the team attempting to resuscitate a critical patient and then extending to the 'family members' (actors) representing the family members of the patient[25]. Programmes that include didactic presentations as well as standardized patients for practise of these communication skills have been developed for EM, and paediatric residents and fellows. In general, these programmes have been successful in developing competency and increasing comfort for the learners[26, 27].

With an increased emphasis on disclosure of errors and transparency with respect to adverse events, there is also a need for healthcare providers to be able to discuss errors and apologize to patients and families of patients. For many physicians, this is an entirely new experience. Many physicians have been advised in the past to avoid contact with families that have been the victims of medical error and never apologize, as this may invite litigation. Physicians now need to learn how to disclose error and apologize, something they may never have previously done. The disclosure and apology, however, are critical to the patient and their family, as well as to the physician for understanding and recovery on both sides[28, 29]. While the use of standardized patients and simulation for the development of communication skills related to the delivery of bad news is becoming an accepted educational method, there has been little use of these tools for the development of skills related to the disclosure of medical error and apology. This is an area for which simulation-based training would offer an important contribution. The incorporation of a critical simulation in which errors occur and the patient is injured would then be followed by the disclosure of error to the 'family members'. This would engender the emotional response, as well as the problem-based response that many physicians rely upon in the case of a mistake.

26.8 **Teamwork and communication training in emergency medicine**

The US Institute of Medicine Report, *To Err is Human* identified the emergency department as the area of the hospital that puts patients at the highest risk for adverse events[30]. The volume of patients, time pressure, and acuity of emergency department patients creates multiple opportunities for medical error. The emergency department shares many of the attributes of other high-risk domains in that:

- problems are ill structured
- information may be incomplete or conflicting
- situation is rapidly changing or evolving
- there may be multiple conflicting goals
- time pressure may be intense
- consequences of error are grave[31, 32].

The Institute of Medicine suggested that simulation training and emphasis on teamwork and standardized communication skills are part of an effective strategy to improve patient safety in this high-risk environment. Crew resource management (CRM) training is often used interchangeably with teamwork training. In reality, CRM represents one area of teamwork training. Teamwork training also includes concepts of standardized communication, situational awareness, target fixation, etc. The adoption of CRM principles and teamwork training is gaining acceptance in a number of high-risk medical specialties. In EM, teamwork training of provider teams has been shown to decrease errors and improve team satisfaction[33]. The essential question is whether the incorporation of simulation training in teamwork training for high-risk endeavours improves performance, increases resilience, and decreases error as compared with teamwork training that does not involve simulation. Given the expense, required resources, and intensive nature of simulation training, the answer is critical. The experience in other high-risk industries that employ simulation (aviation, nuclear power plants) suggests that the investment of time and assets in this type of training is worthwhile. However, the evidence is not entirely clear in many areas of medicine. Demonstration and proof of concept courses of simulation based multidisciplinary teamwork training have been developed and implemented in EM[34, 35]. The participants believed that these courses were useful and would aid them in clinical care, but no clinical outcomes were measured.

Another study evaluated the additive effect of 8 hours of simulation-based training compared with that of a conventional emergency team coordination course. This study demonstrated a trend towards improvement of team behaviour, but this trend did not achieve statistical significance in this study ($p = 0.07$). Participants did rate the addition of simulation training to the conventional course as valuable[36].

A subset of the emergency care team, the trauma team, has also participated in simulation-based training. Military trauma teams participated in simulation-based training and evaluation during a 28-day clinical refresher course. The teams demonstrated an improvement in trauma management skills during this period. However, additional clinical experience was ongoing at this time for all the teams, and so the study does not address the additional benefit of simulation as compared with a didactic or apprentice model of education[37]. Another randomized study did compare the performance of surgical interns trained on a simulator as compared with those trained on moulaged patients. This study did demonstrate a statistically significant improvement in single event and overall performance for those interns that participated in simulation-based trauma training as compared with those who participated in the conventional moulaged patient training[38]. Intuitively, it seems logical that those participants who are able to actually assess important physical findings, such as decreased breath sounds or diminished pulses, and then perform the procedures that will remedy these problems will achieve a higher level of skill than those who merely 'walk through' or describe the process. Experiential learning theory would also support this finding. Learning in an environment as similar as possible to the actual clinical environment promotes acquisition of skills and behaviours as well as an improved ability to use these skills.

Despite the dearth of evidence that simulation-based teamwork training is valuable in particular to EM, there is evidence from other domains that this type of training should be incorporated into EM education. There are skills and teamwork behaviours that are inherent to EM and for which simulation would seem to be the ideal method of training. For example, one can understand the concept of an authority gradient and an assertive statement. One can present videos or role play the use of an assertive statement. However, in a simulation one can recreate the situation, the crisis, and the emotions associated with an assertive statement. We have used the following simulation scenario on multiple occasions to embed this concept.

> A multidisciplinary team is caring for a 5-year-old boy with a severe head injury that requires rapid sequence intubation, and the team leader is scripted to insist upon using succinylcholine 'no matter what'. One of the nurses learns from the patient's mother that this child has a contraindication for using succinylcholine and needs to share this with the team and suggest an alternative medication. If the nurse is not able to convince the physician team leader to use an alternative medication, the patient suffers a ventricular arrhythmia secondary to hyperkalaemia. Eighty percent of the time the nurses do not succeed in successfully asserting their concern on their first experience with this scenario.

In debriefing this scenario, we find that the nurses inevitably describe great emotional difficulty in 'speaking up' to a physician. This is eye-opening to the nurses and the physicians. It allows for sharing of potential solutions around this type of issue as well as the opportunity to practise the behaviour in a safe setting. It is doubtful that education about the authority gradient and assertive statements in a traditional didactic setting would engender the same degree of realism or urgency and, more importantly, allow for the practise of this important behaviour.

Simulation is also an optimal way to train for resilience: the mitigation of and recovery from team errors. Though patient safety initiatives have tended to emphasize the reduction and even the elimination of errors, a sole emphasis on this aspect of safety ignores the reality that as human beings we will make mistakes. High reliability organizations, such as air-traffic control, and nuclear power plants, emphasize a preoccupation with failure and concepts such as 'cross checking' to capture and mitigate errors as well as recover from errors[39]. As specialists studying human factors begin to look at healthcare, opportunities to develop and practise these skills are beginning to emerge from the study of actual events, including near misses[40]. Simulation scenarios provide an opportunity to 'plant' mistakes and errors, and allow emergency teams to develop the skills of cross checking, discovery of, and mitigation of errors. Emergency simulation scenarios can include such features as broken equipment (bag valve masks, blood pressure monitors, cables) or incorrectly labeled medications or blood products. While these defects may appear obvious to the observer, the team in the midst of a crisis may take some time to identify and rectify these issues. The addition of these features to the emergency team simulations acknowledges the importance of vigilance in looking for failure and the responsibility of every team member's contribution to the identification and recovery from mistakes. With respect to simulation and safety training Salas *et al.* have written:

> The use of content-valid scenarios is critical in environments (such as healthcare) where errors if not corrected in a timely manner can have catastrophic consequences... Scenarios may also be crafted so

that trainees can experience these errors and observe the consequences so that those behaviours can be recognized in the future[41].

This also promotes team problem solving and coordination when faced with a medical error as opposed to team paralysis when faced with unexpected difficulties.

26.9 Human factors and the emergency department

Time work studies have been used in other industries to assess the efficiency of personnel and the optimal placement of equipment. Though in its infancy for this application, simulation is now being used to assess the clinical environment and the equipment that is used in the emergency department suite. A recent article describes the use of simulation to assess the usability and equipment placement in a new emergency department prior to opening for patient care. During the simulations, eighteen concerns were identified related to equipment placement or absence, communication systems, and procedural space. Fourteen of these issues were corrected before opening the unit for patient care[42]. A similar intervention is the use of *in situ* simulation, simulation occurring in the clinical setting. The goals of this type of simulation can include evaluation of teamwork, readiness, systems, and resources in the clinical setting[43].

Human factors expertise and simulation can also be used to evaluate health information technology prior to implementation in the healthcare setting, though this has not occurred in a frequent or routine manner. Koppel and Han describe an increase in medication errors and an increase in mortality, respectively, associated with the implementation of computerized order entry systems in their institutions[44,45]. The use of simulation to evaluate the weaknesses of this type of technology would conceivably avoid these types of unintended consequences related to these implementations. In an emergency department caring for multiple patients simultaneously, this type of rigorous testing prior to implementation would potentially avoid errors and injury to patients.

Additionally, new equipment being considered for use in the emergency department or modifications to existing processes and the introduction of new processes are also opportunities for the use of simulation. In our own institution, we have identified difficulties with a particular defibrillator monitor's design prior to its introduction in our department. In several simulations we observed that the synchronization button was not readily apparent to the user and resulted in defibrillation rather than cardioversion of a patient with supraventricular tachycardia. Working with clinical engineers we highlighted the synchronization button to ensure it was more visible to the clinical user.

26.10 Mass casualty incidents

An important aspect of emergency care in which teamwork and coordination is vital is that of multiple simultaneous patients or mass casualty situations. Traditionally, training for these types of disasters has been confined to tabletop or computer simulations supplemented by the delivery of moulaged patients to various hospitals and aid stations. This training suffers from a lack of realism. Healthcare providers are limited to triaging moulaged patients and describing how the patients would be handled. While this qualifies as simulation, it occurs at a very low level and does not promote the critical decision making or allow for practice of the skills and behaviours necessary to handle this type of crisis.

In Israel, simulation has been used to develop and assess the skills necessary for the management of multiple casualties. Skills such as endotracheal intubation and intraosseous line placement are performed on simulated patients by healthcare providers wearing full chemical protective gear[46,47]. This training provides an element of realism that is not matched in other mass casualty exercises. It also provides regional and national planners with a more realistic assessment of the timeframe and resources necessary should such an event occur.

26.11 Certification and credentialing

Baker and Salas have recommended that the various licensure and board certification organizations should assess and regulate the physician's knowledge of the 'components of a team' as well as requiring the physician to 'demonstrate competence in team leadership, mutual performance monitoring, back up behaviour and adaptability'[17]. In the aviation industry, simulation has been used to assess this type of competency. The line operational evaluation (LOE) 'requires pilots and copilots to demonstrate acceptable teamwork skills during this critical certification event'. Further, this type of training and evaluation is mandated during initial certification as well as during periodic recertifications conducted in simulators. The importance of ongoing reinforcement and assessment of technical competence and teamwork behaviours is a major factor in the evolution of aviation as a high reliability industry[17].

The Australasian College for Emergency Medicine has recently introduced a proposal to require simulation-based certification of EM practitioners[48]. In this case it is following the lead of the Australian and New Zealand College of Anaesthetists[49]. In the USA, the American Board of Anesthesiology has also recently decided to require simulation-based recertification of all boarded anaesthesiologists beginning in 2008[50]. Individual institutions have also started to require simulation-based training as part of their requirements for maintenance of medical staff privileges and performance-based credentialing. Many institutions have based these requirements on emerging data that demonstrates a decreased risk of litigation for high-risk specialties like EM that complete periodic simulation training. The optimal length and interval between such training is not clear at this time. It does appear that this represents a trend for simulation-based training from individual specialty boards and institutions that will only increase as simulation becomes more available.

26.12 Conclusion

As in many areas of healthcare the use of simulation in EM is just beginning to be explored. Clear applications for the use of simulation for the education of technical skills exist in EM as in other specialties. However, the use of simulation for non-technical skills, including teamwork training, is rapidly being recognized as equally important. However, the field is immature and there is little evidence directly linking simulation training to improved patient outcomes. Emergency medicine, as many other high-risk areas in healthcare, is still defining the optimal ways of incorporating simulation for education and safety. It does appear that there are specific needs in EM that may only be adequately addressed through simulation, including the evaluation of clinical environments, systems and equipment and training for mass casualty incidents. As expertise evolves, it is likely that additional applications will be identified for simulation in EM.

References

1. Directors American Board of Emergency Medicine (2003). Model of the Clinical Practice of Emergency Medicine 2003 [cited February 7, 2007]; Policy Statement]. Available from: http://www.acep.org/webportal/PracticeResources/PolicyStatements/meded/ ModeloftheClinicalPracticeofEM.htm

2. Society of Academic Emergency Medicine (2007). Model Curriculum for Emergency Medicine Residency Training [cited January 31, 2007]; available from: http://www.saem.org/SAEMDNN/ LinkClick.aspx?link=model.doc&tabid=57&mid=1020

3. McLaughlin SA, Doezema D, Sklar DP (2002). Human simulation in emergency medicine training: a model curriculum. *Acad Emerg Med* **9**(11): 1310–8.

4. Binstadt ES, Walls RM, White BA, *et al.*(2006). A comprehensive medical simulation education curriculum for emergency medicine residents. *Ann Emerg Med* Dec 8.

5. Kneebone R, Kidd J, Nestel D, Asvall S, Paraskeva P, Darzi A (2002). An innovative model for teaching and learning clinical procedures. *Med Educ* **36**(7):628–34.

6. Kneebone RL, Nestel D, Darzi A (2002). Taking the skills lab onto the wards. *Med Educ* **36**(11): 1093–4.

7. Kneebone RL, Kidd J, Nestel D, *et al.* (2005). Blurring the boundaries: scenario-based simulation in a clinical setting. *Med Educ* **39**(6): 580–7.

8. Graber MA, Wyatt C, Kasparek L, Xu Y (2005). Does simulator training for medical students change patient opinions and attitudes toward medical student procedures in the emergency department? *Acad Emerg Med* **12**(7): 635–9.

9. Reznek MA, Rawn CL, Krummel TM (2002). Evaluation of the educational effectiveness of a virtual reality intravenous insertion simulator. *Acad Emerg Med* **9**(11): 1319–25.

10. Mueller MP, Christ T, Dobrev D, *et al.* (2005). Teaching antiarrhythmic therapy and ECG in simulator-based interdisciplinary undergraduate medical education. *British Journal of Anaesthesia* **95**(3): 300–4.

11. Education AcoGM (2005). Simulation and rehearsal. *ACGME Bulletin*. http://www.acgme.org/acwebsite/bulletin/bulletin12–05. pdf.

12. Reznek M, Harter P, Krummel T (2002). Virtual reality and simulation: training the future emergency physician. *Acad Emerg Med* **9**(1): 78–87.

13. Satish U, Streufert S (2002). Value of a cognitive simulation in medicine: towards optimizing decision making performance of healthcare personnel. *Qual Saf Health Care* **11**(2): 163–7.

14. Satish U, Streufert S, Marshall R, *et al.* (2001). Strategic management simulations is a novel way to measure resident competencies. *American Journal of Surgery* **181**(6): 557–61.

15. Education AcoGM (2006). Emergency Medicine Guidelines [cited December 15 2006]; available from: http://www.acgme.org/acWebsite/RRC_110/110_guidelines.asp

16. Group SfAEMSI (2006). Simulation Case Library. [cited November 20, 2006]; available from: http://www.emedu.org/simlibrary/

17. Baker DP, Salas E, King H, Battles J, Barach P (2005). The role of teamwork in the professional education of physicians: current status and assessment recommendations. *Jt Comm J Qual Patient Saf* **31**(4): 185–202.

18. Gisondi MA S-CR, Harter PM, Soltysik RC, Yarnold PR (2004). Assessment of resident professionalism using high-fidelity simulation of ethical dilemmas. *Acad Emerg Med* **11**(9): 931–7.

19. American College of Emergency Physicians (2001). ACEP emergency ultrasound guidelines-2001. *Ann Emerg Med* **38**(4): 470–81.

20. Mateer J, Plummer D, Heller M, *et al.* (1994). Model curriculum for physician training in emergency ultrasonography. *Ann Emerg Med* **23**(1): 95–102.

21. Bordley WC, Travers D, Scanlon P, Frush K, Hohenhaus S (2003). Office preparedness for pediatric emergencies: a randomized, controlled trial of an office-based training programme. *Pediatrics* **112**(2): 291–5.

22. Subbarao I, Bond WF, Johnson C, Hsu EB, Wasser TE (2006). Using innovative simulation modalities for civilian-based, chemical, biological, radiological, nuclear, and explosive training in the acute management of terrorist victims: A pilot study. *Prehospital Disaster Med* **21**(4): 272–5.

23. Subbarao I, Johnson C, Bond WF, *et al.* (2005). Symptom-based, algorithmic approach for handling the initial encounter with victims of a potential terrorist attack. *Prehospital Disaster Med* **20**(5): 301–8.

24. Orledge JD SR (2006). Integration of high-fidelity simulation into the advanced disaster life support class. *International Trauma Care (ITACCS)*: 34–41.

25. Bowyer MW, Rawn L, Hanson J, *et al.* (2006). Combining high-fidelity human patient simulators with a standardized family member: a novel approach to teaching breaking bad news. *Studies in Health Technology and Informatics* **119**: 67–72.

26. Greenberg LW, Ochsenschlager D, O'Donnell R, Mastruserio J, Cohen GJ (1999). Communicating bad news: a pediatric department's evaluation of a simulated intervention. *Pediatrics* **103**(6 Pt 1): 1210–7.

27. Quest TE, Otsuki JA, Banja J, Ratcliff JJ, Heron SL, Kaslow NJ (2002). The use of standardized patients within a procedural competency model to teach death disclosure. *Acad Emerg Med* **9**(11): 1326–33.

28. Wears RL, Wu AW (2002). Dealing with failure: the aftermath of errors and adverse events. *Ann Emerg Med* **39**(3): 344–6.

29. Goldberg RM, Kuhn G, Andrew LB, Thomas HA, Jr (2002). Coping with medical mistakes and errors in judgment. *Ann Emerg Med* **39**(3): 287–92.

30. *To Err is Human: Building a Safer Health System*. Washington, DC: National Academy Press, 2000.

31. Flin R GR, Maran R, Patey R (2004). Framework for Observing and Rating Anaesthetists' Non-technical Skills. November 2, 2004 [cited May 1, 2006]; available from: http://www.abdn.ac.uk/iprc/papers%20reports/Ants/ANTS_handbook_v1.0_electronic_access_version.pdf

32. Flin R GR, Maran R, Patey R (2004). ANTS System-observation and Rating Sheet. November 2, 2004 [cited May 1, 2006]; available from: http://www.abdn.ac.uk/iprc/papers%20reports/Ants/ANTS%20System%20Observation%20Rating%20Sheet.doc

33. Morey JC, Simon R, Jay GD, *et al.* (2002). Error reduction and performance improvement in the emergency department through formal teamwork training: evaluation results of the MedTeams project. *Health Serv Res* **37**(6): 1553–81.

34. Reznek M, Smith-Coggins R, Howard S, *et al.* (2003). Emergency medicine crisis resource management (EMCRM): pilot study of a simulation-based crisis management course for emergency medicine. *Acad Emerg Med* **10**(4): 386–9.

35. Small SD, Wuerz RC, Simon R, Shapiro N, Conn A, Setnik G (1999). Demonstration of high-fidelity simulation team training for emergency medicine. *Acad Emerg Med* **6**(4): 312–23.

36. Shapiro MJ, Morey JC, Small SD, *et al.* (2004). Simulation based teamwork training for emergency department staff: does it improve clinical team performance when added to an existing didactic teamwork curriculum? *Qual Saf Health Care* **13**(6): 417–21.

37. Holcomb JB, Dumire RD, Crommett JW, *et al.* (2002). Evaluation of trauma team performance using an advanced human patient simulator for resuscitation training. *J Trauma* **52**(6): 1078–85; discussion 85–6.

38. Lee SK, Pardo M, Gaba D et al. (2003). Trauma assessment training with a patient simulator: a prospective, randomized study. *J Trauma* **55**(4): 651–7.

39. Salas E, Rhodenizer L, Bowers CA (2000). The design and delivery of crew resource management training: exploiting available resources. *Hum Factors* **42**(3): 490–511.

40. Ebright PR, Urden L, Patterson E, Chalko B (2004). Themes surrounding novice nurse near-miss and adverse-event situations. *Journal of Nursing Administration* **34**(11): 531–8.

41. Salas E, Wilson KA, Burke CS, Priest HA (2005). Using simulation-based training to improve patient safety: what does it take? *Jt Comm J Qual Patient Saf* **31**(7): 363–71.

42. Kobayashi L, Shapiro MJ, Sucov A et al. (2006). Portable advanced medical simulation for new emergency department testing and orientation. *Acad Emerg Med* **13**(6): 691–5.

43. Hunt EA, Hohenhaus SM, Luo X, Frush KS (2006). Simulation of pediatric trauma stabilization in 35 North Carolina emergency departments: identification of targets for performance improvement. *Pediatrics* **117**(3): 641–8.

44. Ammenwerth E, Talmon J, Ash JS, *et al.* (2006). Impact of CPOE on mortality rates–contradictory findings, important messages. *Methods of Information in Medicine* **45**(6): 586–93.

45. Koppel R, Metlay JP, Cohen A, *et al.* (2005). Role of computerized physician order entry systems in facilitating medication errors. *JAMA* **293**(10): 1197–203.

46. Berkenstadt H, Ziv A, Barsuk D, Levine I, Cohen A, Vardi A (2003). The use of advanced simulation in the training of anesthesiologists to treat chemical warfare casualties. *Anesthesia and Analgesia* **96**(6): 1739–42, table of contents.

47. Vardi A, Berkenstadt H, Levin I, Bentencur A, Ziv A (2004). Intraosseous vascular access in the treatment of chemical warfare casualties assessed by advanced simulation: proposed alteration of treatment protocol. *Anesthesia and Analgesia* **98**(6): 1753–8, table of contents.

48. Sweeney M (2006). Director of Education, Medicine Australian College for Emergency Medicine. *Advanced and Complex Medical Emergencies Course.* Personal communication electronic mail December 17, 2006.

49. Weller JM, Morris R, Watterson L, *et al.* (2006). Effective management of anaesthetic crises: development and evaluation of a college-accredited simulation-based course for anaesthesia education in Australia and New Zealand. *Simulation in Healthcare: The Journal of the Society for Simulation in Healthcare* **1**: 209–14.

50. Hurford W (2007), Chair of Anesthesia, University of Cincinnati College of Medicine. personal communication January 9, 2007.

Chapter 27

Cardiopulmonary bypass simulation

Richard Morris and Andy Pybus

Overview

◆ The use of simulators in cardiopulmonary bypass training can be justified using very similar arguments to those that are used to justify the use of flight simulators.

◆ Current approaches to the use of simulators in cardiopulmonary bypass training include: simple hydraulic systems, computer models and animal models.

◆ The potential roles for a high fidelity perfusion simulation system include: skill training and certification of perfusionists, the development and practice of crisis management protocols and the evaluation of novel perfusion equipment or techniques.

◆ The Orpheus high fidelity perfusion simulation system is a computer-controlled hydraulic simulator, which can be used in combination with the institutional heart–lung machine and monitoring systems.

◆ Orpheus incorporates sophisticated drug and blood gas modelling and can reproduce a wide variety of critical incidents.

27.1 Rationale for the use of simulators in cardiopulmonary bypass training

Cardiopulmonary bypass (CPB) is characterized by a relatively low frequency of rapidly evolving but potentially serious critical incidents. In a recent American study, Stammers and Mejak[1] surveyed the results of over 650,000 perfusions carried out at nearly 800 institutions, and reported that serious injury resulting from perfusion-related incidents occurred in approximately 1 in 2000 cases.

Similarly, in an earlier Australasian study by Jenkins et al.[2] the overall rate of death or serious injury complicating perfusion-related incidents was estimated at 1 in 2500 cases. These findings confirmed previous studies in the USA[3] and UK[4], and demonstrated the occurrence of a wide variety of incidents.

Jenkins et al. found that the average perfusionist reported six critical incidents per year and went on to suggest that the management of these incidents might be improved by training. The most frequently experienced categories of incident reported in the Jenkins study are shown in Table 27.1.

During the response to time-critical problems there is little opportunity for reflection or analysis. Rather, effective care is based on the ability to initiate practised, appropriate, pre-planned responses. In addition to a theoretical understanding of the problem, these responses demand a mix of technical and non-technical skills, which are enhanced by rehearsal.

Table 27.1 Most frequently reported incidents by a group of 101 perfusionists in an 18-month period[2]

Incident	Respondents (%)
◆ Heater-cooler failure	43
◆ Urgent circuit re-set-up after disposal	38
◆ Oxygenator leak	35
◆ Hospital power failure	31
◆ Drug related incidents	29
◆ Inability to raise the activated clotting time to 400	29
◆ Accidental cannula displacement	28
◆ Air in circuit not reaching patient	24
◆ Gas supply failure	23

There is little research that examines the performance of perfusionists during the management of critical incidents. However, it seems likely that while the frequency of serious incidents in perfusion is high enough to present a real risk to patients, it is probably too low to permit the development of the high-level skills that are required to deal with any specific problem.

In many ways, significant parallels can be drawn between perfusion and aviation. Both the perfusionist and pilot operate complex machines but are only rarely confronted with critical events (to which they must usually respond very rapidly), both operate as part of teams, and both may have a limited range of responses in any given situation.

In commercial aviation, most of the inputs that are necessary for making in-flight decisions are provided by physical sensors and displayed on instruments. Furthermore, the performance of the aircraft itself can be realistically modelled. It is probably for these reasons that simulators have a long history of use in this domain and that they now fulfil a vital role in the initial and ongoing training of pilots.

This is in contrast to, say, anaesthesia, where some of the most important management decisions are made as a result of direct observation of the patient's physical signs (such as cyanosis and muscle tone), which limit the fidelity of simulators using current technologies.

Within the healthcare domain, perfusion most closely approximates aviation because the crucial input data are also largely provided by physical sensors (pressure, flow, saturation, temperature etc), realistic models of cardiorespiratory performance[5] and drug kinetics[6] are well described, and the hydraulic characteristics of the circulation are quite easy to reproduce. However, at the present time, few high fidelity perfusion simulators are available, and simulation technology has only recently been incorporated into perfusion training schemes.

In the USA during the decade 1993–2003, the rate of coronary artery bypass grafting fell from 16.3 to 11.8 per 10,000 of population, while the rate of coronary artery stenting rose from 20.5 to 30.5[7]. Given this trend towards a reduction in operative caseload and societal pressures to implement the 'shorter working week' it is evident that it will become increasingly difficult for perfusion trainees to acquire the experience deemed necessary for safe practice within a reasonable length of time.

Typically, the number of cases which must be 'logged' by trainee perfusionists before they can proceed to registration ranges between 75 cases (USA) and 200 cases (Australasia) (Table 27.2).

Using Stammers serious incident rate of 1 per 138 cases[1], a trainee in the USA would have only around a 50% chance of witnessing such an incident during the course of his or her training. In contrast, current crisis management simulation courses frequently run six critical

Table 27.2 Number of cases required to be undertaken by a trainee perfusionist before he or she may proceed to certification

Certifying authority	Number of cases
◆ American Board of Cardiovascular Perfusion	75
◆ European Board of Cardiovascular Perfusion	100
◆ College of Clinical Perfusion Scientists of Great Britain	150
◆ Australian Board of Cardiovascular Perfusion	200

incident scenarios in a single day. Thus, a high fidelity perfusion simulator would seem to have an obvious application in the *ab initio* training of perfusionists.

27.2 Current approaches to the use of simulators in cardiopulmonary bypass training

Current approaches to the use of simulators in CPB training include the use of:

- ◆ simple hydraulic systems,
- ◆ screen-based simulations, and
- ◆ animal models.

In the laboratory, the use of a primed circuit with an arteriovenous loop and venous reservoir has traditionally been used for the preliminary training of perfusionists. This permits initial familiarization with the bypass machine, ancillary equipment and bypass circuit.

A simple closed-loop hydraulic circuit has been enhanced with simulated monitor displays for training in paediatric extracorporeal membrane oxygenation (ECMO)[10]. This enables the generation of complex scenarios in a realistic paediatric intensive care environment.

More sophisticated versions of this circuit are used for teaching and equipment testing. For example a heat exchanger, oxygenator and reservoir have been assembled to act as the patient for equipment testing in a simulated environment[8].

Screen-based computer simulations intended for use in perfusion training have been described, but are not in widespread use[9]. Similarly, numerical modelling has been used in the study of the hydraulic behaviour of the circulation. However, these models have not been elaborated to provide teaching tools for perfusionists.

A recent American study of paediatric ECMO training at 32 centres showed that all used lectures, 88% a closed-loop circuit and 16% used an animal laboratory[10].

Large animal models such as sheep and pigs are useful as they provide a detailed and realistic simulation of a patient[11]. However, while these models are realistic, the cost of such models, the expertise needed to undertake them and the ethical issues surrounding animal experimentation limit their usefulness. The difficulties associated with the use of these models have highlighted the need for a realistic, high fidelity perfusion simulation system.

27.3 Potential role of a high fidelity perfusion simulation system

The possible applications of a high fidelity simulation in perfusion include:

- ◆ Skill training of perfusionists.
- ◆ Certification and accreditation of perfusionists.
- ◆ Development of crisis management protocols.

- Practise of crisis and crew resource management.
- Evaluation of new or existing perfusion equipment.
- Evaluation of novel techniques.

27.3.1 Skill training of perfusionists

Skill training of perfusionists involves the practice of specific activities. For new trainees this might simply mean going on and off bypass, administering cardioplegia or dealing with perturbations in patient physiology.

In this context, the most basic bypass sequence can be defined as the:

- initiation of bypass
- administration of a vasopressor
- application of a cross-clamp
- administration of cardioplegia
- release of a cross-clamp
- weaning from bypass.

This minimal sequence can be performed in less than 5 minutes using a simulator, and, furthermore, can be repeatedly practised. In contrast, a real (single) coronary artery graft usually occupies a perfusionist for 3–4 hours, during which time only one bypass sequence is undertaken.

For more advanced trainees, skill training in areas such as the use of centrifugal pumps, soft-shell reservoirs or assisted venous drainage can be undertaken.

27.3.2 Certification and accreditation of perfusionists

At the present time, no regulatory authority uses simulation in the training or recertification of perfusionists. Typically, trainees are required to undertake a formal course of study, keep a logbook of cases managed and pass some form of written and/or *viva voce* examination. In the UK, the trainee is also observed during the conduct of a single case.

The major regulatory authorities have also implemented some form of recertification requirement into their programmes. Typically, recertification is granted if the applicant can show that he or she has undertaken a minimum annual caseload and fulfilled certain ongoing educational commitments. None of the authorities require a minimum annual caseload of more than 30 cases and thus it is unlikely that a perfusionist will have been exposed to a major perfusion incident during such a minimum recertification period.

In contrast, simulators have a long history of use in complex, technical domains such as the aviation and nuclear power industries and, in these endeavours, fulfil an essential role in both the initial and ongoing training of participants and as part of the recertification process. Satisfactory performance during simulation checks is a mandatory requirement for recertification of all commercial pilots and has been for many years.

27.3.3 Development of crisis management protocols

Protocols are a vital tool in the effective management of perfusion incidents and most authorities recommend the use of protocols. For example, the Australian and New Zealand College of Anaesthetists suggest that[12]:

- Basic clinical management protocols for extracorporeal perfusion and anticoagulation should be established in consultation with perfusion, anaesthesia, and surgical staff, and be regularly reviewed.

- Protocols for management of critical events should be distributed and regularly practised by all perfusion staff.
- Such protocols must cover gas leaks or failure, blood circuit leaks or rupture, pump failure, oxygenator, filter or heat exchanger malfunction, and the detection of clots in the circuit.

The replacement of a leaking or clotted oxygenator requires the disconnection, reconnection and priming of multiple circuit components and subsequent checking and de-airing of the system during a period of circulatory arrest. Clearly, the outcome of this process is directly related to the accuracy with which it is performed, the duration of the arrest and the tolerance of this period of arrest by the patient.

It is inevitable that a protocol describing the management of oxygenator replacement will be a relatively complicated document. (The protocol in current use at St George Hospital describes 36 discrete steps.) Such documents are most easily developed and tested using high fidelity simulators. Furthermore, using simulation, the effect of subtle changes to protocol can be judged by measuring not only the time required for execution of the procedure, but by examining more sensitive markers of efficiency such as the nadir of mixed venous or tissue PO_2, or the macroembolic or microembolic load created as a result of the replacement.

27.3.4 Practise of crisis and crew resource management

The ability to handle crises promptly and effectively is a *sine qua non* of any healthcare professional. Given that catastrophic perfusion incidents are relatively uncommon[1], it is apparent that this ability cannot be acquired easily through experience. Rather, some form of practice is essential.

Scenario training, or 'full mission rehearsal' in military parlance, involves the establishment of a detailed environment with extensive props, actors playing supporting roles and a scripted series of events or challenges. It provides an ideal opportunity for the members of a cardiac surgical team to hone their skills in the management of a specific perfusion incident.

The scenario is usually preceded by a discussion of the underlying theoretical issues and a presentation of the response protocol and followed by a debriefing in which the actions of the participants and the response of the patient are analysed in detail. An example of a scenario plan relating to the failure of gas supply to the oxygenator is presented below.

27.3.5 Evaluation of new or existing perfusion equipment

Traditionally, the introduction of any new form of perfusion equipment into an institution occurs under the guidance of an experienced company representative or other expert. Following a period of 'acclimatization' (which varies in length according to the complexity of the equipment) the perfusionist then begins to use the device in an unsupervised manner. This process is expensive in terms of both time and money therefore the length of the supervisory period could be significantly reduced if some initial experience were gained on a realistic simulator.

It should also be remembered that some forms of equipment evaluation simply cannot be undertaken clinically for ethical reasons. Thus, for example, the air-handling characteristics of different oxygenators cannot be examined *in vivo* and can only be evaluated using some form of more-or-less complex simulation system[13,14].

Similarly, the problems associated with the use of nonocclusive, centrifugal pumps (in particular the propensity to backflow) are better demonstrated using a simulation system.

27.3.6 **Evaluation of novel techniques**

As with the evaluation of new perfusion devices, a simulator can also be used to evaluate novel perfusion techniques. So, for example, Munster *et al.* developed their vacuum assisted venous drainage system using a simple simulator[15].

27.4 **Orpheus® – a new high fidelity perfusion simulation system**

Orpheus® is a high fidelity patient simulator (manufactured by Ulco Medical, Sydney Australia) specifically intended for use in the domain of CPB practice. It is a 'hybrid' system comprising a computer-controlled hydraulic model of the human circulation and a suite of real-time computer models which continuously calculate various cardiorespiratory, thermal and pharmacodynamic parameters within the patient. In addition, the system supervisor (trainer) can use the simulator control program to initiate a variety of systemic failures (power, gas, circuit and oxygenator) or to deliver a series of audiovisual cues to the perfusionist (trainee). The system is designed to interface with any modern heart–lung machine (HLM), patient monitoring system, and CPB circuit.

27.4.1 **Description of the Orpheus® perfusion simulation system**

The principal components of the Orpheus® perfusion simulation system are the:

- hydraulic simulator
- electronic control unit
- simulator control software
- failure devices
- trainee screen
- recording system.

These components are shown in Figs. 27.1 and 27.2.

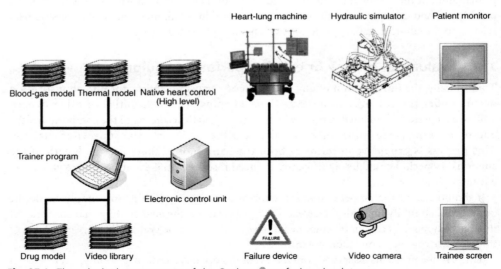

Fig. 27.1 The principal components of the Orpheus® perfusion simulator.

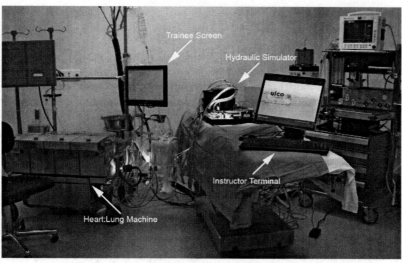

Fig. 27.2 The Orpheus® simulator. The electronic control unit is under the operating table and is not well seen.

The hydraulic simulator is a 'single' circulation comprising two chambers (atrium and ventricle) together with appropriate resistances and capacitances. In addition, the device includes a thermal mass which corresponds roughly to the size of a 70 kg patient, a myocardium that can be perfused with a cardioplegic solution, and a pleural cavity that can accumulate lost blood. The hydraulic simulator can be physically connected to any CPB circuit, HLM and patient monitoring system.

The electronic control unit (ECU) is the interface between the trainer's computer and the hydraulic simulator. It translates commands from the trainer's computer into activity in the hydraulic simulator or the failure devices. In addition, it provides the basic behaviour of the simulator including the cardiac rhythm, myocardial contractility and atrial activity.

The principal functions of the simulator control program include the:

- running of the real-time drug, cardiorespiratory and thermal models
- control of the hydraulic simulator
- streaming of audiovisual prompts
- recording of the trainee's responses
- recording of the physiological and hydraulic data
- initiation (and termination) of system failures.

The control program can either be run on the host computer or on a remote, networked device.

The drug model used by the system continually updates effect compartment concentrations by solving a set of differential equations describing a three compartment pharmacokinetic model. The model allows for the administration of bolus doses or infusions of the following drugs:

- metaraminol
- phenylephrine
- adrenalin
- atropine

- sodium nitroprusside
- heparin
- protamine.

The drugs can be administered as bolus doses or as infusions.

The cardiorespiratory model is a software module which replicates the behaviour of the respiratory gases and metabolic acids under the instantaneous conditions of blood flow, lung ventilation and temperature.

A freestanding, screen-based version of the model which receives its input data through a user interface rather than directly from the hydraulic unit is also available.

Data from the model are presented to the user in the form of arterial and venous blood gas analyses. These data can either be viewed as printed reports or as the output of a continuously updating intravascular blood gas electrode system similar to the Terumo CDI^{TM}. The model consists of a 'single' ventricular circuit which allows for the inclusion of an artificial lung in parallel with the native lung of the patient. Both lungs behave as 'open glottis' systems, which are connected to the atmosphere when not ventilated.

Fig. 27.3 shows the outcome of an exercise which is designed to explore the impact of ventilatory failure (induced by disconnection) in either the natural or the artificial lung on PaO_2. The results of two separate experiments have been superimposed onto a single graph. This exercise demonstrates the usefulness of the simulator as an experimental system for students to test various hypotheses.

Under similar nominal conditions*, ventilation to the natural lung (red) or gas flow to the artificial lung (blue) ceases at time zero. In the case of the artificial lung, note how quickly PaO_2 falls. Note also, that when the PaO_2 approaches the mixed venous point, the decline proceeds

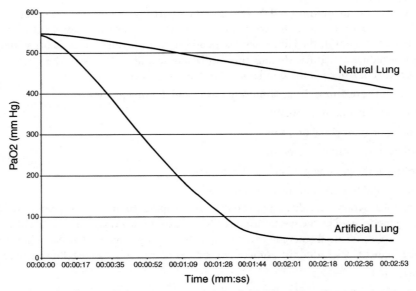

Fig. 27.3 The decline in PaO_2 following disconnection of the oxygen supply to the oxygenator compared with cessation of ventilation to a natural lung under the same nominal conditions. Temperature 37°C; Blood flow 4.25 L/min; FiO2 1.0; Haematocrit 30%; VO_2 200 ml/min.

more slowly. This aspect of the model's function has been validated against that described by Hardman *et al.*[16]

An exercise such as this can be used to teach trainees several important points about artificial lungs and cardiopulmonary bypass. First, the exercise can be used to demonstrate that the functional residual capacity (FRC) of an oxygenator is not large and that, unlike the natural lung, it contains only a small reserve of oxygen. As a result, if gas supply fails in the face of continuing blood flow, then the effluent blood rapidly attains the composition of the incoming venous blood.

Second, the exercise can be used to illustrate the role of the mixed venous blood as a potential oxygen store and the importance of the maintenance of blood flow to the patient – even in the presence of failing oxygenation. The concept of oxygen delivery can be developed and strategies for optimizing the relationship between oxygen delivery and oxygen utilization can be explored.

Finally, the exercise can also be used to highlight the problems associated with monitoring gas flow through an artificial lung. In particular, it can be used to emphasise the point that a visible indication of flow (such as a moving rotameter bobbin) does not necessarily imply continuity of gas supply to the oxygenator.

The benefits of using exhaust gas monitoring as confirmation of gas supply to the oxygenator can then be discussed and the relative merits of the various forms of gas supply monitoring can be examined.

Using data drawn from the simulation system and from other sources, a hierarchy of utility in the detection of gas supply disconnection can be established. This hierarchy is shown in Table 27.3, which shows the time that typically elapses after disconnection before certain sentinel events become evident.

The data represent the case of a patient at 28°C who is perfused at a blood flow rate of 4.25 L/min with a haematocrit of 30%, a basal metabolic rate of 200 ml/min (at 37°C), and in whom 100% oxygen has been supplied to the artificial lung before disconnection.

The table demonstrates that, at one end of the spectrum, side stream, exhaust gas analysis is able to detect gas line disconnection within a few seconds (DAP, personal observation). In comparison, an inline, intravascular blood gas electrode will detect a rise in $PaCO_2$ from, say, 36 mmHg to 40 mmHg within 30 seconds and a fall in PaO_2 from, say, 600 mmHg to 540 mmHg within 1–2 minutes. However, a measured fall of 5% in either the arterial or mixed venous saturation will not be evident until about 5 minutes after disconnection, and visible desaturation (the presence of 3 g/dL of desaturated haemoglobin in the arterial blood) will not be present

Table 27.3 The time required for occurrence of a particular sentinel event after the oxygen supply is disconnected at the oxygenator

Monitor	Criterion	Time to event
Exhaust gas analysis (side stream)	Step change in PO_2 or PCO_2	~ 10 seconds
Intravascular $PaCO_2$	Rise in PCO_2 >10%	~ 30 seconds
Intravascular PaO_2	Fall in PO_2 >10%	~ 1.5 minutes
Arterial saturation (measured)	Fall in saturation >5%	~ 5 minutes
Venous saturation (measured)	Fall in saturation >5%	~ 5 minutes
Visible desaturation[18]	Desaturated Hb >3 g/dL	~ 10 minutes
Oxygen rotameter	Change in indicated flow rate	∞
Inspired oxygen	Change in O_2 concentration	∞

until about 10 minutes after disconnection (DAP, personal observation). Finally, no form of 'upstream' monitoring of gas supply will ever suggest the presence of disconnection.

The cardiorespiratory model is loosely based on the work of C J Dickinson that has been described in the book *A Computer Model of Human Respiration*[17].

27.4.2 **Other functions of the simulator control program**

The simulator control program is also used for high-level control of the hydraulic model. It can be used to change parameters such as myocardial contractility, systemic vascular resistance, pulse rate and cardiac rhythm.

A library of audiovisual clips can be streamed to the trainee's screen by the simulation controller. The clips show the surgeon undertaking manoeuvres such as cannulation, decannulation and aortic cross-clamping. The simulator incorporates a real-time MPEG4 videorecording system, which records the trainee's responses and a physiological and hydraulic data recording system which outputs to an Excel™ spreadsheet.

A wide variety of system failures can be initiated (and terminated) by the simulation controller. These failures include:

- oxygen supply failure
- oxygenator failure
- electrical supply failure to the HLM, heater/cooler and patient monitor
- air-locking of the venous line
- kinking of the venous line
- occlusion of the arterial line.

The trainee screen is a touch-screen terminal that is attached to the HLM. The terminal provides:

- the results of blood-gas analysis
- the results of activated clotting time measurement
- a drug administration interface
- a view of the surgical field.

The system has been designed to allow for the future inclusion of an intra-aortic balloon pump (IABP), venovenous extracorporeal membrane oxygenator (ECMO), a left ventricular assist device (LVAD) or the inclusion of a real-time two dimensional echo sector scan.

The Orpheus® perfusion simulator is distributed with a series of scenarios that have been developed for use with the system. The following scenario is based on accidental disconnection of the gas supply at the oxygenator.

27.4.3 **Sample scenario**

27.4.3.1 **Overview**

The scenario is one of unexplained hypoxaemia, occurring during the course of aortic valve replacement, which has been caused by an unrecognized disconnection of the gas supply to the oxygenator. The disconnection occurs when the aorta has been opened, so that withdrawal from CPB is not a management option. Other problems are explored in the debriefing and can be run as alternate forms of the scenario with more advanced participants or as part of a training sequence on this topic.

27.4.3.2 Learning objectives

+ Recognition of hypoxia on bypass.
+ Differential diagnosis of hypoxia on bypass.
+ Management of hypoxia on bypass.
+ Effective use of second colleague for support in troubleshooting.

27.4.3.3 Faculty roles

+ Simulation manager in the control room.
+ Actor surgeon.
+ Actor anaesthetist.

27.4.3.4 Participant roles

+ Primary perfusionist.
+ Second perfusionist (available to be called in to assist).

27.4.3.5 Simulator set-up

+ Normal systemic vascular resistance.
+ Cross-clamp on.
+ Activated clotting time 700 seconds.
+ Temperature 28°C.
+ Haematocrit 30%.
+ Basal metabolic rate (37°C) 200 ml/min.

27.4.3.6 Room and equipment set-up

+ HLM circuit set up and primed.
+ Simulator draped on operating table connected to HLM and patient monitor.
+ Main arterial pump flow 4.25 L/min.
+ Oxygenator FiO_2 1.0.
+ Oxygenator gas flow 3.0 L/min.
+ Gas supply line to oxygenator is disconnected between the rotameter and the oxygenator.

27.4.3.7 Initial scenario

The following information is supplied to the trainee:

You are asked to go into theatre to relieve a perfusionist who needs to take a short break. The departing perfusionist tells you that:

+ *The patient is an otherwise fit 45-year-old with severe aortic stenosis and a bicuspid aortic valve, who is undergoing aortic valve replacement. He has no other significant comorbidities.*
+ *The surgeon is somewhat irritable, as the case has proved unexpectedly difficult. He has asked for various pieces of equipment (including the HLM) to be repositioned or adjusted several times.*

- *The activated clotting time is >700 seconds.*
- *You are on full bypass (4.25 L/min) at 28°C.*
- *The cross-clamp is on and cardioplegia has just been administered.*
- *Blood gas analysis (just performed) shows:*

PaO_2	*657 mmHg*
$PaCO_2$	*35 mmHg*
pH	*7.50*
HCT	*30%*
SaO_2	*100%*

27.4.3.8 Scenario sequence

- As the relieving perfusionist takes the chair, the simulation manager 'fails' the gas flow to the oxygenator.
- When the oxygen supply is reconnected to the oxygenator the simulation manager 'restores' the gas flow to the oxygenator.

27.4.3.9 Expected response of perfusionist

Once the perfusionist has detected an abnormality, he she should:

- confirm that the FiO_2 is 1.0
- confirm rotameter flow
- confirm the integrity of the gas supply connection to the oxygenator
- confirm the absence of obstruction to exhaust gas from the oxygenator
- check the inlet and outlet pressures of the oxygenator
- inspect the oxygenator for clot
- perform a blood gas analysis
- request that the other perfusionist return to theatre
- advise the surgeon and anaesthetist.

27.4.3.10 Evaluation criteria

Several evaluation criteria can be used in the assessment of the trainee. The objective criteria include the:

- time taken to recognize that there was a problem
- time taken to restore gas flow
- nadir of PaO_2.

  The subjective assessment can be based on the:

- performance of a handover check
- demonstration of a systematic approach to problem solving
- demonstration of the effective use of assistance in handling the event
- demonstration of effective communication with the surgeon and anaesthetist.

27.4.3.11 Questions to the trainee during debriefing

◆ Defusing:

What did you think had happened?

How did you feel when the saturation started to fall?

◆ Technical:

What was your differential diagnosis?

What was your plan for each of them?

What extra equipment would have been useful?

Would a checklist have been any help?

◆ Non-technical:

Who could have helped you?

How could you get them to buy in?

Could you have divided the tasks up differently?

How was the communication with the surgeon/anaesthetist/second perfusionist?

What other resources were available?

27.4.3.12 Instructor notes

◆ The utility of various forms of monitoring in detecting disconnection of the gas supply can be discussed with the trainee (Table 27.3).

◆ The effect of temperature on the evolution of hypoxaemia can be explored (Fig. 27.4).

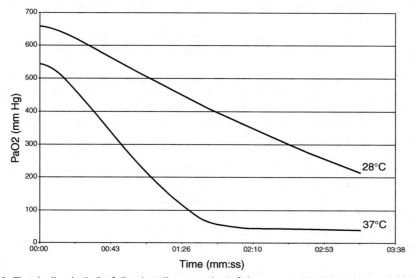

Fig. 27.4 The decline in PaO_2 following disconnection of the oxygen supply to the oxygenator at two different temperatures. The disconnection occurs at time zero from otherwise identical nominal conditions. The PaO_2 at 28°C has not been temperature corrected (i.e. is reported at 37°C).

◆ A more challenging alternative to the 'oxygen line disconnection' scenario is to have the oxygenator itself fail. This will involve the more difficult problem of actually changing out part of the circuit during circulatory arrest. This can be run as a subsequent scenario building on the learning from the first scenario.

This scenario provides an example of how a new high fidelity simulator can be used to enhance learning of cardiopulmonary bypass. The use of simulation for the training of perfusionists is particularly suited to the nature of this work environment, the tasks undertaken and the types of critical incidents encountered.

The Authors declare a commercial interest as part of the research and development team of the Orpheus simulator described in this chapter.

References

1. Stammers AH, Mejak BL (2001). An update on perfusion safety: does the type of perfusion practice affect the rate of incidents related to cardiopulmonary bypass? *Perfusion* **16**: 189–98.

2. Jenkins OF, Morris RW, Simpson JM (1997). Australasian perfusion incident survey. *Perfusion* **12**: 279–88.

3. Kurusz M, Conti VR, Arens JF, Brown W, Faulkner SC, Manning JV (1986). Perfusion Accident Survey. *Proc Am Acad Cardiovasc Perfusion* **7**: 57–65.

4. Wheeldon DR (1986). Safety during cardiopulmonary bypass. In: Taylor KM ed. *Cardiopulmonary Bypass: Principles and Management*. London: Chapman & Hall: 399– 422.

5. Dickinson CJ (1972.) A digital computer model to teach and study gas transport and exchange between lungs, blood and tissues ('MacPuf'). *J Physiol (Lond)* **224**(1): 7P–9P

6. van Meurs WL, Nikkelen E, Good ML (1998). Pharmacokinetic-pharmacodynamic model for educational simulations. *IEEE Trans Biomed Eng* **45**(5): 582–90.

7. Health, United States (2006). *Chartbook on Trends in the Health of Americans.*. National Center for Health Statistics. DHHS Publication No. 2006–1232: Table 99.

8. Schreur A, Niles S, Ploessl J (2005). Use of the CDI blood parameter monitoring system 500 for continuous blood gas measurement during extracorporeal membrane oxygenation simulation. *J Extra Corpor Technol* **37**(4): 377–80.

9. Austin J, Riley J, Calkins J (2003). Competency assessment and analysis of cardiovascular perfusionists using a scenario-based cardiopulmonary bypass simulator. *International Meeting on Medical Simulation*. San Diego, CA.

10. Anderson JM, Boyle KB, Murphy AA, *et al.* (2006.) Simulating extracorporeal membrane oxygenation emergencies to improve human performance. Part 1: methodologic and technical innovations. *Simul Healthcare* **1**: 220–7.

11. Terry B, Gunst G, Melchior R, *et al.* (2005). A description of a prototype miniature extracorporeal membrane oxygenation circuit using current technologies in a sheep model. *J Extra Corpor Technol* **37**(3): 315–7.

12. Professional Standards Document PS27 (2007). *Guidelines for Fellows who Practise Major Extracorporeal Perfusion*. Australia and New Zealand College of Anaesthetists.

13. Beckley PD, Shinko PD, Sites JP (1997.) A comparison of gaseous emboli release in five membrane oxygenators. *Perfusion* **12**(2): 133–41.

14. Rider SP, Simon LV, Rice BJ, Poulton CC (1998). Assisted venous drainage, venous air, and gaseous microemboli transmission into the arterial line: an in-vitro study. *J Extra Corpor Technol* **30**(4): 160–5.

15. Munster K, Andersen U, Mikkelsen J, Pettersson G (1999). Vacuum assisted venous drainage (VAVD). *Perfusion* **14**(6): 419–23.

16. Hardman JG, Wills JS, Aitkenhead AR (2000). Factors determining the onset and course of hypoxemia during apnea: an investigation using physiological modelling. *Anesth Analg* **90**(3): 619–24.

17. C J Dickinson (1997). *A Computer Model of Human Respiration*. First Edition, MTP Press.

18. JF Nunn (1993). *Nunn's Applied Respiratory Physiology*. Fourth Edition. Butterworth Heinemann: 294.

Chapter 28

Simulation for military medical training

Mark W Bowyer and E Matt Ritter

Overview

- Training for both civilian and military trauma care is challenging.
- Training for military environments or care in civilian austere environments must take into account the potential for long delays to definitive care and environmental stressors.
- Simulation applications ranging from physical models to virtual reality computers are either available or being developed to improve trauma skills training.
- The major advantage to using simulation for military training is the ability to practice in a safe environment without risk to patient or provider.
- Currently available validation studies have shown simulation based training to be at least as good as and often better than traditional training strategies.
- Simulation will play an expanding role in trauma skills training in the future.

28.1 Introduction

The care of patients with multiple severe injuries as a result of trauma requires extensive training for all involved. Every member of the trauma team must possess both the individual knowledge and skill to care for the patient as well as understand their role in the overall team. For civilian trauma in the urban setting, where pre-hospital transport times are frequently less than 10 minutes, training for trauma skill management can be focused in specialized trauma centres where interventions such as definitive airway management, control of haemorrhage, performance of tube thoracostomy for haemothorax or pneumothorax, or establishment of intravenous access for fluid resuscitation are typically performed. The care of combat casualties during war time differs in many respects. The transport time from time of injury to definitive care can range from less than an hour when there is air superiority but can be as long as 72 hours. Therefore, it is essential to have a number of pre-hospital providers able to perform these kinds of potentially life saving interventions in the field, and often under austere conditions while engaged in combat. This requires extensive training of not only military doctors and nurses, but a large cadre of battlefield medics who will be called on to provide cutting edge trauma care in some of the worst conditions imaginable.

To help meet this need for extensive, high-quality trauma skills training, the US military has developed a growing interest in the application of emerging simulation technologies to trauma skills training. The goal of incorporating these simulation technologies is not to replace current training, but to augment it. Though to date there has been little study of the use of simulation technology for the training of combat skills, it is logical that lessons learned from other disciplines might well apply. For example, in the field of minimally invasive surgery, both physical and computer based simulators have been shown to predict and improve actual performance in the operating room[1,2]. This is achievable by using simulation solutions that provide feedback to trainees through carefully structured performance metrics, and by requiring training on these simulators until some objectively assessed level of performance is achieved. While simulation for the skills required to manage the trauma patient is more challenging than for minimally invasive surgery, the potential benefit is great.

The paragraphs that follow will review the simulation applications and simulators currently available (or being developed) for both trauma skills task training and trauma team training.

28.2 Task training for trauma and combat casualty care

It is well known that traumatic injuries kill in a predictable fashion, and early recognition and timely treatment are often keys to survival. Trauma training emphasizes an 'ABCDE' approach based on the fact that airway problems (A) result in rapid mortality if not recognized and treated in a timely fashion, while breathing problems (B) and circulatory problems (C) will also lead to death, if not treated, but in a more delayed fashion. Improved outcomes have been recognized when healthcare providers are well versed in these basic concepts. The advanced trauma life support course (ATLS) was developed by the American College of Surgery in 1980 to address perceived deficiencies in the early management of traumatically injured patients. Class II and class III data exists that there are improvements in the care of injured patients following implementation of ATLS programmes with decreases in injury mortality[3,4]. ATLS training has been shown to improve the knowledge base, the psychomotor skills and their use in resuscitation, and the confidence and performance of doctors who have been students in this highly successful programme taught around the globe[5,6].

Unfortunately members of the military often have little opportunity to practise these life saving skills. Until very recently, the skills taught in ATLS courses were performed on animals, which are poor surrogates for human anatomy. In addition, the use of animals does not allow for repetitive practise, due to logistics and expense, and is complicated by ethical issues. Recent advances in simulation technology, have led the development of tools which can teach these vital life-saving skills. These simulators range from inexpensive low fidelity models to high fidelity complex virtual reality trainers. Simulators allow several advantages over traditional educational tools. A learner can practice, new procedures on a simulator repetitively until he/she is judged to be proficient without endangering patients. As the students skills progress, the simulator can also present the learner with cases of increasing complexity. The most valuable aspect of the simulator is that gives the learner 'permission to fail', without killing an animal or human, and then learning from mistakes made.

The American College of Surgeons has recently adopted a mannequin to be used for teaching the surgical skills associated with ATLS. This mannequin, TraumaMan® (manufactured by Simulab, Seattle, WA) is a life-sized human torso with thoracic and abdominal cavities and a simulated neck/trachea for teaching trauma essential skills such as cricothyroidotomy, chest tube insertion, pericardiocentesis, diagnostic peritoneal lavage, and cut down for venous access on a separate ankle model (Fig. 28.1) Preliminary experience with this model was well received by students[7], and has led to widespread replacement of animals and cadavers in over half of all ATLS courses being currently taught. The major advantage of the TraumaMan® is that it obviates the need for an animal, making this course available in places that do not have animal lab facilities. Other clear advantages are the accurate human anatomy and the ability to perform the

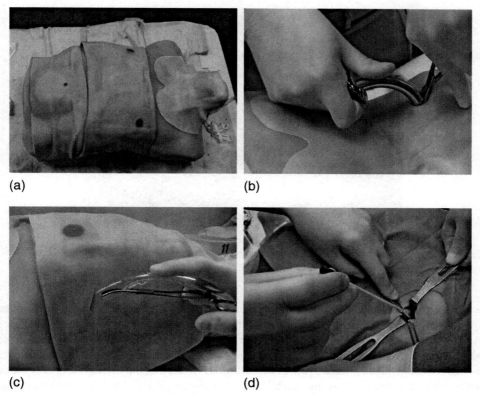

(a)　　　　　　　　　　　(b)

(c)　　　　　　　　　　　(d)

Fig. 28.1 The TraumaMan® (manufactured by Simulab, Seattle, WA) provides a non-animal non-cadaver alternative to teaching trauma skills. It is comprised of a human-like torso (a), with replaceable parts allowing for cricothyroidotomy (b), chest tube insertion (c), and diagnostic peritoneal Lavage (d), as well as pericardiocentesis (not shown).

procedures in the order that they are taught in the course (i.e. doing the airway first), which was the terminal event in the animal model. The mannequin has lungs in the chest and is connected to an air generator that circulates air through the upper airway and the lungs, so that there is fogging of the tube with cricothyroidotomy, and the student will be able to feel the lung when placing a finger into the chest during chest decompression. The major disadvantage of this model is that the cost still remains high, as there is only one such device approved for ATLS courses, and the ability to practise the procedures repetitively becomes cost prohibitive. In addition, static models such as this do not allow for variations in anatomy and physiology that occur in real-life practice.

The military has recognized the need for better training models for their medics and physicians, and therefore several part-task trainers have been developed to meet this need. Several part-task trainers are currently available or under development, and several such examples are listed below.

28.2.1 **Airway part-task trainers**

The earliest airway simulators can be traced back to the pioneering work of Peter Safar on cardiopulmonary resuscitation in the late 1950s[8]. Working with Norwegian doll maker Asmund Laerdal, a full-size training mannequin for mouth-to-mouth ventilation was developed, and served as the springboard for additional airway simulator development[9]. Simulators have been

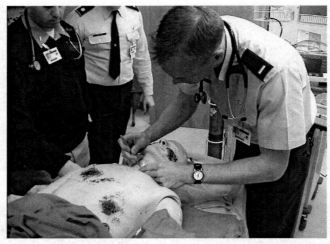

Fig. 28.2 Student performing a surgical airway/cricothyroidotomy on a high fidelity human patient simulator (SimMan® from Laerdal).

used with great success to teach basic airway management. Low fidelity intubation mannequins provide ample opportunity for learners to learn the skills necessary for basic airway management. In head-to-head comparison, models with hard surfaces tend to be less realistic than those with flexible 'skin' such as the Little Anne made by Laerdal[10]. On the other end of the spectrum are high cost high fidelity human patient simulators (HPS) such as the Laerdal SimMan®, which can be intubated, but also has the capability to have obstruction of the airway with laryngeal oedema, pharyngeal oedema, tongue swelling, and trismus. The learner can then perform a surgical airway on the mannequin in an anatomically correct area through replaceable skin (Fig. 28.2). The HPS has been used with great success in teaching emergency airway skills[11,12].

Though both low fidelity and high fidelity mannequins are useful teaching tools they are limited by the inability or limited ability (in the case of the HPS) to alter anatomy. A recent evaluation of the SimMan® concluded that the simulator's airway is generally acceptably realistic, but that it differed from the human airway in important aspects[13]. Students who use this and other simulators must be aware of the differences in order to obtain maximum benefit from training.

Advances in computer technology have led to early development of virtual reality simulators for management of airway problems. One example is a cricothyroidotomy simulator under development in our lab[14]. This simulator combines a graphical user interface with a haptic device that allows the learner to find by palpation the cricothyroid membrane on the screen and make an incision with visible bleeding, and dilate and cannulate the resultant cricothyroidotomy. In the current military conflict in Iraq, it has been the experience of this author that medics are ill prepared to perform this procedure when called upon to do so under fire, with the resultant failed procedure with high potential for loss of life. This cricothyroidotomy simulator was developed specifically to meet the perceived need of the combat medic to provide additional training and familiarity with this high stakes, low frequency procedure. This simulator is currently fielded to Iraq, and is being used to teach combat medics the basics of the procedure, and longitudinal studies of effectiveness will be conducted (Fig. 28.3).

The potential for simulators such as this is great. There is no need for replaceable parts or instruments, and the skill can be practised over and over again merely by resetting the program. The other distinct advantage of simulators such as this is that once developed it is a

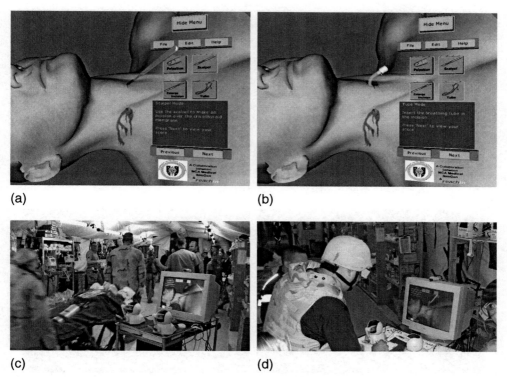

Fig. 28.3 Virtual Reality Cricothyroidotomy simulator combines graphical interface seen above with a haptic interface such that the user feels appropriate tactile feedback when palpating the cricothyroid membrane, making the incision (a), enlarging the incision, and cannulating the trachea (b). This simulator is currently being used to train military medics in a military hospital in Iraq (c) allowing soldiers to practice the skill over and over (d).

straight-forward matter to change the anatomy and body habitus of the virtual patient. Increasing levels of difficulty and complications can be added, with the ability to track performance and provide feedback and opportunities for remediation. For instance, the neck can be altered to represent that of a patient with a short fat neck, or one with an expanding haematoma.

Simulators are becoming an increasing part of integrated curricula, and it is in this role (a part of the curricula) that they seem to be most effective. In the case of teaching airway skills the introduction of simulation into an existing airway management curriculum makes logical sense and improved outcomes in a recent study of flight crews[15].

28.2.2 Simulators for breathing problems

Thoracic trauma is a significant cause of mortality. Many thoracic trauma patients die after reaching the hospital and many of these deaths could be prevented with prompt diagnosis and treatment[16]. Most patients sustaining life-threatening thoracic trauma can be managed with chest tube placement, therefore this skill is essential to teach all healthcare providers to reduce correctable mortality[17]. Teaching this skill to military medics is also of great importance, as treatment of pneumothorax has been identified as one of the things that will improve survival from battlefield injuries[18]. Current simulators for chest tube training are limited. Traditional training has most commonly occurred using cadavers and animals, with the challenges and costs

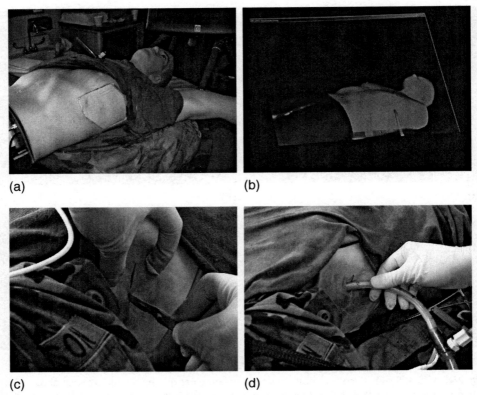

(a)   (b)

(c)   (d)

Fig. 28.4 The VIRGIL chest tube simulator, combines a realistic human form (a) with a graphical user interface (b) that provides instruction and metrics, as well as playback of performance. The student is able to make an incision (c) and place a chest tube (d) through materials that provide realistic resistance and either air or blood upon chest entry.

inherent to both of these modalities. The human patient simulators available from both Laerdal and Medical Education Technologies Inc (METI) offer a portal for chest tube insertion, but both lack realistic resistance of chest wall musculature, and rib detail. Of the part task trainers available for chest tube insertion the TraumaMan® offers the most realistic 'pop' of the clamp entering the chest, and also has 'lungs' within the chest cavity that move against the interrogating finger when placed in the chest.

Responding to the needs of the military, a chest tube simulator was developed by the Center for Integration of Medicine and Innovative Technology in Boston. This simulator, the VIRGIL™ Chest Trauma Training System, combines sophisticated 3D anatomical models generated from CT scans of actual human anatomy with a mannequin built from these models (Fig. 28.4). A touch-screen computer interface leads trainees through a self-directed or instructor led tutorial that covers basic first aid and the management of tension pneumothorax, haemothorax, and haemopneumothorax using either a chest dart and/or a chest tube. All the proper steps of the procedure such as infiltration with local anaesthesia, incision (Fig. 28.4B), clamp insertion, and insertion of the chest tube (Fig. 28.4C) can be performed, and are tracked for immediate feedback. The instruments used with VIRGIL™ are tracked with a software package that follows the motion of the instrument relative to the anatomy. When the trainee completes the procedure, the system automatically plays back the path of the tube or dart showing whether or not the treatment was successful (Fig. 28.4D).

VIRGIL™ has undergone some preliminary validation studies with the finding that the simulator is at least equivalent to an animal model if not better for teaching medical students to insert chest tubes (Bowyer, MW unpublished data). The replaceable portals used with VIRGIL™ have realistic skin, soft tissue, muscle, and rib materials with a fairly reasonable approximation of the resistance encountered when inserting a chest tube in a human. The limitation of this particular simulator is that it is not yet commercially available and the cost for the replaceable portals is still high.

28.2.3 Simulators for circulatory problems

One rapidly life-threatening condition associated with thoracic trauma is cardiac tamponade. This can occur with either blunt or penetrating trauma to the chest, and the accumulation of blood in the sac around the heart leads to compromise of circulation with resultant hypotension and death if not corrected[16,17]. Prompt recognition and treatment of this condition should be accomplished before addressing other circulatory concerns as it can be rapidly fatal. Recent advances in bedside ultrasound technology have made this historically difficult at times diagnosis much easier to make. Prompt evacuation of pericardial blood is a lifesaving manoeuvre and is most simply achieved by performing pericardiocentesis[19]. Traditionally the animal model has been used in ATLS courses to teach pericardiocentesis, but are limited by the distinct differences in anatomy. The use of cadavers is also unsatisfying as the ability to instill fluid around the heart is limited. The TraumaMan® simulator provides realistic human anatomy with fluid return if performed properly (Fig. 28.5A). The HPS from METI also allows for performance of a pericardiocentesis. Virtual reality pericaridocentesis simulators are currently under development by Immersion Medical (Gaithersburg, MD), and also by the National Capital Area Medical Simulation Center (Fig. 28.5B) of the Uniformed Services University (Bethesda, MD)[20]. Both systems incorporate a graphical user interface with haptics such that the trainee gets tactile feedback as the needle is inserted in the chest. The advantage of such systems is that the student can practise over and over again with or without faculty at low cost.

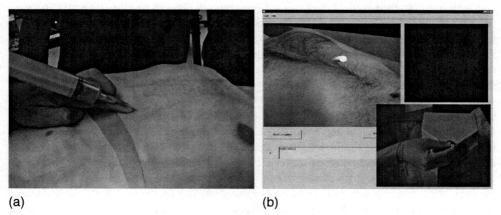

(a) (b)

Fig. 28.5 Pericardiocentesis being performed with return of blood on the TraumaMan® (a) and a Virtual Reality Simulator (b) where the movements of the needle at the haptic interface are translated to the computer screen.

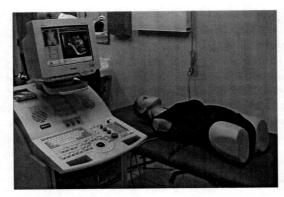

Fig. 28.6 The UltraSim® simulator for ultrasound training.

Haemorrhage is the most common cause of shock in the trauma patient[21] and extremity haemorrhage specifically is the leading cause of potentially preventable death on the battlefield[22]. When dealing with disorders of circulation, trainees must be able to recognize and control haemorrhage, and replace the intravascular fluid deficits that arise.

The first step in the management of haemorrhage is recognition, which is not always as straightforward as it seems. While life-threatening bleeding from an extremity is often visible, bleeding from other sites may not be directly seen. Unlike the extremity, intra-abdominal bleeding can be subtle, and the ability to rapidly and reliably assess the peritoneal cavity for bleeding is an essential skill. The most common method of assessing the abdomen of a haemodynamically stable trauma patient is with a CT scan, but this is typically not an option for the unstable trauma patient or the military patient in the field. For these patients, the diagnostic modalities of choice are either ultrasonography with the Focused Assessment with Sonography for Trauma (FAST) exam, or a diagnostic peritoneal lavage (DPL). Simulation applications are available to train both of these skills.

To perform a FAST exam, providers must correctly image and interpret four anatomic locations, looking for blood. The UltraSim® (MedSim USA, Ft Lauderdale FL) is a computer based simulation application available to facilitate this training (Fig. 28 6). The computer software recreates actual patient images that correlate with the orientation of probe placement on a simulated patient mannequin. Trauma related modules in the UltraSim® software recreate a normal, negative FAST exam as well as positive findings in all areas of investigation. In addition, fluid accumulation over time can be simulated so that while the initial FAST exam is negative, positive findings will be present on subsequent exams.

Only a single study is available comparing UltraSim® training *versus* live patient training for the performance of the FAST exam[23]. This study consisted of a group of surgical residents who were trained on the simulator and a similar group trained using live patients who demonstrated both negative and positive findings. Both groups significantly improved their abilities to perform and interpret the FAST exam and no differences were detectable in the groups after either mode of training. This showed that simulation can replace the cost and inconvenience of using real patients. While training time in both groups of this study was limited to 1 hour, the additional training made possible by the availability afforded by the simulator may have resulted in additional skills improvement with continued practice.

An important adjunct to the management of trauma patients is the DPL. This procedure involves placing a catheter into the abdomen and instilling fluid into the abdomen and then

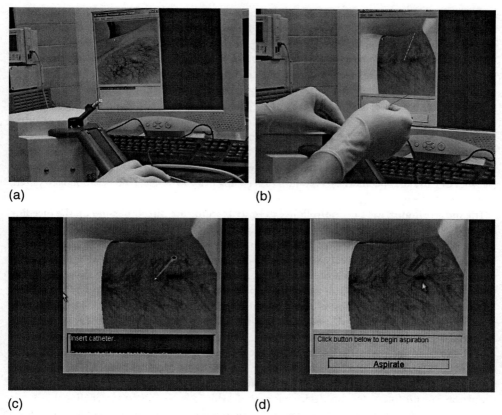

(a) (b)

(c) (d)

Fig. 28.7 The SimPL, a simulator for Diagnostic Peritoneal Lavage training consists of a haptic enabled graphical user interface (a) in which motions made on the interface are seen in real time on the computer screen (b). The student is taken through all steps of the procedure such as inserting the catheter (c) and aspiration (d) with a report of performance generated.

withdrawing it. If blood in a certain amount is recovered the lavage is considered positive and the patient likely to need surgical intervention[24]. Advances in ultrasound technology have lead to the use of small portable devices at the bedside for trauma and have all but replaced DPL in most trauma centres[25]. In spite of the widespread existence of small ultrasound devices, they are not universally available and the need to teach DPL remains and continues to be part of the ATLS course. This is particularly true in the military setting where the usual tools may not be available, and therefore it is important that military providers be facile with DPL. Given the fact that DPL is infrequently performed in most current clinical settings, the need for adequate training is magnified. Traditionally, this skill has been taught using an animal model with all of the associated anatomical and ethical difficulties. Both a physical simulation and computer based simulation application for training this skill currently exist.

The TraumaMan® simulator allows for the practice of DPL (Fig. 28.7A), but has the limitation of cost and anatomical invariability previously discussed. A computer based simulator for diagnostic peritoneal lavage, SimPL, has been developed by the National Capital Area Medical Simulation Center (Uniformed Services University, Bethesda, MD)[26]. SimPL is a haptic enabled, needle based, graphical user interface that can be used to teach the requisite skills of

DPL (Fig. 28.7B). This simulator has undergone a validation study during which training on SimPL was compared to training on an animal in a prospective randomized trial. After completing either arm of training, subjects performed a DPL on the TraumaMan® mannequin and had their performance scored by a blinded senior trauma surgeon. The SimPL group out-performed the animal group with respect to site selection and execution for the steps of the Seldinger technique[27]. Unfortunately, the SimPL is not commercially available at this time.

Whether the source of haemorrhage is in the abdomen or extremities, once it is recognized, it must be controlled. Control of intra-abdominal haemorrhage for trauma typically requires a celiotomy, and almost universally required in the military combat setting. Currently no simulation application exists to train the skills required to perform a trauma celiotomy and this is a procedure that should only be performed by a fully trained surgeon at an appropriately equipped facility. For extremity haemorrhage, control of bleeding prior to surgical intervention is required, and can often be life saving.

The most common ways of controlling extremity bleeding are direct pressure on the bleeding site, and use of a tourniquet. While most minor bleeding will cease with direct pressure, rapid or poorly exposed sites of bleeding will not be controllable with this method. The rapid and correct application of a tourniquet in this setting can be life saving. Traditionally, training for the control of extremity haemorrhage has been done using anaesthetized animals, typically the swine. While under general anaesthesia, a limb is severed and vessels divided. The trainee must then control the bleeding through application of direct pressure and/or a tourniquet. Problems with this type of training model are multiple and include differences in anatomy, differences in the force required on the tourniquet to arrest bleeding, ethical concerns for the animals, and lack of repeatable training as erroneous management frequently results in death of the animal. To address these problems and improve training, the US Army Medical Research and Material Command has funded the development of a computer based Exsanguinating Limb Hemorrhage simulator. The prototype for this device has been developed by SimQuest International in Silver Spring Maryland and consists of a sensored haptic interface device shaped like a generic limb married to a software package. It allows for physics based pulse and blood flow, and accurately measures the constricting force applied to the limb to give the user the sense of the forces required to arrest bleeding from a human limb in various physiological conditions. While this simulator is still under development, it holds great promise for training future providers.

After haemorrhage is recognized and hopefully controlled, the final step is restoration of intravascular volume to allow for adequate cardiovascular function. This fluid is most commonly replaced via direct intravenous administration. This direct route, however, requires placement of an intravenous cannula, preferably of large diameter in a peripheral vein. The technique of peripheral venous access is an absolutely essential skill for those providers caring for traumatically injured patients and is currently taught to all levels of providers from the first responder in the field to the surgeon in the trauma centre. Traditionally this skill has been taught on patients (i.e. the student received didactic instruction on the procedure, observed a few procedures, and then began to perform the procedure on actual patients who required venous access). While this method has been an effective way to learn, it comes at the expense of the patients we are trying to help. Luckily over the past few decades there have been developed several simulation applications to aid in the training of this technique.

The most basic class of simulation trainer is the 'rubber arm' (Fig. 28.8a). This product which is available from multiple manufacturers is essentially a recreation of a human arm. Deep to the synthetic skin is a series of fluid filled tubes to simulate veins. When the needle accesses the tubing, a 'flash' of blood is simulated and the catheter may be advanced into the tubing. While this type of simulator does allow for practise of the steps of the procedure, the feel produced by the

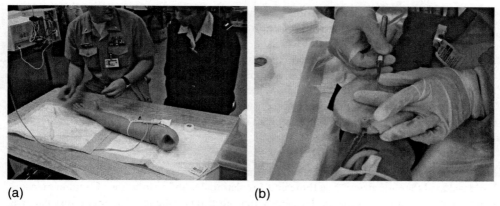

(a)   (b)

Fig. 28.8 A typical 'rubber arm' simulator for teaching intravenous cannulation (a) and the ACF Antecubital Fossa Pad (b).

synthetic tissue often causes difficulty, there is no objective feedback provided on performance, and any feedback that is received requires a trained observer to be present throughout the procedure. Additionally the arm doesn't allow trainees to learn to prepare patients for the procedure through communication, and is difficult in incorporate into combined trauma training scenarios. A slight but significant twist on the 'rubber arm' theme that helps overcome some these short-comings is the Ante Cubital Fossa (ACF) Pad (Limbs and Things, Bristol UK). This device shown in Fig. 28.8B is a pad that can be applied with a Velcro strap to a real arm. The pad contains a fluid filled series of veins based on the anatomy of the antecubital fossa. It can be connected to an external fluid reservoir to allow for blood draws and actual fluid administration, thus in addition to placing the catheter, fluids can be administered to determine if the catheter is truly functional. This device can be directly applied to simulated patients for incorporation into mass casualty and other trauma training scenarios, and has performed well in our experience using the device to train and assess our military medical students during field exercises.

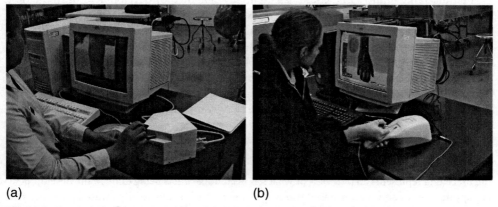

(a)   (b)

Fig. 28.9 The CathSim® IV trainer (a) and the Virtual-IV trainer® (b) both incorporate a haptic interface with graphical representation of a patient with actions on the interface reproduced on the computer screen.

In addition to the physical simulation applications, computer based simulation applications have also been developed. The two best know of these are CathSim® (Immersion Medical, Gaithersburg MD) (Fig. 28.9A) and Virtual-IV® (Laerdal Medical, Gatesville TX) (Fig. 28.9B). Both of these computer based simulators combine a software application with a haptics interface device to virtually recreate the procedure. Since the entire procedure is virtual, more robust performance feedback data can be obtained from these simulators than with the physical simulators. This along with the ability to practice repeatedly without incurring additional cost makes training until achievement of a level of skills proficiency a major benefit of this type of simulation[28].

28.2.4 Simulators for disability

Simulation applications for the detection, treatment, and prevention of disability are somewhat less developed than for airway, breathing and circulation. Disability in terms of trauma management usually equates to neurological disability, but can also be expanded to other injury patterns that can result in disabling injury such as ocular injury or major orthopaedic trauma.

Eye injuries have been historically noted in 5–10% of all combat casualties, and also occur in civilian trauma[22]. In contrast to civilian trauma, military casualties are subject to long transport times to a facility equipped with ophthalmological capabilities. In Vietnam, nearly 50% of all penetrating eye injuries resulted in globe loss[22]. Currently, in an effort to decrease the rate of globe loss, ophthalmic operative microscopes are available at Level IV and some Level III military medical facilities. While the equipment often required for globe salvage is now more readily available, current practices of surgeon sub-specialization means that many ophthalmologists may not routinely perform intraocular procedures in their peacetime practices, and thus not be confident in their technical abilities to perform such procedures in the trauma setting. There is currently one simulation application available that may aid military ophthalmologists in maintaining these skills and thus possibly improve the globe salvage rate. The EYESI (VRMagic, Mannheim Germany) is a computer based virtual reality simulator for training intraocular surgical skills. The software package includes modules for fundamental psychomotor skills training as well as performance of vitrectomy and intraocular membrane manipulation. Like most other computer based simulators, robust performance metrics can be generated to guide training. Currently, no trials have demonstrated the benefit of EYESI for intraocular training, but those studies are planned.

Other disabling injuries that could be potentially benefited by development of simulation training applications include management of extremity fractures, identification and treatment of compartment syndrome, and identification and treatment of intracranial bleeding. The US Army's Telemedicine and Advanced Technology Research Center (TATRC) is either funding or seeking to fund development of simulation applications to address all of these issues. Work to this end is currently underway in both the National Capital Area Medical Simulation Center and elsewhere. One such project (a military thigh trauma simulator) is being developed by Touch of Life Technologies using a virtual environment based on the Visible Human Project[29].

28.3 Future directions

The preceding represents an overview of what has been done and is being done in the development and application of simulation-based training to the care of traumatically injured patients. The 'simulators' range from simple rubber mannequins to complex virtual reality computer systems. As the simulation effort in trauma moves forward, we will see advances in two main areas, the technology of the simulation, and the application of the simulation to training.

The first area of advancement, improving technology, is what we see around us every day. Computers and machines are constantly becoming smaller, faster, more reliable, and less expensive. As this technology improves, we will see an increasing shift away from the physical simulation applications such as mannequins and rubber arms and increased use of virtual reality and other computer based platforms. The benefits of completely virtual training are multiple and include the ability to create unlimited training scenarios, the ability to repeatedly try and fail in a consequence free environment, and preservation of animal life. Additionally, when training is conducted in a virtual environment, every step that is performed is essentially data. Every movement a trainee makes is reproduced by the computer, and thus the computer can track and record each and every movement. This abundance of data makes it possible to create very robust performance metrics not obtainable in the physical world. Through these metrics, performance can be quantified to a level never before achievable.

By requiring trainees to reach an objectively established performance goal or proficiency level, variability in post-training performance can be significantly reduced, improving the overall quality of the trainee. As technology improvements allow good performance to be better quantified, correct application of simulation based training will result in an improved level of care.

While improvements in technology, training and simulators will surely happen, there is undoubtedly a myriad of unknown happenings that will help shape how simulation based training is conducted in the future. Caring for the traumatically injured patient can be one of the most challenging undertakings in all of medicine. The need for military medics to care for the traumatically injured combat casualty will undoubtedly continue and simulation in some form will undoubtedly aid in the training of those providers who rise to meet the challenge.

References

1. Seymour N, *et al.* (2002). Virtual reality training improves operating room performance: results of a randomized, double-blinded study. *Ann Surg* **236**: 458–64.
2. Grantcharov T, *et al.* (2004). Randomized clinical trial of virtual reality simulation for laparoscopic skills raining. *Brit J Surg* **91**: 146–50.
3. Ali J, *et al.* (1993). Trauma outcome improves following Advanced Trauma Life Support program in a developing country. *J Trauma* **34**: 890–9.
4. Williams MJ, Lockey AS, Culshaw MC (1997). Improved trauma management with Advanced Trauma Life Support (ATLS) Training. *J Accid Emerg Med* **14**: 81–3.
5. Ben Abraham R, *et al.* (1997). The impact of Advanced Trauma Life Support Course on graduates with non-surgical medical background. *Europ J Emerg Med* **4**: 11–14.
6. Firdley FM, *et al.* (1993): Advanced Trauma Life Support: Assessment of cognitive achievement. *Milit Med* **158**: 623–7.
7. Block EF, Lottenburg L, Flint L, Jakobsen, Liebnitzky D (2002). Use of a human patient simulator for the advanced trauma life support course. *Am Surg* **68**: 648–51.
8. Safar P (1958). Ventilatory efficacy of mouth-to-mouth artificial resuscitation: Airway obstruction during manual and mouth-to-mouth artificial respirartion. *JAMA* **157**: 335–41.
9. Grenvik A, Schaefer J (2004). Advances in human simulation education: From Resusci-Anne to Sim-Man: The evolution of simulators in medicine. *Crit Care Med* **32**: S56–7.
10. Rosenthal E, Owen H (2004). An assessment of small simulators used to teach basic airway management. *Anaesth Inten Care* **32**: 87–92.
11. Mayo PH, Hackney JE, Mueck JT, Ribaudo V, Schneider RF (2004). Achieving house staff competence in emergency airway management: results of a teaching program using a computerized patient simulator. *Crit Care Med* **32**: 2422–77.

12. Good ML (2003). Patient simulation for training basic and advanced clinical skills. *Med Educ* **37**: S14–21.

13. Hesselfeldt R, Kristensen MS, Rasmussen LS (2005). Evaluation of the airway of the SimMan full-scale patient simulator. *Acta Anaesthesiol Scan* **49**: 1339–45.

14. Liu A, Bhasin Y, Bowyer M (2005). A haptic-enabled simulator for cricothyroidotomy. *Stud Health Tech Inform* **111**: 308–13.

15. Davis DP, *et al.* (2007). The effectiveness of a novel, algorithm-based difficult airway curriculum for air medical crews using human patient simulators. *Prehosp Emerg Care* **11**: 72–9.

16. Poole G, Myers RT (1980). Morbidity and mortality rates in major blunt trauma to the upper chest. *Ann Surg* **193**: 70–5.

17. Pezzella AT, Silva WE, Lancey RA (1998). Cardiothoracic trauma. *Curr Prob Surg* **35**: 649–50.

18. Bellamy RF (2000). History of surgery for penetrating chest trauma. *Chest Surg Clin N Am* **10**: 55–70.

19. Callahan M (1984). Pericardiocentesis in traumatic and non-traumatic cardiac tamponade. *Ann Emerg Med* **13**: 924–45.

20. Kaufmann C, Liu A (2001). Trauma training: virtual reality applications. *Stud Health Tech Inform* **81**: 236–41.

21. American College of Surgeons COT (2004). *Advanced Trauma Life Support for Doctors.* Chicago: American College of Surgeons.

22. Army Medical Department Center & School FSH (2004). Texas and the Borden Institute WRAMC, Washington DC. Emergency War Surgery. Washinton DC: Borden Institute.

23. Knudson M, Sisley A (2000). Training residents using simulation technology: experience with ultrasound for trauma. *J Trauma* **48**: 659–65.

24. Root HD (1990). Abdominal trauma and diagnostic peritoneal lavage revisited. *Am J Surg* **159**: 363–4.

25. Rozycki GS (1995). Abdominal ultrasonography in trauma. *Surg Clin N Am* **75**: 175–91.

26. Liu A, Kaufmann C, Ritchie T (2001). A computer-based simulator for diagnostic peritoneal lavage. *Stud Health Tech Inform* **81**: 279–85.

27. Bowyer MW, Liu AV, Bonar JP (2005). Validation of SimPL – a simulator for diagnostic peritoneal lavage training. *Stud Health Tech Inform* **111**: 64–7.

28. Bowyer M, et al (2005). Teaching intravenous cannulation to medical students: comparative analysis of two simulators and two educational approaches. *Stud Health Tech Inform* **111**: 57–63.

29. Reinig K, *et al.* (2006). The United States military's thigh trauma simulator. *Cin Orthop Relat Res* **442**: 45–56.

Chapter 29

Incorporating simulation into the medical school curriculum

Randolph Steadman and Rima Matevosian

Overview

- This chapter reviews the use of simulators in undergraduate medical education. Our experience since 1996 starting and enhancing the simulation programme for medical students at UCLA is presented.

- Successful medical student simulation programmes spark interest in the school, and its departments.

- Simulation programmes provide unique teaching opportunities for faculty, and afford medical students an earlier exposure to role models and clinical material.

- Simulation is well suited to demonstrate the clinical application of previously introduced concepts.

- Students appreciate simulation sessions that have well chosen objectives that are meaningful in the context of the course and the overall curriculum.

- The role of simulation in medical student assessment is just beginning and will undoubtedly grow.

- Medical school simulation programmes must plan (target audiences and courses) and budget (equipment and personnel) in order to sustain successful programmes.

- A significant time commitment can be required of the simulation programme director, who may need relief from clinical duties to grow and maintain the programme.

- Instructors that facilitate student discovery, rather than provide answers, optimize the experiential learning that simulation affords.

29.1 Introduction: definition and scope of simulation

Simulation for medical students encompasses a wide array of interactive, experiential learning techniques, including:

- standardized patients (actors coached to portray a patient)
- screen-based computer programs (realistic physiology, pharmacology and/or a combination of both incorporated into a clinical scenario)

- part-task trainers (models for intravenous catheter insertion, prostate examination, newborn delivery, etc)
- computerized full-scale high fidelity mannequins designed to incorporate the benefits of computer-based physiological modeling with life sized, interactive mannequins that breathe, have pulses, produce an electrocardiogram and respond to medications.

The common aspect unifying these modalities is the reproduction of a state that allows the learner to systematically and deliberately rehearse tasks and/or thought processes associated with clinically relevant objectives. The role of deliberate practice, or *rehearsal*, in domains such as athletics and music, has been identified as important for medical training. Accrediting bodies recently expressed support for simulation as a risk free, standardized modality that promotes practice[1].

The repetition of procedures has been documented to improve competency. Forty-seven tracheal intubations, 60 brachial plexus blocks, and 90 epidurals were needed for novices to achieve an 80% success rate in the respective procedure[2]. Whether simulated experiences are as effective as clinical experience is unknown. However, models that permit the novice to learn from their mistakes have an intrinsic appeal, as such experiences are difficult, if not unethical, in the clinical setting. It is expected that the public will, over time, come to expect a certain level of proficiency in the simulated environment before a trainee approaches the bedside.

Simulation is not just for procedures. Imagine a fourth year medical student at the bedside of a status asthmaticus patient ... the student simultaneously begins assessment and treatment, and manages the entire patient encounter independently. Or consider a final year medical student evaluating and managing a general anaesthetic for a patient with coronary artery disease undergoing an emergency appendectomy without input from a supervising physician. Far fetched? In real life, yes. Yet simulation permits medical students to experience decision-making challenges generally reserved for interns, residents, and fully trained practitioners. The planned simulation experience also includes a structured opportunity for reflection, and repetition if needed, something which the demands of the clinical setting seldom allow.

Simulation-based learning is not just for fourth year students. In this chapter we will review the rationale for starting a programme for medical students, outline practical issues that affect a programme's success, consider appropriate simulation-based learning objectives for students in the preclinical and clinical years and define the core elements of a successful programme. Also we will describe the simulation curriculum of the David Geffen School of Medicine at UCLA, and conclude with a review of the evidence supporting simulation as an educational tool for medical students. Hopefully, this will stimulate your imagination and help you fashion a School of Medicine simulation-based programme that is right for your institution.

29.2 **Rationale for starting a programme**

The primary reason for starting a programme is to provide experiential training in a risk-free environment. This experience can be standardized to permit a reliable, reproducible experience. Such consistency is important for training, and mandatory for assessment.

A successful programme increases departmental visibility, both within and outside the institution. Prospective applicants are often interested in the simulation programme and the institutional commitment to learning that it represents.

Simulation broadens career choices by exposing students to clinicians earlier in their education.

From the standpoint of the instructor, simulation-based training is an opportunity to observe without the need to intervene. The open-ended format identifies gaps in knowledge that are obscured by explicit direction in clinical settings. Minus the distractions of the clinical environment, instructors can focus on teaching. Students appreciate the attention and frequently reward instructors with laudatory evaluations.

29.3 Practical issues

A thorough knowledge of the existing course schedule is mandatory when incorporating simulation-based material as *proper timing of the material is key*. Simulation exercises that trail, or precede, the topic in the course curriculum by a week or more are considered poorly integrated by the students' standards and will be viewed as parenthetical offerings. In particular, if testing on the topic has already occurred, the simulation-based exercise is viewed as irrelevant. Proper timing alone does not guarantee success, or even understanding, but is a prerequisite to success.

The medical terms used during the simulation-based sessions should be standardized with the terms used within the remainder of the course, particularly for first year courses, when knowledge of medical terminology is scant. For instance, first year students may not recognize 'congestive heart failure' as 'pump failure'. Understanding such details requires discussions with lecturers, a review of lecture notes or lecture attendance.

Deciding where to place the first simulation offering into the school of medicine curriculum can be a difficult decision. Who are the advocates for interactive learning at your institution? The Dean of Education will usually gladly serve this role, or point you to the proper individuals. The medical education committee of the school (termed curricular committee by some schools) deals with school of medicine curricular reform; the chairman of this committee is generally aware of the school's needs. Instructors for poorly received courses frequently welcome liaisons that update their teaching methods.

A discussion with student class representatives (most schools have students from each year on the curricular committee) will provide information regarding opportunities for improvement.

Do not underestimate the high-stakes nature of your first simulation-based foray into the curriculum. First impressions are important. You should be confident that you're ready to deliver the agreed upon objectives, that the scenario has been piloted, that ambiguities have been eliminated and that learning objectives are clearly defined and appropriate.

Select topics based upon the natural strengths of the chosen simulation format. For instance, mannequin-based simulation is particularly engaging for cardiac and pulmonary pathophysiology and pharmacology. Equally valuable topics include medical errors, giving bad news, working as teams, and dealing with disruptive family and/or staff.

Always consider the student perspective when developing learning objectives. We have been consistently impressed by students' willingness to approach complicated simulated clinical scenarios with zeal (and a disregard for the possibility of embarrassment) when such experiences afford them the opportunity to exercise their clinical reasoning ability in a risk-free environment.

Similarly, the faculty perspective must be considered and addressed prior to imposing a new, touted technique on experienced teachers. Requiring that instructors leave behind the comfort of a well-rehearsed slide show for the unknown of simulation makes new demands on instructors. Rarely will scenarios evolve in as predictable a manner as a slide-based lecture. Instructors must not only be comfortable with the application of the subject matter, but also comfortable with the increasing technical nature of the prop they are using.

However, the hardest, and most foreign, aspect for the instructor is standing by idly while the student flounders or commits frank errors. Yet it is this experience that is so powerful and unique, as it illustrates the unintended consequences of their decisions. Instructors who use simulation must have an understanding and appreciation of the power of self-discovery, and avoid interrupting the process, which shortcuts the students' experience.

29.4 **Learning objectives of a simulation-based programme for medical students**

Simulation-based programmes offer a chance for clinicians to teach applied physiology and pharmacology to preclinical students, complementing the course material developed by the school's basic science departments. The application of knowledge in these areas places complex material into a practical framework, and introduces first year students to the clinical relevance of the subject matter. Students can experience the clinical setting before they see their first patient and develop clinical reasoning and problem solving. For specific topics and an example of the structure and format used at UCLA, please see below. Other institutions have published their first/second year simulation curriculum[3].

For students in their final (clinical) years of medical school, the number of appropriate topics is extensive. Ideal topics to consider are the diagnosis and treatment of vital sign abnormalities (hypotension/hypertension, bradycardia/tachycardia, and dysrhythmias), hypoxamic states, situations incorporating equipment (physiological monitors, bag-valve mask devices, intravenous lines, ventilators, defibrillators), infusions of vasoactive medications, and teamwork skills, to name a few.

29.5 **Essential elements for a medical student simulation programme**

The following elements are suggested for a successful programme:

- Simulation-savvy clinician, typically the centre director, who serves as the liaison to the course director
- Instructors who understand that simulation-based learning involves discovery (trial and error) on the students' part
- Content experts who set the objectives of simulation exercise
- Technical support personnel who are able to assist clinicians in scripting the scenario, programing the simulator, and running the simulator during the training exercise
- Educational objectives that are coordinated with the course content, have an appropriate degree of complexity for the level of the trainee and use the simulator's capabilities (interaction with the mannequin and physiological monitoring)
- A script that incorporates an appropriate group size (all students are involved to varying degrees)
- Clinically relevant equipment
- A standardized orientation to the environment, including the simulator (Table 29.1).

Supplemental elements (to be added as the programme grows) include:

- Isolated areas for orientation, the simulation encounter and the debriefing
- Capability of videotaping, which allows reflection and analysis of performance. Though there is no proven benefit to the learner, videotaping allows research to be conducted without the need for data collection 'on the fly'[4]. Videotaping is also invaluable for instructor standardization.

29.6 **The UCLA simulation curriculum**

The UCLA simulation programme serves approximately 600 medical students (150 per year).

Table 29.1 Simulation orientation checklist

Welcome

- Acknowledge/minimize performance anxiety
- Indicate whether participants' performance will be assessed

Session format

- Indicate that scenarios are designed unfold in a predetermined manner based upon actual case files, or a composite of several cases
- The evolution of the scenario may be modified by the participants' management
- Indicate the level of training expected of participants during the scenario (e.g. "Behave as if you are an intern")
- Describe the format for the session (e.g. "Each participant will be the primary provider for one case and serve as an observer and/or first responder for the remaining cases")
- Describe the role of first responders (e.g. "Responders should provide input as asked and not take control of the case")
- Describe the approximate duration of each scenario
- Describe the approximate duration of the debriefing for each scenario
- Instruct participants to speak out loud/verbalize thoughts (to facilitate the debriefing)
- Indicate whether sessions will be videotaped for use during the debriefing, as time permits
- Videotapes will not be used for evaluation unless specifically stated
- Videotapes will not be used for research unless you consent
- Please do not reveal the scenario content or diagnoses to others

Simulator interaction

- During orientation, assess the simulator capabilities by:
  - Listening to the heart and lung sounds
  - Palpating pulses
  - Practising mask ventilation and intubation, as appropriate
- Point out the simulator's limitations: for example, cannot display skin changes or move
- Describe how to administer medications and fluids
- During the session speak in a loud and clear voice so we input your treatment correctly
- During the session describe what you hear when listening to the hear or breath sounds (so ambiguities can be corrected if needed)
- Treat the simulated patient as if you were treating a real patient
- Indicate whether charting is required during the scenario

Monitor and other equipment

- Orient participants to physiological monitor
- Orient participants to other necessary equipment
- Describe how (and from whom) to request additional equipment if needed

29.6.1 **Year 1**

For first year students, the creation of an elaborately realistic environment can be more of a distraction than a benefit, so only the specifically required equipment is available. Videotaped debriefings are not typically used during the first year sessions.

29.6.1.1 Prematriculation motorcycle accident

This scenario was introduced into the curriculum prior to the start of the simulator programme, and is a good example of how content developed for a small group, problem-based learning format can be supplemented with simulation. This case was originally presented in two problem-based learning sessions held over the course of a week. The simulation session follows the first session.

The scenario is designed to encourage incoming first year students to think critically. The students are at the scene of the accident, where they witness a motorcycle swerve to avoid debris in the road. The driver has a head injury, flaccid lower extremities and a partial airway obstruction. Ultimately, he is found to have a cervical fracture, and a spinal cord injury with paraplegia. The passenger has pain in the chest and leg. She is found, after emergency department evaluation, to have fractured ribs, a ruptured spleen, and a lower leg fracture.

Learning objectives include ethical issues (are you required to render assistance?), legal issues (what is your legal exposure? what's the Good Samaritan law?), first aid (leave the victims in the road or move them to safety?), triage (which victim requires assistance first?), pre-hospital care (what steps should be taken prior to transport? What are the in-the-field treatment priorities?), and how the emergency department affects care. The learning objectives for the simulation session include an introduction to realistic physiological monitors, and an introduction to the primary and secondary trauma surveys.

29.6.1.2 Cardiac, pulmonary, renal block: shock scenario

Students are asked to interpret marginal vital signs (mild hypotension and tachycardia) and answer the question of whether shock exists. Students describe the types of shock (cardiogenic, hypovolaemic and distributive) and indicate whether the vital signs can be used to distinguish between these aetiologies. The concept of preload, afterload and cardiac output, which had been discussed in lectures, are illustrated in a clinical context using the pulmonary artery (PA) catheter and, if desired, transoesophageal echocardiograph. The simulated advancement of the PA catheter through the right heart is accompanied by the students' interpretation of the pressure tracings displayed on the monitor. The three types of shock are modeled during three separate scenarios. Illustrations from the students' textbook, enlarged and laminated, serve as visual tie-ins to the course. Twelve students attend each 75-minute session. If time permits, the effect of dysrhythmias such as atrial fibrillation on blood pressure, heart rate, cardiac output, preload, and afterload are discussed. Students wear nametags and each is asked, by name, to contribute.

29.6.1.3 Cardiac, pulmonary, renal block: hypoxaemia scenario

In the respiratory session, students are asked to describe the clinical changes that accompany hypoxaemia, such as changes in respiratory rate, heart rate, auscultatory findings, pulse oximetry tone, and waveform. Additional diagnostic studies such as chest X-ray, blood gases, and spirometry are provided for each specific diagnosis.

29.6.1.4 Cardiac, pulmonary, renal block: acid–base disturbances

The 75-minute acid–base session session reenacts four scenarios that illustrate the usefulness of blood gases: an exacerbation of chronic obstructive pulmonary disease (respiratory acidosis with compensatory metabolic alkalosis), an acute asthmatic episode (acute respiratory alkalosis, progressing to respiratory acidosis), an acute cardiac arrest resulting from ventricular tachycardia (respiratory and metabolic acidosis), and primary hyperaldosteronism suggested by a hypokalaemic alkalosis found on a venous sample sent for routine electrolytes.

29.6.2 **Year 2**

29.6.2.1 Cardiac, pulmonary, renal block (second year): adult respiratory distress syndrome (ARDS) scenario

This scenario unfolds over two sessions, with time in between for students to research self-identified learning issues. During the initial discussion session, students elicit the history of a 62-year-old patient with diabetes, hypertension and coronary artery disease who is admitted with abdominal tenderness and stable vital signs after a motor vehicle accident. Imaging shows significant intraperitoneal fluid and a small amount of intrapericardial fluid. When the patient deteriorates, students are asked to manage the ensuing shock. At the conclusion of the first session, the students are given citations that address the value of pulmonary artery catheters in critically ill patients.

The simulator session follows the first discussion session. The session starts with the patient in the operating room. Students must manage haemorrhagic shock due to splenic rupture. Over time the pericardial effusion increases, causing tamponade, which must be recognized and treated. Lastly, this unlucky patient experiences anaphylactic shock from antibiotic administration. He leaves the operating room intubated, which sets the stage for the discussion of non-cardiogenic ARDS during the second discussion session.

29.6.3 **Year 3**

The third year of medical school begins with a 2-week orientation called *Clinical Foundations*, which serves as an introduction to the clinical years. The simulation topics are airway management and cardiac arrhythmias. Sessions use partial task-trainers and full-scale patient simulators to introduce students to life-saving skills.

29.6.3.1 Clinical foundations

The airway workshop portion of *Clinical Foundations* provides each of the 170 third year medical students 2 hours of hands-on experience in airway management skills. This time is divided into 30 minutes at each of four stations (bag-valve mask ventilation, tracheal intubation, introduction to alternate airway devices, and a simulated patient encounter).

The simulation station integrates the skills introduced in the other three stations. The simulator exercise emphasizes the cognitive aspects of patient management, including when, and whether, to use their newly learned skills. The scenario begins with the student called into a surgical patient's room. The patient becomes unresponsive and the students, anxious to put their freshly acquired skills to use, begin bag-valve mask ventilation and generally proceed to intubation. Students who search for an underlying cause discover an opioid overdose. Students are taught that consideration of the differential diagnosis can lead to targeted treatment, which may preclude the need for endotracheal intubation.

The dysrhythmia portion of *Clinical Foundations* is divided into three 20-minute stations. One station addresses rhythms requiring defibrillation and other pulseless rhythms (asystole, pulseless electrical activity). The second station demonstrates dysrhythmias with pulses, such as stable supraventricular tachycardia, heart blocks and bradycardia. Students learn to recognize dysrhythmias on an oscilloscope, to assess the patient clinically (establish unresponsiveness, assess chest rise, check for pulses) and to use the defibrillator and transcutaneous pacer. The third station integrates these skills using the patient simulator. A team of students is asked to manage a cardiac arrest due to ventricular fibrillation. Everyone is given a role during the simulation.

29.6.3.2 Surgery clerkship

During the third year *Surgery Clerkship* students, in groups of 6–8, attend a simulator session, involving the case of a 50-year-old cholecystectomy patient who becomes hypotensive on postoperative day 1. During the 2-hour session students ask for and receive clinical information (presence/absence of râles, jugular venous distention, fever, etc) consistent with the aetiology of the patient's condition. Alternate groups can be given different diagnoses as desired by varying the clinical findings. Plausible aetiologies include haemorrhage, fluid overload (exacerbated by the patient's diuretics failing to be resumed postoperatively) or biliary sepsis (from a retained common duct stone). This session is not designed as an assessment, as this is done through an oral examination.

29.6.4 Year 4

29.6.4.1 Colleges foundation week

At the start of the final year of medical school, UCLA students participate in a weeklong course called *College Foundations*, which is specific for the students' chosen career tracks. Each of the four colleges (Acute Care, Applied Anatomy, Primary Care and Medical Specialists' College) has its own *College Foundations* curriculum, which specifically focuses on the core skills for that college. The number of students per simulation session is kept relatively constant at 6–8 students, a smaller number than for sessions in the preclinical years. This reflects the goal of increased student autonomy during the later years.

The Acute Care College incorporates 3 days of simulation that are integrated with the week's didactics, cadaver labs, and small group discussions. After an orientation to the simulation sessions' format, each student is individually given a unique 5–7 minute scenario that focuses on the day's topic, **altered vital signs**. While one student is in the 'hot seat' the other students observe their colleagues while waiting their turn. During the mid-week session, scenarios relate to the topics of **dyspnoea** and **acute abdominal pain.** On the last day of the week, each student manages a unique case based upon one of the earlier didactic topics. For each of these sessions, students are debriefed using pre-assigned case checklists specific for each scenario. During the final session of the week, students are videotaped and undergo an individualized debriefing using the videotape. Examples of the cases including cardiac arrest, congestive heart failure, urosepsis, dissecting aneurysm, ruptured spleen, abdominal aortic aneurysm, anaphylaxis, drug overdose, pneumothorax, and pulmonary embolism. Many of the week's other activities augment, enhance or supplement the simulation experience. The list of cases for each of the Acute Care College's session is included in Table 29.2, a sample checklist is in Table 29.3. The remaining colleges focus on critical care skills specific to their colleges' focus.

29.6.4.2 Subinternships and evening seminars

In addition to the *College Foundations* simulation sessions, senior medical students also have the opportunity to practise their skills on the simulator throughout the year. Anaesthesia subinternships and college evening seminar workshops provide supplemental hands-on experiences.

Anaesthesia subinternship students practise intubation on mannequins and intravenous insertion on simulated arms. Screen-based simulations familiarize students with the induction and maintenance of anaesthesia. During mannequin-based sessions, students demonstrate their skills on 3–4 cases. Examples include the management of hypoxaemia in the recovery room, a sudden cardiac arrest in a critical care unit, congestive heart failure after surgery, and a difficult airway in

Table 29.2 Fourth year medical student scenarios

Session 1	Session 2	Session 3
◆ Cardiac arrest (ventricular fibrillation)	◆ Abdominal aortic aneurysm	◆ Asthma in an adolescent
◆ Lower gastrointestinal bleeding	◆ Ruptured spleen	◆ Pneumothorax
◆ Head injury	◆ Small bowel obstruction	◆ Anaphylaxis to bee sting
◆ Unstable supraventricular tachycardia	◆ Ruptured ectopic pregnancy	◆ Chronic obstructive pulmonary disease
◆ Urosepsis	◆ Asthma in a child	◆ Tension pneumothorax
◆ Cardiogenic shock	◆ Spontaneous pneumothorax	◆ Pulmonary oedema
◆ Sick sinus syndrome	◆ Narcotic overdose in drug user	◆ Postoperative patient-controlled analgesia overdose
◆ Dissecting aneurysm	◆ Anaphylaxis to antibiotics	◆ Anaphylaxis from drug reaction
◆ Cardiac arrest (pulseless ventricular tachycardia)		◆ Expanding neck haematoma

the operating room. These sessions include students from a number of medical schools who have varying degrees of familiarity with simulation, so an orientation to the mannequin and the session's objectives is important (see Table 29.1).

29.7 Evidence supporting simulation-based learning for medical students

Teaching critical thinking skills using a lecture format suffers from a number of limitations. These include difficulty teaching cognitive and psychomotor skills, a lack of engagement due to the non-interactive nature of lectures and inability to assess whether students incorporate the material into patient care[5]. Simulation clearly addresses each of these limitations. The University of Pittsburgh has described a third and fourth year medical school curriculum that emphasizes the evaluation and management of patients with respiratory distress and cardiovascular events (chest pain, arrhythmias and pulselessness)[6].

Despite the theoretical advantage of simulation, there are no data supporting error reduction through the use of simulation. However, improved patient outcomes are a tall order for any educational endeavor. If this level of evidence is applied to continuing medical education (CME) programmes, none could fulfill this criterion. Let's take a closer look at where and how simulation's value has been assessed.

29.7.1 Surveys addressing the value of simulation

Numerous published surveys have shown that medical students value simulation. Specifically, students have found the simulated learning environment realistic and capable of meeting their learning objectives[7–9]. Most students were comfortable in the simulator setting, though a quarter of students in one study indicated they were not[7]. In another survey, 85% of students rated the session excellent or very good, and 80% thought simulator-based training should be required for

Table 29.3 Sample checklist

Chest pain/cardiogenic shock scenario (35 pts)

History (8 pts)

☐ Pain (1 pt)

    ☐ Pattern (1 pt)

    ☐ Quality (1 pt)

    ☐ Radiation (1 pt)

    ☐ Severity (1 pt)

    ☐ Temporal aspects (1 pt)

☐ Other symptoms (nausea, shortness of breath, syncope)? (½ pt)

☐ Past medical history: history of similar event? (½ pt)

☐ Medications (½ pt)

☐ Allergies (½ pt)

Physical Exam (14 pts)

☐ Assess airway (air movement or stridor or phonation) (1 pt)

☐ Assess breath sounds (3 pts)

☐ Assess pulse oximetry (3 pts)

☐ Assess respiratory rate (1 pt)

☐ Cardiac exam: S3, murmurs? (3 pts)

☐ Abdominal evaluation (1 pt)

☐ Extremity oedema? (1 pt)

☐ Skin evaluation (warm/cool, colour, dry/moist) (1 pt)

Diagnostic Evaluation (9 pts)

☐ Evaluate rhythm, 12 lead EKG (3 pts)

☐ Chest X-ray (1 pt)

☐ Pulmonary artery catheter (1 pt)

☐ Cardiac enzymes (3 pts)

☐ Electrolytes, haematocrit, prothrombin time or platelets (1 pt)

Management (4 pts)

☐ Oxygen (3 pts)

☐ Aspirin (1 pt)

---

medical students[10]. Another survey, completed by 90 medical students who encountered simulation during an internal medicine clerkship, showed similar results. Ninety-four percent felt the simulator should be incorporated permanently into the clerkship[11]. Important aspects of simulation sessions, identified during surveys, include 'being put on the spot' and an integrative session at the completion of the scenario[11]. The integrative analysis, also known as a debriefing, allows for 'discharging of emotions' and 'capturing of learning'[12].

29.7.3 **Screen-based simulation for medical students**

Computer-based simulation has been used for medical students in a number of areas, including teaching trauma skills (no improvement compared to seminar-based training)[13], and pharmacokinetics (improvement over a control group that had less contact time with material)[14]. An advantage of computer-based technology is that it can be 'the equivalent of a teacher's best day' in the classroom[15]. Computer-based technology can be made readily available, but the user interface and the personal nature of such programs have led to limited acceptance in the classroom. Students who desire a more extensive exposure to a particular topic use screen-based simulation to supplement classroom material.

29.7.4 **Mannequin-based simulation for medical students: is it effective?**

Mannequin-based simulation, used to teach trauma skills to interns, resulted in improved scores when compared with moulage-trained interns[16]. Both groups were tested in both the simulation and moulage environments. Others, using mannequin-based simulation, have not shown a difference when comparing simulation-based training with lecture-based instruction[17]. Of note, this study used a written pre-post test format to assess outcomes. Written test scores, when compared to simulation-based skills, have not correlated well[18], a fact conceded by the authors and others[19,20]. This is expected, as written testing measures knowledge, not the application of knowledge which simulator-based training emphasizes.

Simulation-based training was compared to videoassisted learning for 144 medical students, and no difference was found[21]. However, using videoassisted learning as the comparator group may have minimized potential outcome differences, and the differences between the groups were further minimized by the design, which allowed the simulator sessions and the video sessions to be paused for faculty discussions[22]. When our group at UCLA evaluated the benefits of simulation-based training in 31 fourth year medical students, simulation-based training resulted in improved assessment and management skills when compared to training using a problem-based learning format[23]. However, others were unable to demonstrate improved skill acquisition using a chest pain scenario[24].

29.7.5 **Using simulation for medical student assessment**

In a study of 40 medical students and first year interns at Washington University in St. Louis, acute care skills were measured using simulation[25]. Interrater reliability was high ($r = 0.95$–0.97), though considerable variability in individual's scores was noted between the various cases. The authors' suggested that the reliability of the assessment could be improved by increasing the number of cases beyond the six scenarios per subjects used in their study. Validity was assessed by correlating time spent in critical care electives with simulator performance results ($r = 0.24$, $p < 0.05$). The correlation of simulation score with total critical care time was higher for several cases (myocardial infarction, cerebral haemorrhage/herniation, 0.41 and 0.48, respectively)[25]. In their study, which used scenarios with well-defined diagnostic and treatment actions, one rater was sufficient.

This contrasts with a study of 135 final year medical students at the University of Toronto, where reliability was improved from 0.77 to 0.86 by the use of pairs of raters[26]. Simulation scores correlated poorly with clinical marks ($r = 0.13$) and written test scores ($r = 0.19$). Written test scores and clinical marks also showed minimal correlation with each other ($r = 0.23$). These authors also noted a wide variation between cases in individuals' scores and suggested that the lack of a gold standard for undergraduate assessment may have contributed. Although medical schools are required to specify the skills expected of its graduates, performance standards for these skills are rarely standardized.

In another study from the University of Toronto, the construct validity of simulation-based testing was demonstrated, as the scores of fully trained anaesthesiologists and residents were higher than that of medical students[27]. These researchers also noted considerable inter-case variability in scores.

Clearly, the content and difficulty of the scenarios must be considered, and scenarios with well-defined and agreed-upon expectations perform best.

29.7.6 Simulation for procedural skills acquisition

One half of all adverse events are a result of an invasive procedure[28]. It follows that trainees desire procedural skills training with simulators. In a survey of 158 trainees, of which approximately one third were medical students, safety and the comfort level of the supervising physician were identified as the major benefits of simulation[29]. Chest tube insertion, central line placement, and tracheal intubation were felt most likely to benefit from simulation (procedures rated less highly, in decreasing order, were peripheral intravenous line insertion, arterial blood gas draw, nasogastric tube insertion, bladder catheterization and venipuncture). The Society of American Gastroenterologists and Endoscopic Surgeons (SAGES) has endorsed a Fundamental of Laparoscopic Surgery (FLS) programme, which is being incorporated into surgical residency training programmes[30]. In a study comparing medical students' intracorporeal knot-tying and suturing skills to those of senior surgical residents, simulator-trained students achieved equivalence in the number of needle manipulations, with nearly a similar number of errors[31].

29.7.8 Virtual reality

Virtual reality implies a computer-generated world, which can be 'entered' and 'explored' using visual, aural and haptic (tactile) senses[32]. This technology has been touted for over a decade as the learning environment of the future, yet little research has been done, presumably due to the cost. Examples of currently available virtual reality simulators include MIST and VIST (Minimally Invasive Surgical Trainer and Vascular International System Trainer, Mentice, Gothenburg, Sweden) and endoscopy trainers (Accutouch, Immersion Medical, Gaithersburg, Maryland, USA). Virtual reality trainers, seldom used for undergraduate medical training, are primarily found in the realm of resident training and continuing medical education.

29.8 Conclusions

As the acuity of hospitalized patients continues to increase, the role of students on the healthcare team has been diminished. Patients with less acute problems, which are traditionally assigned to students, are now cared for in ambulatory settings, and are less accessibel to students. Both of these trends have resulted in fewer learning opportunities. Simulation addresses these shortcomings and provides students a risk-free setting in which to apply physiology and pharmacology and to learn teamwork skills.

The evidence supporting simulation continues to accrue, although it is not yet clear that proficiency in simulated settings consistently translates to proficiency in clinical settings and no one has shown that improved patient outcomes result from simulation-based learning. However, no other learning modality meets that lofty goal.

Despite this lack of evidence, educational organizations support the concept of deliberate rehearsal and practise for skill acquisition, and students recognize and appreciate the opportunity that simulation affords. As the safety initiative changes patients' expectations, it is unlikely that trainees will continue to be directed to the bedside of patients to learn using the apprenticeship methods of the past.

Simulation is here to stay. As the technology evolves, more life like and realistic replicas of human anatomy, physiology and behaviour will be ushered into undergraduate medical education. Accrediting agencies and specialty societies have already embraced the idea that simulation is a necessary component of training, and soon, the use of simulation for assessment will follow. As educators further define the role and scope of rehearsal in medical training, the integration of simulation into undergraduate medical education will undoubtedly continue.

References

1. Simulation and Rehearsal. ACGME; 2005 [updated 2005; cited June 6, 2005]; Available from: http://www.acgme.org/acWebsite/bulletin/bulletin12_05.pdf.
2. Konrad C, Schupfer G, Wietlisbach M, Gerber H (1998). Learning manual skills in anesthesiology: Is there a recommended number of cases for anesthetic procedures? *Anesth Analg* **86**: 635–9.
3. Euliano, TY (2001). Small group teaching: clinical correlation with a human patient simulator. *Adv Physiol Educ* **25**: 36–43.
4. Savoldelli, GL, Naik VN, Joo HS, *et al.* (2006). Evaluation of patient simulator performance as an adjunct to the oral examination for senior anesthesia residents. *Anesthesiology* **104**: 475–81.
5. Rogers, PL (2004). Simulation in medical students' critical thinking. *Crit Care Med* **32**: S70–1.
6. McIvor WR (2004). Experience with medical student simulation education. *Crit Care Med* **32**: S66–9.
7. Cleave-Hogg D, Morgan PJ (2002). Experiential learning in an anaesthesia simulation centre: analysis of students' comments. *Med Teach* **24**: 23–6.
8. Weller, JM (2004). Simulation in undergraduate medical education: bridging the gap between theory and practice. *Med Educ* **38**: 32–8.
9. Zirkle, M, Blum R, Raemer DB, Healy G, Roberson DW (2005). Teaching emergency airway management using medical simulation: a pilot programme. *Laryngoscope* **115**: 495–500.
10. Gordon, JA, Wilkerson WM, Shaffer DW, Armstrong EG (2001). "Practicing" medicine without risk: students' and educators' responses to high-fidelity patient simulation. *Acad Med* **76**: 469–72.
11. McMahon GT, Monaghan C, Falchuk K, Gordon JA, Alexander EK (2005). A simulator-based curriculum to promote comparative and reflective analysis in an internal medicine clerkship. *Acad Med* **80**: 84–9.
12. Stafford F (2005). The significance of de-roling and debriefing in training medical students using simulation to train medical students. *Med Educ* **39**: 1083–5.
13. Gilbart MK, Hutchison CR, Cusimano MD, Regehr G (2000). A computer-based trauma simulator for teaching trauma management skills. *Am J Surg* **179**: 223–8.
14. Feldman RD, Schoenwald R, Kane J (1989). Development of a computer-based instructional system in pharmacokinetics: efficacy in clinical pharmacology teaching for senior medical students. *J Clin Pharmacol* **29**: 158–61.
15. McGee JB, Neill J, Goldman L, Casey E (1998). Using multimedia virtual patients to enhance the clinical curriculum for medical students. *Medinfo* **9**(2): 732–5.
16. Lee SK, Pardo M, Gaba D, *et al.* (2003). Trauma assessment training with a patient simulator: a prospective, randomized study. *J Trauma* **55**: 651–7.
17. Gordon JA, Shaffer DW, Raemer DB, Pawlowski J, Hurford WE, Cooper JB (2006). A randomized controlled trial of simulation-based teaching versus traditional instruction in medicine: a pilot study among clinical medical students. *Adv Health Sci Educ Theory Pract* **11**: 33–9.
18. Schwid HA, Rooke GA, Michalowski P, Ross BK (2001). Screen-based anesthesia simulation with debriefing improves performance in a mannequin-based anesthesia simulator. *Teach Learn Med* **13**: 92–6.
19. Maatsch JL (1981). Assessment of clinical competence on the Emergency Medicine Specialty Certification Examination: the validity of examiner ratings of simulated clinical encounters. *Ann Emerg Med* **10**: 504–7.

20. Schuwirth LW, van der Vleuten CP (2003). The use of clinical simulations in assessment. *Med Educ* **37**(Suppl. 1): 65–71.

21. Morgan PJ, Cleave-Hogg D, McIlroy J, Devitt JH (2002). Simulation technology: a comparison of experiential and visual learning for undergraduate medical students. *Anesthesiology* **96**: 10–6.

22. Gaba DM (2002). Two examples of how to evaluate the impact of new approaches to teaching. *Anesthesiology* **96**: 1–2.

23. Steadman RH, Coates WC, Huang YM, *et al.* (2006). Simulation-based training is superior to problem-based learning for the acquisition of critical assessment and management skills. *Crit Care Med* **34**: 151–7.

24. Schwartz LR, Fernandez R, Kouyoumjian SR, Jones KA, Compton S (2007). A randomized comparison trial of case-based learning versus human patient simulation in medical student education. *Acad Emerg Med* **14**: 130–7.

25. Boulet JR, Murray D, Kras J, Woodhouse J, McAllister J, Ziv A (2003). Reliability and validity of a simulation-based acute care skills assessment for medical students and residents. *Anesthesiology* **99**: 1270–80.

26. Morgan PJ, Cleave-Hogg DM, Guest CB, Herold J (2001). Validity and reliability of undergraduate performance assessments in an anesthesia simulator. *Can J Anaesth* **48**: 225–33.

27. Devitt JH, Kurrek MM, Cohen MM, Cleave-Hogg D (2001). The validity of performance assessments using simulation. *Anesthesiology* **95**: 36–42.

28. LeapeLL, Brennan TA, Laird N, *et al.* (1991). The nature of adverse events in hospitalized patients. Results of the Harvard Medical Practice Study II. *N Engl J Med* **324**: 377–84.

29. Greene AK, Zurakowski D, Puder M, Thompson K (2006). Determining the need for simulated training of invasive procedures. *Adv Health Sci Educ Theory Pract* **11**: 41–9.

30. Peters JH, Fried GM, Swanstrom LL, *et al.* (2004). Development and validation of a comprehensive programme of education and assessment of the basic fundamentals of laparoscopic surgery. *Surgery* **135**: 21–7.

31. Van Sickle KR, Ritter EM, Smith CD (2006). The pretrained novice: using simulation-based training to improve learning in the operating room. *Surg Innov* **13**: 198–204.

32. Hoffman H, Vu D (1997). Virtual reality: teaching tool of the twenty-first century? *Acad Med* **72**: 1076–81.

Chapter 30

Surgical simulation

Roger Kneebone and Fernando Bello

Overview

- Surgical practice demands a complex mixture of knowledge, judgement, technical skill,and effective teamworking. But surgical practice is changing dramatically, with greatly curtailed training time.

- Simulation offers the opportunity to practise within a learner-centred environment that meets criteria for educational effectiveness yet avoids risk to patients.

- Simulation-based training should allow regular context-based practice, providing feedback within a supportive, learner-centred milieu. A theory-grounded curriculum should underpin surgical training and ensure a connection between clinical and simulation-based experience.

- Surgical simulators include physical models, virtual reality computer systems, and hybrids that combine the two.

- Increased computational power and advanced 3D modelling techniques make possible the combination of an individual patient's anatomy and pathology to generate personalized simulations.

- The context of learning is inseparable from the skills that are learned. Each surgical learning experience is unique and must be related to the specific needs of the learner.

- The relationship between fidelity of a simulation and its effectiveness is not a simple one. Levels of realism should be tailored to meet educational goals within practical constraints of cost and technical feasibility.

- Any new technology needs to be validated. The acid test for simulation is whether it maps onto clinical performance and leads to improved outcomes.

- Future developments include patient specific simulation (uploading individual clinical data into simulations) and patient focused simulation (using actors to play the part of patients within simulations and provide feedback from the patient's perspective).

- Multiscale integrative simulation from the nano to the macro scale, requiring trainees to deal with all currently available information about a patient and her state of health, represents the next big challenge in medical simulation.

30.1 **Introduction**

Simulation is now firmly established within mainstream surgical training. We start this chapter by painting a broad picture of what surgical simulation can offer and why it is widely used. After summarising key contributions from educational theory, we give an overview of currently available simulators. Finally we highlight areas of likely growth and speculate about where these might lead in the future.

Technical expertise is so obviously essential to surgery that it tends to steal the limelight. For example, much high fidelity virtual reality (VR) simulation has focused on surgical techniques. However, technical skill is only one component of safe surgical practice, and there are dangers in focusing too narrowly on technique. Knowledge, decision making, communication and an awareness of clinical risk are equally important.

One of our aims in this chapter is to highlight this wider landscape of clinical context, so that surgical simulation centres can decide where to position themselves along the spectrum of realism and complexity. However, individual constraints and opportunities will shape the range of simulation which any centre can offer.

We distinguish between 'simulators' (apparatus designed for practising techniques) and 'simulation' (the wider universe within which simulators may be used). Although these terms are sometimes used interchangeably, in our view this leads to confusion.

30.2 **Background**

Surgery is an area where the arguments for simulation are very compelling. It seems obvious that novices should learn the basics of their craft on inanimate models before being let loose on patients. It is also evident that surgeons in training should continue to refine their techniques by practising within a safe environment. Perhaps the most powerful argument for simulation is the absence of an acceptable alternative.

Traditional approaches to surgical training involved extended apprenticeships stretching over many years. But healthcare is changing dramatically, working hours are being curtailed and traditional ways are being overturned. Political and public pressure is mounting to make surgical training transparent, and patients are no longer willing to be practised on. Simulation offers the opportunity for safe, focused learning to complement and reinforce clinical experience.

Yet these apparently obvious truths conceal a more complex reality. Of course technical skill is an essential component of any surgeon's work. Yet technical procedures are only a part of the story, and too much emphasis on technique can divert attention from other important aspects. Surgery, after all, begins with the first preoperative encounter, and extends beyond the operation to postoperative care, discharge and follow-up. Teamworking, communication, decision making and a host of other qualities are essential for providing safe, high quality clinical care.

Moreover, there is no such thing as a generic 'surgical learner'. A novice struggling to master the basics of minimal access surgery (MAS) will have very different needs from an experienced consultant perfecting a new technique in their specialized field. An awareness of what simulation can – and cannot – offer is therefore essential. Areas include:

◆ acquisition of technical skill

◆ application of skills within a clinical context

◆ learner-centred, patient-focused education and training.

30.3 **Simulation components**

We start with an overview of what we consider are the components of surgical simulation. Most simulation centres focus on a selection of these, depending on demand and resources.

30.3.1 **The procedure or operation**

This area is dominated by simulators. Much development and investment focuses on apparatus for practising specific surgical techniques across a range of complexity. Later in the chapter we offer a classification of simulators, with a guide to current products.

In recent years there have been major advances in technology, especially with the realism of virtual reality computing[1] and customized human–computer interfaces. Until recently, however, simulators focused on specific procedures and offered a relatively limited range of variants within in a given intervention. Minimal access procedures, for example, relied on repeated performance of the same set of tasks. This raised concerns that learners would 'play the simulator' without necessarily gaining skills that would improve their performance with patients. Many VR simulators now offer levels of challenge, with a range of anatomical variants.

An exciting development is patient-specific simulation. Using advanced image processing algorithms and 3D modelling techniques, it is now possible to combine scanned images of an individual patient's anatomy and pathology to generate individual simulations[1]. At present, this is being developed to allow specialists to plan and rehearse challenging cases before an actual operation. It seems likely that this technology will have a trickle down effect, providing a rich set of resources for more basic training (especially in minimal access procedures). This realistic unpredictability will increase the scope of simulator based training.

30.3.2 **The professional setting**

Surgeons do not operate in isolation, but as members of a complex team. Effective functioning within the team is as important to a satisfactory outcome as technical expertise. Communication with anaesthetic, nursing and other team members is essential to decision making and high quality care[2,3,4]. Many of the stresses of operative surgery relate to the professional environment rather than purely technical problems[5].

Extremely high levels of realism can now be achieved within simulated operative settings, and simulated operating theatres are becoming increasingly widespread. This builds on the pioneering work within anaesthesia over recent decades[6,7,8]. Later in this chapter we will discuss the importance of context upon learning.

The potential to create complex, convincing scenarios is attractive. But such scenarios are difficult to set up and costly to run and will not be appropriate to all learners. So, again, each simulation centre must make decisions based on its desired outcomes. Moreover, not all surgical procedures take place in the operating theatre. Context-sensitive simulation offers possibilities here, recreating a range of professional environments within which teams can practise and review their performance.

30.3.3 **The patient experience**

Clinician–patient communication is crucial to all healthcare practice, and surgery is no exception. Even when a procedure itself is to be performed under general anaesthetic, the patient will

---

[1] Defined here as the use of computer software and hardware to generate an immersive and interactive simulation of either reality-based or imaginary images and scenes.

require explanation before and afterwards. This demands high levels of sensitivity and awareness on the part of the clinician.

Increasingly, however, invasive procedures are carried out under local anaesthesia, sometimes with light sedation. Such patients are conscious for at least part of the surgical procedure. Procedures include operations (ranging from simple skin surgery and hernia repair to prostatectomy and carotid endarterectomy) and invasive investigations and therapeutic interventions (e.g. cardiological and vascular procedures).

Traditionally, surgical simulation has not addressed patient communication during procedures. Instead, it has focused on techniques as they would be performed under general anaesthesia. Innovative work by our research group has combined inanimate models and VR simulators with simulated patients (professional actors) to create scenarios for practising operations and other procedures (see below)[9,10,11,12,13]. This focus on the patient's perspective – including feedback from the patient's viewpoint – adds an additional dimension to what simulation can offer.

30.3.4 **Educational theory**

In order to understand what simulation can achieve, and what its limitations are, some educational theory will be helpful[14]. If theory is ignored, there is a risk of providing simulators without proper educational support. Although some learning will take place in such cases, there is a real danger that it may not be effective. In each of the following categories, a brief overview of key theories is followed by a discussion relating to surgical simulation.

In a nutshell, surgical simulation needs to be actively managed and to have specific aims. Simulator technology is only part of a wider picture, with simulators being necessary but not sufficient for effective simulation. It is important to pay attention to the conditions required for acquiring expertise, to provide tutor support when needed, to ensure that simulation-based experience maps onto actual clinical practice, integrating well within the curriculum, and to create a supportive, learner-centred environment.

30.3.5 **Expertise**

The acquisition of technical skill is perhaps the most obvious use for simulation. The literature on expertise is enormous. Much of it is drawn from domains outside surgery, such as sport and the performing arts. It is clear that the key to gaining expertise is sustained deliberate practice over a prolonged period. In the case of elite performers in other domains, a minimum of 10 years is required[15,16].

Yet simple repetition of a task is not sufficient. Practice has to be driven by a motivation to improve. Each learner needs a clear vision of what they are aiming for, together with the opportunity to practise repeatedly and gauge the effect of their practice. Knowledge of results and expert feedback is crucial here, if learners are not to develop bad habits.

It is clear that some forms of practice are more effective than others. Distributed practice (divided into limited sections) achieves better results than blocked practice (extended continuous periods). Moreover, newly gained skills are easily lost if not regularly reinforced. Episodic exposure to simulators is unlikely to be effective unless it takes place within a carefully structured programme which ensures that skills are consolidated.

Simulation can offer some of the conditions for sustained deliberate practice. Learners can practise repeatedly until they have gained technical mastery. They can consolidate their learning through structured programmes and they can experiment and explore the consequences of action (or inaction) without jeopardizing real patients. But there are limits to what can be achieved without expert guidance.

30.3.6 Tutor support

Of course much surgical learning takes place by observation, by experience and by doing. Yet a skilled tutor can help this process enormously. The work of Lev Vygotsky is helpful here[17,18]. Vygotsky (a Russian psychologist in the first half of the 20th century) developed the concept of the 'zone of proximal development' (ZPD). In the ZPD, a learner can solve problems 'in collaboration with more capable peers' even if unable to do so unassisted. Later descriptions of *scaffolding* and *contingent instruction* have developed this idea further, elaborating the concept of help which is there when needed but which fades away when no longer required[19,20,21].

This process is clearly seen in the operating theatre, with one to one teaching. But it can also take place within simulation. Tutor support may be personal, or it may involve educational technology (e.g. from a VR simulator computer).

Together with more recent authors, we suggest that each learner's ZPD can be thought of as a space where supported learning takes place[22]. This requires active engagement of both learner and tutor, but can be augmented by aids such as simulators, such that within the ZPD there are *learning resources* (e.g. simulators, books, computer programs) and *tutors* (who provide individual feedback and guidance).

The learning which takes place within the ZPD is seldom linear. For a tutor, the art is to establish a sensitive, responsive relationship with each learner, ensuring a balance between support (especially at the early stages of learning) and space (where the learner can consolidate learning without intrusion). Feedback lies at the heart of this process.

The implications for simulation are clear. Simply providing simulators is not enough. Simulators must form part of a curriculum which combines equipment with expert tuition. Most important of all, simulation needs to connect with the clinical reality it is designed to mirror. So how can this be achieved?

30.3.7 The context of learning

Surgical simulation has a very practical aim – to improve patient care. So we must consider how the simulated universe maps onto the clinical one. For unless there is a clear connection between the two, simulation-based practice risks being out of touch with reality. If this should happen, technical skills may be learned in isolation but never applied.

Most surgical learning takes place within a clinical setting such as the operating theatre. Simulation must complement workplace learning, not supplant it. It is therefore important to understand how learning in the workplace happens.

Apprenticeship lies at the heart of surgical learning. According to the traditional model, a learner sits at the feet of a master and learns directly from him or her by a slow absorptive process lasting many years. A more contemporary view, based on the concept of communities of practice, sees learning as an integral part of social practice[23,24]. In such communities, newcomers learn by joining a group of professionals who share a common aim. Relations between peers are quite as important as relations between apprentice and master. Indeed, the learner gains as much from being part of the community of practice of which the master is a part, as directly from the master himself. According to this view, apprenticeship is as much about conferring legitimacy and establishing a professional identity, as about the transmission of knowledge and skill. Surgical care offers many such communities of practice, with the operating theatre being perhaps the most obvious example.

It follows from this that the context of surgical learning is crucial. If skills are practised out of context and there is no opportunity to apply them clinically, they will not feed into the communities of practice where clinical learning takes place. Moreover, learning will not form part of that growing pattern of professional development which interweaves technical skill with other key elements such as teamworking, communication, professionalism, and decision making. There is a danger that simulation will be seen as an amusement arcade activity, requiring dexterity and adroitness but no awareness of the bigger picture.

Therefore simulation must deliberately set out to be relevant to the clinical activity in which learners engage after leaving the skills centre. Ideally, it should offer opportunities for 'just in time' learning, triggered by day to day clinical experience. This has implications for where simulation centres are sited and how they are designed.

30.3.8 **The climate of learning**

Unlike the clinical environment, simulation is designed for the benefit of the learner. Rather than fitting learning opportunities around clinical care, the learning itself takes the spotlight.

Teachers have a responsibility to set up a simulated environment to be as effective as possible. We know that the affective component of learning has a powerful impact on participants. The effect of inspiring teachers can last for decades, and so can humiliating experiences. Here again, it is not enough simply to provide simulators. We must ensure that they are used within an environment which provides the conditions for effective learning. This requires a supportive, learner-centred setting where all participants behave with respect and professionalism.

Such a supportive climate is especially important in giving feedback. Timely, focused feedback is crucial to effective learning but is often lacking from simulated procedures. Networked videomonitoring technology can be helpful here as it provides a means for assessors to observe and rate performance within the simulated environment remotely. Participants can then access summary information about their performance and review videorecordings in their own time. Our ICFAS (Imperial College Feedback and Assessment System) combines this technology with a custom designed assessment management system that integrates multiple assessment sources to generate secure, web-based feedback offering participants graphical summaries and detailed information about their individual performance within hours[10].

30.4 **Simulator technology**

Simulation is now used across the whole range of surgical experience[25]. Four key levels can be identified:

- **Clinical procedures** include models for venepuncture, inserting IV infusions, urinary catheterization. Competence in these procedures is required by a wide range of clinicians at different stages of training (medical, nursing and others).

- **Basic surgical skills** include handling surgical instruments, making and closing wounds, performing bowel and vascular anastomoses.

- **Minimal access skills** include port insertion, tissue dissection, haemostasis and intracorporeal suturing.

- **Specialized procedures** with established simulations include urology, cardiology, ENT and orthopaedics.

Although only part of the wider picture outlined above, simulator technology plays a vital role in each of these levels. We will now outline three main types of simulator currently available, presenting the pros and cons of each. We write from a UK perspective, where the use of live animals for training has been prohibited for more than a century. We therefore do not cover live animal simulations in our discussion The final selection of which simulator(s) to use will depend on individual requirements and the proposed curriculum.

30.4.1 Physical models

Benchtop models are widely used within surgical training, especially at undergraduate and early postgraduate levels. These models are made from a variety of plastic and latex materials. They address a range of clinical procedures (e.g. venepuncture, cannulation, urinary catheterization, basic suturing) as well as bowel and vascular anastomosis, hernia repair and other commonly performed surgical tasks. They have the advantage of being able to interact directly with instruments and to show a range of tissue handling characteristics.

Box trainers allow minimal access surgery procedures to be practised using endoscopic instruments. A covering of artificial skin allows port insertion and basic camera management, and a variety of tasks can be presented within the box. These include object transfer and other manipulative tasks. Box trainers are especially helpful during the early stages of training, since basic techniques such as camera handling, tissue dissection and endoscopic suturing can be rehearsed repeatedly. Dead animal tissue can be used for practising more advanced procedures.

Advances in materials technology have improved the realism of such models, which fulfil a useful function by allowing novices to practise tasks repeatedly. In comparison with VR computer simulators, physical models are relatively cheap. A major drawback is that models are divorced from their clinical context and can lead to a reductionist approach to learning. They also do not incorporate facilities for objective performance assessment.

30.4.2 Virtual reality computing

A rapidly expanding range of computer-generated simulations can now recreate many surgical procedures with a high degree of realism, allowing learners to interact with a convincing computer-based environment. Minimal access procedures lend themselves especially to such simulations, as manipulating objects with surgical instruments while watching a 2D screen reflects the reality of minimal access surgery.

Such simulators consist of a manipulation station (using instruments which resemble those used in surgical procedures), a screen and a computer. Learners choose procedures from a menu of varying levels of difficulty. Performance metrics (e.g. time taken, bleeding encountered, errors made) and the procedure itself can be recorded automatically. Feedback based on these metrics is normally provided after the procedure, with or without a tutor's input.

The first generation of VR simulators focused on training basic skills by performing isolated tasks (e.g. pick and place, navigation) using abstract scenes and 2D representations of geometric solids. Systems like MIST-VR have an established record of efficacy and have been extensively validated.

The second generation focused also on basic skills, but attempted to achieve this by using more realistic procedural tasks, such as clipping blood vessels or intracorporeal knotting. In these programs, the background to the simulation looks much more like that of a real operation, with deformable tissues and realistic organ responses. Surgical Science's LapSim® was one of the first systems using this approach.

The current generation allows entire procedures (e.g. laparoscopic cholecystectomy) to be simulated. Anatomical variants can create a range of difficulty levels. This is a significant advance in creating an environment which moves beyond psychomotor skill and begins to include decision making in a complex world. The LapMentor® from Simbionix is a force feedback enabled laparoscopic training simulator offering trainees the possibility to train on either the basic skills or perform full blown laparoscopic cholecystectomy procedures.

However, the more complex a simulation and the more variables it offers, the greater the computing power it requires. There is a trade-off between high visual fidelity on the one hand and the program's ability to respond in real time on the other. For example, some simulators combine high quality graphics with miniature servo motors to provide haptic feedback (the sensation of interacting with tissue while operating) in order to increase fidelity. This in turn increases the demand for computing power even further, and most existing haptic feedback devices are not yet robust and reliable enough to be used routinely.

A major drawback of these simulators is their cost and their need for specialised support. Before investing in such equipment it is important to define the training need they are expected to meet.

30.4.3 Hybrid simulators

These are perhaps the most interesting development, as they offer great potential for recreating the clinical context of practice. Hybrid simulators combine a physical model (replicating the instruments as well as the anatomy interface) with a computer program (which creates interactive settings within which learning can take place). A key advantage of such technology is its potential for team training and for moving beyond the practice of isolated technical skills.

Sophisticated patient mannekins (Laerdal's SimMan®, METI's iStan®) are computer driven full scale model humans which present a range of pathophysiological variables and can respond to the administration of drugs, as well as give immediate feedback to a range of interventions. They are well established within anaesthetic training, for example, and are becoming increasingly common within other domains including advanced life support training, operating room training and paediatrics. Such simulators may be used within a dedicated educational facility (e.g. a training centre or simulated operating theatre) but also in the field. Portable mannekins allow realistic disaster scenarios to be mounted in a range of authentic settings, enabling clinical assessment and casualty evacuation.

Hybrid endoscopy simulators (Immersion's Endoscopy AccuTouch®, Simbionix's GI Mentor®) combine an authentic interface (the endoscope) with realistic VR displays of the endoluminal view seen by the operator. They simulate a range of diagnostic and therapeutic endoscopic procedures, including upper and lower gastrointestinal flexible endoscopy. A collection of virtual patient cases offers different levels of difficulty, allowing novice and intermediate learners to gain the basics of manipulative skill through repeated practice. Performance metrics are captured by the software and presented to the learner after each procedure. A range of pathological conditions and technical challenge levels is offered.

Hybrid interventional endovascular simulators (Immersion's Endovascular AccuTouch®, Mentice's VIST®, Simbionix Angio Mentor®) use sophisticated computer graphics and modelling techniques to produce synthetic live fluoroscopy images and simulate the interaction between vascular walls, catheters and guidewires. Custom-made hardware interfaces using real catheters reproduce the crucial force feedback involved in such procedures. Current simulators offer a variety of cases covering a range of vascular procedures including coronary, neurovascular, renal, SFA and iliac artery interventions, and carotid stenting. The decision-making process is enhanced during the simulation by the display of vital signs, haemodynamic wave tracings and patient responses that appropriately reflect the physiology.

The range of simulators on the market continues to expand, both in terms of functionality and the range of procedures covered. It seems likely that specialised programs making use of simulator technology will become established in most major surgical specialties. Table 30.1 summarizes the currently available commercial surgical simulators at the time of going to press, grouping them according to the above classification and briefly commenting on their functionality. It should be borne in mind that simulator development is a fast moving field, and that the life cycle of individual simulators is often shorter than a book's production time. This makes it all the more important to have a clear educational strategy in place before selecting expensive items of equipment.

Table 30.1 Summary of existing commercial surgical simulator systems

Simulator	Comments
Physical	
◆ Beating Heart Model (The Chamberlain Group)	Physical model of a beating heart including pump
◆ Suture Tutor (Limbs & Things)	Skin pad & multimedia instruction CD-ROM for practising basic wound closure
◆ Bowel and vascular trainers (Limbs & Things)	Benchtop models for anastomosis practice
Virtual reality computing	
◆ MIST-VR (Mentice)	Low fidelity key laparoscopic surgical techniques and high fidelity suturing
◆ LapSim (Surgical Science)	High fidelity basic laparoscopic skills plus suturing and dissection. Gynaecology module available
◆ SEP (Simsurgery)	Basic laparoscopic skills and procedure related tasks
◆ SIMENDO (Simendo Systems)	Low fidelity laparoscopic basic skills trainer including knot tying and suturing
◆ SkillsSetPro (Verefi Technologies)	Comprehensive solution to laparoscopic basic skills training including several modules for training eye–hand coordination, laparoscopic suturing, basic laparoscopic motor skills and competitive/collaborative tasks
◆ LAP Mentor (Simbionix)	Basic laparoscopic skills and those required for cholecystectomy. Incorporates force feedback and high fidelity graphics
◆ SIMENDO Arthro (Simendo Systems)	Low fidelity arthroscopy basic skills trainer
◆ Procedicus VA (Mentice)	Arthroscopy simulator comprised of a base platform, customized haptic device, and modules for various joints and procedures including shoulder and knee
Hybrid	
VIST-VR (Mentice)	Vascular interventional procedures, such as coronary, carotid and renal stenting, plus pacemaker lead placement. Incorporates force feedback
Angio Mentor (Simbionix)	Interventional endovascular basic skills and complete procedures
mini Angio Mentor (Simbionix)	Portable, integrated training solution for basic skills practice of angiographic procedures. Includes modules for training interventional endovascular procedures
Endoscopy AccuTouch (Immersion)	Percutaneous coronary and peripheral interventions and cardiac rhythm management
Virtual IV (Laerdal)	System for training intravenous catheterization
Mediseus Epidural (MedicVision)	Full procedure epidural simulation with integrated core curriculum
PERC Mentor (Simbionix)	Percutaneous access procedures using fluoroscopy
URO Mentor (Simbionix)	Cystoscopy and ureteroscopy procedures with real-time fluoroscopy. Flexible and rigid scopes

Continued

Table 30.1 (continued) Summary of existing commercial surgical simulator systems

GI Mentor (Simbionix)	Endoscopy simulator for colonoscopy and gastroscopy. Includes modules for ERCP practice
Accutouch/Cathsim (Simbionix)	Endoscopy and cardiac catheterization simulators
ProMIS (Haptica)	Basic skills and techniques of minimally invasive surgery
ProMIS LC (Haptica)	Laparoscopic colectomy simulator
EYESI (VRmagic)	Simulator for intraocular surgery
METIMan, SimMan, MedSim (METI)	Intelligent anaesthetic, ultrasound and emergency scenario dummies already used in some universities

30.4.4 **Fidelity**

Fidelity is a key issue, especially when deciding on the level of investment to make. Researchers are constantly developing new simulation technologies and making serious efforts toward the construction of high fidelity systems. But further work is needed to determine the actual requirements of simulators to make an effective training tool. It is widely believed that higher fidelity in simulation will improve training, but this may not be the case. A recently published conceptual framework for laparoscopic VR simulators[26] considers VR simulation as a didactic means to meet different training needs, using a range of resources: fidelity resources, teaching resources and assessment resources. Using this framework, simulator design and selection can be considered as an optimization task between available resources to meet a specific training need. Thus, fidelity is considered alongside all other simulator functionalities, in the context of a specific training curriculum. This view acknowledges that no single level of realism will meet all needs, and effective decisions will require a closer collaboration between users and designers/manufacturers.

30.4.5 **Simulator evaluation and validation**

Simulators allow trainees to practice repeatedly with permission to fail and to experience the consequences of error without endangering patients. Moreover the conditions which typically lead to erroneous behavior can be recreated to support error prevention strategies, Such an environment has clear educational, economic and efficiency advantages. However, not all simulators are equally effective. Successful simulation demands a symbiotic relationship between users and developers. For end users (surgical trainers and trainees), simulators must meet educational needs and improve clinical practice. For simulator developers, however, technical development and profitability are key drivers. This tension can lead to unhelpful confusion about who is leading and who is following. This may divert attention from the key tasks of identifying training needs and working collaboratively towards reliable and valid systems which satisfy them.

While it is widely acknowledged that VR simulators offer obvious benefits as formative tools for training and are extensively used for this purpose already, the place of this type of simulators for summative assessment has yet to be confirmed. The problem is not that of obtaining performance metrics, but in validating simulators as proxies for surgical performance[27]. In the validation process, objective studies are used to demonstrate resemblance to a real world task (face validity) and to measure an identified and specific situation (content validity). Simple tests, such as construct validation, may show that an expert performs better than a novice in the model under test, while more complex, randomized controlled studies (concurrent validation) correlate the new method with a gold standard, such as apprenticeship. Simulator-based competence should improve over time and with increasing operative experience, and it should be possible to discriminate between surgically naive and more experienced subjects.

Ultimately, if simulators are to be valid measures of operative ability, a surgeon's competence in a simulator should correlate with actual performance in the operating theatre. Predictive validity evaluates the impact on performance in a real procedure. Although several studies have demonstrated the feasibility, reliability and validity of simulators as training aids in laparoscopic surgery, very limited work has been done in studying the transfer of simulator training into operative performance.

30.5 **Future developments**

The rapid pace of development in the fields related to simulator technology makes the prediction of the future very hard. Nevertheless, we believe that there will be further symbiosis between users of simulators and their developers. Together with the acceptance and insistence by the public that all surgery professionals reach a required level of competence using simulation-based training before treating a patient, this symbiosis will serve as a catalyst for the more widespread use of surgical simulators. To support this use, simulator technology will become more portable and cheaper.

We consider patient-specific simulators (PPS) and patient-focused simulation (PFS) to be two exciting major trends in the coming years.

30.5.1 **Patient-specific simulation**

Simulators permitting the uploading of patient-specific models and data will become the norm, allowing surgeons to practise preoperatively, combining scanned images of a patient's anatomy and pathology with computerized simulations of the procedure itself (augmented reality – Fig. 30.1). Increased awareness of the importance of context will result in a move away from task-based simulators to complex simulator systems supporting a more team-based approach. Hybrid simulator technology will continue to develop, expanding into all areas of

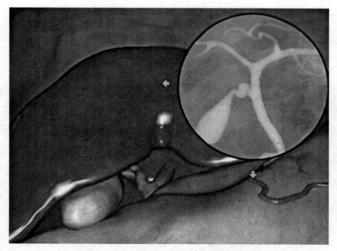

Fig. 30.1 Simulator combining 3D models of anatomy with scanned images of the patient. (Simbionix LAP Mentor. Reproduced with courtesy of Simbionix).

surgical practice and providing clinical challenges within a realistic yet safe environment. Such simulators will also support teams, enabling both individuals and teams to explore the consequences of their actions or decisions.

The use of PSS is not just confined to education and training; it can also serve as an aid in treatment planning and rehearsing before operating on the patient as well as be extended to provide real time guidance during interventional procedures.

30.5.2 **Patient-focused simulation**

Simulation has traditionally been used to practise isolated elements of surgical technique. There are attractions in focusing on one component of a procedure, without the confounding effect of real-world complexity. Yet there is also a danger of oversimplification. Increasingly, surgical simulations are taking place within a professional context such as a simulated operating theatre. But there is little in the literature about including patients in procedural tasks, even though many procedures are carried out on conscious patients.

Procedures on conscious patients require a sophisticated mixture of simultaneous skills, including effective communication with the patient. Not only is it necessary to perform each procedure while interacting with the patient, but the clinician must have enough confidence and skill to recognize if the procedure is going wrong and take steps to remedy the situation. This requires far-reaching expertise in several dimensions, backed up by the ability (usually based on personal experience) to recognize early warning signs and act on them promptly.

In the past, such expertise was born out of endless years of practice – practice at the bedside, in the clinic and in the operating theatre. In the current climate of reduced clinical exposure, how can clinicians gain that unconscious mastery which blends technical and non technical expertise while remaining sensitive to the unexpected?

PFS offers a possible solution, by placing the patient at the centre of the procedure. Pioneered by our research group, PFS uses an imaginative combination of inanimate training models with simulated patients (SPs), professional actors trained to play a role during clinical procedure scenarios (Fig. 30.2). Although the clinician performs the technical procedure on the simulator, the presence of a human 'patient' taps into real world experience, creating a powerful illusion of reality and forcing clinicians to combine technical and interpersonal skills. Feedback from multiple perspectives is key to PFS. Each procedure is watched by a clinical expert who provides focused feedback after the procedure[10,13]. The SP provides the patient's perspective, which highlights different aspects of performance.

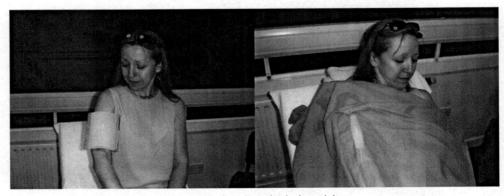

Fig. 30.2 Patient-focused simulation example using physical models.

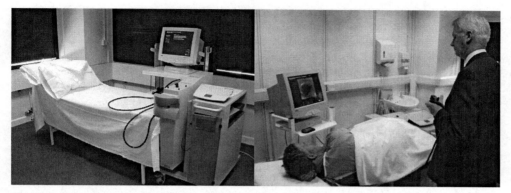

Fig. 30.3 Patient-focused simulation example using hybrid simulator.

Early work with simple clinical scenarios led to more complex procedures such as endoscopy (using hybrid flexible sigmoidoscopy and colonoscopy simulators within a simulated procedure suite – Fig. 30.3) and vascular interventions (e.g. carotid endarterectomy under local anaesthetic, within a simulated operating theatre)[5,12]. Such scenarios can be created without elaborate facilities and at a modest cost. Many existing physical models and VR simulators can be combined with SPs to create procedural scenarios.

30.6 **Conclusion**

Simulation seems certain to be a mainstay of surgical training in the future. These are exciting times, and the pace of change is breathless. Advances in computing and materials technology will increase the realism of skills-based simulators. A growing awareness of context will highlight the importance of teamworking and professionalism within the surgical environment. PSS will offer tailor-made experiences based on individual cases. Patient focused simulation can make the context of learning as authentic as possible.

Yet a major challenge for any simulation centre is to ensure that learners' needs come first. Without a curriculum, there is a danger that technology will dominate learning and that educational goals will be eclipsed. Clear vision is essential to make wise use of simulation's enormous potential, and to ensure an equal partnership between pedagogy and technology.

Acknowledgements

We wish to acknowledge the work of our colleague Dr. Debra Nestel in developing patient-focused simulation and many other aspects of simulation referred to in this chapter.

References

1. Vidal FP, Bello F, Brodlie KW, et al. (2006). Principles and applications of computer graphics in medicine. *Comput Graph Forum* **25**: 113–37.
2. Lingard L, Reznick R, Espin S, Regehr G, DeVito I (2002). Team communications in the operating room: talk patterns, sites of tension, and implications for novices. *Academic Medicine* **77**(3). 232–7.
3. Lingard L, Espin S, Whyte S, et al. (2004). Communication failures in the operating room: an observational classification of recurrent types and effects. *Qual.Saf Health Care* **13**(5): 330–4.
4. Musselman LJ, MacRae HM, Reznick RK, Lingard LA (2005). You learn better under the gun: intimidation and harassment in surgical education. *Med Educ* **39**(9): 926–34.

5. Wetzel CM, Kneebone RL, Woloshynowych M, *et al.* (2006). The effects of stress on surgical performance. *Am J Surg* **191**(1): 5–10.

6. Bushell E, Gaba D (2002). Anesthesia simulation and patient safety. *Problems in Anaesthesia* **13**: 506–14.

7. Gaba D, Howard S, Fish K, Smith B, Sowb Y (2001). Simulation-based training in anaesthesia crisis resource management (ACRM): a decade of experience. *Simulation and Gaming* **32**(2): 175–93.

8. Gaba DM (2004). The future vision of simulation in health care. *Qual.Saf Health Care* **13** (Suppl. 1): i2–10.

9. Kneebone R, Kidd J, Nestel D et al. (2005). Blurring the boundaries: scenario-based simulation in a clinical setting. *Medical Education* **39**: 580–7.

10. Kneebone R, Nestel D, Yadollahi F, et al. (2006). Assessing procedural skills in context: exploring the feasibility of an Integrated Procedural Performance Instrument (IPPI). *Med Educ* **40**(11): 1105–14.

11. Kneebone R, Nestel D, Wetzel C, et al. (2006). The human face of simulation: patient-focused simulation training. *Acad Med* **81**(10): 919–24.

12. Kneebone R, Nestel D, Moorthy K, et al. (2003). Learning the skills of flexible sigmoidoscopy – the wider perspective. *Medical Education* **37**(Suppl. 1): 50–8.

13. Kneebone R, Kidd J, Nestel D, Asvall S, Paraskeva P, Darzi A (2002). An innovative model for teaching and learning clinical procedures. *Med Educ* **36**(7): 628–34.

14. Kneebone RL (2005). Clinical simulation for learning procedural skills: a theory-based approach. *Academic Medicine* **80**(6): 549–53.

15. Ericsson KA (2004). Deliberate practice and the acquisition and maintenance of expert performance in medicine and related domains. *Academic Medicine* **79**(10): S70–S81.

16. Ericsson KA (1996). *The Road to Excellence: the Acquisition of Expert Performance in the Arts and Sciences, Sports and Games.* Lawrence Erlbaum Associates, Mahwah, New Jersey.

17. Vygotsky LS (1978). *Mind in Society.* Harvard University Press, Cambridge, Massachusetts.

18. Wertsch JV (1985). *Vygotsky and the Social Formation of Mind.* Harvard University Press, Cambridge, Massachusetts.

19. Bruner JS (1960.) *The Process of Education.* Harvard University Press, Cambridge Massachusetts.

20. Bruner JS (1967). *Toward a Theory of Instruction.* Harvard University Press, Cambridge, Massachusetts.

21. Wood D (1998). *How Children Think and Learn.* Second edn, Blackwell, Oxford.

22. Guile D, Young M (2001). Apprenticeship as a conceptual basis for a social theory of learning. In: C. Paechter *et al.*, eds. *Knowledge, Power and Learning.* Paul Chapman Publishing Ltd, London: 56–73.

23. Lave J, Wenger E (1991). *Situated Learning. Legitimate Peripheral Participation.* Cambridge University Press, Cambridge.

24. Wenger E (1998). *Communities of Practice. Learning, Meaning, and Identity.* Cambridge University Press, Cambridge.

25. American College of Surgeons (2006). *Technical Skills Education in Surgery.* http://www.facs.org/education/technicalskills/foreword/foreword.html.

26. Lamata P, Bello F, Kneebone R, Aggarwal R, Lamata F, Gomez E (2006). Conceptual Framework for Laparoscopic VR Simulators. *IEEE Computer Graphics & Applications* **26**: 69–79.

27. Carter FJ, Schijven MP, Aggarwal R, *et al.* (2005). Work Group for Evaluation and Implementation of Simulators and Skills Training Programmes 2005, Consensus guidelines for validation of virtual reality surgical simulators. *Surg Endosc* **19**(12): 1523–32.

Chapter 31

Creating virtual reality medical simulations

A knowledge-based design and assessment approach

Dale C Alverson, Thomas P Caudell, and Timothy E Goldsmith

Overview

- Our virtual reality simulation development is based upon the concept of providing a distributable simulator environment in which individual trainees and instructors can work together virtually as teams despite physical separation at different locations.

- Using a multiplayer collaborative participatory environment, enabled over advanced internet networks, offers a platform for 'just-in-time' team training, training on demand, refreshment training, and performance assessment, that can compliment onsite simulation

- As in other forms of simulation, virtual reality also can be applied to individuals, as well as teams, and the simulator technology or user interface matched with the goals of the simulation, needs of the learners/trainees and their best learning style.

- Virtual reality simulations provide a means for interactive, experiential, problem-based learning and integrated into simulation centres, an overall curriculum or training milieu, creating safe environments to make mistakes, a sense of presence, and engagement to enhance learning.

- Virtual reality simulation should be matched with the specific training goals and objectives; it may be designed for skill training, cognitive assessment and decision making, or both.

- In our initiatives, virtual reality simulations are based upon a rules-based artificial intelligence engine developed in conjunction with subject matter experts (SMEs) and computer programmers that dynamically governs changes in physiology, physical findings, movement and events, as well as responses to the user.

- Important concepts can be embedded into the virtual reality simulation scenario applying a knowledge-based design using the SME's knowledge structure as a gold standard.

- In addition, the expert knowledge structure can be used to compare the novice learner to the expert, provide a measure of the effect of the simulation in improving the learner's knowledge structure, and progression toward becoming an expert.

- Virtual reality simulation development requires a coordinated, collaborative transdisciplinary team of subject matter experts, computer scientists, engineers, graphic and sound artists, communication network specialists, educators, cognitive psychologists, and evaluators.

Overview *(continued)*

♦ Virtual reality can include high fidelity graphics and animation that can be changed to match the needs of the simulation scenario.

♦ Virtual reality can also enable reification of abstract concepts that provides a method wherein those abstractions can be perceived, rendered and visualized as something concrete with which the users can interact.

31.1 **Introduction**

This chapter describes the step-by-step approach to creating a virtual reality (VR) simulation for medical education, training, and performance assessment, as well as an example of the tools and methods that can be applied. VR simulations can be used onsite as part of a simulation centre or independently offsite, by individual learners or teams of learners, as well as used interactively by teams over distance at different sites in distributed VR environments. VR allows students and trainees to be uniquely immersed and engaged in lifelike situations where they can learn without suffering the consequences that may occur due to lack of experience[1]. With VR, as with simulation in general, students are offered a type of experiential training that would otherwise be impossible to achieve, a safe environment to make mistakes and improve performance through practice. Simulation training is especially important in medical education where students are expected to learn how to react in high-risk situations where human lives are potentially at stake. VR simulation for training and education represents 'serious games' that provide an opportunity for students to apply important concepts while thinking on their feet without endangering themselves or others, opportunities to improve understanding, gain confidence in application of their knowledge and skills. In addition, through a process called reification, VR can create environments in which participants could not normally interact, environments that are not normally accessible but that could be produced for improving comprehension of otherwise abstract concepts, making them appear concrete with which the learner can interact[2]. Virtual reality simulations of complex or abstract concepts offer powerful tools to improve human comprehension and understanding of those concepts, through the process of 'reification' in which those abstractions can be made to appear concrete and with which the learner can interact. In this manner, the individuals can use their senses to perceive better the relevance of important concepts, entering virtual worlds outside of normal experience, interacting through 'perceptualization', a combination of visualization, sound, touch and perhaps even taste and smell. These principles have been applied in developing a 'fantastic voyage' into the human kidney, in which the 'voyager' can interact and manipulate the important elements in the virtual world, and thus begin to grasp the important abstract concepts that are often difficult to learn, understand and teach.

Developing ways to increase student competence and comprehension is an ongoing pursuit in medical education as attempts to decrease medical errors and improve quality of care have been brought to the forefront of curricula in medical schools across the country[3,4]. Simulations are also being used in several other domains as a method to enhance learning, training, and assessment of competence[5–7]. Similarly, using advanced communication networks, VR can create environments for distributed team training independent of distance or location. These types of team interactions further represent the actual type of situation in which interdisciplinary medical teams need to work together. Distributed VR simulations also can allow 'just in time' training or education on demand without requiring participants to be at the same physical location.

Several studies have been carried out under the auspices of Project TOUCH (Telehealth Outreach for Unified Community Health), a multi-year collaboration between The University of

Hawaii and The University of New Mexico. Previous TOUCH investigations determined whether medical students could work as a team within a virtual problem-based learning environment. These studies concluded that team performance within the VR environment was as good as in real life team sessions[1,8]. Another study investigated whether medical student learning could be objectively demonstrated within VR training[9]. The study found evidence of significant learning as a function of a single VR training experience. Education is shifting from developing the ability to remember and repeat information to developing the ability to find information and use it in a timely, effective, and appropriate manner[10]. Educational methods are much more learner-centred to promote learning with understanding, and more importantly, enhance the ability to transfer learning to other settings[11]. These principles apply to the broad arena of healthcare education where acquiring and maintaining, the knowledge and skills to become a competent healthcare professional are a significant challenge[3].

People understand and process information in different ways, but they learn by making sense out of their experiences[10]. How much and how well they learn has to do with how successfully their learning experience matches their individual learning style[11]. Virtual simulations provide experiential learning environments that appeal to the four basic learning styles, but particularly, promote learning through doing, sensing and reacting. One of the most important benefits of simulations occurs through the learner interacting with objects within the virtual environment, which fosters the discovery process through interaction and exploration as opposed to didactic instruction[12]. This adds significant value to virtual teaching and learning environments[13].

Dramatic advances in information technology, including high performance computing, interactive simulations, visualization, VR and collaborative networks, and artificial intelligence offer a unique opportunity for enhancement of learning.

The creation of a VR simulation requires that a development team combine the elements of high performance computing, computer science and engineering, visualization and perceptualization, VR, coding for artificial intelligence, high fidelity graphics and 3D models, knowledge-based design, health sciences expertise, evaluation, education, and advanced communication networking, as well as students related to those various domains. In fact, several students have completed their research requirements or received advanced degrees related to initiatives involved in these VR simulation projects. Subject matter experts (SMEs) pertinent to the content material and learning goals and objectives in the simulation are key participants.

This chapter captures these concepts and lays out a process for developing VR simulation including describing specific steps, methods, and tools. It also provides a method for evaluating the impact of VR stimulation on learning and performance. Finally, it gives specific examples of VR simulation and suggests future approaches to research and development.

31.2 Knowledge structure approach

Underlying much of our work in designing and evaluating VR simulations is the idea of an explicit representation of knowledge, and in particular the representation of knowledge by a human expert. By knowledge representation we mean a set of core concepts and their corresponding interrelationships. It is this type of expert knowledge structure that guides our VR research and serves as a basis for evaluating student learning.

Our thinking in this area has been influenced by several decades of research in cognitive science showing that not only do experts acquire a vast amount of domain-specific knowledge but they represent this knowledge in long-term memory in highly structured ways[14–16]. Over the past decades, an impressive literature has accumulated showing that the structural properties of domain knowledge are closely related to domain competence[17]. How a person has the central concepts of a domain organized in memory reflects his knowledge. Experts share a particular structural organization of concepts, and as a consequence, are more likely to see certain relevant, abstract relationships and connections[10]. Studies have shown that experts in various domains, such as physics and computer programming, organize the central concepts along semantic dimensions, whereas novices organize their knowledge along surface level characteristics[18]. It is this organization of domain knowledge, that reflects an individual's degree of conceptual understanding in a domain.

There have been various attempts to elicit individuals' knowledge structures beginning in the 1970s[19–21]. Much of this work had an educational focus where students' knowledge structures were used to assess how much they understood about a studied topic. Our own work uses a three-phase method for eliciting and evaluating an individual's knowledge structure:

- elicit some behavioural index of an individual's organization of domain concepts
- represent these elicited data as a formal representation (e.g. network) that captures the important structural properties of the knowledge
- evaluate the goodness or level of expertise of the derived representation.

The elicitation phase begins by identifying a master set of terms and concepts from textbooks, manuals, reports and SMEs. We then ask SMEs to rate the centrality or relevance of these terms to the knowledge domain. From these averaged relevance ratings we pare down the list to around 25–30 terms. The SMEs then rate the relatedness of each pair of terms, and it is an average of these pair-wise relatedness ratings of the central concepts that serve as the basis for deriving a single expert knowledge structure. There exists a long history of research and theory in psychology that justifies using concept ratings as a measure of semantic structure[22–24].

During the second phase, the relatedness ratings are transformed into a form that elucidates the underlying structure of the concept relations. This resulting representation should:

- capture the structural relations among concepts
- be easy to comprehend
- capture all relevant (e.g. predictive) latent structure
- be data-driven.

In previous research, we evaluated several different scaling algorithms—including multidimensional scaling[25], hierarchical clustering[26], and untransformed proximity data – and found that the Pathfinder algorithm[27] best met these criteria[28,29]. Pathfinder generates a connected graph, or knowledge network, that depicts local concept relationships as directly linked nodes in the graph. Pathfinder knowledge networks were found to predict well students' classroom performance[30].

Finally, in the evaluation phase, a person's knowledge structure (i.e. Pathfinder knowledge network) is evaluated to assess its level of competence. We use a referent-based evaluation to compare a student's knowledge structure to a corresponding expert knowledge structure[31]. A similarity index based on the commonality of directly linked concepts between the two networks provides the best predictor of student performance. This measure is referred to as structural similarity. Using this measure we find that experts have more similar knowledge structures to one another than do less experienced people, and the degree of similarity between a student's knowledge structure and an expert's is an index of how much the student knows about the domain. A second, referent-free method of evaluation called coherence, measures the internal consistency of a set of ratings by examining how well sets of ratings satisfy a generalized triangle inequality law. Coherence has been shown to increase with levels of domain expertise. Both structural similarity and coherence exist on a 0–1 scale.

Using the above methods we derive for each VR simulation an expert knowledge structure. This knowledge structure is obtained by averaging concept ratings across a group of SMEs and then using Pathfinder to derive a single network. The resulting expert knowledge structure is used for two purposes: to guide the development of the VR simulation and to serve as a gold standard against which to assess students' learning of the domain.

31.2.1 Assessing student learning in VR

A principal goal in creating a VR simulation is to foster student learning of the simulated domain. To assess this, we obtain knowledge structures from students for the same set of concepts that occur in the expert knowledge structure. We acquire these knowledge structures two times, once before the student experiences the VR simulation and then immediately after VR training. Students rate the relatedness of concepts before and immediately after training, and Pathfinder is applied to both sets of ratings to derive two network representations per student.

We then compute the structural similarity between each student's knowledge network and the expert's network. The change in pre/post-training similarities is viewed as an index of VR learning. The pre/post change in knowledge structures serves as an immediate and objective index of the effect of VR simulation on students' understanding of the domain. Learning is assumed to have occurred if students' similarity scores significantly improve over the course of VR training[9]. Further, these sorts of knowledge structures are particularly appropriate for assessing complex, conceptual understanding[32], exactly the type of knowledge that is the focus of our VR simulations.

However, we acknowledge that there are other and perhaps even more valid measures of student learning, such as how well knowledge transfers to other courses of study or how well it transfers to a clinical setting. In future work, we plan to examine how well the acquired conceptual knowledge transfers to novel tasks. We hypothesize that participants receiving simulation training will not only develop improved conceptual understanding of the domain, but that this understanding will transfer to tasks requiring the application of knowledge.

31.3 Methods: creating the VR simulations and processes for development

31.3.1 Knowledge-based design approach

In this section of the chapter, we describe what we believe to be a unique approach to designing VR simulations. The essence of the approach is to use the core concepts and relationships of the expert knowledge structure to guide the design of the simulated environment. As part of this process, the VR development team brainstorms with SMEs to identify multiple approaches for representing conceptual relationships; from this process storyboards emerge. The development team creates prototypes in a visualization tool or game engine, initially using coarse models, animations and sounds. SMEs then help refine elements of the simulation that best represent their conceptual understanding of the structure and process being simulated. A concept audit is conducted for each potential simulated environment to ensure that critical associations in the expert knowledge structure occur within the simulation. An initial rule-based artificial intelligence (AI) is also created to capture the general interactions of conceptual elements using SME-validated rules.

We also use student learning to refine the VR simulation. The change in students' knowledge structures as a result of VR training serves as an immediate and objective index of training effectiveness.

We examine what aspects of the students' knowledge structures change over the course of training, or more importantly what aspects do not change. As an example, assume that domain experts have concepts A, B, and C tightly linked together as a meaningful substructure in their knowledge network. Assume further that these links are absent from students' knowledge structures after VR training. We would want to examine how these concepts and their relationships are represented in the simulation and how this representation can be altered to make their associations more salient. Hence, achieving agreement between students' and experts' knowledge structures serves as an objective goal for guiding and refining the simulation.

The VR simulation design team iteratively refines game content and rules to arrive at the validity level required to begin learning experiments. Human subjects' knowledge structures are measured before and after system exposure and statistically compared to those of the SMEs. Changes are correlated with representational elements from the audit matrix to determine how they potentially contributed to the changes. Designers use the analysis to evolve or redesign the representation and possibly reevaluate which key concepts are included. The process is repeated until post-exposure subject performance best matches that of the experts. Detailed steps of the VR simulation are as listed:

0 – Identify subject matter experts (SMEs) and refine topic domain, source material collected

1 – Collect a superset of conceptual terms from as many SMEs as is possible for the topic domain.

2 – Perform analysis to down select a smaller set of key concepts ~30, validation by SMEs.

3 – One SME gives a 1-hour in-service explaining the key concepts to the team and how they relate to the topic, ranking of degree of difficulty of overall problem.

4 – Representation design formally begins; brainstorming, multi-forked approaches encouraged, storyboards created.

5 – For each completed representation design, make weighted association between each representational element and key concepts (a matrix), as well as ranking the degree of 'reification' and implied degree of VR immersion.

6 – Several representations are fleshed out and prototyped in a VR tool.

7 – Best representation is selected by SME panel and team.

8 – Selected representation validation by SMEs *vis-à-vis* key concept matrices, with constructive feedback.

9 – Iterative refinement (back to item 7) until deemed stable enough to test.

10 – Knowledge structure evaluation experiment, pre and post exposure, with knowledge-level filtered subjects.

11 – Analysis of knowledge structural changes and correlation with representational elements (from matrix), determining what elements potentially contributed to the changes.

12 – If time, repeat items 4 to 10 with varying degrees of either reification or immersion.

13 – If time permits, repeat items 0 to 12 with varying degree of overall problem domain difficulty.

14 – Document the results.

31.3.2 Validation of the VR simulations

Each VR simulation should be subjected to various levels of validation: face, content, construct, concurrent, and predictive.

31.3.2.1 Establishing face validity

SMEs review the VR simulation to determine whether the representation of the material and concepts matches their expected appearance of the content. Through an iterative process with the SMEs, the VR representation is refined.

31.3.2.2 Establishing content validity

The VR scenario and treatment algorithms are assessed for content accuracy to ensure that the curriculum goals have been incorporated, as well as for degree of fidelity and detail. Each scenario is evaluated in depth to determine if it is appropriate and situation specific. The scenario, simulation algorithm and content are then revised as needed.

31.3.3.3 Establishing concurrent validity

Each simulation scenario's outcomes related to measures of student learning are compared to an established 'gold standard' teachning method to assess whether learning goals have been met, with the ultimate objective to assure comparable outcomes or favourable enhancement of the teaching program when using the VR simulations.

31.3.2.4 Establishing construct validity

Scenarios are evaluated to ensure that performance in the VR simulation discriminates among novice, intermediate, and expert users based on prior assessment of the participant as to their level of knowledge or skills before the simulation experience. Performance criteria that differentiate those skill or knowledge levels should be demonstrable and measurable within the VR simulation and not based on competency in using the VR simulation tools alone.

31.3.2.5 Determining predictive validity

Scenarios can also be evaluated according to how well they predict subsequent performance or knowledge transfer to other real or simulated scenarios. The effects of pre-training and didactic information given to subjects prior to VR training can be evaluated by examining performance, stress level, and knowledge retention. Retention will be assessed at specified intervals, evaluating the effect of mastery upon the ability to transfer knowledge in a manner that is retained over time.

31.3.3 VR simulations tools

31.3.3.1 Flatland: a computer software platform and lattice for VR simulation

Flatland serves as the software infrastructure and is the platform, performance stage and lattice for visualization and the virtual reality application development environment. It was created at the University of New Mexico[33]. As a perceptualization and virtual environments development tool, Flatland allows software authors to construct, and users to interact with, arbitrarily complex graphical and aural representations of data and systems. It is written in C/C++ and uses the standard OpenGL graphics language to produce all graphics. In addition, Flatland uses the standard libraries for window, mouse, joystick, and keyboard management. It is object oriented, multi-threaded and uses dynamically loaded libraries to build user applications in the virtual environment (VE). As an open source code, Flatland can be run on a variety of operating systems including: IRIX, Linux, Unix, Mac OSX, and Windows. The end result is a VR immersive environment with sight and sound, in which the operator using joy wands and virtual controls can interact with computer-generated learning scenarios that respond logically to user interaction.

Virtual patients can be simulated in any of several circumstances, with any type of disease or injury.

31.3.3.2 VR simulation artificial intelligence

The artificial intelligence (AI) is a forward chaining IF-THEN rules-based system and contains knowledge of how objects interact within the VR simulation. The rules, which are determined by subject matter experts, are coded in a C computer language format as logical antecedents and consequences, and currently have limited human readability. The AI loops over the rulebase, applying each rule's antecedents to the current state of the system, including time, and testing for logical matches. Matching rules are 'fired', modifying the next state of the system. Time is a special state of the system that is not directly modified by the AI, but whose rate is controlled by an adjustable clock. Since the rate of inference within the AI is controlled by this clock, the operator is able to speed up, slow down, or stop the action controlled by the AI. The simulation AI engine dynamically governs changes in physiology, physical findings, movement and events, as well as responses to the user. This allows the participant user to make mistakes and repeat a scenario as a way to aid learning from those mistakes.

31.3.3.3 Tracking in the Flatland VR environment

Flatland is designed to make use of any position-tracking technology. A tracker is a multiple degree of freedom measurement device that can, in real time, monitor the position and/or orientation of multiple receiver devices in space, relative to a transmitter device. In the standard Flatland configuration, trackers are used to locate hand held wands and to track the position of the user's head. Head position and orientation are needed in cases that involve the use of head mounted displays or stereo shutter glasses.

User interaction is a central component of Flatland, and as such, each object is controllable in arbitrary ways defined by the designer. Currently there are four possible methods for the control of objects:

- pop-up menus in the main viewer window
- the keyboard
- 2D control panels either in the environment or separate windows
- external systems or simulations.

In the future there will also be available 3D menus and controls in the virtual environment, as well as possible voice recognition.

The immersed user or avatar interacts with the virtual patient or other virtual objects using a joy wand equipped with a six degree of freedom tracking system, buttons, and a trigger. The wand's representation in the environment is a virtual human hand. The user may pick up and place objects by moving the virtual hand and pulling the wand's trigger. Multiple user avatars can participate in the virtual environment simultaneously and interact with each other independently of location or distance (Fig. 31.1)[34,35]. The avatars can also interact verbally while in the VR environment.

The immersive 3D environment allows real-time exploration, examination, and manipulation of 3D objects and images. The interactive patient simulation engine allows students to dynamically determine the direction of the case scenario. The AI engine is coupled to the virtual environment to represent a virtual patient that manifests the signs and symptoms of the medical scenario. Students, who are fully immersed are represented within the virtual environment as avatars and can be observed by others from outside the virtual world via computer monitor or on a projection screen. Immersed students wear a head-mounted display associated with the

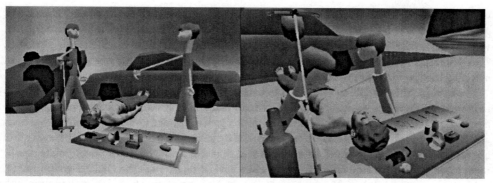

Fig. 31.1 Students at different locations interacting together as full body avatars in the virtual environment as they perform diagnostic evaluation and management of a virtual patient.

trackers, allowing them a sense of presence and interaction within the virtual environment. Team members within the virtual environment will be able to see each other as full human figures and interact as if they were physically present, even when those students are separated by significant distances. Immersed students can examine the virtual patient by independently controlling their viewpoint and motion within the virtual world. The ratio between real time and virtual time can be varied to allow events to progress slower or faster. The immersed users can work with others in a learning group to gather information and initiate interventions. During the simulation process, the students and tutor can discuss the case as it unfolds, pause the scenario as appropriate in order to talk about their observations, hypothesize, and generate learning issues (Fig. 31.2).

31.3.4 **Establishing user competency to operate the VR system**

The ability to manipulate objects in, and navigate within, the virtual environment significantly impacts user competence. A user must be able to function at different levels within the virtual environment, and it is likely that users from the videogaming generation will find it easier to navigate than users with little videogame experience. This leads to a potential confounding variable

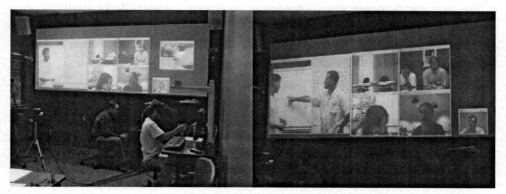

Fig. 31.2 Using the Access Grid the students and a tutor at different locations can observe the simulation, discuss the case as it unfolds, and pause the scenario as appropriate in order to talk about their observations, hypothesize, and generate learning issues.

when considering a participant's ability to navigate within the virtual environment. The 'expert' group may have subject matter expertise but be novices at navigating virtual environments, whereas the 'novice' group may have navigation expertise but be true novices in the subject matter. This potential variable can impact the ability to discriminate between novice and expert in assessing true performance with respect to the training or education objectives.

To overcome this, all subjects will need to have a period of orientation and training in how to manipulate objects and navigate within the virtual Flatland environment before participating in a scenario. This training should be continued until a predetermined level of competence has been achieved. It can take place in a 'sanitized' virtual environment in which no details of the scenario are revealed or a 'partially sanitized' environment that will allow the user to manipulate equipment associated with a simulation scenario while navigating through the Flatland environment. Subjects can be trained to meet a preset criterion, such as completing tasks in a certain time with an acceptable rate of errors. Levels for minimum competent performance can be defined by examining the distribution of performance indices, such as time to complete the sanitized or partially sanitized scenario and number of errors committed. Once those criteria for satisfactory competence for using the simulation tools have been established, each participant can be tested to assure reaching that minimal performance standard in using the system prior to the actual simulation training scenario. Ideally, all participants should train to a minimal level of competence in the totally sanitized environment and/or the partially sanitized environment prior to the actual VR simulation experience that is being used for training or education. In this manner one can judge better the effects of the actual simulation scenario on learning or skill attainment as opposed to measuring skills only related to the ability to use the simulation system.

31.4 **Preliminary studies of VR simulations**

Our initial efforts in VR research and development simulation have been in collaboration with the University of New Mexico, University of Hawaii, and our high performance computing centres, the Pacific Telehealth and Technology Hui at Tripler Army Medical Centre/VA, and the Uniformed Service University National Capital Area medical simulation centre, through the multi-year initiative Project TOUCH. Over the last several years we have developed an integrated, fully immersive, interactive VR system designed for medical education and training implemented in Flatland. These efforts have, in turn, led to iterations of the system to improve practical applications to meet specific user requirements. An interdisciplinary team has been participating in the ongoing planning, development and implementation of these virtual reality simulation projects. Our preliminary experiments in problem-based learning (PBL) setting have demonstrated that:

- virtual collaboration within VR is possible with multiple participants independent of distance
- students accept use of VR for education and training
- participants state they felt more engaged in VR
- students also felt they learned best from their mistakes in VR.

In comparative experiments, post-testing performance was similar between VR and non-VR groups, as well as distributed and non-distributed groups, indicating VR or distance distribution 'does no harm', demonstrating concurrent validity with standard text-based case methods[36].

Perhaps most significant was the evidence of improvement in knowledge structure after the VR simulation experience in a select group of learners with initial lower levels of knowledge structure correlation with that of experts[5]. Knowledge structure relatedness ratings were significantly improved in those students with lower pre-VR relatedness ratings which indicate the potential value of simulation in learning, particularly for those students with lower levels of knowledge of the concepts being learned. In general, the results suggest that the method used for eliciting, representing and evaluating knowledge structure offers a sensitive, objective and valid means for determining learning in virtual environments. More research is needed using controlled studies to determine specifically what aspects of the learning event produced the changes in knowledge.

Two simulations were developed:

- a virtual patient head injury case
- the reified nephron, a representation of the complex physiological functions of the kidney.

31.4.1 The virtual patient: a case of head trauma – 'Mr Toma'

In the Mr Toma case, a student arrives at an accident scene where paramedics have removed a victim from a car and prepared him for treatment[37]. The task is to diagnose the patient's injury and stabilize him for transport. The player can apply a range of instruments, bandages, and drugs at will. The rule-based AI system controls the behaviour of every internal patient element, including the patient's physiology, treatment responses, and drug effects. Knowledge from subject matter experts populates the AI system, which mirrors the way the experts cognitively structure this knowledge. Using our knowledge structure assessment methods, we have demonstrated that trainee VR immersion effectively increases students' level of understanding (Fig. 31.3)[9].

31.4.2 Reified models: nephron project

The renal simulation focuses on one of the microscopic multicellular filtering systems in the kidney: the nephron[2]. Students can control the flows, filtres, and functionality of each subcomponent of

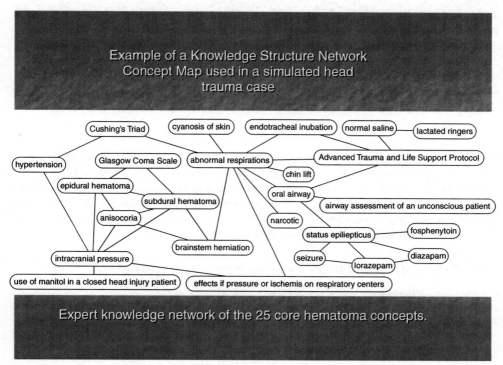

Fig. 31.3 An expert knowledge network can be used as the standard against which the novice learner can be compared. (Reprinted from: Westwood JD et al.(2005). Virtual reality training improves students' knowledge of medical concepts. *Medicine Meets Virtual Reality* **13**: 519–25. Reproduced with permission of IOS Press.)

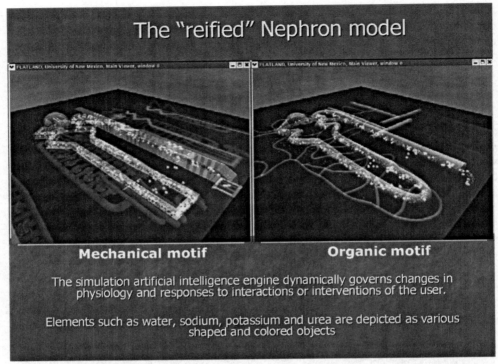

Fig. 31.4 The reified nephron represented in the virtual environment with which participants can interact and explore to better understand physiological concepts. (Reprinted from: Westwood JD *et al.* (2006). Reification of abstract concepts to improve comprehension using interactive virtual environments and a knowledge-based design. *Medicine Meets Reality* **14**: 13–18. Reproduced with permission of IOS Press.)

the nephron. They can zoom in and flow along with the various molecular components, and even rebuild the nephron to study the sensitivity of its functioning to its structure. In addition, a student may morph the graphical representation between a reified plumbing model and an anatomically correct model to help with orientation[38]. Again, a rule-based AI system derived from kidney experts' knowledge structure assessments controls all of the nephron physiology, component functionality, and their reaction to various drugs (Fig. 31.4).

31.5 Future VR simulation developments and next steps

Future VR simulations are likely to offer users a variety of interfaces to enhance usability and functionality, such as systems projected on standard monitors or screens without head mounted displays, as well as VR gloves or other types of user interfaces found in standard gaming devices (Fig. 31.5). The acceptance and familiarity of these types of systems, their ease of use, decreased complexity, and affordability should help advance the adoption of VR simulation.

Integration of other sensory modalities, such as sound[39], touch and even smell can enhance the sense of presence for the participants and the feeling of being there as opposed to being there in the real world. In addition, the degree of immersion and the level of fidelity necessary to

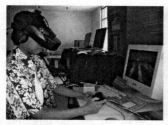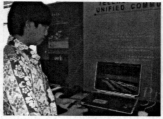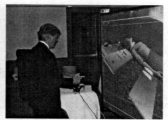

Fig. 31.5 A variety of user interfaces can be incorporated for interaction in the virtual reality environment with or without a head mounted display, rendered on a monitor or projection screen, and using different gaming-type devices. (Reprinted from: Westwood JD *et al.* (2007). The effect of degree of immersion upon learning performance in virtual reality simulations for medical education. *Medicine Meets Reality* **15**: 155–60. Reproduced with permission of IOS Press.)

provide for adequate user engagement and sense of presence could be studied in the development of the most effective forms of simulation that are also cost effective.

High level architecture (HLA) for interoperability and sharing simulations independent of platforms offers more wide spread usage but remains a challenge as the simulations user and developer communities address the balance between protecting intellectual property versus making simulations widely accessible.

Potential user acceptance should increase as outcome studies provide evidence of enhanced learning. We envision more general adoption and the creation of a library of simulations that can be integrated into curricula and training programs in a manner that can be modified to meet specific learning goals and objectives of a variety of trainees. Following the establishment of a production algorithm, it will be possible to create on-demand VR simulations. In this regard, partnering with the digital media and gaming industry offers the promise of high quality productions that can better meet the consumer demand and broader range of needs.

In accomplishing these goals, more interdisciplinary and inter-institutional collaboration in research, development, and evaluation of outcomes on learning, training and performance must be conducted in order to advance the field of VR simulation.

31.6 **Conclusions**

This chapter described a step-by-step approach for creating a VR simulation for medical education, training, and performance assessment, as well as a discussion of the tools and methods needed to create VR simulations.

VR simulation can be complementary to other simulation methods, offering educational capabilities that are currently unattainable with mannequins, live-actor simulation, and other traditional methods. Virtual patients can be animated, enabling visualization of signs and behaviours, such as convulsions, vomiting, coughing, tearing, and cramping, as well as exhibit behaviours consistent with clinical signs and emotional states, such as, fright, sadness, anxiety, pain, and lethargy. Virtual patients can dynamically change their appearance to visualize cyanosis, rashes, lesions, and other skin manifestations. VR simulations can be interactive, with lifelike conversation and behaviour, for reporting of symptoms and events, as well as allow the participant to be mobile, moving about the scene in a purposeful manner. These representations can be readily altered to represent the range of human diversity including gender, ethnicity, age, race, or other cultural variations. VR simulations can be duplicated, allowing practise of triage in a mass casualty simulation individually or as teams.

A simulation-based approach offers the opportunity to learn in a relatively realistic problem-solving environment, to practice skills without danger, to explore real and artificial situations, to modify the time-scale of events, and to interact with simplified versions of the process or system being simulated.

The initial research and development of virtual reality simulations require significant time and resources through an extensive iterative process requiring ongoing evaluation and improvements. Although our studies did not evaluate cost–benefit, we anticipate that with continued experience, production time and cost should diminish. In addition, we speculate that by using these simulations for distributed team training, students would avoid travel costs and time, and training scenarios could be more consistent.

Combining the elements of high performance computing, artificial intelligence, human-computer interface, perceptualization, high fidelity graphics, 3D models and knowledge-based design distributed over the next generation of the internet, creates the rubric of VR simulation that can enhance human understanding and learning. These efforts, which complement the development of advanced computing, digital media and gaming expertise, are converging to develop new models for interdisciplinary research and education that can provide tools for improving human understanding in a complex virtual world, a truly 'fantastic voyage'.

Acknowledgements

The project described was supported partially by grant 2 D1B TM 00003–02 from the Office for the Advancement of Telehealth, Health Resources and Services Administration, Department of Health and Human Services. Its contents are solely the responsibility of the authors and do not necessarily represent the official views of the Health Resources and Services Administration.

The project was also partially made possible by grant number W81XWH-04–1–0875 from the USAMRAA. Its contents are solely the responsibility of the authors and do not necessarily represent the official views of USUHS, the US Department of Defense, or the Henry M. Jackson Foundation for the Advancement of Military Medicine, Inc.

References

1. Alverson DC, Saiki SM Jr, Caudell TP, *et al.* (2005). Distributed immersive virtual reality simulation development for medical education. *Journal of International Association of Medical Science Educators* **15**: 19–30.
2. Alverson DC, Saiki SM Jr, Caudell TP, *et al.* (2006). Reification of Abstract Concepts to Improve Comprehension Using Interactive Virtual Environments and a Knowledge-based Design: A Renal Physiology Model. In: JD Westwood, RS Haluck, HM Hoffman, GT Mogel, R Phillips, RA Rob, KG Vosburgh, Eds. *Medicine Meets Virtual Reality 14; Accelerating Change in Health Care: Next Medical Toolkit, Volume IV Studies in Health Technology and Informatics.* IOS Press, Amsterdam, The Netherlands: 13–18.
3. Windish DM, Paulman PM, Goroll AH, Bass EB (2004). Do clerkship directors think medical students are prepared for the clerkship years? *Academic Medicine* **79**: 56–61.
4. Committee on Quality of Health Care in America (2001). *Crossing the Quality Chasm: A New Health System for the 21ˢᵗ Century.* Institute of Medicine, Washington DC, National Academy Press.
5. Winn WD (1993). A conceptual basis for educational applications of virtual reality. *Human Interface Technology Laboratory Technical Report TR-93–9.* Seattle, WA: Human Interface Technology Laboratory, University of Washington.

6. Champion HR, Higgins GA (2000). Meta-analysis and planning of SimTrauma: medical simulation for combat trauma training. *USAMRMC TATRC Report*, No.00–03.

7. Satava RM, Jones SB (1999). The future is now: virtual reality technologies. In: Tekian A, McGuire CH, McGaghie WC and Associates, eds. *Innovative Simulations for Assessing Professional Competence: from Paper-and-Pencil to Virtual Reality*. (12) University of Illinois at Chicago, Department of Medical Education: 179–93.

8. Alverson DC, Saiki SM, Jacobs J, *et al.* (2004). Distributed interactive virtual environments for collaborative experiential learning and training independent of distance over Internet2. In: JD Westwood, RS Haluck, HM Hoffman, GT Mogel, RPhillips, RA Rob, Eds. *Medicine Meets Virtual Reality 12; Building a Better You: The Next Tools for Medical Education, Diagnosis, and Care. Studies in Health Technology and Informatics B. Volume 28*. IOS Press, Amsterdam, The Netherlands: 7–12.

9. Stevens SM, Goldsmith TE, Summers KL, *et al.* (2005). Virtual reality training improves students' knowledge Ssructures of medical concepts. In: JD Westwood, RS Haluck, HM Hoffman, GT Mogel, R Phillips, RA Rob. *Medicine Meets Virtual Reality 13; The Magic Next Becomes the Medical Now, Volume III Studies in Health Technology and Informatics*. IOS Press, Amsterdam, The Netherlands: 519–25.

10. Bransford J, Brown AL, Cocking RR (2000). *How People Learn: Brain, Mind, Experience and School*. Washington DC: National Academy Press.

11. Kolb DA (1983). *Experiential Learning: Experience as the Source of Learning and Development*. Upper Saddle River, NJ: Prentice Hall.

12. Dalgarno B (2002). *The potential of 3D virtual learning environments: A constructivist analysis*. Available as a PDF document at http://www.usq.edu.au/electpub/e-jist/docs/Vo15%20No2/Dalgarno %20-%20Final.pdf.

13. Winn WD (1999). Learning in virtual environments: A theoretical framework and considerations for design. *Education Media International* **36**(4): 271–9.

14. Chase WG, Simon HA (1973). The mind's eye in chess. In: WG Chase, Ed. *Visual Information Processing*. New York: Academic Press.

15. Chi MTH, Feltovich P, Glaser R (1981). Categorization and representation of physics problems by experts and novices. *Cognitive Science* **5**: 121–52.

16. Ericsson KA, Smith J (1991). *Toward a General Theory of Expertise: Prospects and Limits*. New York, NY: Cambridge University Press.

17. Glasser R (1986). On the nature of expertise. In: Klix F, Hagendorf H, Eds. *Human Memory and Cognitive Capabilities: Mechanism and Performances*. North Holland: Elsevier Science.

18. Chi MTH, Glaser R, Rees E (1982). Expertise in problem solving. In: Sternberg RJ, ed. *Advances in Development of Human Intelligence, Vol. 1*. Hillsdale, NJ: Lawrence Erlbaum Assoc.

19. Fillenbaum S, Rapoport A (1971). *Structures in the Subjective Lexicon*. New York: Academic Press.

20. Geeslin WE, Shavelson RJ (1975). Comparison of content structure and cognitive structure in high school students learning of probability. *Journal of Research in Mathematics Education* **6**: 109–20.

21. Shavelson RJ, Staton GC (1975). Construct validation: methodology and application to three measures of cognitive structure. *Journal of Educational Measurement* **12**: 67–85.

22. James W (1983). *The Principles of Psychology*. Cambridge, MA: Harvard Univiversity Press: 434.

23. Shepard RN (1987). Toward a universal law of generalization for psychological science. *Science* **237**: 1317–23.

24. Tversky A (1977). Features of similarity. *Psychological Review* **84**: 327–52.

25. Kruskal JB (1964.) Multidimensional scaling by optimizing goodness of fit to a nonmetric hypothesis. *Psychometrika* **29**: 1–27.

26. Johnson SC (1967). Hierarchical clustering schemes. *Psychometrika* **32**: 241–54.

27. Schvaneveldt RW, Ed. (1990). *Pathfinder Associative Networks: Studies in Knowledge Organization*. Norwood, NJ: Ablex Publishing Corporation.

28. Johnson PJ, Goldsmith TE, Teague KW (1994). Structural knowledge assessment: Locus of the predictive advantage in Pathfinder-based structures. *Journal of Educational Psychology* **86**: 617–26.

29. Johnson PJ, Goldsmith TE, Teague KW (1995). Similarity, structure, and knowledge: A representational approach to assessment. In: Nichols, Chipman and Brennan, eds. *Cognitively Diagnostic Assessment*. Hillsdale, NJ: Lawrence Erlbaum Assoc: 221–49.

30. Goldsmith TE, Johnson PJ, Acton WH (1991). Assessing structural knowledge. *Journal of Educational Psychology* **83**: 88–96.

31. Goldsmith T, Davenport D (1990). Assessing structural similarity of graphs. In: Schvaneveldt R, Ed. *Pathfinder Associative Networks: Studies in Knowledge Organization*. Norwood NJ: Ablex Publishing Corporation.

32. Trumpower DL, Goldsmith TE (2004). Structural enhancement of learning. *Contemporary Educational Psychology,* **29**: 426–46.

33. Caudell T, Summers KL, Holten IV J, *et al.* (2003) Virtual patient simulator for distributed collaborative medical education. *The Anatomical Record (Part B: New Anat.)* **270B**: 23–9.

34. Mowafi M, Summers KL, Holten J, *et al.* (2004). Distributed interactive virtual environments for collaborative medical education and training: Design and characterization. In: Westwood JD, Haluck RS, Amsterdam H, Eds. *Medicine Meets Virtual Reality 12; Building a Better You: The Next Tools for Medical Education, Diagnosis, and Care, Volume 98. Studies in Health Technology and Informatics*. Amsterdam, the Netherlands: IOS Press: 259–61.

35. Childers L, Disz TL, Hereld M, *et al.* (1999). Active spaces on the grid: the construction of advanced visualization and interaction environments. In: B Engquist, L Johnsson, M Hammill, F Short, Eds. *Parallelldatorcentrum Kungl Tekniska Högskolan Seventh Annual Conference (Simulation and Visualization on the Grid), vol. 13, Lecture Notes in Computational Science and Engineering*. Stockholm, Sweden: Springer-Verlag: 64–80.

36: Alverson DC, Saiki SM, Jacobs J, *et al.* (2004). *Distributed Interactive Virtual Environments for Collaborative Experiential Learning and Training Independent of Distance over Internet2. (abs) Medicine Meets Virtual Reality 12*. Newport Beach, CA.

37. Jacobs J, Caudell T, Wilks D, *et al.* (2003). Integration of advanced technologies to enhance problem-based learning over distance: Project TOUCH. *Anat Rec (Part B:New Anat)* **270B**: 16–22.

38. Winn WD (2002). Current trends in educational technology research: The study of learning environments. *Educational Psychology Review* **14**(3): 331–51.

39. Panaiotis, Vergara V, Sherstyuk A, *et al.* (2006). Algorithmically generated music enhances VR nephron simulation. In: JD Westwood, RS Haluck, HM Hoffman, GT Mogel, R Phillips, RA Rob, KG Vosburgh, Eds. *Medicine Meets Virtual Reality 14; Accelerating Change in Health Care: Next Medical Toolkit Volume IV Studies in Health Technology and Informatics*. IOS Press, Amsterdam, The Netherlands: 422–7.

Chapter 32

Respiratory medicine and respiratory therapy

Brian Robinson

Overview

- Clinical simulation-based education and training is becoming established in respiratory care for competency skills assessment, and developing critical thinking.
- Training in the areas of respiratory assessment are well catered for, with a variety of computer and mannequin based breath-sound simulators, and computer-based arterial blood gas training programmes.
- Opportunities exist using a variety of patient simulators, mannequins, part-task trainers and lung/breathing simulators for training respiratory care skills.
- Respiratory care skills include oxygen administration, airway management, respiratory support, and ventilation.
- Mannequins and other technologies also available for chest drain insertion and care, and the use of flexible fibreoptic bronchoscopy.
- No single simulation device currently exists for the training and assessment in all aspects of respiratory medicine and associated therapies.
- Combinations of devices, and clinical training and assessment techniques are required to provide comprehensive coverage.
- Future features of simulators may include integration of these features into the one mannequin.

32.1 Introduction

Simulation-based education and training is becoming established in respiratory care[1] and recognized to enhance competency skills assessment[2]. Clinical simulation is considered an important strategy for developing critical thinking in respiratory care training, and in the intensive care setting[3,4].

The aim of this chapter is to provide examples for using simulation and skills based teaching methods focusing on the respiratory care of patients. It is intended for all health specialties that provide respiratory care of patients, and provides examples to facilitate undergraduate and postgraduate learning. These may extend to multidisciplinary or inter-professional learning, and provide opportunities for certification or credentialing assessments.

When looking through catalogues and websites, there is a vast array of part-task clinical trainers, mannequins, and simulators applicable for clinical training and respiratory care. The issue that often confronts the trainer, the teacher or instructor is selection of the most suitable device. The frequent problem is the gap that exists between the learning objectives and the capabilities of the device. Often the role of a clinical training facilitator is to bridge those gaps. Although an array of respiratory care mannequins or training devices exists, effective learning will occur when use is appropriately matched to intended learning outcomes.

The following sections describe the varieties of part-task trainers, mannequins, and simulators available for clinical respiratory teaching and training. These have been divided into three sections focusing on learning outcomes: respiratory assessment, clinical respiratory skills and therapies, and clinical decision-making regarding the care of a patient. Because there is a large and expanding range of training devices and software on the market, it is likely that some devices may not be described here. The training devices, software, and methods described are provided as examples and are by no means comprehensive.

32.2 **Respiratory assessment**

32.2.1 **Breath sounds**

Teaching interpretation of breath sounds could be considered a core skill for respiratory assessment. In considering training in breath sounds there are three major features.

32.2.1.2 **Recognition of the breath sound**

Trainees have a need to know how breath sounds are produced, use of a stethoscope, and normal patterns and phases of sounds. This is most easily taught on the trainees themselves. For teaching recognition of abnormal breath sounds, several training devices are available. A variety of breath sound generators are available from manufacturers such as Laerdal (e.g. VitalSim® with auscultation module) and LifeForm (e.g. Heart and Lung Sounds Mannequin, Auscultation Simulator) that have audiospeakers, and may also have listening points for auscultation with stethoscope. These sound generators can also be connected to mannequins for auscultation on the chest (e.g. Laerdal Nursing Anne). There is also a canine model available for training veterinary professionals (Rescue Critters K9 Breathsound and Heartsound Simulator). Compact discs, such as the 3M Learning Lung Sounds, Cardionics Learning Lung Sounds or the Kyoto Kagaku Lung Sound Auscultation Trainer (LSAT), are interactive training programmes that are run on personal computers. These programmes display sonograms synchronized to each breath sound, and they have the advantage of being useful for group learning and tuition, but also provide self-directed learning packages. Cardionics also produce the PneumoSim Digital Breath Sound simulator that allows recorded and simulated breath sounds to be edited and altered for students to obtain better understanding of the inspiratory and expiratory components of the sound. There are also online open source sounds files that can be accessed through the internet. Generally the quality of inbuilt computer speakers is far from desirable for listening to breath sounds, and may be improved using speakers with lower frequency response or head-phones (Fig. 32.1).

32.2.1.2 **Where to listen to breath sounds**

The major issue of teaching this skill is appropriate placement of the stethoscope to listen to breath sounds. The computer CD programs have instructional diagrams indicating where auscultation should be made. This may not equate to actually placing the stethoscope on a patient's chest and can be one potential advantage to using a mannequin. However most breath sound training mannequins are recumbent and can usually be auscultated in four areas, generally the left and right anterior chest, and midaxillary regions corresponding to the size and placement of

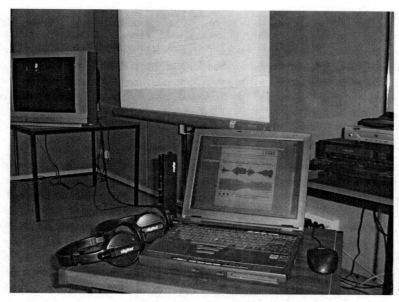

Fig. 32.1 Using lung sound CD for training. 3M Learning Lung Sounds run on computer with infra-red head phones for multiple tangle free users and sonograms projected onto screen.

speakers for manufacturing ease rather than clinically ideal regions. The LifeForm Auscultation Trainer and SmartScope®, and the Kyoto Kagaku LSAT are trainers comprising adult chests that allow for the auscultation in up to 17 positions, including the posterior chest wall, and differentiate between listing locations. These trainers do not have respiratory movement to identify specific inspiratory and expiratory breath sounds. The LifeForm Auscultation Trainer is a stand alone unit that requires the use of the electronic SmartScope®. The Kyoto Kagaku LSAT uses standard stethoscopes, is connected to a personal computer that combines a screen-based training package. Harvey (University of Miami) is also a simulator that enables breath sounds to be linked with cardio-respiratory signs.

32.2.1.3 Interpretation of the breath sound

In the context of other clinical signs, this is perhaps the final step in this process. The interpretation of inspiratory and expiratory breaths sounds associated with chest movement should be an advantage of the high and intermediate fidelity patient simulators over the static part-task trainers. Currently, however, the breath sounds can only be auscultated on a limited number of anterior and midaxillary positions in patient mannequin simulators, and it is fair to say that the breath sounds available are of limited quality and quantity. The small speakers placed in mannequins are generally of the type that have higher frequency ranges than associated with breath sounds, and this does not aid learning or interpretation. The breathing movements mechanisms of mannequin simulators are generally achieved by hinged anterior rising and falling of the chest rather than in combination with lateral chest expansion. Instructors and their trainees frequently report confusion by the extraneous sounds generated from simulator respiratory mechanisms and respiratory movement. These provide opportunities for future simulator refinement.

32.2.2 **Percussion**

Percussion of the chest wall is one other clinical skill used in respiratory assessment. Mannequins tend to have chest walls that do not lend itself to teaching these skills or allowing any form of interpretation. One simple but elegant method for teaching this skill is the use of 2 litre plastic paint tubs that are empty (to sound hyper-resonant), filled with large polystyrene beads (to sound normal) or filled with rolled oats (to sound dull). Percussing the lids allows students to learn to distinguish sounds[5].

32.2.3 **Blood gas interpretation**

During respiratory management courses run in our simulation centre, the training of arterial blood gas interpretation is generally run as problem-based learning scenarios, and we have found that this complements skill stations and scenarios in terms of adult interactive learning. Simulated blood gas physiology is available in patient simulators and personal computer programmes. Currently the Medical Education Technologies Inc. Human Patient Simulator (METI-HPS®) provides calculations of P_aCO_2, P_aO_2, pH and SaO_2, but not HCO_3^- or base excess. The values are indicative of the gases within the simulator lungs generated by minute ventilation, linked O_2 consumption and CO_2 production, and a 'shunt factor' that is an approximation of lung ventilation and blood flow mismatch. The values are not adjusted for metabolic, renal, haemoglobin or temperature affects on blood gas physiology, and therefore should be used cautiously for teaching. Several screen-based blood gas simulation programmes based on physiological models are available. Blood Gases from Mad Scientist Software provides a tutorial programme suited to self-directed learning. The Nottingham Physiological Simulator is a sophisticated and detailed programme suited for research or teaching at the very advanced level[6]. Either of these programmes may be useful for generating blood gas results when running clinical simulations.

32.3 **Clinical respiratory skills and therapies**

32.3.1 **Oxygen administration**

Teaching oxygen administration allows an opportunity to distinguish between the different oxygen delivery modes and the effect of patient respiration. The high fidelity patient simulators, such as the METI-HPS®, have sophisticated pulmonary mechanisms that replicate oxygen uptake and carbon dioxide production. This can be controlled to create patient pathologies and ventilatory changes (e.g. patients with congestive heart failure or asthma) as well as an adjustable functional residual capacity (e.g. the affect of pregnancy or morbid obesity). The METI-HPS® has internal gas analysis can be accessed to demonstrate, at the alveolar level, differences between oxygen delivery though nasal prongs or the various face masks, and the effects of increased or decreased minute ventilation.

These effects may also be demonstrated with volunteers, usually the course participants, by measuring end tidal oxygen concentrations. We have used an anaesthetic gas analyser with fast oxygen analysis (e.g. paramagnetic) with gases sampled from nasal prongs worn by a volunteer. Placing different face masks with various oxygen flows on a volunteer allows inspired and expired oxygen concentrations to be displayed. Instructing the volunteer to breathe as usual, or to hyperventilate or hypoventilate for short periods can demonstrate the effect of oxygen delivery and interaction with respiration. When providing these demonstrations it is important to recognize that sampling expired nasal gases does not reflect actual alveolar concentrations; this method is qualitative rather than quantitative.

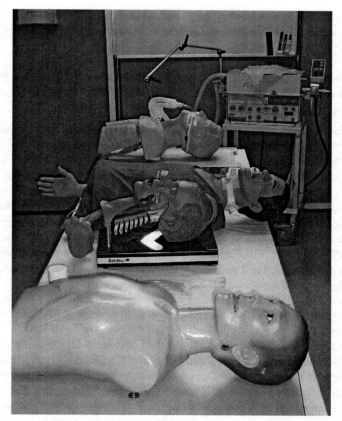

Fig. 32.2 Airway skills management work station. Scopin II Broncho Boy Trainer and Ambu Airway Management Trainer are used for nasopharyngeal airway insertion. Laerdal airway mannequins are used for training tracheostomy open suction and endotracheal tube closed suction (attached to ventilator tubing).

32.3.2 Airway management

The opportunities for airway management in the setting of respiratory care may involve, but is not restricted to, the following:

32.3.2.1 Nasopharyngeal airway (NPA)

This commonly used therapy requires training with appropriate mannequins. The cut-away head mannequins such as the Ambu Airway Management Trainer® (Fig. 32.2) allow the nasopharyngeal vault to be visualized, and is ideal for demonstrating positioning of the NPA, the importance of appropriate NPA size selection, and the correct and incorrect insertion techniques. Most airway management mannequins can be used for training NPA placement, although mannequins with more accurate nasal anatomy, as in the Scopin II Broncho Boy Trainer®, are often preferred.

32.3.2.2 Endotracheal and tracheostomy tube management.

Suctioning of secretions from the endotracheal and tracheostomy tube is a skill frequently taught and assessed. Appropriately intubated mannequins can be used in conjunction with suction, catheters (using both the simple catheter and closed suction systems), and gloves. Applying tracheal suction to the mannequins with exposed lungs such as the Laerdal Airway Management Trainer® generates small reductions of the lung volumes and can demonstrate the concept of suction on the alveoli.

32.3.3 Respiratory support: bi-level positive airway pressure (BiPAP), continuous positive airway pressure (CPAP) and intermittent positive pressure breathing (IPPB)

Nursing and allied health professionals are increasingly more involved in providing noninvasive respiratory therapy. These therapies require a good seal between the patient and facemask, and one limitation frequently encountered is the difficulty in obtaining a quality seal between masks and the silicon or plastic face of mannequins. Despite this limitation, the high fidelity patient simulators with pulmonary mechanics (e.g. METI-HPS®) can be used to demonstrate noninvasive respiratory techniques. It is important that the instructor is practiced in the technique of placing the face mask on the mannequin to obtain a suitable seal, and the students are aware that there will be subtle differences to using this technique on patients. Laerdal do not recommend using high flow devices such as CPAP or BiPAP devices on their simulators (e.g. SimMan®). Mannequins can be used to demonstrate equipment static set-ups, and we have found the Laerdal ALS Baby® with its soft face and nose useful for demonstrating the set up for paediatric nasal CPAP.

Alternatively, course participants can also be used for demonstration of the device set-up, correct attachment of facemask, and settings of equipment. Brief periods of CPAP, BiPAP or IPPB are generally tolerated.

Biomedical equipment test devices can also be used in clinical skills training. One example is the ALS 5000 Breathing Simulator® produced by Ingmar Medical. This is a computer controlled low resistance large volume piston that simulates the respiratory air flows of spontaneous breathing and can also be manually ventilated. It has sophisticated lung modelling that replicates pressure flow curves associated with changes in respiratory compliance (e.g. pneumothorax) and airway resistance (e.g. bronchospasm). Ingmar Medical also produce the QuickTrigger® which, when coupled to other test lungs (e.g. Ingmar RespiTrainer® or QuickLung®) can also be used to simulate spontaneous breathing.

32.3.4 Ventilation

Manual ventilation is often used to loosen secretions in the intubated and ventilated patient in the intensive or critical care setting. A high fidelity simulator (e.g. METI-HPS®) can be used the for this purpose as it allows programming of reduced lung and chest wall compliance, and raised airway resistance to provide the appropriate lung dynamics of the ICU patient. Training can use either the self-inflating resuscitation bag or the passive filling anaesthetic bag connected to a 'T-Piece' type circuit, depending on local practices. In our centre the aim of the sessions is to coach therapists to obtain as high peak expiratory flows as possible but to avoid generating peak inspiratory pressures that could cause patient complications such as a pneumothorax. In clinical practice in our organization, technique also involved the use of an airway pressure manometer to keep peak pressures below 40 cm H_2O. We have found that connecting a spirometer (Fig. 32.3) to the resuscitation bag allows airway pressure and flow to be continuously shown to trainees. This increases their understanding of the concepts of peak pressure, plateau pressure, and peak expiratory flows.

The high fidelity simulators, such as the METI-HPS®, were developed originally for use in anaesthesia, and as a result have sophisticated mechanisms generating lung compliances appropriate for healthy patients and patients with respiratory dysfunctions or pathologies. This allows

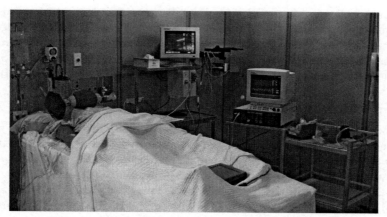

Fig. 32.3 Manual ventilation for respiratory physiotherapy in intensive care patients. A high fidelity simulator (METI HPS®) is ventilated by resuscitation bag and monitored with intensive care monitor. A separate monitor on right (Datex AS3, Instrumentarium, Helsinki, Finland) displays airway pressure and airway flow measured using spirometry.

application of intermittent positive pressure ventilation (IPPV) on the simulator to be ventilated using modern electronic controlled ventilators. The intermediate fidelity simulators such as the METI-ECS® or Laerdal SimMan® have lungs that do not have these mechanisms; instead they have simple lungs (i.e. passive filling bags) that, when inflated, result in chest rise. The compliance of these lungs is restricted by the weight of the mannequin chest wall and elastance of chest skin. This compliance is typically very low at around 25ml/cm H_2O (or approximately one third the compliance of the usual adult human at 70 ml/cm H_2O). Ventilating these intermediate fidelity simulators using a modern ventilators with typical patient settings results in activation of high peak pressure and low tidal volume alarms. These compliances are acceptable and not discernable when manually ventilated with a resuscitation bag[7]. Faced with the cost of purchasing the more expensive high fidelity simulator, several remedies include connection to a biomedical test lung through a 'T' connection in the breathing circuit, or the recalibration of the ventilator controls. Ingmar Medical produce the RespiTrainer® which comprises an adult head that can be ventilated *via* endotracheal tube or face mask, a lung that can be adjusted for airway pressure or compliance, and displays respiratory rate, peak pressure and tidal volume wirelessly on a pocket personal computer.

32.3.4 Chest drain insertion and management

There are a variety of training devices for the treatment and management of pneumothorax. These range from stand alone devices that can be used for training needle thoracotomy (e.g. Simulaids Pneumothorax Simulator®, Laerdal Pneumothorax Trainer®) through to devices for chest drain insertion, securing and dressing (e.g. LifeForm Chest Tube Mannequin®, SimCentral Super Annie II®, Simulab TraumaMan®, Pharmabotics Chest Drain Simulator®). The METI and Laerdal range of simulators also allow for needle thoracotomy and chest drain insertion procedures to be performed. Several of these mannequins (LifeForm Chest Tube Mannequin®, SimCentral Super Annie II®) can also be used for training in the care and trouble shooting of the chest drain by connection to underwater seal drains, and demonstration of swinging and bubbling associated with normal and abnormal chest drain function. This not only provides training opportunities but also creates opportunities to assess students' understanding of chest drain function, critical patient management and diagnostic skills. Several professional organisations also provide online training resources for self-directed learning in chest tube insertion and thoracic drain management (e.g. http://www.thoracic.org.au/intercostal.html).

32.3.5 Bronchoscopy

Flexible fibreoptic bronchoscopy (FOB) is generally associated with the respiratory physician, ear, nose and throat surgeon, anaesthetist, and intensive care specialist. It is often used to assess patients in the intensive or critical setting, and in some health systems FOB is also performed on the intubated patient by non-medical health professionals. Because FOB is a difficult clinical skill to acquire it lends itself to simulation and part-task trainers, and there are a variety of methods for training in this technique with several anatomical and non-anatomical training devices available. Examples of anatomical training devices are all airway management trainers to which a bronchial tree can be added (e.g. Laerdal Airway Management Trainer®, SimMan® and AirMan®, Scopin II Broncho Boy Trainer® and TruCorp AirSim®). Non-anatomical training devices (Pharmabotics Oxford Training Box®, Replicant Dexter Endoscopy Training System®) focus on the acquisition of learning the psychomotor skills required for FOB. The Endoscopy AccuTouch® system (manufactured by Immersion Medical) consists of a personal computer, an interface device, proxy bronchoscope, and software modules providing training scenarios using computer-generated airways. The advantage of the Replicant and Immersion Medical devices is that they are provided with self-directed learning modules, and can potentially provide assessment of endoscopy skills prior to patient contact[8,9].

32.4 Decision-making in clinical skills assessment and team work in respiratory care: putting together scenarios for clinical education

The design of scenarios has been covered elsewhere in this book (see Chapter 12), and two examples highlighting decision making and team work issues are presented here (Examples 1 and 2). It is important to provide students and course participants with all information to enable reasoned decisions to be made. This may require appropriate laboratory and clinical tests such blood gas and electrolytes results, ECG printouts, chest X-rays etc. Decision making is considered an important proficiency in respiratory care, and both case studies and clinical simulation are potentially important strategies towards making better decisions[3]. In the future, respiratory care will probably involve more procedures, and health professionals will require more extensive training, so competency assessments will become common[10]. The opportunities that exist for respiratory medicine and respiratory care are strongly weighted in favour of using simulation, as it has the potential to be used in training as well as competency skills and decision making assessments.

32.4.1 Example 1: Introduction of CPAP training

The arrival of simulation in our organization in the late 1990s coincided with research indicating that nursing led triage influenced early CPAP intervention and this lead to reductions of patient intubation and assisted ventilation[11]. It was apparent that a demand for CPAP therapy would increase, and structured training programmes were required. With patient simulation available, an ideal opportunity for training existed and advanced acute care nursing study days comprising discrete clinical skills sessions were established. In addition to didactic lectures, skills sessions and problem-based learning sessions consisted of:

- respiratory assessment
- oxygen therapy
- blood gas interpretation
- airway management
- setting up CPAP equipment
- patient scenarios.

The patient scenarios, generally 40 minute pause and discuss sessions, relating to respiratory distress or respiratory failure, consolidated the learning process and were constructed around a patient with a defined pathology (e.g. congestive heart failure) to include these topics:

- Patient assessment: history, respiratory and cardiovascular functions, hydration status, consciousness, pain etc., and repeating these assessments within a dynamically changing scenario
- Oxygen therapy: matching appropriate oxygen delivery with oxygen demand
- Blood gas interpretation: determining the respiratory and metabolic status of the patient and potential management plan(s)
- Airway management: anticipating and planning appropriate airway management for loss of consciousness or preparation for elective rapid sequence intubation and controlled ventilation
- Medication: planning for the administration of appropriate drug therapies
- Applying CPAP therapy: ensuring the equipment set-up is understood, used appropriately, and effective communication with the patient regarding the course of the treatment
- Team management: allocation of a team leader, verbalization of patient care plan and management, allocation of team members to specified areas of responsibility, clear direct communication within the team, and anticipation and planning.

32.4.2 Example 2: Positive pressure ventilation in ICU setting

Changes to weekend rostering in our institution required general respiratory physiotherapy cover for the intensive care unit. Respiratory physiotherapists are responsible for clearing lung secretions in this setting. As a result a skills competency programme was introduced, and clinical skills sessions based on core competencies were established for this technique and consisted of:

- Airway management: open and closed suction of the endotracheal tube
- Intermittent positive pressure ventilation to clear secretions.

The IPPV skills training session runs on a high fidelity (i.e. METI-HPS®) and focussed on:

- Manual IPPV technique
- Equipment used for IPPV
- Potential complications and considerations for the causes of increased airway pressure during IPPV: failure of equipment, migration of tube to endobroncheal intubation, mucus plug in lung or tube, or pneumothorax
- Airway management: anticipating, recognizing concomitant physiological changes (e.g. oxygen saturation, heart rate, blood pressure), and planning appropriate management in response to increased airway pressure.

32.5 **Future developments**

It is important to recognize that applying simulation to respiratory care training and assessment is not a new concept. The first commercially available resuscitation training mannequin, the Laerdal Resusci Anne®, was manufactured around 50 years ago for the purpose of training and assessing airway management and ventilation skills in addition to cardiac compression. SimOne®, the first computer-controlled patient simulator, was developed in the mid 1960s and initially focused on training and assessment of skills acquisition in anaesthesiology residents[12,13]. SimOne® was reported to be useful in the training of ventilator use and patient ventilation in medical, nursing and allied health professionals and students[14].

Today, manufacturers are developing new products and applications for respiratory care. Models of patient care will also change; patients' length of stay in hospital will reduce while the intensity of in-hospital treatment will increase, and patient care will move from the hospital to the home. Clinical educators and trainers need to consider who will be providing patient care, and the setting of that care. It will be important to match training and simulation technology to clinical skills with development of appropriate assessment methods.

There will be developments in the range of products for training in respiratory assessment and care. Some of the advances may include the colour changes to skin and mucosa, lung and airway secretions or improving chest movement to indicate respiratory difficulties that were the planned additional features for SimOne® [10]. There may be the integration of existing technologies and the development of new technologies. We may see self-directed learning and automated training assessment similar to those available for resuscitation training. It will be fascinating to observe both technical advances and professional development with the use of simulation and skills training over the next 50 years.

Acknowledgments

Many of the workstations and scenarios described here were developed in conjunction with Jane MacGeorge, Robyn Lange, Julie Little, Camille Lamond and Sue McCullough. Dr Andy Wearn shared the method for percussion training.

References

1. Weinstock PH, *et al.* (2005). Towards a new paradigm in hospital-based pediatric education: the development of an onsite simulator program. *Pediatr Crit Care Med* **6**: 712–3.
2. Tuttle RP, *et al.* (2007). Utelizing simulation technology for competency skills assessment and a comparison of traditional methods of training in simulation-based training. *Respiratory Care* **52**: 263–70.
3. Hill TV (2002). The relationship between critical thinking and decision-making in respiratory care students. *Respiratory Care* **47**: 571–7.
4. Sinz EH (2004). Partial-task-trainers and simulation in critical care medicine. In: Dunn WF, Ed. *Simulators in Critical Care and Beyond*. Society of Critical Care Medicine, Des Plaines: 33–4.
5. Wearn A (2007) Teaching, learning and assessing clinical skills: Does one size fit all?. *Second International Clinical Skills Conference*. Monash Centre, Prato, Italy.
6. Hardman JG, *et al.* (1998). A physiology simulator: validation of its respiratory components and its ability to predict the patient's response to changes in mechanical ventilation. *Br J Anaesth* **81**: 327–32.
7. Gough JE, *et al.* (1999). Tactile assessments of lung compliance are not reliable. *Acad Emerg Med* **6**: 761–4
8. Ost D, *et al.* (2001). Assessment of a bronchoscopy simulator. *Crit Care Med* **164**: 2248–55.
9. Martin KM, *et al.* (2004). Effective non-anatomical endoscopy training produces clinical airway endoscopy proficiency. *Anesth Analg* **99**: 938–44.

10. Hess D (2005). Training and education challenges for the twenty-first century: respiratory care competency and practice. *Respir Care Clin N Am* **11**: 531–42.

11. MacGeorge JM, *et al.* (2003). The experience of the nurse at triage influences the timing of CPAP intervention. *Accid Emerg Nurs* **11**: 234–8.

12. Denson JS, *et al.* (1969). A computer-controlled patient simulator. *JAMA* **6**: 712–3.

13. Abrahamson S, *et al.* (1969). Effectiveness of a simulator in training anesthesiology residents. *J Med Educ* **44**: 515–9.

14. Hoffman KI, *et al.* (1975). The 'cost-effectiveness' of Sim One. *J Med Educ* **50**: 1127–8.

Useful product websites

http://www.laerdal.com/
http://www.enasco.com/
http://www.rescuecritters.com/
http://solutions.3m.com/
http://www.cardionics.com/
http://www.kyotokagaku.com/
http://www.crme.med.miami.edu/harvey_changes.html
http://www.METI.com/
http://www.madsci.com/
http://www.ambuusa.com/
http://www.adam-rouilly.co.uk/
http://www.ingmarmed.com/
http://www.simcentral.com.au/
http://www.simulab.com/
http://www.pharmabotics.com/
http://www.simulaids.com/
http://www.trucorp.co.uk/
http://www.dexterendoscopy.com/
http://www.immersion.com/

Chapter 33

Role of cognitive simulations in healthcare

Usha Satish and Satish Krishnamurthy

Overview

- Simulations allow healthcare providers to hone their skills without endangering the patient or hurting their self confidence. A number of simulations are available and their use enhances safety of patient care.

- Cognitive simulations provide a realistic replication of a healthcare professional's workday that involves several complex demands that have to be processed simultaneously. Cognitive simulations help assess and train the underlying process variables of medical decision making, including planning, strategy, multitasking, critical thinking and overall perspective.

- Healthcare provider is often challenged by VUCAD (volatility, uncertainty, complexity, ambiguity, and by problems with delayed feedback such as test results) when decisions have to be made. Healthcare providers need to have the ability to respond to complex challenges by processing information optimally in addition to factual content knowledge necessary to respond to the task at hand. Strategic management simulations (SMS) provide an optimal opportunity to acquire both.

- SMS assesses and trains 'how' we think.

- Standard testing of cognitive parameters are usually performed individually and the interaction of various parameters are extrapolated to real life subsequently. SMS simultaneously evaluates multiple cognitive parameters simultaneously in a 'real-life' situation. This real world atmosphere allows for a more realistic (ecologically relevant) assessment of competency.

- In addition, SMS can also help both the learners and teachers to understand performance in the simulation in relation to a number of well-validated factors as well as help in retraining. SMS can be used for individual or team evaluation or training.

- SMS has been used to evaluate generic thinking in a wide variety of subjects. SMS successfully differentiates performance among normal subjects (superior functioning managers *versus* average functioning managers; better medical residents *versus* average or poorly functioning residents). SMS is effective in evaluating a change in functioning due to medications or environmental chemicals, or due to disordered brain function.

- SMS can demonstrate milder deficits in head injured patients in the relative absence of deficits in standard neuropsychological tests.

- SMS technology provides a strong compliment to existing simulator technologies, which greatly enhance specific procedural or algorithmic skills.

33.1 **Introduction**

"High-quality learning is impossible in the absence of high-quality patient care; likewise, high-quality patient care is impossible without high-quality learning. Attention to both is needed." Leach and Philibret, 2006.

A number of constituencies are becoming increasingly interested in measuring the performance of physicians in their day-to-day clinical practices, especially since the Institute of Medicine's report suggested that the quality of care may often be less than optimal[1]. Purchasers of healthcare services, for instance, are concerned about the effects of suboptimal care on workforce productivity, and seek to maximize the quality of care provided. Consumers of care also want to be able to identify high-quality physicians and institutions but lack the effective means to do so. Although some groups have measured and reported quality of care for individual medical groups and physicians, these efforts have been limited[2]. Both patients and healthcare purchasers desire more effective means of identifying excellent clinicians, and a number of organizations have begun discussing and implementing plans for assessing the performance of individual clinicians and the settings in which they choose to practice.

The combination of changes in healthcare delivery, shortened hospital stays, more home and ambulatory care, variations in care not explained by science, declining reimbursements and, above all, the inexorable and visible failure of the current system to deliver safe care, has been described as the 'perfect storm'. Safer and more predictable care is needed. Paul O'Neill has said that he knows of no other industry that accepts a 38% reimbursement on amounts billed. McGlynn *et al.*[3] has said that we deliver care known to be best only 54% of the time. These numbers may be related[4].

Simulation enhances both safety and predictability. Every patient deserves a competent physician every time. The domains of simulation and rehearsal in medicine encompasses non-computer-dependent modalities such as human cadavers, animal models and standardized patients, along with various forms that rely on electronic technology to create situations and scenarios. They range from simple electronic models and mannequins, personal computer screen-based approaches to high-technology, high fidelity interactive patient simulators for individuals and teams of participants. Simulation scenarios can encompass procedural tasks, crisis resource management, and introduction of learners to clinical situations.

33.1 **Definition**

The Society for Simulation in Healthcare[5] uses the following definition of simulation in healthcare: Simulation is a technique – not a technology – to replace or amplify real patient experiences with guided experiences, artificially contrived, that evokes or replicates substantial aspects of the real world in a fully interactive manner[6].

Artificial environments such as flight simulators for the training of airline pilots, the USS Enterprise's Holodeck, movie set-like towns and alleys for military to train within, computer models of weather prediction using 'what if' scenarios or hospital drills come within this definition[5]. All of these techniques for learning and training have been successful in improving pattern recognition thought process, specific skills, outcomes, and post-encounter evaluations.

Despite this plethora of simulation options, medicine as a whole is a relative newcomer to simulation, when compared with domains such as aviation and one medical specialty – anaesthesiology. Yet in the span of a few years, robust evidence of its benefits has moved simulation from the vanguard to the cutting edge of validated practice in medical education and the professional development of practising physicians[7].

Widespread use of computers has enabled simulating real environments and its application to the field of healthcare possible. There are several attractions in applying simulations to the field of healthcare. Healthcare providers whether they are in training or already trained are constantly learning how to provide better care for patients. Maintenance of certification which includes lifelong learning and audit of one's practice is a requirement for physicians from all specialties. Various tasks involved in taking care of a patient, namely clinical skills, algorithmic management of emergent conditions, surgical procedures, thinking skills, and teamwork have all been successfully simulated with good results.

The recipient of care, subjects covered, skills learnt, time required and the cost of simulation vary widely. Literature search using either general search engines or Medline generates several hundred articles. A variety of institutions have a centre for simulation, several societies and journals devoted to simulation exist, reflecting an explosive interest in this area. The prime goal for all these simulations appears to be improved patient safety. Simulations allow healthcare providers to hone their skills without endangering the patient or hurting their self confidence. Simulation has the potential for the evolution of a new teaching paradigm for the new millennium[8]. These techniques do not depend on hospital encounters and can be re-run, stopped, or otherwise altered to enhance educational value. Thereby, creating a non threatening learning environment where multiple options could potentially be tested, worked through and mastered. "Every patient deserves a competent physician every time. Every resident deserves competent teachers and an excellent learning environment. Simulation serves both of these core principles."[4]

33.2 Underlying principles: the need for simulations

In *To Err Is Human: Building a Safer Health System* the Institute of Medicine encouraged the medical community to reach out boldly to other domains for insight and inspiration for different models of performance and teaching[1]. Effective use of simulation technology is a substantial contributor to making commercial air transportation the safest available mode of travel.

Human error is routinely blamed for disasters in the air, on the railways, in complex surgery, and in healthcare generally[9]. While one action or omission may be the immediate cause of an incident, closer analysis usually reveals a series of events and departures from safe practice; each influenced by the working environment and the wider organizational context. Understanding the characteristics of a safe and high performing system, therefore, requires research of the context, the development and maintenance of individual skills, the role of high technology, the impact of working conditions on team performance, and the nature of high performance teams. Simulation is an essential tool in the learning and understanding of high performing systems. Safety in these high reliability organizations (HROs) is ultimately understood as a characteristic of the system – the sum total of all the parts and their interactions[10].

This cultural evolution required the creation of a continuous improvement process. This process includes firstly, an event reporting system that processes data into meaningful knowledge, creating opportunity for meaningful change within an organization. Secondly, it required simulations to study systems and to implement changes within an organization. The importance of effective teamwork in aviation is critical to safety.

Human beings make mistakes. Until crew performance was studied in simulation, the captain was God in the cockpit; and his crew disagreed with him at their peril. In this tradition or 'culture', the airplane, passengers, and crew were exposed to the captain's potential errors while deprived of the knowledge and skill that resided among the remaining members of the crew. Simulation studies demonstrated that airplanes could be more safely and reliably operated if the knowledge and skills of the entire crew were applied to the flight tasks. Techniques and procedures were developed in simulation that preserve and enhance the captain's authority and effectiveness by enhancing the flow of information among the entire crew[10].

Contemporary airline safety is in significant measure the product of this loop of operational reporting, analysis in simulation, and training in simulation. State-of-the-art airline crew training, the Advanced Qualification Program (AQP), emerged out of simulation studies during which reported actual events were recreated in simulation. AQP identified specific team skills that enhance safety through effective use of all available resources – human, hardware, and information. The process achieved a greater degree of integration of the team skills in part because AQP team training and practice increases awareness of human and system error, and provides techniques and skills that will minimize their effects. This is accomplished through awareness of crew member attitudes and behaviour, and the use of practical management skills[10].

An important variant of simulators are cognitive simulations. These simulations have the intrinsic capability of replicating several aspects of a learner's environment simultaneously. This provides a realistic replication of a healthcare professional's workday that involves several complex demands that have to be processed simultaneously. In other words, cognitive simulation technologies, help assess and train the underlying process variables of medical decision making, including but not limited to planning, strategy, multitasking, critical thinking and overall perspective. This technology provides a strong compliment to existing simulator technologies, which greatly enhance specific procedural or algorithmic skills.

33.3 Requirements for effective medical decision making

Competency in professional endeavours may require much more than finding a single 'correct' response to some particular situation[11,12]. There are task situations where a single correct action or where multiple correct actions will solve the problems at hand, but not all challenges fit that pattern. Complex tasks – including medical decision making tasks – can generate unpredictable dynamics that defy treatment with standard content knowledge approaches[13,14]. Factual (content) knowledge can be gained from reading books or from memorizing lecture notes, and from repeating successful prior actions in response to repetitive challenges that led to success. When a task is highly challenging and does not fit a memorized or documented pattern, an additional set of skills is necessary; adequate competency in information processing is essential[15].

Just as factual knowledge must be learned, information processing skills are also subject to learning and training although this form of training cannot be transmitted through books or lectures[16]. In fact, modern learning theorists clearly distinguish the processes involved in the acquisition and use of specific content knowledge and the acquisition and use of intellectual processing skills that are free of specific knowledge content[17]. The latter skills represent cognitive strategies that an effective decision maker uses to regulate his or her own processes of attending, learning, remembering and thinking[18], involving external (incoming) information as well as internal or remembered information and concepts[19]. These 'information processing strategies' are not fixed; they must adjust to changes in task challenges – for example, different patients with different sets of morbidities and conditions – and they must adjust to gains in knowledge over time[20]. Learning to apply such processing strategies requires guided personal experience.

We respond to an environmental stimulus based on our interpretation of 'normal' for the situation we are in. Our sense of normal depends on extent of exposure to that particular situation, our knowledge, and our ability to learn. Response to a stimulus depends on our alertness, ability to focus (without distractions akin to sterile areas in the cockpit where no one is allowed to distract the pilot and the co-pilot during take-off or landing), knowledge of the context, accurate interpretation of the stimulus and threshold level for a response. Last but not the least, the execution of the

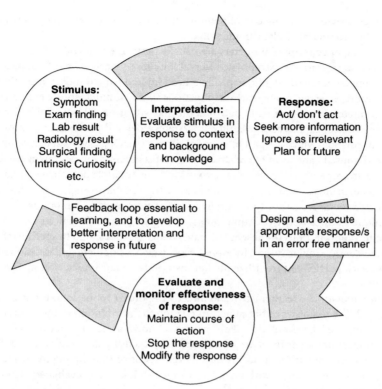

Fig. 33.1 Stimulus-Response-Feedback loop.

response needs to be error free. The results need to be monitored for desired outcome and the response is modified if the outcome is deviating from the optimum (Fig. 33.1)

In addition, the physician or medical team is often challenged by VUCAD (volatility, uncertainty, complexity, ambiguity and by problems with delayed feedback such as test results)[15] when decisions have to be made. How can we make sure that physicians will effectively manage a network of interrelated problems that involve ambiguity, inconsistency, novelty and surprise[21]? We have known for some time that learning, transfer of knowledge and ability are impacted by both *task structure* and *task complexity*, and by the *structural information processing competence* of the individual (physician) involved[22]. We need to ensure that medical personnel have the factual content knowledge needed to respond to the task at hand, but we also need to make sure that they can respond to complex challenges by processing information optimally. Simulations, if used as part of an appropriate training system, provide an optimal opportunity to acquire both.

33.4 Fundamental concepts of strategic management simulations and its relevance to healthcare and HROs

Cognitive simulations have the intrinsic capability of replicating several aspects of a learner's environment simultaneously. This provides a realistic replication of a healthcare professional's workday that involves several complex demands that have to be processed simultaneously.

This technology provides a strong compliment to existing simulator technologies which greatly enhance specific procedural or algorithmic skills.

Standard testing of cognitive parameters are usually performed individually and the interaction of various parameters are extrapolated to real life subsequently. The true impact of a mild memory loss and a decreased attention span in a head injured patient might mean that s/he will not be employable. Strategic management simulations (SMS) simultaneously evaluates multiple cognitive parameters simultaneously in a 'real life' like situation. This 'real life' like situation means that the subject experiences volatility, uncertainty, delayed feedback and ambiguity with inadequate information, which are part of everyday decision making. SMS can demonstrate milder deficits in head injured patients in the relative absence of standard neuropsychological deficits[23]. The real world atmosphere of the task and setting, involving multiple potentially interactive components of task demands as well as multiple and interactive options to engage in various aspects of behavior allows for a more realistic (ecologically relevant) assessment of competency.

SMS is unique in the absence of requirements to engage in specific actions or to make decisions at specific points in time, the absence of stated demands to respond to specific information, the freedom to develop initiative, and freedom for strategy development and decision implementation allows each participant to utilize his/her own preferred or typical action, planning and strategic styles.

Most of the simulations are interactive and directly responsive to the actions taken by the subject. SMS records the responses of the subject in relation to the evolution of the scenario but does not alter the course of the simulation. This feature is known as quasi experimental simulation and allows comparison of performance of different subjects using the same scenario. This property has allowed determination of norms for different levels of functioning in normal subjects. Comparison of a subject with or without a drug or medication can be evaluated. Reported studies include effects of caffeine[24], alcohol[25] etc.

SMS described below go beyond simply recreating the learner's complex environment and allowing the learner to practice or be evaluated. In addition, SMS can also help both the learners and teachers to understand performance in the simulation in relation to a number of well-validated factors as well as help in retraining[26].

SMS has been used to evaluate generic thinking in a wide variety of subjects. SMS successfully differentiates performance among normal subjects (superior functioning managers *versus* average functioning managers[27]; better medical residents *versus* average or poorly functioning residents[28]). SMS is effective in evaluating a change in functioning due to medications[29] or environmental chemicals, or due to disordered brain function[23]. It is commonly known in the managerial world that a CEO who is successful in selling cars can be successful in selling any other widget. This implies that successful managers think differently and this 'how of thinking' is important in addition to specific knowledge of cars or the specific widget.

Whereas team task analysis as detailed by Burke *et al.*[30] focuses on designing a simulation for a specific situation, SMS evaluates generic thinking processes. As mentioned previously, both content specific knowledge as well as generic decision making competencies is essential for optimal functioning. Further, SMS uses several different scenarios all of which evaluate the same generic thinking processes, effect of learning from repetition is eliminated. Effectiveness of focused training of areas of deficiencies in a subject can be objectively evaluated using SMS.

33.4.1 **Description of the SMS**

SMS assess both basic cognitive and behavioural responses to task demands as well as cognitive and behavioural components that are commonly subsumed under the rubric of executive functions. High levels of predictive validity, reliability and applicability of the SMS simulations to real world settings have been repeatedly demonstrated both in North America and Europe [26,31]. The method provides more than 80 computer gathered and calculated measures of functioning, loading on 12 reliable factors (based on factor analytic varimax rotation for more than 2000 prior subjects). Among others, simulation data predict success on indicators such as 'job level at age', 'income at age', "number of persons supervised', and 'number of job promotions during the past 10 years' (corrected for industry, location, etc)[26]. These simulations can be administered to both individual participants as well as teams. While individual simulation runs offer feedback to a participant on their individual decision making pattern, group performances yield rich data on how teams function together. Further team evaluations also provide detailed information on each of the individual team participants thereby enhancing the feedback and improvement potential. These are particularly important performance of teams of physicians and other healthcare providers. Potential applications for team performance include handling of mass casualties and disastrous situations.

During a simulation, participants make decisions during a one half-hour task period. The absence of requirements to engage in specific actions or to make decisions at specific points in time, the absence of stated demands to respond to specific information, the freedom to develop initiative, and freedom for strategy development and decision implementation allows each participant to use his/her own preferred or typical action, planning and strategic styles. The real world atmosphere of the task and setting, involving multiple potentially interactive components of task demands as well as multiple and interactive options to engage in various aspects of behaviour allows for a more realistic (ecologically relevant) assessment of competency.

33.4.2 SMS measurement outputs

Data in response to the factors listed in Table 33.1 are captured and provided via computer generated scores and represented in two primary output modalities. These outputs are used for feedback and potential training as required.

Table 33.1 Definition of SMS Measures

Measures	Definitions
◆ Activity level	Overall level of activity (measures both focused activity that is directed to a specific context and activity that is directed toward overall goals)
◆ Response speed	Speed of responses both in terms of emergent and non-emergent situations
◆ Task orientation	Ability to focus on a task at hand and also focus on 'larger' goals
◆ Initiative	Ability to generate activity without an overt external stimulus that would aid in successful task completion. Elements pertaining to initiative in context and strategy are also measured
◆ Information management	Ability to seek and use information efficaciously
◆ Strategy	Ability to form systematic plans and actions that are optimally sequenced and goal directed in the long term
◆ Breadth of approach	Ability to think along multiple dimensions and find different solutions to problems
◆ Planning	Ability to make task oriented plans in the short and long term
◆ Emergency responses	Ability to think critically and strategically under conditions of emergency and stress

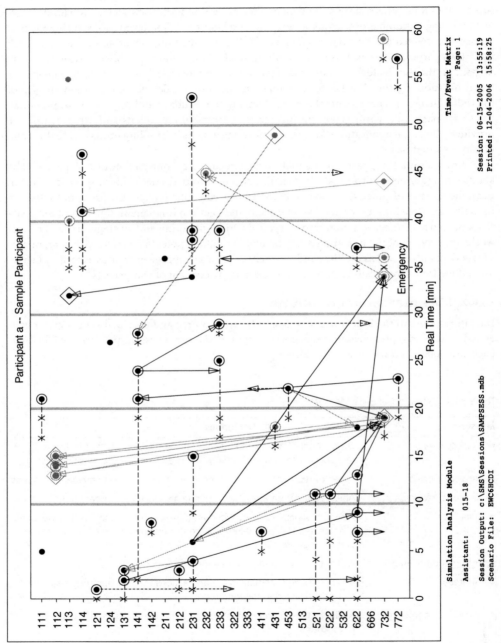

Fig. 33.2 Time-event matrix.

33.4.2.1 Time event matrix (Fig. 33.2)

These are direct graphic representations of performance, and are captured during the performance period. A good analogy to describe this complex output is like a magnetic resonance imaging scan of decision making. These graphs are represented with various combinations of lines and symbols that represent different aspects of decision making. Based on appropriate interpretation these graphs accurately predict the 'underlying process' of thinking in a participant.

In general, richer performance by the subject during the simulation is indicated by a more complex graph. Time during the simulation is plotted on the horizontal axis and the vertical axis represents the variety of decisions made by the participant. Individual actions are represented by a point, placed vertically above the time when the action occurred and horizontally in line with the particular decision code. Information provided or incoming information is denoted with a star. If an action corresponds to incoming information, one or more stars (depending on the number of pieces of information) are placed on the same horizontal level where the action is located, with stars placed at the point when each item of information was received. The action is circled to indicate that it was responsive to an event or a message.

If the participant thinks and acts strategically, these actions are connected with diagonal lines. Different strategies used (visionary or opportunity based) are represented by different colors. The ability to create plans is also similarly captured. In addition, there are several other symbols and line formations that represent elements of critical thinking such as initiative, multitasking and sustained planning, among others.

A serious emergency is introduced at some point in all the strategic management simulation scenarios. The emergency requires rapid and decisive action. Performance patterns during this time point can be compared to other time points in the simulation to judge both the effectiveness of crisis handling as well as preparation for a crisis and recovery patterns after crisis.

33.4.3.2 Profile (Fig. 33.3)

This profile represents the 12 factors listed above in terms of percentile scores. The scores reflect low, moderate and high levels of performance based on normative data. These profiles are used to ascertain the performance pattern of a participant in the various parameters of decision making. Further since these measures are fine tuned in terms of the definition of a given parameter and its implications in the real world, it helps make the training more focused and thereby time effective.

33.4.3 SMS and healthcare applications

David Leach outlines several reasons why simulations should be used for medical education[4]. To ensure patient safety, clinical skills have to be learnt as far away from the patient as possible. Simulations allow actions to be planned, studied and debriefed to allow safer patient care.

Simulation is a great tool for educating residents. Simulations can be used as a formative tool for resident development. Simulation can be used to expose mastery of both rules and values. Familiarity with protocols becomes clear during simulations. At the same time, it is also possible to require improvization as the learner manages emerging situations. Rules are either demonstrated or not; improvization calls forth adaptive expertise. Improvisation exposes values. It is an efficient and safe way to explore competence. Residents can intentionally make mistakes and learn about their consequences during simulations.

Simulation can determine how residents respond in different contexts. Simulation can be used to populate a portfolio of assessed experiences that enable residents to demonstrate their abilities. Simulation offers a controlled way to learn systems based practice. Simulations can be constructed

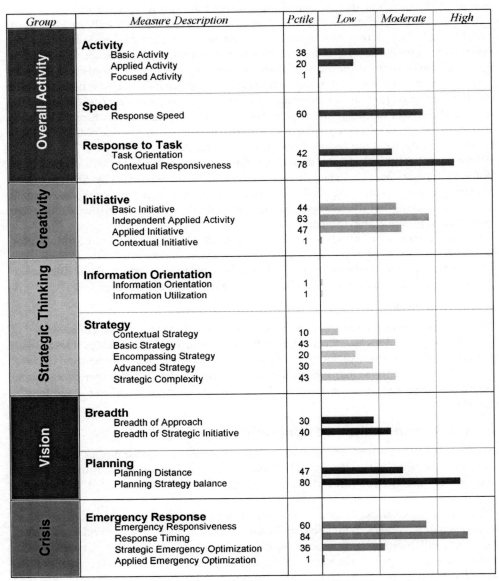

Fig. 33.3 Strategic management simulation profile chart.

that involve multiple interdependent variables. Simulation can document how residents think, as well as what they think. Every resident deserves competent teachers and an excellent learning environment[4].

The complexity of medicine is best demonstrated in the fact that frequently there is inadequate information, rapidly changing conditions, delayed feedback, uncertainty of results with the same treatment in different individuals and multiple providers involved in the care of a single patient. These challenges are best addressed using complex cognitive simulation scenarios where participants can actually think through all the possibilities and arrive at appropriate solutions.

Clearly, simulations have the distinct advantage of providing 'real world' experiences to the learner without causing harm to patients or learners. Simulations can be designed to replicate virtually all complex realities and offer training and retraining using well-standardized paradigms. Simulations are increasingly used for training in and evaluation of procedural skills in surgery and anaesthesia, for example. We believe that simulation can also be a highly effective way to evaluate decision-making and leadership skills in medicine, providing students and residents with insights into their own abilities and needs, and assisting faculty in reliably assessing competence in these areas.

The complexity of teaching the art and science of medicine is a quest that will be a continued challenge to healthcare professionals. However, it would be wise to bear in mind the virtue of constant learning and improvement as noted by Mahatma Gandhi's words of wisdom, "Live as if you were to die tomorrow, Learn as if you were to live forever."

References

1. Kohn, L, Corrigan, J, Donaldson M, Eds. (2000). *To Err is Human: Building a Safer Health System.* National Academy Press, Washington, DC: 146.

2. Landon BE, Normand ST, Blumenthal D, Daley J (2003). Physician Clinical Performance Assessment: Prospects and Barriers. *JAMA* 290: 1183–9.

3. McGlynn EA, Asch SM, Adams J, et al. (2003). The quality of healthcare delivered to adults in the United States. *N Engl J Med* **348**(26): 2635–45.

4. Leach D (2005). Simulation: it's about respect. *ACGME Bulletin* December 2005.

5. http://www.ssih.org/about%20ssh/ssh-what-is-sim.html

6. Gaba DM (2004). The future vision of simulation in healthcare. *Qual Saf Health Care* **13**(Suppl. 1): i2–i10.

7. Editor's Introduction (2005). *ACGME Bulletin* December 2005.

8. Dunn WF (2004). *Simulators in Critical Care Education and Beyond.* Society of Critical Care Medicine: Introduction.

9. Reason J (1990). *Human Error.* New York: Cambridge University Press.

10. Hamman W, Rutherford W (2005). The language of aviation simulation training: Relevance for medical education. *ACGME Bulletin* December 2005: 5–7.

11. Breuer K, Streufert D (1996). Authoring of complex learning environments: design considerations for dynamic simulations. *J Struct Learn* **12**: 315–21.

12. Scandura JM, Stone DC, Scandura AB (1986). An intelligent role tutor CBI system for diagnostic testing and instruction. *J Sruct Learn* **9**: 15–61.

13. Streufert S (1970). Complexity and complex decision making: convergences between differentiation and integration approaches to the prediction of task performance. *J Exp Soc Psychol* **6**: 494–509.

14. Hall N (1993). *Explaining Chaos: a Guide to the New Science of Disorder.* New York: W W Norton.

15. Streufert S, Streufert SC (1978). *Behavior in the Complex Environment.* New York: John Wiley.

16. Streufert S, Swezey R (1985). *Complexity, Managers and Organizations.* New York: Academic Press.

17. Gagné RM (1985). *The Conditions of Learning and Theory of Instruction.* New York: Holt Rinehart and Winston.

18. Breuer K (1992). Cognitive development based on process-learning environments. In: Dijstra S, Krammer HPM, van Merrienboer JJG, Eds. *Instructional Models in Computer Based Learning Environments*. Berlin: Springer Verlag.

19. Tennyson RD, Thurlow K, Breuer K (1987). Problem oriented simulations to develop and improve higher order thinking strategies. *Comput Hum Behav* **3**: 151–65.

20. Toffler D (1980). *Zukunftschance*. Munich: Deutscher Taschenbuch Verlag.

21. Isenberg DJ (1984). How senior managers think. *Harvard Bus Rev*: 84608.

22. Buss AR (1972). Learning, transfer and changes in ability factor: a multivariate model. *Psychol Bull* **80**: 106–12.

23. Satish U, Streufert S, Eslinger PJ (1999). Complex decision making after orbitofrontal damage. *Neurocase* **5**: 355–64.

24. Streufert S, Satish U, Pogash R, *et al.* (1997). Excess coffee consumption in simulated complex work settings: detriment or facilitation of performance? *J Appl Psychol* **82**(5): 774–82.

25. Streufert S, Pogash RM, Roache J, *et al.* (1992). Effects of alcohol intoxication on risk taking, strategy, and error rate in visuomotor performance. *J Appl Psychol* **77**(4): 515–24.

26. Streufert S, Nogami G, Swezey RW, *et al.* (1988). Computer assisted training of complex managerial performance. *Computers Hum Behav* **4**: 77–88.

27. Streufert S, Pogash R, Piasecki M (1988). Simulation-based assessment of managerial competence: reliability and validity. *Personnel Psychol* **41**: 537–57.

28. Satish U, Streufert S, Marshall R, *et al.* (2001). Strategic management simulation is a novel way to measure resident competencies. *Am J Surg* **181**: 557–61.

29. Streufert S, DePadova A, McGlynn T, Pogash R, Piasecki M (1988). Impact of beta blockade on complex cognitive functioning. *Am Heart J* **116**(1 Pt 2): 311–5.

30. Burke CS, Salas E, Wilson-Donnelly K, Priest H (2004). How to turn a team of experts into an expert medical team: guidance from the aviation and military communities. *Qual Saf Health Care* **13**(Suppl. 1):i96–i104.

31. Breuer K, Satish U (2003). Emergency management Simulations: An approach to the assessment of decision-making processes in complex dynamic crisis environments. In: *From Modeling to Managing Security*. Norwegian Academic Press, Norway: 145–55.

Chapter 34

Effective management of anaesthetic crises
Design, development and evaluation of a simulation-based course

Jennifer Weller

Overview

- The need for effective crisis management training in anaesthesia is well recognized. The Effective Management of Anaesthetic Crises (EMAC) course was developed to address this need.

- Collaboration between the Australian and New Zealand College of Anaesthetists (ANZCA) and the simulation centres has resulted in a uniform, 2.5-day simulation-based course in crisis management for all anaesthetists.

- The EMAC course is attended by both specialists and trainees, and is now an integral component of the anaesthesia training programme, and the ongoing professional development of specialist anaesthetists in Australia and New Zealand.

- EMAC has explicit standards for facilities, resources, instructors and teaching methods. These standards are maintained though ANZCA governance.

- The need for doctors to respond effectively to clinical emergencies is not limited to anaesthesia but is also a requirement for many other acute care specialities.

- This description of the EMAC course may provide a useful template for those contemplating similar initiatives in different countries, and in different domains of clinical care.

34.1 Introduction

Establishing a new course within an existing curriculum or training programme can be challenging. Implementing a programme on a national or international level, while maintaining and controlling course standards and uniformity presents specific advantages and particular challenges. This chapter describes the development, design and implementation of a course in crisis management and its incorporation into the anaesthesia training programme across three countries. Our experiences in this course may assist others considering similar initiatives.

The Effective Management of Anaesthetic Crises (EMAC) course grew from collaboration between the Australian and New Zealand College of Anaesthetists (ANZCA) and simulation centres in Wellington, Melbourne, and Sydney. The new course was established to address a deficiency in anaesthesia training in crisis management, capitalizing on technological advances in computerized patient simulators.

34.2 Rationale for simulation in training for emergencies

Training in anaesthesia relies heavily on clinical experience, and exposure to a range of patients and interventions. This apprenticeship model works well for routine cases, but anaesthetists may have limited experience in uncommon, life-threatening events. Crises occur rarely and unpredictably, and cannot be scheduled, repeated, or presented in varying degrees of complexity to suit the level of trainee. In an emergency, time is limited, there are multiple tasks to perform simultaneously and the cause of the problem is often unclear. A good outcome relies on rapid and effective actions by the anaesthetist. In a crisis, the trainee will rarely have the chance to take a leadership role, as the most experienced clinician will take control in the interests of patient safety. This limits the development of expertise during training, and the maintenance of this expertise as a specialist, and may compromise optimal patient care.

Simulation, using computerized patient mannequins, provides an innovative means to address this deficiency. Within the safe environment of a simulation centre, emergencies can be scheduled and repeated, the level of difficulty can be varied, and the simulations can be designed to address a range of learning objectives from simple application of algorithms, to dealing with the aftermath.

The leaders in the simulation centres recognized the opportunity to improve training, and looked for a means to ensure all anaesthetists received training in crisis management.

34.3 The educational environment

By fortunate coincidence, ANZCA was redefining its role in education and was open to a proposed collaboration. Previously the role of ANZCA had been limited to that of an accrediting body, conducting Fellowship Examinations and making determinations on specialist accreditation. In Australia and New Zealand, anaesthesia trainees must pass Part 1 and Part 2 Fellowship Examinations, show evidence of appropriate clinical experience, and complete a formal project in order to gain specialist status. A number of trainees in Hong Kong and Malaysia also choose to register for training with ANZCA. ANZCA also oversees and accredits the Maintenance of Professional Standards (MOPS) programme, accrediting activities and managing yearly MOPS returns from specialists. Increasingly, however, ANZCA has taken a more active role as an educational provider, with the appointment of a Director of Education, the development of a written curriculum, and provision of training for supervisors. The College recognized the value of providing training in crisis management, and was in a position to consider a proposal for a course, developed by and for anaesthetists, that would be a become part of the ANZCA training programme.

With the growth in the number of suitable simulation centres in Australia and New Zealand, widespread access to appropriate facilities was possible. Individuals from different simulation centres agreed to co-operate on the project and presented a proposal to the ANZCA Council to develop a course in crisis management.

The Council accepted this proposal and established a working party to oversee course development and implementation.

34.4 Course development

ANZCA hosted a number of 2-day workshops for the simulator group and College representatives to establish the course philosophy, main aims, and overall format. The course was divided

Table 34.1 The EMAC modules

Day 1	am	Human performance
	pm	Cardiovascular emergencies
Day 2	am	Airway emergencies
	pm	Anaesthetic emergencies
Day 3	am	Trauma

into five distinct modules: human performance, cardiovascular emergencies, airway emergencies, anaesthetic emergencies, and trauma (Table 34.1). Individual members of the group took responsibility for each module, and developed the curriculum, learning outcomes, teaching methods and the teaching materials.

Over the course of the next 2 years, alongside course development, the regulations governing the course were developed and approved by College Council. The course manual was written, and a comprehensive instructors' manual developed, which contained all the information and written materials required to run the course.

Eventually, the EMAC course emerged; a 2.5-day course, underpinned by a comprehensive participants' manual, and taught using a range of interactive teaching methods, making much use of simulation, skills stations, case-based discussions, videos and games.

Two pilot courses held in 2001 were observed by College Councillors and the College Director of Education, and course participants completed evaluations of each module and the overall course. A report was produced by the Director of Education and submitted to ANZCA Council for approval.

The EMAC course was approved by College Council as a component of training for Fellowship of ANZCA and courses were offered from the simulation centres in Melbourne, Sydney and Wellington from early 2002.

Although initially developed for a target group of anaesthesia trainees in their second year of training, it soon became apparent that the course had considerable appeal to specialist anaesthetists. The College recognized the value of specialist participation in EMAC and accredited the EMAC course for its MOPS programme in 2002. Not only are MOPS points awarded for participants, but the College recognized the professional value of instructing on the EMAC course, and EMAC instructors are also awarded MOPS points. The EMAC course now plays a significant role in maintenance of professional standards for many specialist anaesthetists, participation in which is a requirement for registration with the New Zealand Medical Council, and strongly encouraged in Australia.

34.5 **Course participation**

Anaesthesia specialists and trainees attend the EMAC course in almost equal numbers. Trainees in their first year are discouraged from attending as they would not have sufficient knowledge or experience to gain maximum benefit from the course. There is an even spread of participation across the other 4 years of training, and courses contain a mix of specialists and trainees. Participation by specialists, who provide supervision to trainees back in the workplace, has important implications for reinforcing lessons learned in EMAC in the actual theatre environment.

The EMAC course is now established as an integral part of the anaesthesia educational environment for both trainees and specialists across Australia, New Zealand, and Hong Kong. It is currently delivered in eight accredited centres across the region.

In the order of 15 courses are run across the region each year. Over 600 trainees and specialists participated in the course in the years 2002 to 2005, and increasing numbers of courses are being offered each year. A significant proportion of the anaesthesia workforce in Australia and New Zealand has now attended an EMAC course, and the concepts of situational awareness, teamwork and leadership, and systematic approaches to problem solving are now widespread.

34.6 Regulation of EMAC

A subcommittee of ANZCA provides governance of the EMAC course. This committee accredits simulation centres to run EMAC. The aim of this accreditation is to maintain consistency of the course across all centres, and ensure each course and course provider meet appropriate and explicit standards. These standards include physical facilities, adherence to course curriculum and methods of course delivery, numbers and training of instructors, availability of models and equipment for each session, and specifications for simulators. Prospective course providers must complete the initial documentation and provide information on facilities, instructors and equipment. A satisfactory submission results in probationary approval to run the EMAC course. This must be followed by an onsite visit by College appointees in the first or second course, which can result in provisional or full approval. The onsite visit is performed by ANZCA Council appointees with appropriate expertise. Each course provider is reviewed at least every 5 years. The EMAC course regulations are published on the ANZCA website at http://www.medeserv.com.au/anzca/edutraining/EMAC/index.htm.

34.7 The EMAC course

The EMAC course follows a simple template that could be applied easily to other acute care specialities. The course consists of five modules delivered consecutively over 2.5 days. There is a maximum of 12 participants per course and a minimum of four instructors at any one time, with additional staff playing roles in scenarios, running simulators or co-ordinating activities. Prior to the course, participants receive a course manual which provides the knowledge-base underpinning the learning objectives in each module.

The overall aim of the course is to develop a systematic approach to the management of medical emergencies, incorporating essential knowledge and skills, strategies for problem solving and problem avoidance, and the principles of crisis resource management as described in the early 1990s[1,2].

During the 2.5 days of the course, participants experience around 20 simulations, five skills stations, and numerous games, case-based discussions, videos and interactive presentations. Essential core knowledge and technical skills are learnt through case-based discussions and skills stations. Participants learn and apply protocols and drills in clinical scenarios using the medium fidelity simulator SimMan® (Laerdal). Full immersion simulations using a high fidelity patient simulator such as the Medical Education Technologies Inc., Sarasota, Florida, Human Patient Simulator (METI-HPS®) or MedSim® (Eagle) simulator, allow application of knowledge and skills in a realistic clinical context, and development of problem solving strategies and behaviours for effective crisis management. Throughout the course the teaching methods aim for maximum participant engagement, and emphasize reflection on practice and the linking of course experiences to real life practice.

The five course modules are Human Performance Issues, Airway Emergencies, Anaesthetic Emergencies, Cardiovascular Emergencies, and Trauma. Each of the modules addresses the broad goals of prevention of and preparedness to respond to clinical emergencies.

34.7.1 Human performance issues module

The human performance module uses a combination of videos, games, simulation and interactive presentations to explore the various factors that affect performance of individuals and healthcare teams, and introduces the key principles of crisis management. The use of games allows the exploration of ideas outside of medical context. For example, the 'Tennis Balls Game' is a graphic illustration of how a situation can slowly escalate and become chaotic when there are too many tasks and no advance planning. Six participants standing in a circle are asked to catch a ball, read out the information on the ball and pass it on to a team member. They cope easily with one ball, or two or three, but as more and more balls are added to the circle, chaos ensues. Reflecting on what happened in this simple exercise, participants identify a number of key issues around crisis recognition, advance planning, task management and leadership. Another example involves an unexpected 'cardiac arrest' that draws the 12 participants to a 'patient' who has collapsed in the adjacent post-anaesthesia care unit. The task for the group is to resuscitate the patient while establishing the cause of the collapse. As no-one has prior 'ownership' of the case, participants grapple with the issues around how leadership is established and the value of making leadership explicit. The wide range of methods used in this session aim to engage participants, demonstrate relevance to clinical practice, and establish basic principles of crisis management, which can then be reinforced throughout the remaining modules of the course.

34.7.2 Airway emergencies module

The airway module focuses on avoiding airway problems through advance planning and preparation, and rehearsing for problems if and when they do arise. Skills stations include a range of airway devices and manoeuvres which may aid ventilation and/or intubation. A surgical airway workshop combines hands-on practice with equipment for transtracheal airway access and ventilation, and the decision-making process behind the choice of the different options. A range of airway problems, including airway obstruction, inadequate ventilation and oxygenation, and unanticipated difficult intubation are presented in a series of six short simulations. Participants' management of these situations is compared with published airway algorithms. Personal stories are encouraged, drawing on the real-life experiences participants bring to the session. These simulations provide an opportunity to apply the skills learnt in the preceding

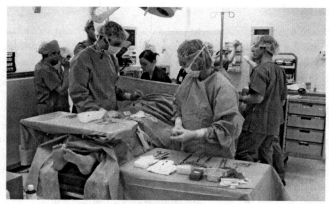

Fig. 34.1 A simulated case of malignant hyperthermia.

sessions and to develop a logical step-by-step approach to airway management, moving from simple manoeuvres to relieve upper airway obstruction to a definitive surgical airway. Videos and interactive discussions draw the content together into a framework of planning for airway emergencies.

34.7.3 Cardiovascular emergencies module

The cardiovascular module addresses acute perioperative derangements in cardiac perfusion, output and rhythm, which require immediate intervention. The module begins with an update on advanced cardiac life support and the underlying rationale for international guidelines. A preliminary case discussion followed by full immersion simulations on the METI simulator explore the management of intraoperative cardiac ischaemia and cardiogenic shock, and provide opportunities to practise crisis management behaviours. A series of short scenarios using the Laerdal SimMan® demonstrate broad complex tachycardia, narrow complex tachycardia, bradycardia, and atrial fibrillation. Participants diagnose and treat the rhythm disturbance, applying vagal manoeuvres, administering drugs, using cardioversion or transcutaneous pacing as required. The simulator is programmed to respond to their interventions, and appropriate management is reinforced by debriefing against accepted published treatment algorithms.

34.7.4 Anaesthetic emergencies module

The anaesthetic emergencies module is an intensive 4-hour session of simulations, focusing on emergencies in anaesthesia where the interface between patient, airway equipment and the anaesthesia machine are of prime importance. Scenarios build on lessons from the previous scenario and reinforce lessons learnt in the preceding modules. The crises present with a generic problem, such as hypoxia or increased airway pressure, and the goal is to develop a systematic approach to the initial diagnosis and management of these common presentations. By incorporating a systematic review of equipment and patient, the aim is to enhance situational awareness and reduce the likelihood of inappropriate early closure on diagnosis from fixation errors and frequency gambling. Again, participants are encouraged to draw on their own experiences, adding rich clinical material to support the lessons in the simulations. The scenarios provide an opportunity to practise and reinforce the principles of crisis management introduced in the human performance module.

34.7.5 Trauma module

The core principles of trauma management based on the primary and secondary patient survey are incorporated into the trauma module to ensure different professional groups are working to the same goals. In the EMAC course, the focus is on the role of the anaesthetist in trauma, with particular attention to airway management and intraoperative care. Following presentations of introductory material, participants apply the primary and secondary survey in a series of simulated trauma cases, emphasizing the need to prioritize in the face of multiple competing tasks, and the need for regular re-evaluation due to the evolving nature of severe trauma. Detection and evaluation of haemothorax or pneumothorax, or detection of misplaced or blocked chest drains may be life-saving. Case discussions are supplemented by skill stations, for example, practical management of chest drains. Management of anaesthesia for the head-injured patient is addressed through case discussion, and a hands-on skills station ensures a logical and safe approach to managing the patient with potential cervical spine injury.

34.8 **Assessment**

ANZCA trainees must complete either an EMAC course or the 'Early Management of Severe Trauma' course as part of their training for Fellowship of ANZCA.

EMAC participants are awarded a Certificate of Completion after attending all five modules. There is no requirement to pass a formal assessment.

Considerable formative assessment takes place during the course in the form of feedback on performance in simulations and skills stations. Inclusion of a formal assessment in EMAC has often been hotly debated.

Core knowledge and some aspects of problem solving could be assessed in written tests or oral vivas. However the College already has a robust mechanism for this in the existing examination process. Demonstrating proficiency in technical skills could also be assessed with relative ease, but this assessment may be feasible and more valid in the workplace or on readily available models. The Part 1 examination for Fellowship of the Royal College of Anaesthetists incorporates simulations, and simulated emergencies are a component of the Israeli national board examination in anesthesiology[3].

Managing a well-defined event with a clear treatment pathway is an important and relatively easily assessed prerequisite to managing a clinical emergency. Conducting such an assessment is clearly feasible, but not within the 2.5 days of the EMAC course, and as with any high stakes assessment, a rigorous process is necessary for a fair and accurate result. Assessing performance in a realistically simulated crisis is more problematic, and for a reliable score, multiple cases and multiple judges are required[4], and issues of validity of simulator performance as a measure of real life performance have not been resolved.

In terms of incorporating an assessment component within the EMAC course, or any similar course, there are additional considerations.

Firstly, in the EMAC course, we encourage participants to try out new behaviours. Fear of assessment would limit experimentation. Secondly, the simulations are already stressful without the additional stress of a formal assessment. Although a small amount of stress can be good for learning, high levels of stress are counterproductive. Thirdly, the EMAC course introduces complex ideas and suggests radical changes in behaviour. It may take attendees some time to work on incorporating these new approaches into their own practice. Fourthly, participants work in teams and some team members are more or less helpful, which makes it difficult to score to a single member of the team. Finally, and significantly, the score from one or two scenarios would be very unreliable. Test theory predicts that 3–4 hours testing time would be required to give a reliable result.

For these reasons, the assessment in EMAC is purely formative at this stage.

34.9 **The ethics of reporting on poor performance in EMAC**

Aside from the issue of incorporating formal assessment into EMAC, another issue arising in EMAC, and in many simulation based courses, is what to do where participants are observed behaving in a way that would put patients at risk.

Participating in a simulation, observed by peers and instructors, is highly exposing and for maximum learning, participants are encouraged to engage with the scenario as if it were real. To promote this buy-in, and recognizing that participants will and do make mistakes, there is a commitment to confidentiality at the beginning of every EMAC course. What then is the ethical responsibility of instructors when they observe unsafe practice? Should the supervisor or head of department be notified?

A number of arguments can be mounted against reporting. Poor performance will be as obvious in the workplace as it is in the simulator, and the responsibility lies with the employer. Observing one or two simulations is not a reliable measure of workplace performance. Participants are working in a team, who may impact positively or negatively on their performance. The purpose of the scenarios is learning not assessment and the necessary standardisation and control of the scenario is insufficient for a high stakes assessment. The implications of informing a supervisor or head of department are significant and potentially damaging. Fear of negative consequences would discourage anaesthetists from attending the course. The alternative argument is that failure to report the practitioner is putting patients at risk, that there is a duty to report poor practice in the workplace and this should extend to a simulated workplace. This is clearly an ethical dilemma. In EMAC, we have resolved that feedback and recommendations will be given to the participants only, and that no participants will be reported to their supervisors or employers.

34.10 Evaluation

Evaluation is an integral part of every EMAC course. Participant evaluations are collected by the College and used as a quality improvement tool, to ensure consistently high standards of the course.

At the end of each of the five modules, and again at the end of the course, participants complete an anonymous evaluation form, rating course components across a five point rating scale (1=strongly agree, 2=agree, 3=undecided, 4=disagree, 5=strongly disagree). As a measure of increased competence, participants also rate their own level of mastery of the material before and after each module. Finally, written comments are invited on key areas of learning and the best and worst aspects of their experience of EMAC.

Over 500 evaluation forms have been analysed at the time of writing. This analysis is fully reported elsewhere[5]. Participants rate the individual EMAC modules and the overall course highly in terms of structure, standard, relevance to practice and learning (Table 34.2).

There was a statistically significant shift in self-assessed scores from 'beginner' to 'master' over the course of the modules ($p \leq 0.001$).

A number of themes emerged from written responses. The simulations had a major impact on participants, and importantly, they were impressed by the collegiality and non-judgemental approach of the instructors and the high standard of instruction. Participants commented that

Table 34.2 Summary course evaluation data from 500 participants

Overall course evaluation	Agree or strongly agree (%)
• The modules were well organized	97
• There was the right amount of information	76
• The course was pitched at the appropriate level	85
• The standard of instruction was high	99
• The course facilities were suitable	94
Responses for individual module evaluations	**Agree or strongly agree – range over five modules**
• I learned a great deal from this module	81–96
• I learned things that were relevant to my practice	91–99
• I will change my practice as a result of this module	71–88

they learnt from each other by working together and watching each other in simulations. A minority noted the stress of the simulations, and some found the course long and tiring, but the vast majority were very positive, and had gained insight into their own performance and felt motivated to improve.

To explore whether this reported learning did translate to subsequent change in behaviour, we conducted a postal survey of a group of anaesthetists who had attended a course some 3–12 months previously, asking them what they had learnt and how they had changed their practice subsequent to the course. Ninety-eight anaesthetists responded (45% response rate). Of these, 99% considered the course had improved their ability to manage anaesthetic emergencies and 86% agreed that attending an EMAC course had changed the way they practised anaesthesia. Ninety-seven percent thought the EMAC course should be a requirement for training.

One of the main themes to emerge from the postal survey was developing a more systematic approach to acute clinical events, including new problem solving strategies such as standing back and making a global assessment, anticipating and planning ahead, constant re-evaluation, avoiding assumptions, verbalising and sharing the problem. Many commented on improved communication and teamwork in a crisis, strategies to improve their leadership in a crisis and the importance of appropriate delegation of tasks to other members of the operating room team.

34.11 Instructors

A key component of success of the EMAC course has been the pool of enthusiastic and talented instructors. These courses are resource intensive, requiring a high instructor–participant ratio. For example, the two EMAC-accredited simulation centres in New Zealand run eight EMAC courses per year, and each course involves around eight instructors, many of whom are present for the whole course. In addition, one or two trainee instructors attend each course. The instructors are anaesthetists from all regions in New Zealand. New instructors must first participate in an EMAC course, then attend a 2-day EMAC Instructor Course, and then participate in two EMAC courses as a trainee instructor and obtain satisfactory evaluations. The responsibility for instructor training rests with the accredited EMAC centres.

Ongoing training for instructors is provided through peer review observed, sessions during an EMAC course using a structure rating form, and regular workshops. Interest in becoming an EMAC instructor is high, with constant demand for instructor courses. Instructor retention is also high, with many of the original instructors still teaching on the course.

34.12 The recipe for success

The EMAC course can be judged a success on the basis of the evaluation and its obvious popularity among anaesthetists and much of this is due to the success of the partnership between the College and the simulation centres. The ANZCA label gives the course legitimacy and encourages participation. The College provides governance for the course, overseeing course standards, uniformity and development. The simulation centres provide the instructors and facilities to run the course and the drive for continuous improvement.

The success is also due to the fact that the course is based on sound educational principles. The course was designed to address a real area of need, has relevant learning outcomes and uses teaching methods that engage and challenge learners and link new learning to clinical practice.

A by-product of this venture is that a large number of anaesthetists have been engaged in formal teaching, attended teaching workshops and developed expertise as teachers. Many have been motivated to take postgraduate education qualifications. This has benefits for the anaesthesia community beyond the confines of simulation.

34.13 **EMAC revision**

A curriculum should be considered as an evolving document, to maintain relevance, freshness, and the interest of its instructors. The EMAC course requires ongoing review and revision. The evaluations revealed specific areas for improvement in individual modules, and new evidence and practice guidelines have been published since the course was first written.

The initial creative enthusiasm for a new course may drive individuals to work extra hours to develop the materials. However, revising and updating a course are less exciting, and more directive strategies and specified resources are likely to be required to obtain the required results. Planning for course maintenance should be included from the outset, and an ongoing curriculum committee to oversee the course is required.

34.14 **Future recommendations**

This course provides a model for training anaesthetists in crisis management. It is, however, merely 2.5 days in a 5-year training programme and is the only such course provided by the College. It is likely that repeated exposure will be more effective than a single course, however intense. Vertical integration of crisis management training throughout the anaesthesia training programme would be desirable.

Participants have identified a number of areas for future simulation-based courses, for example, a course for novice anaesthetists, obstetric emergencies, paediatric emergencies and advanced airway skills. This could be the basis of a programme of training in crisis management throughout the 5 years of training, and like the current EMAC course, could appeal to specialists as well as trainees.

34.15 **Conclusion**

The need for effective crisis management training in anaesthesia has been recognized for many years, and there is considerable evidence to support its formal inclusion in the curriculum[1,6–8]. EMAC is one of only a few such initiatives world-wide. Østergaard describes a compulsory, 4-day course in Anaesthesia Crisis Resource Management in Denmark[9], but in general, crisis management training has been offered through local initiatives without coordination by accrediting bodies. The formal involvement of ANZCA in the EMAC course has resulted in widespread involvement of anaesthetists across three nations in a uniform course in crisis management, with explicit course standards, and shared learning outcomes.

Clinicians are called on to respond rapidly and effectively to emergencies in many areas of medical practice. Implementation of programmes similar to EMAC in other acute care specialities is proceeding in the region, with the development of a course for emergency medicine physicians and clear opportunities for intensive care training.

The description of the EMAC course may provide a useful template for those contemplating similar initiatives in different regions and across different domains of clinical care.

References

1. Howard S, *et al*. (1992). Anesthesia crisis resource management training: teaching anesthesiologists to handle critical incidents. *Aviation, Space and Environmental Medicine* **63**: 763–70.
2. Gaba D, Fish K, Howard S (1994). *Crisis Management in Anesthesiology*. 1st ed. Churchill Livingston: 290.
3. Berkenstadt H, *et al*. (2006). Incorporating simulation-based objective structured clinical examination into the Israeli national board examination in anesthesiology. *Anesthesia and Analgesia* **102**(3): 853–8.

4. Weller J, *et al.* (2005). Psychometric characteristics of simulation-based assessment in anaesthesia and accuracy of self-assessed scores. *Anaesthesia* **60**(3): 245–50.

5. Weller J, *et al.* (2006). Effective management of anaesthetic crises: development and evaluation of a College accredited simulation-based course for anaesthesia education in Australia and New Zealand. *Simulation in Healthcare* **1**(4): 209–15.

6. Garden A, *et al.* (2002). Education to address medical error – a role of high fidelity patient simulation. *New Zealand Medical Journal* **115**(1150): 133–44.

7. Holzman R, *et al.* (1995). Anesthesia crisis resource management: real-life simulation training in operating room crises. *Journal of Clinical Anesthesia* **7**: 675–87.

8. Kurrek M, J Fish (1996). Anaesthesia crisis resource management training: an intimidating concept, a rewarding experience. *Canadian Journal of Anaesthesia* **43**(5): 430–4.

9. Østergaard D (2004). National Medical Simulation Training in Denmark. *Critical Care Medicine* **32**(2 Suppl.): S58–S60.

Chapter 35

Simulation in high-stakes performance assessment

Leonie Watterson

Overview

- There are numerous potential applications of simulation to assessment of clinical competence; however, it has not been widely supported within the healthcare community to date.

- Concerns about the application of simulation to performance assessment mirror those that have been identified previously with other assessment methods. In particular, there are competing tensions between the dual goals of achieving both high reliability and high validity, because these appear to require mutually exclusive test conditions. Experimental studies have demonstrated that moderate levels of reliability and validity can be achieved simultaneously with mannequin simulators if test conditions are appropriately managed.

- Like other assessment methods, simulation should not be used in isolation to make a determination about a practitioner's overall performance. It should instead be incorporated into a broader multifaceted programme. Lessons from medical education and registration boards should be observed. These are presented in this chapter.

- The New South Wales Medical Board incorporates simulation methods into its 'high-stakes' performance assessment programme.

35.1 Introduction

'High-stakes' performance assessment generally refers to that which leads to an overall judgment about a previously qualified practitioner's professional performance for the purpose of renewing practice privileges. It may involve a standardized screening exercise for routine recertification, or a tailored exercise in response to specific concerns that his or her clinical performance is substandard.

35.2 Why conduct assessment in a synthetic environment?

Incorporating simulation-based methods into high-stakes assessment has a number of potential benefits.

Many of these mirror the commonly cited benefits of simulation as an educational tool:

- Employing actual patients may be unethical or unacceptable.

- Access to sufficient numbers of patients may be limited.

- Exposure to infrequently occurring cases is limited.
- Patient variability may reduce ability to standardize methods and conditions.

Situational factors relevant to assessment offer several additional reasons:

- Some practitioners may be on extended leave from clinical practice and hence it is not logistically possible to observe their care of patients.
- The workplace may present an unreasonably difficult environment for assessment. For instance, a practitioner's clinical responsibilities may have been revised and he or she is unfamiliar with their new roles and working environment.
- Assessment conducted in the clinical service environment may be conspicuous to patients and staff and hence disruptive to clinical service, patients' perceptions of the safety of the care they receive, and the practitioner's reputation.
- Some practitioners may be suffering stress or other psychological disorders, contributed to by the assessment or the events leading up to it. The practitioner's psychological well being may be better monitored and managed in a synthetic environment.

Finally, developing assessment methodologies deployed in synthetic environments will benefit the validation of educational activities delivered in these environments. The latter are rapidly increasing along with demands by employers and funding bodies to show evidence of training transfer and training effectiveness.

35.3 **Status of simulation-based performance assessment**

35.3.1 **Existing programmes**

Despite these potential benefits the use of simulation in assessment of performance is limited, especially high-stakes assessment of clinical performance. Two centres have published descriptions of assessment for anaesthetists in conjunction with high-stakes performance assessment[1,2] and one for dentists recuperating from physical injury[3]. There are no published reports of simulation being used for recertification. However, mannequin simulators have been piloted as a component of assessment in conjunction with lower stakes certification for anaesthesia trainees[4] and final year medical students[5]. In addition, cardiology simulators are now routinely incorporated into some internal medicine certification exams[6]. A survey of simulation centres conducted in 2002 provides evidence of unpublished use of high fidelity mannequin simulators for assessment. Fifteen percent of responders in this survey indicated their centres used this medium for practice assessment and 49% agreed that simulation should be used for certification testing[7]. The author has unpublished experience with its use in peer assessment and appraisal of specialist anaesthetists reentering clinical practice following voluntary leave, and assessment and remediation of junior doctors following critical incidents.

35.3.2 **Validation studies**

35.3.2.1 Reliability and validity

Assessment methods have been traditionally assessed according to their measurement properties[8]. Reliability is the extent to which test results will be reproduced by different raters (inter-rater reliability), by a candidate on different occasions (test retest reliability) or by subsets of the same test (internal consistency). Reliability is considered best achieved by standardizing as many components of tests as possible (e.g. case design and delivery, scoring criteria and raters). This requires exclusion of as many variables as possible. Validity is the extent to which the outcomes of

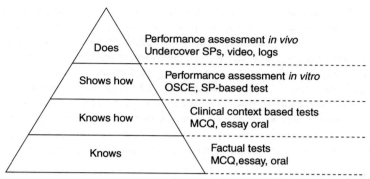

SP = simulated patients; OSCE = Objective Structured Clinical Examination; MCQ = Multiple Choice Examination

Fig. 35.1 Miller's model of competence[8]. (Reprinted from Wass V, Van der Vleuten C, Shatzer J, Jones R (2001). Assessment of clinical competence. *Lancet* **357**: 945–49. Reproduced with permission of Elsevier.)

a test faithfully reflect the tasks and traits it is intended to. We generally accept a test has high content validity if experts have been adequately consulted about relevant competencies; construct validity if candidates' scores increase with their level of experience; and concurrent validity if candidates' scores on the test correlate with those of other tests which assess the same tasks and traits. High validity is achieved in part by retaining as many variables as possible so as to preserve the realism of the cases.

The latter is a central assumption of assessment conditions conducted at the 'does' level of Miller's hierarchical performance assessment model[9]. This model proposes that clinical performance can be assessed at different levels of deconstruction. The base of the triangle assesses foundation knowledge (knows) whereas the apex represents the performance of clinical tasks under the same conditions in which they are provided in the workplace (Fig. 35.1) Work-based assessment is distinguished from competency-based assessment. The latter measures what doctors can do in controlled representations of professional practice, such as an objective structured clinical examination (OSCE)[10].

Several published studies have demonstrated that adequate levels of validity and, or reliability can be achieved when simulation is used to assess components of clinical competence, provided test conditions and methods are appropriate. Acceptable reliability has been demonstrated in tests employing the OSCE method and standardized patients[11] and the Harvey simulator[12]. In these studies, contextual factors (and hence realism) were reduced and performance criteria were highly deconstructed into component competencies. It is widely believed that these conditions will contribute to reliable scoring. However, tests designed in this manner are considered to achieve only moderate levels of validity, equating to Miller's 'shows how' level of performance[10]. In contrast, studies employing high fidelity mannequin simulators designed the assessment case scenarios to reproduce a number of contextual factors characteristic of the workplace. These include a realistic clinical environment, team-mates who interact with the candidate, and situations, such as telephone calls, which require the candidate to divide his or her attention. These studies have consistently demonstrated that two experts can achieve high inter-rater reliability when using subjective rating instruments to observe contextually rich scenarios[4, 5,13,14,15,16]. Several of these have demonstrated a correlation between test scores and increasing experience.

The author used this finding to conclude that the studies achieved both acceptable reliability and construct validity. To date, no authors have propositioned where this increased level of realism sits according to Miller's model. It has been previously opined that assessment at the 'does' level requires testing in actual clinical service environments where realism is wholly intact[10]. Thus, mannequin simulators can reasonably claim to assess performance at a level approaching, but not achieving Miller's 'does' level when contextually rich scenarios are provided. These recent developments with mannequin simulators represent an important advance in this field.

Reviewers of these studies conclude that while the results are encouraging, there is still insufficient evidence to support the use of mannequin-based simulation for high-stakes performance assessment[17,18]. These reviews, written nearly a decade apart, reveal that progress with this topic remains slow.

35.3.2.2 Acceptability

The above reports of high-stakes assessments of anaesthetists[1,2] concluded that using simulation positively contributed to conducting a fair and meaningful assessment with several of the specialists subsequently undergoing remediation training tailored to their identified needs. However, it is predictable that the acceptability of simulation-based assessment will be influenced by the consequences of assessment as perceived by practitioners. For example, a recent survey of anaesthetists indicated that while 75% were willing to undergo testing of their own volition, 65% were not in favour of compulsory recertification[19]. Meanwhile, use of simulation under lower stakes conditions has been reported to be highly acceptable to trainee anaesthetists[4,15] and final medical students[5]. Subjects in these pilots indicated that the assessment scenarios achieved high face validity in that they were highly realistic and representative of their performance. This suggests that the perceived consequences of high stakes assessment may be unnecessarily slowing progress with this medium.

35.4 Barriers to acceptance – lessons from non-simulation assessment methods

The recent history of test validation using simulated technologies shares many similarities with assessment methods in general. Numerous non simulation methods of assessment have existed for some time, including written examinations, 'long' and 'short' patient cases, OSCE, objective structured assessment of technical skills (OSATS), and mini clinical exercise (mini-CEX). However, research has yet to identify any single method of assessment that is considered wholly valid as a sole method of assessing performance[20]. Reasons for this include the following.

35.4.1 Test psychometrics

There is an apparently irresolvable tension created by the dual aims to achieve both high reliability and high validity in test design. Until now, test designers been unable to resolve the competing interests of high standardization *versus* high realism required to achieve high reliability and validity, respectively[10].

35.4.2 Selection of competencies as markers of performance

There is uncertainty regarding what competencies should be assessed. The scope of competencies – or at least the open expression of these – expected of modern health professionals is continually broadening. Clinical knowledge, previously the cornerstone trait of a competent practitioner, is now commonly presented as but one component of a suite of items in modern competency frameworks[21,22]. This has created considerable challenges for educators, employers and regulators who have the task of developing appropriate curricula and assessment methods. Unfortunately, the development and validation of performance markers and assessment tools has lagged behind.

35.4.3 Understanding human performance

Our understanding of performance is also undergoing considerable change. Miller's model is widely accepted as a reasonable representation of performance across the health professions. While this model remains popular, several key constructs regarding performance have recently been elaborated.

- Performance at the 'does' level involves not only integrated performance of single tasks, but also the execution of multiple interdependent, team-based tasks. Hays describes three performance domains defining doctors as 'managers of patient care', 'managers of their environment' and 'managers of themselves'[23]. Numerous other models describe components of work-based practice, each calling for appropriate assessment methods[24].

- Valid assessment of performance also requires measurement of habitual practice. Several studies have shown that there are differences between what doctors can do in controlled high stakes situations and what they really do in actual practice away from the scrutiny of test conditions[10].

- Performance deficiencies are multifactorial, some reasons include inadequate training and support, poor motivation, behavioural misconduct, a stressful workplace, poor relationships within a clinical team and physical or mental ill health[25].

- Medical practitioners' performance is not consistent either within or between episodes of patient care. Patient safety research describes numerous factors that contribute to errors or degraded performance. Some of these reflect individual factors (e.g. fatique) while others reflect conditions under which the individual performs (e.g. heavy workload, production pressure and ambient conditions)[26,27].

35.5 Key principles of high-stakes global performance assessment

The concerns and issues raised above have not prevented global performance assessment from occurring. No definitive solutions have been identified, however there is sufficient published work in this area to formulate a few guiding principles. Much of this work has been generated by medical licensing bodies and universities[8,10,28–37].

35.5.1 Selection

It should be reserved for a small subset of practitioners for whom other forms of regulation have failed, including: self-regulation, professional regulation and organizational performance management.

35.5.2 Governance

It should have an appropriate governance framework with fair and transparent processes for selection, decision-making, appeal, remediation, reassessment, and ongoing monitoring and management.

35.5.3 Interim practice privileges

In some instances it will be appropriate to place temporary restrictions on the practitioner's privileges until the assessment is completed.

35.5.4 **Preparation**

The overall process should be made clear to the practitioner including reasons for, and purpose of assessment, possible consequences, assessment activities, assessment criteria, appeal processes and time frame.

35.5.5 **Individualized programmes**

These should be tailored to individual practitioners' workplace responsibilities and privileges, perceived deficiencies and other factors relating to logistics, fairness of process and defensibility.

35.5.6 **Structure**

The components of assessment should be coherently linked to the purpose and consequences of the assessment. Selection of competencies and attributes to be tested should:

- be selected appropriately to measure different components of performance relevant to the practitioner's discipline.
  - An appropriate discipline-specific competency framework may be used a guide. For example, the ability to perform effectively during time-critical emergencies is ranked higher for practitioners working in critical care environments than those who do not.
- sample across a wide range of clinical cases that are representative of the scope of the practitioner's workplace responsibilities and practice privileges.
  - This is referred to as 'domain sampling'. Assessing small numbers of cases has been consistently demonstrated as a key cause of poor reliability in assessment of performance. The scope of the practitioner's responsibilities and privileges can be obtained by interviews with the practitioner and employers.
- assess against the level of autonomy the practitioner is expected to achieve.
  - Practitioners whose medical registration allows them to practice independently must be able to demonstrate they can perform effectively in relatively poorly supported, adverse environments, without relying upon capable nursing staff or colleagues to buffer them. So it is reasonable to build criteria into test designs that reveal the level of support the practitioner needs. This is often gleaned from interviews with colleagues; however, mannequin-based simulation is considered a potentially ideal tool for this.
- include tests which measure habitual practices in contrast to performance witnessed on one occasion.
  - Examples include medical record review, audit, prescribing practices and quality of documentation.
- endeavour to assess the practitioner's insight into his or her ability, and how they are perceived by patients and colleagues.
  - Also assess their capacity and willingness to learn and modify practice, if required. This can be achieved by interviewing the practitioner and undertaking 360-degree assessment.
- endeavour to assess whether psychological or personality factors may be degrading an individual's performance or the potential for them to remediate.
  - Psychometric tests and interviews with the practitioner, colleagues and employer can address this.
- assess extrinsic factors which may be degrading an individual's performance including environmental, systems factors, team factors and workplace culture.

- Difficulties with interpersonal relationships may influence the practitioner's performance. Generally this is done through interviews with the practitioner, colleagues and management. Conversely, testimonies from colleagues may be prejudiced and unreliable. This risk will be reduced by increasing the number of colleagues interviewed.

35.5.7 Standards against which performance is measured

These must be clear to the test designers, assessors and practitioners. It must be clear what is considered acceptable versus unacceptable practice. This in turn is matched with the purpose and consequence of the assessment. Different standards may apply to a practitioner being assessed to practice under different conditions such as: subspecialty *versus* community practitioner; after-hours emergencies *versus* elective cases; supervised or supernumary *versus* independent practice; isolated *versus* supported facility; procedural *versus* non-procedural duties.

35.5.8 Selection of appropriate methods

Given the limitations inherent in any single assessment method, assessment of global performance should be based on triangulated data. That is, multiple raters or sources of evidence, obtained on different occasions, using multiple methods.

35.5.9 Rating tools

The appropriateness of rating methods varies with test design. Tests based on direct observation, particularly those with high levels of realism, favour global rating scales. These can be supported by checklists and should be criterion rather than norm-based. Ratings should collectively incorporate a judicious blend of quantitative and qualitative outcome measures to compensate for the identified limitations of any single test.

35.5.10 Assessors

Assessors should be content experts given they will use global rating instruments. They should have recognized good standing within the professional community and be screened to exclude conflicts of interest. They must also be appropriately trained to administer and score the tests. This requires calibration of their personal standards to the pre-determined standards established by the governing body.

35.5.11 Test conditions

Test conditions need to be fair and reflective of the workplace. If not, they have reduced concurrent validity. The level of case difficulty must be appropriately controlled by test designers, administrators and participating actors. If the designers wish to faithfully reproduce a workplace that is recognized to be challenging, then the scoring standards must take this into consideration. The provision of diagnostic information and prompts should also be controlled as these can introduce threats to validity by disrupting diagnostic cues or the normal level of prompting that practitioners obtain from teammates.

35.5.12 Risk management

Candidates undergoing performance assessment are at risk of a number of events including personal stress, loss of income, detriment to reputation and loss of referrals. Given the potential consequences, they may also behave in a litigious manner. The performance assessment programme should build in risk reduction strategies for practitioners and assessors.

Strict conditions should be placed regarding the release of information and participants should be monitored and followed up. Assessors should be indemnified.

35.6 Lessons from reports of assessment employing simulation

Closer examination of the methods described in mannequin-based simulation assessment reveals some common practices which appear to increase the validity of tests conducted with this medium. In programmes to date[1,2,4,5] the simulation-based methods:

- were integrated with a larger multifaceted programme, overseen by a medical regulatory body, specialty college or university assessment process
- specified the competencies being assessed; these were predominantly integrated clinical management of critical care patients
- employed a battery of test scenarios that sampled a relevant and sufficiently broad range of clinical management tasks, including emergency *versus* non-emergency situations.

Additionally, test conditions used in these programmes, as well as experimental studies[13–17,38]:

- managed threats to construct validity by achieving a level of realism somewhere between an OSCE and real-world conditions.
- managed threats to reliability by controlling the conditions under which the scenarios were delivered. These included: carefully scripted cases, keeping the simulators' vital signs within pre-set parameters, providing instructions to actors regarding the delivery of important diagnostic cues and the degree to which they prompted or supported the candidates.
- used criterion-based, subjective global rating scales in at least some of the scoring instruments.

35.7 Case description: the New South Wales Medical Board performance assessment programme

35.7.1 Overview

In 2000, the author, in collaboration with the New South Wales Medical Board (NSWMB) and Sydney Medical Simulation Centre[1] (SMSC) developed a methodology for high-stakes simulation-based assessment of anaesthetists as an integral component of the board's Performance Assessment Programme (PAP).

35.7.2 Context

In order to practise medicine Australian doctors must be registered with their relevant state or territory's medical registration board. Like their international counterparts, each board has an established process for responding to complaints and notifications about the safety and quality of a doctor's practice.

Currently, each state's regulatory processes are individualized. In NSW, the regulatory process is enshrined within the legislation of the NSW Medical Act, 2002. It operates on a coregulatory model, where two independent bodies, the NSWMB and NSW Health Care

---

1 The Sydney Medical Simulation Centre is a synthetic training facility, located in the state of NSW, Australia. It houses a range of simulators – specializing in high fidelity mannequin-based systems – and conducts training, assessment and research relevant to multi-professional healthcare teams and professional groups.

Complaints Commission work together to deal with complaints against medical practitioners. The seriousness of complaints about doctors varies widely; some are unsubstantiated while others warrant their removal from the medical register. To ensure dealings are fair and transparent key determinations are made in stages, according to formulated processes, and often by independent groups of people. In the preliminary phase, serious issues are identified and subsequently directed along one of three discrete pathways. Broadly these deal with conduct related matters, impairment due to illness or drug and alcohol and professional performance.

Doctors are directed along the professional performance pathway if there is a concern that their clinical performance is substandard. This process is overseen by the NSWMB's Performance Committee. A subset of practitioners will be referred by this committee on an 'as needed' basis to undergo an individualized performance assessment according to the PAP's established methodology. The simulation-based assessment described in this chapter is an integral component of the PAP and is employed exclusively for specialist anaesthetists. Approximately, one to three anaesthetists undergo assessment each year.

The results of this assessment are reported in writing to and considered by the Performance Committee which may refer the matter for a further review by a specially convened Performance Review Panel (PRP). The PRP, consisting of two medical and one lay member, provides the practitioner with the opportunity to respond to the assessment report and make submissions. If the panel finds that the practitioner's professional performance is unsatisfactory, it will make one of the following recommendations:

- Conditions should be placed on the practitioner's registration.
- The practitioner should complete a specified educational course.
- The practitioner should report on their medical practice.
- The practitioner should seek and take advice from specified persons.
- A complaint should be made. This option is recommended if there appears to be a significant issue of public health or safety, or indications of a case of professional misconduct or unsatisfactory professional conduct.

35.7.3 Purpose and goals

The PAP's purpose is to investigate concerns regarding individual practitioners' performance and make recommendations to ensure the public is kept safe. Its broad goal is to identify performance deficiencies with a view to remediation, however, as explained above, this process may potentially conclude with restrictions being placed on registration.

Australian anaesthetists are trained as generalist anaesthetists, commonly providing a wide range of services, often on a locum basis, at multiple hospitals. Being listed on the NSWMB's register provides a practitioner with considerable latitude, placing no restrictions on the sub-specialty type of anaesthesia they administer or the type of hospital facilities in which they practice. Restrictions regarding practice privileges are generally the responsibility of the medical specialist appointments committees of individual hospitals. One specific objective of the PAP is to assess whether the anaesthetist is excessively buffered by colleagues as this assists in predicting whether he or she will perform safely and autonomously in an unfamiliar less supportive environment. Practitioners who are considered to have rectifiable deficiencies, but who are not currently able to perform safely as independent practitioners, may have temporary restrictions placed which prohibit them providing certain types of services. For anaesthetists restrictions may be placed to prohibit after-hours emergency, subspecialty anaesthesia, and services delivered in private hospitals, the latter generally not providing back up peer support. The performance committee and PRP consider the assessors' conclusions in their final determinations. However, assessors are not involved in this step.

Table 35.1 PAP performance criteria and grades*

Unsafe

- Failed to comply with recommendations for minimum safe practice as published in professional documents by the Australian and New Zealand College of Anaesthetists
- Generally failed to convey knowledge or demonstrate practices of sufficient standard to maintain safe conditions for the patient
- Failed to respond to a serious event with a standard of care expected of an independent practising anaesthetist
- Made a serious error
- Failed to maintain a safe environment for the staff

Questionable practice

Not unsafe but practice not well justified or supported in terms of usual criteria for practice
- Published best practice guidelines
- Customary practice
- Awareness of contemporary practice and attitudes
- Evidence-based literature

Acceptable practice

Practice which is not unsafe (as above) and which is well supported using criteria listed under 'questionable practice'

Not assessable

Insufficient opportunity to assess this domain

*The grade awarded is based on the professional judgment of the assessors. This is supported by performance indicators provided separately for each case. The performance indicators represent expert opinion.

35.7.4 Standards

An acceptable standard of performance is that which is reasonably expected of a practitioner of an equivalent level of training or experience. For instance, a community anaesthetist is expected to demonstrate the knowledgebase and currency equivalent to a peer of good standing, rather than a recently graduated Fellow of the Australian and New Zealand College of Anaesthetists (ANZCA). The assessors consider a number of standards when they grade the anaesthetist in the various exercises included in the PAP (Table 35.1).

35.7.5 Assessors

Assessors are practicing anaesthetists of high standing within the profession who have a good knowledge of ANZCA processes, such as standards documents and training and examination processes. In addition, they have expertise assessing within a simulation environment. They work on a regular basis with the board. The assessors assigned to any one practitioner comprise two specialist assessors plus the director of the PAP. In addition, a medical simulation expert is assigned as a third non-assessing assessor. The role of this person is to design a tailored assessment programme for the practitioner and monitor the process.

35.7.6 Assessment methods

Assessment methods follow principles described previously with an emphasis on multiple, triangulated sources of data and appropriately wide sampling of cases (Table 35.2). These can be

Table 35.2 Components of the performance assessment programme

Assessment exercises	Attributes or tasks measured
NSWMB	
Review of incident reports of specific trigger events	Assessor's understanding of the incidents and contributing factors
Interview and review of reports submitted by complainants	Assessor's understanding of the complainant's concerns, their perceptions of trigger events and other events used to support complaint
Interview with practitioner	Assessor's understanding of the practitioner's: ◆ previous training, continuing professional development activities ◆ working patterns (e.g. hours and sessions) ◆ awareness of standards of practice ◆ perceptions of trigger events Assessor's understanding of: ◆ factors affecting the practitioner's performance, including their attitudes to patients, colleagues and work duties ◆ the impact of the notification on the practitioner's psychological well-being
Neuro-psychiatric assessment (in selected cases)	Practitioner's: ◆ Cognitive function and mental health
Workplace	**Practitioner's:**
Observation of patient care	◆ Clinical competence ◆ Standards (e.g. universal precautions) ◆ Currency and appropriateness of practice
Medical record review	◆ Habitual practice ◆ Routine standards of documentation ◆ Currency and appropriateness of practice
Interviews with colleagues and managers	◆ Habitual practice ◆ Clinical competence ◆ Standards of practice (e.g. universal precautions) ◆ Vigilance ◆ Frequency of critical incidents ◆ Ability to recognize and respond to critical events and level of support required from team ◆ Team communication
Simulation environment*	**Practitioner's:**
Interview	◆ Understanding of complainant's concerns, their perceptions of trigger events and other events used to support complaint
Oral viva (pre-scenario interview)	◆ Applied knowledge
Observation of skills using procedural simulators	◆ Procedural skills
Preparation of equipment and environment prior to anaesthesia	◆ Routine checking practice ◆ Knowledge of equipment ◆ Interaction with colleagues

Continued

Table 35.2 (continued) Components of the performance assessment programme

Simulation environment*	Practitioner's:
Scenarios involving actor patients (e.g. pre-anaesthetic consultation)	◆ Patient-doctor communication ◆ Case planning
OSCE scenarios using mannequin simulators (low context)	◆ Management of single tasks ◆ Recognition critical events and application of emergency drills
Graded immersive scenarios on mannequin simulators (high context)	◆ Management of multiple tasks ◆ Non-emergent clinical anaesthesia practice ◆ Non-emergent technical skills ◆ Recognition and management of critical events ◆ Crisis behaviours ◆ Stress coping ◆ Level of support and cueing required from team
Post-scenario interview	◆ Verification of events ◆ Understanding of events ◆ Situation awareness and cognitive processing relevant to decision-making ◆ Insight
Critique of videobased cases by third-party teams	◆ Professional and ethical behaviours ◆ Systems factors ◆ An alternative method to scenarios

*Exercises are not represented in the order they are conducted and the selection of exercises varies with practitioners

broadly categorized into 'NSWMB', 'workplace', and 'synthetic environment' according to the location in which the exercises are conducted

35.7.6.1 Aims

The simulation-based exercises have two broad aims:

◆ To verify the findings of assessments conducted in the workplace (concurrent validity).

◆ To undertake assessments not easily completed in the workplace, for reasons described in Section 35.2.

35.7.6.2 Specific objectives

The component conducted in the synthetic environment has the following specific objectives:

◆ Assess previously identified performance deficits.

◆ Screen practice across the scope of the anaesthetist's expected responsibilities and practice privileges.

◆ Assess the anaesthetist's capacity to recognize and manage key life-threatening complications that can occur in any type of anaesthetic, for example cardiopulmonary collapse.

◆ Diagnose specific competency deficits to guide remediation, for example, clinical knowledge, technical skills, communication and professional practices.

◆ Identify factors that substantially degrade his or her performance, for example case complexity, decreased attention span, reduced time to formulate plans and decisions, high workload, time pressure, distracting events, and conflict.

◆ Predict the level of autonomy that is appropriate for the anaesthetist by assessing the level of support he or she needs from colleagues.

35.7.6.3 Structure

The simulation component is tailored to individual needs and circumstances. It is commonly conducted over a single day. Practitioners are asked to change into anaesthetic attire and choose to bring any cognitive aids or references they would reasonably employ in their workplaces. They may also bring a support person, however that person doesn't observe any exercises. The practitioner is familiarized with the mannequins and other simulators to their satisfaction.

A range of simulation modalities is employed. Technology and methods are selected to suit individual assessment exercises as shown in Table 35.2. Most exercises are built on case management scenarios using high fidelity mannequin simulators.

35.7.6.4 Scenario design

A range of cases is selected from the anaesthetist's usual scope of practice. The cases are graded in difficulty including routine and emergency events and have variable focus according to the specific objective(s) targeted in that scenario. Each scenario is of 30–90 minutes duration, and is conducted in three phases representing the pre-, intra- and post-anaesthetic phases of practice.

Preliminary interview (15–30 minutes) this is an oral viva. On occasion an actor patient will be used to enable observation of the preoperative patient consultation. The assessors are provided with a scripted case, including patient information and relevant investigation results. The assessors ask predetermined questions but may undertake unscripted questioning, at their judgment. This enables assessment of patient doctor communication and patient assessment including history taking, examination and some professional behaviours (e.g. patient centredness), preoperative case planning and applied knowledge.

Observed scenario (15–30 minutes) this is conducted under conditions previously described for training with mannequin simulators[39]. The assessors generally observe this component of the scenario remotely. Realism is embedded in the scenario by adding contextual factors. Context is added by recreating a realistic operating theatre environment, providing actors to play the roles of teammates, increasing clinical complexity and introducing nonclinical situations in parallel with the clinical issues. The amount of context used varies between scenarios according to the specific objectives. For example, a low context scenario may have a single clinical event, no parallel situations and minimal equipment to work with. This is considered useful for assessing management of a single sequenced task, such as a resuscitation drill. The reduced context then requires test administrators to be in the room with the anaesthetists and provide some prompts. It is conducted in a manner not dissimilar to an OSCE. Conversely, a high context scenario may present more complex clinical issues which assess the anaesthetist's ability to interpret clinical events from multiple systems and manage multiple clinical tasks simultaneously. Scripting in other situations, such as a telephone call or equipment problem places further loads on the anaesthetist's attention. Scripting in interactions with teammates can be used to focus on communication and teamwork issues. In actual clinical practice teammates (from supportive teams) usually offer some prompts to medical practitioners, for example by pointing out irregular events. So reasonable degrees of prompting are allowed. However on some occasions the actors who play colleagues are briefed to reduce the level of support they provide as a means of assessing the anaesthetist's ability to function independently, as they would with an unsupportive team. Overall, the scenarios are graded and monitored for difficulty as a set. It is not customary in actual clinical practice for an anaesthetist to experience a battery of overly complex and difficult cases in an average day. To present these under assessment conditions would reduce the assessments concurrent validity. This practice is avoided.

Post-scenario interview (15–30 minutes) the assessors interview the anaesthetist immediately following each observed component using previously described debriefing methods[39]. We consider this a critical component of the assessment as it provides an opportunity to clarify events and explore the anaesthetist's situational assessment and decision making.

35.7.6.5 Rating methods

The assessors provide the NSWMB with a joint report of the proceedings of the simulation-based component of the assessment. The report makes conclusions about the anaesthetist's standard of practice, addressing the specific objectives. The report contains a series of quantified numeric scores for different activities conducted, a written narrative appraisal citing examples to justify their conclusions and videorecordings of the scenarios. The two assessors come to their overall conclusions by discussing their individual scores and achieving consensus.

Each activity is scored using the performance grades listed in Table 35.1. Each assessor will make an independent assessment of the anaesthetist's performance against 16 dimensions (Table 35.3).

Table 35.3 Example of a numeric scoring sheet

Grade legend:			
'U' Unsafe	'Q' Questionable	'A' Acceptable	'NA' Not assessed

Broad dimension of performance	Case 1	Case 2	Case 3	Case 4
Knowledge				
1. Basic knowledge				
2. History taking				
3. Case planning				
4. Preparation				
5. Specific knowledge relevant to the primary management plan				
6. Knowledge relevant to emergency clinical management				
7. Preparation				
Observed performance				
ROUTINE CONDITIONS				
8. Baseline clinical practice				
9. Basic airway management skills				
10. Non-emergency communication and psychosocial skills				
EMERGENCY CONDITIONS				
11. Recognition of serious event				
12. Clinical management during activated emergency				
13. Advanced procedural management skills				
14. Decision-making and problem-solving under emergency conditions				
15. Emergency communication skills				
16. Appropriate recruitment of assistance				

The latter provides a framework for the assessor's discussions and a guide to remediation. They are presented hierarchically as a progression from knowledge-based attributes toward practice-based attributes. An additional guide to scoring is provided for each scenario which provides performance markers for specific scenarios.

35.8 Conclusion

Paraphrasing Finnucaine *et al.*, the utility of any assessment tool critically depends on its level of acceptance by those on whom the assessment impacts[40]. Performance assessment impacts on three distinct groups: patients /consumers, practitioners, and employers. Presently, practitioners' acceptance of simulation for high-stakes assessment is low. However, simulation has numerous potential benefits. Potentially, practitioners may consider high-stakes assessment more acceptable if it incorporated simulation. This would necessitate changes in the steps that precede high-stakes assessment, including initial certification, practitioner-led continuing professional development, recertification, and performance management. Ideally, practitioners would be exposed to simulation in each of these steps.

Acknowledgements

The simulation assessment programme described in this chapter was developed in collaboration with the following individuals: Dr Michele Joseph, Consultant Anaesthetist, The Alfred Hospital, Melbourne; Dr Alison Reid, Medical Director and Head PAP, NSW Medical Board, Dr Richard Walsh, Consultant Anaesthetist, Royal Prince Alfred Hospital, Sydney, and Ms Suzanne Wulf, Technical Operations Manager, SMSC. The author also wishes to acknowledge their contribution to the preparation and review of this manuscript.

References

1. Cregan P, Watterson L (2005). High stakes assessment using simulation – an Australian experience. *Stud Health Technol Inform* **111**: 99–104.
2. Rosenblatt MA, Abrams KJ (2002). The Use of a Human Patient Simulator in the Evaluation of and Development of a Remedial Prescription for an Anesthesiologist with Lapsed Medical Skills *Anesth Analg* **94**: 149–53.
3. Raborn GW, Carter RM (1999). Using simulation to evaluate clinical competence after impairment *J Can Dent Assoc* **65**(7): 384–6.
4. Berkenstadt H, Ziv A, Gafni N, Sidi A (2006). Incorporating simulation-based objective structured clinical examination into the Israeli National Board Examination in Anesthesiology. *Anesth Analg* **102**: 853–8.
5. Morgan PJ, Cleave-Hogg DM, Guest CB, Herold J (2001). Validity and reliability of undergraduate performance assessments in an anesthesia simulator *Can J Anaesth* **48**(3): 225–33.
6. Hatala R, Kassen BO, Nishikawa J, Cole G, Issenberg SB (2005). Incorporating simulation technology in a canadian internal medicine specialty examination: a descriptive report. *Acad Med* **80**: 554–6.
7. Morgan PJ, Cleave-Hogg D (2002). A worldwide survey of the use of simulation in anesthesia. [see comment]. *Can J Anaesth* **49**: 659–62.
8. Wass V, Van der Vleuten C, Shatzer J, Jones R (2001). Assessment of clinical competence *Lancet* **357**: 945–49.
9. Miller GE (1990). The assessment of clinical skills / competence performance. *Acad Med* **65**(Suppl.): S63–S67.
10. Rethans JJ, Norcini JJ, Baro'n-Maldonado N, *et al.* (2002). The relationship between competence and performance: implications for assessing practice performance *Med Educ* **36**: 901–9.

11. Regehr G, Freeman R, Robb A, Missiha N, Heisey R (1999). OSCE performance evaluations made by standardized patients: comparing checklist and global rating scores. *Acad Med* **74**(10; Oct RIME Suppl.): S135–S137.

12. McGaghie WC, Issenberg SB, Gordon DL, Petrusa ER (2001). Assessment instruments used during anaesthetic simulation. [Letter] *B J Anaesth* **87**(4): 647–8.

13. Devitt JH, Kurrek MM, Cohen MM, *et al.* (1997). Testing the raters: inter-rater reliability of standardized anaesthesia simulator performance. *Can J Anaesth* **44**: 924–8.

14. Weller JM, Bloch M, Young S, *et al.* (2003). Evaluation of a high fidelity patient simulator in assessment of performance of anaesthetists. *Br J Anaesth* **90**(1:) 43–7.

15. Weller JM, Robinson BJ, Jolly B, *et al.* (2005). Psychometric characteristics of simulation-based assessment in anaesthesia and accuracy of self-assessed scores. *Anaesthesia* **60**(3): 245–50.

16. Devitt JH, Kurrek MM, Cohen MM, *et al.* (1998). Testing internal consistency and construct validity during evaluation of performance in a patient simulator. *Anesth Analg* **86**: 1160–4.

17. Wong AK (2004). Full scale computer simulators in anesthesia training and evaluation *Can J Anaesth* **51**(5): 455–64.

18. Byrne AJ, Greaves JD (2001). Assessment instruments used during anaesthetic simulation: review of published studies. *Br J Anaesth* **86**: 445–50.

19. Riley RW, DH, Freeman JA (1997). Anaesthetists' attitudes towards an anaesthesia simulator. A comparative survey: USA and Australia. *Anaesth Intensive Care* **25**: 514–9.

20. Hutchinson L, Aitken P, Hayes T (1992). Are medical postgraduate certification processes valid? A systematic review of the published evidence *Med Educ* **36**: 73–91.

21. General Medical Council, Good Medical Practice. http://www.gmc uk.org/guidance/good_medical_practice/GMC_GMP.pdf [Last accessed May 30 2007]

22. Accreditation Council of General Medical Councils, Outcome Project. General Competencies http://www.acgme.org/outcome/comp/compMin.asp [Last accessed May 30 2007]

23. Hays RB, Davies HA, Beard JD, *et al.* (2002), Selecting performance assessment methods for experienced physicians *Med Educ* **36**: 910–17.

24. Norcini JJ (2005). Current perspectives in assessment: the assessment of performance at work. *Med Educ* **39**: 880–9.

25. Chief Health Officer (2006). Assessing Clinical Practice. In: *Good Doctors, Safer Patients*. Department of Health Publications, Chapter 5: 96.

26. Cooper JB, Newbower RS, Long CD, *et al.* (1978). Preventable anesthesia mishaps: A study of human factors. *Anesthesiology* **49**: 399–406.

27. Eastridge BJ, Hamilton EC, O'Keefe GE, *et al.* (2003). Effect of sleep deprivation on the performance of simulated laparoscopic surgical skill. *Am J Surg* **186**: 169–74.

28. Short JP (1993).The importance of strong evaluation standards and procedures in training residents. *Acad Med* **68**(7): 522–25.

29. Southgate L, Hays RB, Norcine J, *et al.* (2001). Setting performance standards for medical practice: a theoretical framework *Med Educ* **35**: 474–81.

30. Schuwirth LWT, Southgate L, Page GG, *et al.* (2002) When enough is enough: a conceptual basis for fair and defensible practice performance assessment. *Med Educ* **36**: 925–30.

31. Van der Vleuten CPM, Schuwirth LWT (2005). Assessing professional competence: from methods to programme mes *Med Educ* **39**: 309–17.

32. Melnick DE, Asch DA, Blackmore DE, Klass DJ, Norcini JJ (2002). Conceptual challenges in tailoring physician performance assessment to individual practice *Med Educ* **36**: 931–5.

33. Hays RB, Davies HA, Beard JD, *et al.* (2002). Selecting performance assessment methods for experienced physicians *Med Educ* **36**: 910–17.

34. Schuwirth LWT, van der Vleuten CPM (2006). A plea for new psychometric models in educational assessment. *Med Educ* **40**: 296–300.

35. Schuwirth LWT, van der Vleuten CPM (2004). Changing education, changing assessment, changing research? *Med Educ* **38**: 805–12.

36. Van der Vleuten CPM, Norman GR, De Graaf E (1991). Pitfalls in the pursuit of objectivity: issues of reliability. *Med Educ* **25**: 110–8.

37. Medical Board Performance Assessment programme http://www.nswmb.org.au/index.pl?page=6 [Last accessed May 7th 2007]

38. Devitt JH, Kurrek MM, Cohen MM, Cleave-Hogg D (2001). The validity of performance assessments using simulation. *Anesthesiology* **95**: 36–42.

39. Howard SK, Gaba DM, Fish KM, *et al.* (1992). Anesthesia Crisis Resource Management Training: teaching anesthesiologists to handle critical incidents. *Aviat Space Environ Med* **63**(9): 763–70.

40. Finucane PM, Barron SR, Davies HA, Hadfield-Jones RS, Kaigas TM (2002). Towards an acceptance of performance assessment. *Med Educ* **36**: 959–64.

Chapter 36

Simulation in sedation training for non-anaesthesiologists

Mordechai Bermann, Bryan L Fischberg, and Malay Rao

Overview

- Demand and usage of sedation outside the operating room is increasing in the USA.
- In the USA, The Joint Commission has enlisted input from the American Society of Anesthesiologists to establish management and training guidelines for non-anaesthetists.
- Simulation is well suited for the training of non-anaesthetist sedation providers, emphasizing monitoring vigilance, team management during emergencies, and agent selection.
- Scenarios include patient evaluation, assessment of sedation, extra procedural complications, anaphylaxis, and airway emergencies.
- Demand for sedation is increasing and simulation methods and products are evolving to meet the related challenges.

36.1 Introduction

Full-scale simulators provide an educational setting where healthcare providers can acquire skills and develop expertise necessary to recognize and manage infrequent life-threatening events[1]; it has the potential to be a well-suited teaching technique for non-anaesthetists providing sedation. This chapter addresses some general considerations, specific examples, and trends in effective use of simulation for sedation training.

There is currently a growing trend in the USA, and worldwide, for non-anaesthesiologists to perform moderate sedation (formerly known as 'conscious sedation') for various medical procedures. Additionally there are an increasing number of procedures and diagnostic tests requiring only moderate sedation.

The relative shortage of available anaesthesiologists, time constraints, scheduling conflicts and cost-containment efforts motivate the need for non-anaesthesiologists to perform intravenous (IV) sedation. The American Society of Anesthesiologists (ASA) recognizes this trend and has laid out the credentialing criteria for non-anaesthesiologists performing IV sedation.[2] In short, we predict that an increasing number of qualified non-anaesthesiologist healthcare providers will need to acquire the skills to recognize, and safely care for patients at, the desired level of sedation (Table 36.1).

Table 36.1 Sedation levels*

Sedation	Responsiveness	Airway	Spontaneous ventilation	Cardiovascular function
Minimal sedation	Normal response to verbal stimulation	Unaffected	Unaffected	Unaffected
Moderate sedation/analgesia	*Respond purposefully** to voice/touch*	*No intervention required*	*Adequate*	*Usually maintained*
Deep sedation/ analgesia	Respond Purposefully** to repeated stimulation/ pain	Intervention may be required	May be adequate	Usually maintained
General anaesthesia	Unarousable	Intervention often required	Frequently inadequate	May be impaired

*Continuum of Depth of Sedation – Definition of General Anaesthesia and levels of Sedation/Analgesia. Adopted at American Society of Anesthesiologists House of Delegates meeting 27 October 2004.

**Reflex withdrawal from a painful stimulus is NOT considered a purposeful response.

36.2 Sedation credentialing guidelines for non-anaesthesiologists (USA)

In the last decade, The Joint Commission (formerly the Joint Commission on Accreditation of Healthcare Organizations or JCAHO) served as the catalyst to establish guidelines for administration of sedation by non-anaesthesiologists at their accredited institutions.[3] The Joint Commission looked to the ASA to develop uniform sedation and analgesia standards for any practitioner in the interest of patient safety.

In practice, the ASA has delineated guidelines to grant privileges to non-anaesthesiologists (physicians, podiatrists, or dentists). These practitioners can both supervise and personally administer moderate sedation only if they have completed the required education and training. This is most commonly implemented via residency training[4] and continuing medical education (CME) where simulation is being utilized.

36.3 Unique elements of simulation in sedation training

The person performing the procedure may be additionally burdened by the responsibility of being a monitoring anaesthetist. The nature of procedures done under moderate sedation requires the ability to divide attention among performing the procedure, monitoring the patient's level of sedation, and following their physiological status blunted by medications. Monitors are routinely relied upon. However, their information needs to be smoothly integrated with clinical observations and procedural details. These patients are often draped and may be in a darkened room hampering direct observation. Sustaining continuous monitoring of haemodynamic status is an additional challenge. Simulating patient responses promotes a unique vigilance that is new to the non-anaesthesia provider. Among our goals is to heighten students' awareness of the newly introduced sedation considerations so that they proactively anticipate problems.

The simulator facilitates an emphasis on interaction within the procedure team. In many cases the physician performing the therapeutic or diagnostic procedure is also supervising other team members. Adjusting the scenarios can alter stress points on various team roles. Since the team composition varies by procedure, discipline, and regulatory agency's requirements common situations that arise can be 'tested' under different circumstances. Teaching medical team performance emphasizes willingness to ask for help, clarity of communication, role loyalty, and resource utilization.

The speed of our simulation was adjusted to illustrate the importance of timing. Several sophisticated human patient simulators actually model the pharmacodyamics in real time. The behavior of short acting agents, like fentanyl, can be easily created in real time in order to give the participant an appreciation of the duration of action and agent selection. Illustrating interactions among comorbidity and medications or intoxicants requires planning and skill from the trainer. Longer term effects of these drugs, like amnesia, are harder to recreate. These issues involve role play more than mannequin simulation. Concepts of longer duration can be addressed effectively by 'fast forwarding' through the monotonous or uneventful sections of the scenario.

In summary, many of the objectives of simulation training in critical care and anaesthesia described elsewhere in this book should guide one in developing a curriculum for this training.

36.4 Implementation of simulation for sedation training

The moderate sedation course at Robert Wood Johnson University Hospital[5] (RWJUH) was assembled as a collaborative effort of the Department of Anaesthesia at UMDNJ-Robert Wood

Johnson Medical School and the Department of EMS and Trauma Education at the core teaching hospital (RWJUH), which operates the ACLS Training Center. This began as an internal programme for about 250 eligible physicians. Since our children's hospital had its own sedation credentialing process, we focused on non-anaesthesiologist physicians who provide sedation to adult patients only. However, this concept could be adapted to diverse healthcare providers administering sedation to varied patient populations[6]. Our bimonthly weekday original offering had three components that took about 4 hours each.

Didactic information was provided to students to prepare in advance of the classroom meetings with instructors. The content mainly covered policy information, various clinical protocols and assessment scales, equipment, and pharmacology. Immediately upon arrival, participants were issued a pre-test on the preparatory material, and a minimum score was required to continue in the classroom session. Instructor-led slide-enhanced presentations followed to clarify and integrate the patient evaluation, equipment checkout, selection of agents, administration of sedation, patient monitoring, handling of intraprocedural emergencies, and discharge evaluation. Participants were then divided into two rotations: one addressed airway emergencies and effective bag-valve-mask (BVM) ventilation that included both small group lecture and mannequin (Laerdal Skillmeter®) practice, and the second station was a full-body mannequin-based simulation (METI HPS, Laerdal SimMan®) of sedation cases. The simulations began with an uncomplicated, uneventful case of sedation to introduce students to the simulation environment.

Subsequent cases then highlighted inappropriate level of sedation, impending hemodynamic changes, arrhythmia, team management, equipment failure, and airway emergencies. The participants then completed a written post-test and a standard course evaluation.

We admitted no more than ten students to each session to ensure that no more than four or five students were present at the mannequin stations.

Flexible case selection is crucial to addressing students' needs (e.g. cardiac laboratory, endoscopy, plastics, radiology, etc.) (Fig. 36.1). All participants are debriefed following the scenario.

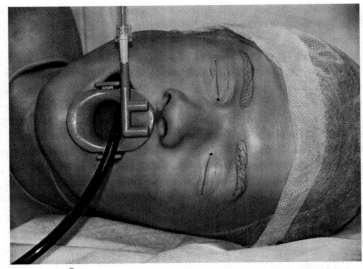

Fig. 36.1 Laerdal SimMan® used for sedation training during upper gastrointestinal endoscopy.

Our cases highlighted the following situations with an emphasis on appropriate team dynamics and crisis resource management principles.

36.4.1 Patient evaluation

Goal Motivate students to appreciate the importance of obtaining and reviewing a focused preprocedural history and physical exam.

Example At the beginning of the simulation case, a limited amount of information is presented, expecting the students to elicit the key elements of preprocedural evaluation. The scenario is guided to highlight the area inadequately evaluated. We commonly direct the case to emergencies with airway, intraprocedural arrhythmia, and anaphylaxis.

For instance, a patient is hastily presented to the student. According to routine nursing protocol, the patient receives one gram of cefazoline after sedation began but prior to the procedure. The sedated patient does not verbalize symptoms, but develops hypotension, tachycardia, and desaturation a few minutes into the procedure. Anaphylaxis points out the incomplete history (missing allergy to cefazoline).

36.4.2 Sedation effectiveness

Goal Motivate students to be continuously aware of the level of sedation. Students must demonstrate familiarity with the various levels of sedation and be able to keep the patient in the intended level of sedation. The Joint Commission defines these levels (Table 36.1).

Example A patient intended to be moderately sedated is suddenly withdrawing from painful stimulation during the procedure. The student is required to demonstrate how he/she is attempting to differentiate the withdrawal as a reflex or purposeful movement and judiciously adjust the level of sedation, if needed.

36.4.3 Hemodynamic events

Goals Motivate student to be aware of presedation H&P, use and interpret haemodynamic monitoring, and clinically prioritize the management of haemodynamic events along with the procedure.

Example A patient with a history of atrial fibrillation being treated with antiarrhythmic and anticoagulant agents begins his procedure in normal sinus rhythm. While the procedure is under way, his rate accelerates to sinus tachycardia then evolves into rapid atrial fibrillation with oxygen desaturation. Students typically focus predominantly on the rhythm change. The student is required to recognize, prioritize, and manage the hypoxia.

36.4.4 Equipment failure

Goal Emphasize the importance of checking monitors, emergency equipment, and support resources to students.

Example It is the last patient of the day. The student relieves a colleague near the end of his shift. The patient desaturates and becomes tachycardic. The desired outcome is for the student to discover that the oxygen tank is empty. This scenario emphasizes the importance of preprocedure equipment checklist, hand-off communication, and how to initiate emergency support resources (oxygen supply, EMS activation).

36.4.5 Airway emergency

Goals sensitize students to the importance of recognizing patients who may be difficult to ventilate or have challenging airway anatomy; reinforce a low threshold to intervene with basic airway manoeuvres; and reinforce proactive assistance.

Example a patient with a history of chin implant for microganthia is undergoing an unrelated procedure under moderate sedation. The patient desaturates during the procedure and BVM ventilation is difficult because the chin anomaly was underappreciated. The desired outcome is for the student to realize help is readily available and consider alternatives to mask ventilation in their environment.

36.5 Trends in sedation training

The demand for sedation by non-anaesthetists will increase as other short-term invasive, diagnostic, and therapeutic procedures are moving out of the traditional operating room and into the non-operating room locations, such as diagnostic suites and private offices. Furthermore, with the introduction of newer (safer) pharmacological agents and monitoring technologies to the ambulatory care arena, the medical severity of the patients undergoing these procedures is escalating. These developments demand the need to preserve a consistent level of care no matter where the procedure is performed. The ASA is actively debating its recommendations for the needed personnel and their qualifications in order to provide safe sedation.

While our course used a full-body patient simulator, other commercial products are also available including a personal computer simulation programme (e.g. AneSoft®). We anticipate that virtual reality will make inroads in this area as well. However, presently we cannot comment on the relative effectiveness of this simulation technique for sedation training. Overall, simulation could play an important roll in facilitating safe sedation training whenever simulation technology is available.

36.6 Summary

Professional and economic pressures are increasing the demand and popularity for non-anaesthetists to safely deliver moderate sedation for procedures outside the operating room. Credentialing often involves CME training in sedation. Simulation is an effective tool for teaching appropriate medical monitoring, vigilance, and safety to these practitioners. It was especially useful to orient sedation practitioners to patient evaluation, sedation planning, intraprocedural emergencies, equipment difficulties, and team member interaction. While we used mannequin-based activities and simulation in our programme, other types of simulation are evolving to fill this need.

References

1. Schwid HA, Rooke GA, Carline J, *et al.* (2002). Evaluation of anaesthesia residents using mannequin-based simulation: A multi-institutional study. *Anaesthesiology* **97**: 1434–44.
2. American Society of Anesthesiologists. Task Force on Sedation and Analgesia by Non-Anaesthesiologists (2002). Practice guidelines for sedation and analgesia by non-anaesthesiologists. *Anesthesiology* **96**: 1004–17.
3. JCAHO (2004). *Comprehensive Accreditation Manual for Hospitals: The Official Handbook*. JCAHO, Oakbrook Terrace, Il.
4. Bermann M, Hammond J, Fischberg B (2004). A new method for teaching a course on sedation and analgesia by non–anaesthesiologists using innovative technologies. *Anaesthesiology* **101**: A1360.
5. IV Sedation & Analgesia Care for the Non-Anesthesiologist. Robert Wood Johnson University Hospital. Bermann M. On the Internet at http://www2.umdnj.edu/anesweb/residency/moderate_sedation.htm
6. Chen MI, Edler A, Wald S, *et al.* (2007). Scenario and Checklist for Airway Rescue During Pediatric Sedation. *Simulation in Healthcare* **2**(3): 194–98.

Chapter 37

Medical educational simulation: a European perspective

Willem van Meurs, Doris Østergaard, and Stefan Mönk

Overview

◆ Simulator-based medical education in Europe and in its global context.

◆ History and mission of the Society in Europe for Simulation Applied to Medicine (SESAM).

◆ Current challenges and opportunities for medical educational simulation in Europe and beyond.

37.1 Introduction

The purpose of this chapter is to highlight selected European contributions to medical educational simulation and briefly describe the Society in Europe for Simulation Applied to Medicine (SESAM). At the time of preparation of the manuscript, the authors were president, vice-president, and immediate past-president of SESAM, respectively.

37.2 Medical educational simulation in Europe

Early records of simulator-based training in Europe go back to the Age of Enlightenment[1]. Educational simulation in acute care and other medical fields draws heavily on a broad range of research: human factors, application of simulation in the aviation and military contexts[2], and modeling of human physiology and pharmacology[3,4], all with deep European roots. Several European teams explored anaesthesia simulation in the early 1990s, often developing simulators that had a similar level of sophistication as their American counterparts[5,6,7]. Here we mention the Leiden anaesthesia simulator[8], PatSIM® [9] and the Sophus anaesthesia simulator[10]. A low cost, but high impact approach to full-body anaesthesia simulation was pioneered by Byrne et al. with the ACCESS system[11]. Screen-based simulators in anaesthesia and intensive care were developed first in the USA[12,13], and were soon followed by European examples[14]. Early European simulation centres that developed their own simulators included Basel, Copenhagen, Leiden, Stavanger, and Swansea. The simulation centre in Brussels first adopted a prototype American system. Simulation centres using commercialized American systems sprang up around Europe in the second half of the 1990s. Here we mention: Bristol, Erlangen, Heidelberg, Mainz, Santander, and Stirling. Only one of the two American manufacturers of full-body, model-driven acute care simulators survived the 1990s. Medical Education Technologies, Inc. (METI) established a European Office in 1998. Laerdal Medical, the leading manufacturer of script-driven full-body simulators, is based in Norway. A small, but vibrant community of simulation and simulator developers, from Europe and beyond, started meeting regularly, and in 1994 created SESAM in Copenhagen. Of the recent European contributions to medical educational simulation, we mention the work by Fletcher *et al.* on a behavioral marker system for non-technical skills in anaesthesia[15], and the study by Draycott *et al.* on the impact of simulator based training in obstetric emergencies on neonatal outcome[16]. Trends in the spread of simulator based training to other clinical areas beyond anaesthesia and intensive care are similar in Europe and the USA. Simulator-based training is now used in civil and military emergency medicine, obstetrics, neonatology, and other areas of acute care medicine. Training of minimally invasive surgical skills is greatly facilitated by virtual reality based simulators. The range of students and healthcare professionals benefiting from simulator-based training has similarly evolved. Representatives of these communities actively participate in SESAM.

37.3 The society in Europe for simulation applied to medicine

Initially SESAM and the SESAM meetings were synonymous. The conferences had an important role providing a European forum for the sharing of information and experience concerning educational concepts, simulation technologies and research methods, in this multidisciplinary field. There was little activity outside the annual conferences. The previous and current executive committees (2003–2007) have made it their task to broaden the range of SESAM services. Meeting organization and society leadership were formally separated. One of the goals of the Society is to encourage high quality, well organized meetings. By having rotating, independent meeting organizers, we stimulate creativity and diversity in terms of national approaches to medical educational simulation and clinical focus areas. Basic policies were established to select meeting sites and support meeting organizers in their task. Membership administration and the financial–legal status of the society were formalized. New activities included revival of the web-page (http://www.sesam.ws) and emailing list, and a society newsletter. Mission and vision statements were established and published in the Autumn 2003 newsletter.

37.3.1 Mission

- ◆ Encourage and support the use of simulation for training, quality assurance, and human factors research in health care.
- ◆ Provide a European forum for the sharing of information and experience concerning educational concepts, simulation technologies and research methods, in this multidisciplinary field. Special attention will be given to new EU member states.
- ◆ Facilitate information exchange between other professional societies, the medical device industry, and government agencies in this field.
- ◆ Develop a vision for – and stimulate the development of – new simulation applications, curricula, technologies, and simulator based training and competency evaluation in this field.

37.3.2 Vision

- ◆ There is an urgent need for grouping, editing, and spreading of information to avoid repeated 're-invention of the wheel' in terms of simulator centre preparation and start-up, educational curricula, competency evaluation methods, inventories of existing simulation, and observation technologies, etc.

♦ In the near future, simulator-based training and evaluation of acute care providers will become part of established curricula. It is our ambition to accompany this intricate process by formulating guidelines, and identifying and removing logistical and methodological stumbling blocks.

♦ Simulator-based training and evaluation is spreading out over various healthcare disciplines. It is vital to SESAM to open up its forum for exchange of information to more medical specialties and healthcare provider functions. Expansion of collaboration with non-medical professionals will be pursued.

♦ There is much room for new simulator based applications, and for innovation concerning curricula, technologies, and simulator-based training and competency evaluation methods. It is our ambition to help identify the needs, and provide stimulation and guidance for new applications and developments.

The histories of SESAM and the Society for Simulation in Healthcare (SSH) are closely intertwined. SSH grew out of the Society for Technology in Anaesthesia (STA) and the Rochester, NY meetings on medical simulation. A European group meeting at one of the STA satellite meetings on medical simulation led to revival of SESAM and the 1998 meeting in Leiden, The Netherlands. Several SESAM members played an important role in organizing international meetings and in the early discussions on an international society. The SSH journal *Simulation in Healthcare* is an affiliate journal of SESAM, and SESAM offers special membership to those who want to be a members of both the European and International/American Society.

37.4 **Challenges and opportunities**

Medical educational simulation faces a number of challenges:

♦ Support to start-up and existing simulation centres.

♦ Validation and improvement of simulators and simulation-based training programmes in a renewed partnership between clinical educators, researchers, and industry.

♦ Adaptation of existing curricula to integrate simulator-based training.

♦ Best evidence medical education[17] supported by rigorous educational impact and clinical outcome studies.

♦ Expansion of the application of simulator-based approaches from training to evaluation to selection of candidates.

♦ Accreditation of centres and programmes.

Due to the variety of national languages and educational and healthcare systems in Europe, meeting those challenges will require specific continental and national approaches. In the same time, this variety also forms a very rich source of experimental conditions and ideas. Building on this diversity and its history, we expect Europe to continue to contribute to the safety culture in healthcare in general, and to simulator based training in particular.

References

1. Le Boursier du Coudray AM (1759). *Abrégé de l'art des accouchements*. Paris, France, Vve. Delaguette.
2. Farmer E, van Rooij J, Riemersma J, Jorna P, Moraal J (1999). *Handbook of Simulator-based Training*. Ashgate, Aldershot.
3. Beneken JE, Rideout VC (1968). The use of multiple models in cardiovascular system studies: transport and perturbation methods. *IEEE Trans Biomed Eng* **15**: 281–9.

4. Hull CJ, van Beem HBH, McLeod K, Sibbald A, Watson MJ (1978). A pharmacodynamic model for pancuronium. *Br J Anaesth* **50**: 1113–23.

5. Denson JS, Abrahamson S (1969). A computer-controlled patient simulator. *JAMA* **208**: 504–8.

6. Gaba DM, DeAnda A (1988). A comprehensive anaesthesia simulation environment: re-creating the operating room for research and training. *Anaesthesiology* **69**: 387–94.

7. Good ML, Gravenstein JS (1989). Anaesthesia simulators and training devices. *Int Anaesthesiol Clin* **27**: 161–6.

8. Chopra V, Engbers FHM, Geerts MJ, *et al*. The Leiden anaesthesia simulator. *Br J Anaesth* **73**: 287–92.

9. Rettedal A, Freyer S, Kleppa R, Larsen P (1996). PatSim – simulator for pactising aneasthesia and intensive care. *Int J Clin Monit Comput* **13**: 147–52.

10. Christensen UJ, Andersen SF, Jacobsen J, *et al*. (1997). The Sophus anaesthesia simulator v. 2.0. A Windows 95 control-center of a full-scale simulator. *Int J Clin Monit Comput* **14**: 11–6.

11. Byrne AJ, Hilton PJ, Lunn JN (1994). Basic simulations for anaesthetists. A pilot study of the ACCESS system. *Anaesthesia* **49**(5): 376–81.

12. JH Philip (1986). Gas Man – an example of goal oriented computer assisted teaching which results in learning. *Int J Clin Monit Comput* **3**: 165–73.

13. Schwid HA (1987). A flight simulator for general anaesthesia training. *Comput Biomed Res* **20**: 64–75.

14. Christensen UJ, Heffernan D, Andersen SF, Jensen PF (1998). resusSim 98 – a PC advanced life support trainer. *Resuscitation* **39**: 81–4.

15. Fletcher G, Flin R, McGeorge P, Glavin R, Maran N, Patey R (2003). Anaesthetists' Non-Technical Skills (ANTS): evaluation of a behavioural marker system. *Br J Anaesth* **90**(5): 580–8.

16. Draycott T, Sibanda T, Owen L, *et al*. (2006). Does training in obstetric emergencies improve neonatal outcome? *BJOG* **113**(2): 177–82.

17. Issenberg SB, McGaghie WC, Petrusa ER, Lee Gordon D, Scalese RJ (2005). Features and uses of high-fidelity medical simulations that lead to effective learning: a BEME systematic review. *Med Teach* **27**(1): 10–28.

Potential conflict of interest

Dr van Meurs receives royalties from the University of Florida for simulator technology licensed to Medical Education Technologies, Inc. (METI). He is a paid consultant to METI. His past research and development was funded in part by grants from METI. Dr Østergaard, is Head of the Danish Institute for Medical Simulation, which has a collaborative agreement with Laerdal AS, and which at present receives a 3-year grant from the Laerdal Foundation. Dr Østergaard is a board member of the Laerdal Foundation. Dr Mönk is working for AQAI Simulation Center in Mainz which provides International Customer Support and other activities for Medical Education Technologies, Inc. (METI). He provides project and research and development work for METI.

Chapter 38

Society for simulation in healthcare

Daniel Raemer

Overview

♦ The Society for Simulation in Healthcare (SSH) is the principal international organization that brings together multidisciplinary and multispecialty professionals to share experience in simulation.

♦ SSH was officially started in 2004, though its roots trace back through several anaesthesiology-based organizations to the early 1990s.

♦ SSH conducts the International Meeting on Simulation in Healthcare each January.

♦ SSH produces the journal *Simulation in Healthcare*, the only multidisciplinary and multispecialty publication devoted to applications of simulation in healthcare.

38.1 Introduction

The Society for Simulation in Healthcare (SSH) is the international association that provides a forum for the simulation community to share ideas, concerns, and interests (Fig. 38.1). By design, SSH is interdisciplinary and multispecialty in its programmes, leadership and membership. From its inception in 2004, SSH was envisioned as an umbrella organization that would provide a central point for regional associations with an interest in simulation to collaborate. As such, a number of organizations, such as the Society in Europe for Simulation Applied to Medicine, and the Australian Society for Simulation in Healthcare, have joint membership agreements with SSH and use the society's journal as an official publication of their own society.

SSH sponsors a number of conferences and symposia, the most widely attended being the International Meeting on Simulation in Healthcare (IMSH) held every January, usually in the southern USA. IMSH features noted speakers, panels on numerous topics, and a wide variety of roundtables and special interest group meetings. Traditionally IMSH invites abstracts for poster and oral presentation that are peer reviewed as well as abstracts for poster presentation of 'works-in-progress'. Since its inaugural meeting date in 2004 where over 500 attendees participated, the IMSH has more than doubled in attendance each year. The meeting has increased the number of offerings proportionately and has added a number of pre-conference courses in starting simulation programmes, and advanced educational techniques. An endowed keynote presentation, the *Michael S Gordon MD Center for Medical Education Honorary Lecture*, is another highlight of IMSH.

In addition to the annual meeting, SSH sponsors symposia that bring together specialty societies, regulatory agencies, and governmental bodies that are interested in how simulation can impact them. The first 'Simulation Stakeholders Summit' was held in November 2006 in Chicago, where 60 organizations were represented. As a working meeting, this body produced some consensus

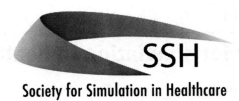

Society for Simulation in Healthcare

Fig. 38.1 Logo of Society for Simulation in Healthcare.

statements about the need for standards and guidelines around the use of simulation as an educational and evaluative tool.

SSH owns and is responsible for the scientific content of the journal, *Simulation in Healthcare* that is published by Lippincott, Williams, and Wilkins, a division of the Dutch publishing house, Wolters Kluwer. The first Editor-in-Chief, David M Gaba MD, was appointed in 2006 and he has led the journal to become the preeminent peer-reviewed publication dealing with every modality of simulation applied to the healthcare domain. The journal features empirical research articles as well as editorials, important meeting abstracts, case discussions, and technical articles.

An active listserv is one modality for sharing ideas and information that has seen heavy usage since it began in 2004. On a daily basis, members place requests for job descriptions, scenario ideas, technological tips, equipment purchase advice, curriculum sharing, research collaboration, and many other needs. In addition, interesting and important discussions develop on the listserv on subject matter such as legal issues around video consent, applications of simulation in patient safety efforts, novel uses of simulation, and other philosophical, ethical, or programmatic topics.

SSH has developed a number of other programmes for education of its members, including reference materials on legislation, summaries of other organization's simulation related symposia, and guidelines for simulation programme accreditation. SSH will continue to be the principal organization providing education, promoting research, and distribution of information for applying simulation to healthcare.

38.2 **History**

The history of SSH dates back to 1995 when simulation was first beginning to be applied to anaesthesiology, and a number of programmes had sprouted up around the world. Hoping to spur collaboration between the centres where mannequin-based simulation had taken root, the University of Rochester sponsored a symposium entitled, *First Conference on Simulators in Anesthesiology Education*, in May of 2005 at Rochester, NY. This conference, though attended by fewer than 100 participants, was considered a rousing success and was repeated the following year. There were a number of conversations among participants at both of those meetings about starting an organization to represent this new field, but nothing materialized. By 1997 an increasing number of abstracts and panel presentations on the subject of the use of simulation in anaesthesiology began appearing at the Annual Meeting of the Society for Technology in Anesthesia (STA). The annual meeting of STA in 1998 chose as its topic *Simulation in Anaesthesia* and the University of Rochester lent its support. The opening of the meeting was anything but smooth as the first presenter, Colin MacKenzie from Baltimore, Maryland, tried to show a videotape of a trauma event and sound was absent. The session chair, David Gaba from Stanford and the STA Meeting Chair, Dan Raemer from Boston, Massachusetts attempted to assist Dr MacKenzie. While readjusting the audio connections smoke and fire emanated from the videoplayer causing an onstage crisis. As the three supposed experts in 'crisis management', 'trauma', and 'engineering' stood helplessly on the stage, the audience could not help but think that an elaborately constructed 'simulation' was being played before them. Ironically, this incident stimulated a relaxed atmosphere and began a tradition of participatory workshops and presentations that has persisted throughout the meeting's history. In spite of the rocky start, the meeting was a success and the board of directors of STA asked Raemer to conduct an email survey of attendees and others interested in simulation based education to see if there was interest in starting a subsection of STA, in a meeting devoted to the topic, and the timing and venue of any future events. With approximately 130 respondents evenly split on whether to form a separate group, a stand-alone society, or some sort of virtual society no further measures were taken. However, during 2000 discussion continued and STA finally decided to host a simulation specific meeting in January of 2001 overlapping with its own annual meeting. Thus, the first International Meeting on Medical Simulation (IMMS) was held on January 15, 2001 in Scottsdale, Arizona at the Princess Hotel. The meeting was very well attended and there were excellent panel discussions and presentations. The IMMS meeting continued as an adjunct to the STA annual meeting for the next 2 years in Santa Clara, California, and San Diego, California, respectively. The attendance of the IMMS meeting grew steadily while the STA annual meeting attendance was relatively stable. From an open discussion from the podium among the attendees of IMMS in 2003 it was decided to start a separate society dedicated to simulation. By unanimous consent, Raemer was asked to form a committee to hold an election for a Board of Overseers to initiate the society that would be called, Society for Medical Simulation (SMS). The first meeting of the Board of Overseers was held in Albuquerque, New Mexico on January 15, 2004. The elected board consisted of William Dunn from Rochester, MN, David Feinstein from Boston, Masachusetts, David Gaba from Palo Alto,California, James Gordon from Boston, Bernadette Henrichs from St. Louis, Missouri, Bosseau Murray from Hershey, Pennsylvania, Dan Raemer from Boston, Elizabeth Sinz from Hershey, and Jeffrey Taekman from Durham, North Carolina (Fig. 38.2).

Raemer was elected Chairman, Sinz was elected Treasurer, and Taekman was elected Secretary. Initial plans for the new society were that it would be incorporated in the State of California, be

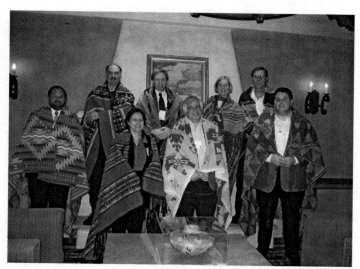

Fig. 38.2 First Board of Overseers in Albuquerque, New Mexico, USA. (back L-R) Dunn, Gaba, Feinstein, Sinz, Murray. (front L-R) Henrichs, Raemer, Taekman.

broadly based in all respects, and be independent of all other organizations. At that meeting it was planned that the newly formed society would hold a 2005 IMMS in conjunction with STA and then consider holding its meeting independently in 2006. During the first year of existence, SMS, under its Board of Overseers developed bylaws, procedures, raised funds, and hired an Executive Director, Beverlee Anderson. Mrs Anderson would prove critical to the success of the new organization, generously contributing her time and expertise with eventual remuneration uncertain. Annual dues were set at $25 and about 300 persons joined.

An agreement was reached in July of 2005 with the publisher, Lippincott, Williams, and Wilkins, to start a new journal entitled *Simulation in Healthcare*. David M Gaba was named the first Editor-in-Chief. Gaba appointed with approval of the Board of Directors, five Associate Editors, Jeffrey Cooper from Boston, Michael DeVita from Pittsburgh, Pennsylvania, Ronnie Glavin from Glasgow, Scotland, and Daniel Scott from Dallas, Texas The first issue of the journal was published in January 2006.

In February, 2006, SMS changed its name to the Society for Simulation in Healthcare (SSH) in order to broaden its appeal to non-physicians. Consequently, the annual meeting became the International Meeting on Simulation in Healthcare (IMSH).

By the last quarter of 2007 membership in SSH had grown to upwards of 2000 persons. The membership is evenly split between physicians, nurses, allied health professionals, educators, and scientists.

38.3 Conclusion

SSH is the principal international organization dedicated to simulation in healthcare. The IMSH is the largest independent conference for persons interested in this field. The journal, *Simulation in Heatlhcare* is the only multidisciplinary and multispecialty publication solely dedicated to simulation.

References

Raemer D (2006). A new name. *Simul Healthcare* **1/2**: 63.

Sinz EH (2007). 2006 Simulation Summit. *Simul Healthcare* **2/1**: 33–8.

Glossary of UK and US medical terms and abbreviations

UK	US	Explanation
	AAP	American Academy of Pediatrics
AB		Antibiotic
ACCESS		Anaesthesia Computer Controlled Emergency Situation Simulator
	ACEP	American College of Emergency Physicians
	ACGME	Accreditation Council for Graduate Medical Education (USA)
ADO	Anaesthesia Technician	Anaesthesia Department Orderly; a trained anaesthesia assistant who does not generally give direct patient care
ACF		Ante-cubital fossa
ACLS /ALS		Advanced (cardiac) life support
ACRM		Anaesthesia crisis resource management
	ACS	American College of Surgeons
	AHA	American Heart Association
AKA		Also known as
Ambulance Officer	Emergency Medical Technician (EMT), Paramedic	A trained professional who delivers emergency pre-hospital care
AI		Artificial intelligence: The study and design of intelligent agents where an intelligent agent is a system that perceives its environment and takes actions.
Adrenaline	Epinephrine ('Epi')	A vasopressor drug used in resuscitation and treatment of anaphylaxis; many English-speaking countries are switching to the United State Pharmacopeia (USP)
Anaesthesia	Anesthesia, Anesthesiology	The practice and science of anaesthesia
Anaesthetist	Anesthesiologist	A physician who administers anaesthesia
ANTS		Anaesthesia non-technical skills
ANZCA		Australian and New Zealand College of Anaesthetists; the fellowship degree is 'FANZCA'
	ATLS	Advanced Trauma Life Support (see EMST)

UK	US	Explanation
A&E (Accident & Emergency); ED (Emergency Department)	ER, Emergency Room	A dedicated area in a hospital for the treatment of emergencies
	APSF	Anesthesia Patient Safety Foundation (USA)
AROM		Artificial rupture of membranes
AV		Audiovisual (equipment or system)
Avatar		A graphical representation of a person participating in a virtual environment whether in the form of a three-dimensional model as used in cyberspace or virtual reality environments.
BEME		Best Evidence Medical Education
BiPAP		Bi-level positive airway pressure
BLS		Basic Life Support
BURP		Backwards, Upwards, Rightwards Pressure (a manoeuvre to improve laryngeal view)
CAE-Link		Canadian Aviation Electronics – Link Corporation – a company synonymous with aviation simulation
CASE		Comprehensive Anesthesia Simulation Environment (Stanford University)
Consultant; Specialist	Attending; Faculty	A medical practitioner who has undergone training in a specialty and is practising in that specialty
	CBC	Complete blood count (full blood count)
CbD		Case-based discussion
CBS		Capillary blood sugar
CCO		Critical Care Outreach
CCTV		Closed-circuit television
CGI		Computer-generated image
CLC		Closed-Loop Communication
CME		Continuing Medical Education: a formal system of further education in a medical, nursing or paramedical field (see also MOPS and CPD)
CMV		Controlled mechanical ventilation
COTS		Commercial off-the-shelf (product)
CPAP		Continuous positive airway pressure
CPB		Cardio-pulmonary bypass
CPD		Continuing Professional Development: a formal system of further education in a medical, nursing or paramedical field
CRM		Crisis Resource Management; Cockpit Resource Management; Crew Resource Management
	CRNA	Certified Registered Nurse Anaesthetist

UK	US	Explanation
CTT		Crisis Team Training
CVC		Central Venous Catheter
CVP		Central Venous Pressure
CXR		Chest X-ray
D5W		5% dextrose in water (IV solution)
DAC		Data Acquisition and Control system
DAM		Difficult airway management
DNR		Do not resuscitate
DOPS		Direct observation of procedural skills
DPL		Diagnostic peritoneal lavage
D/W		Discussed with
EAR		Expired air resuscitation
	ECFMG	Educational Commission for Foreign Medical Graduates (USA)
ECG	EKG	Electrocardiogram
ECMO		Extra-corporeal membrane oxygenation
ECS		Emergency Care Simulator (a METI product)
ED		Emergency Department (see A&E)
EJ		External jugular (vein or catheter)
ELT		Experiential Learning Theory
EM		Emergency Medicine
EMD		Electro-mechanical dissociation; now known as pulseless electrical activity
EMS		Emergency Medical Service
EMST	ATLS	Emergency Management of Severe Trauma (EMST) and Advanced Trauma Life Support (ATLS) course are similar trauma courses
EMAC		Effective Management of Anaesthetic Crises course (Australian and New Zealand College of Anaesthetists' course)
EN		Enrolled Nurse
ETCO$_2$		End-tidal carbon dioxide
ETI		Endotracheal intubation
ETT		Endotracheal tube
EHA		European Heart Association
	FAA	Federal Aviation Authority
FAST		Focussed Assessment with Sonography for Trauma
FBC/ FBP		Full blood count / picture
FOI		Fibreoptic intubation; freedom of information
FRC		Functional residual capacity

UK	US	Explanation
GAS		Gainesville Anesthesia Simulator
GMC		General Medical Council (UK)
GP		General (Family) Practitioner
Haptics		Relating to devices or systems which provide a user force feedback; a sense of touching or feel ing an object represented in a virtual environment, in particular relating to the perception and manipulation of objects.
HLM		Heart–lung machine
House Officer		A first, second or third year medical graduate who has not commenced specialty training
HPS		Human Patient Simulator (a METI product)
HRO		High reliability organization
HTA		Hierarchical task analysis
IABP		Intra-aortic balloon pump
IAFSTA		International Airline Flight Simulator Technical Association
IATA		International Air Transport Association
IBM		International Business Machines
IC		Integrated circuit
ICAO		International Civil Aviation Organization
ICP		Intracranial pressure
IMSH		International Meeting on Simulation in Healthcare
Intensive Therapy Unit (ITU)	Intensive Care Unit (ICU) /Critical Care Unit (CCU)	Dedicated ward for the care of critically ill patients
Intensive Care Physician	Intensivist	Medical specialist in Intensive Care Medicine
Intern	Intern, or First Year Resident	A first year medical graduate
	Internist	Internal Medicine Physician
IJ		Internal jugular (vein or catheter)
ILCOR		International Liaison Committee On Resuscitation
IPPB / IPPV		Intermittent positive-pressure breathing/ventilation
IPPI		Integrated Procedural Performance Instrument (Kneebone R)
IV		Intravenous (line, catheter, cannula)
	JCAHO	Joint Commission on Accreditation of Healthcare Organizations (USA)

UK	US	Explanation
Lignocaine	Lidocaine	A local anaesthetic drug, also used in treatment of arrhythmias; many English-speaking countries are switching to the United State Pharmacopeia (USP)
	LPN	Licensed Practical Nurse (USA)
LMA		Laryngeal mask airway
LOFT		Line Oriented Flight Training
Lux		The SI unit of illuminence
LVAD		Left ventricular assist device
MCC		Medical Council of Canada
MCQ		Multiple choice question (or examination)
MET or MERT		Medical Emergency Team; Medical Emergency Response Team
Mini-CEX		Mini clinical exercise
Mini-PAT		Mini peer assessment tool
MOPS (Maintenance of Professional Standards)	CME (Continuing Medical Education)	A formal system of further education in a medical, nursing or paramedical field
MSF		Multi-source feedback
MSR		Israel Centre for Medical Simulation
	NASCAR	National Association of Stock Car Auto Racing
	NASA	National Aeronautics and Space Administration
Nor-adrenaline	Nor-epinephrine	A vasopressor drug used in resuscitation and treatment of cardiovascular emergencies
NMB		Neuromuscular blockade
NOTSS		Non-technical skills in surgery
NPA		Nasopharyngeal airway
NS		Normal saline (IV solution)
NTS		Non-technical skills
Nurse Anaesthetist	CRNA, Certified Registered Nurse Anesthetist (often shortened to Anesthetist)	A nurse who has completed graduate education in the field of anaesthesia
	OB/GYN	Obstetrics and Gynaecology; 'Obs & Gobs'
Obs / Observations	Vital signs	A set of clinical measurements of a patient: temperature, pulse, respirations (rate), blood pressure (and perhaps pain score)
ODA		Operating Department Assistant
ODD		Oesophageal detector device
OT, Operating Theatre, Operating Suite	OR, Operating Room	A dedicated area where surgery is performed
OSATS		Objective Structured Assessment of Technical Skills

UK	US	Explanation
OSCE		Objective Structured Clinical Examination
	PACU	see Recovery room
PALS		Paediatric Advanced Life Support
PBL		Problem-based learning
PC		Personal computer (also 'politically correct')
PEA		Pulseless electrical activity; formerly EMD (Electro-mechanical dissociation)
Pethidine	Meperidine (Demerol®)	An opioid drug
PFS		Patient-focused simulation
PHTLS		Pre-Hospital Trauma Life Support course
Physiotherapist	Physical Therapist	A person trained in physiotherapy
PICU		Paediatric Intensive Care Unit
PPH		Post-partum haemorrhage
PRP		Performance Review Panel
PSS		Patient-specific simulation
RA		Right atrial
Radiographer	X-ray Technician	A person trained to safely operate X-ray apparatus
R&D		Research and development
Reification		Making an abstract concept appear as something concrete with which a person can interact or creating a data model for a previously abstract concept.
Respiratory Technician	Respiratory Therapist (RT)	A person trained in respiratory and ventilator care, responsibilities are different between countries
Registrar	Resident	A trainee in a medical specialty
	Residency	A medical specialty training programme
RN		Registered Nurse
Royal College of Anaesthetists	American Board of Anesthesiologists	The medical specialty organization responsible for accrediting specialist anaesthetists
RR, Recovery Room	Post-Anesthesia Care Unit (PACU)	A dedicated ward that receives patients following anaesthesia and/or surgery
	RRC	Residency Review Committee
RRT		Rapid Response Team
ROSC		Return of spontaneous circulation
RSI		Rapid-sequence induction (also known as crash induction)
RS232		An electrical engineering communication standard ('Recommend Standard number 232')
SAD		Supraglottic airway device

UK	US	Explanation
SAED		Semi-automatic external defibrillators
	SAEM	Society for Academic Emergency Medicine
Salbutamol	Albuterol	A common bronchodilator drug
SESAM		Society in Europe for Simulation Applied to Medicine
SME		Subject matter expert
SMS		Strategic Management Simulations
SP		Standardized patient
SpO$_2$		Oxygen saturation – measured by a pulse oximeter
SPOT		Student perception of teaching
SPRAT		Sheffield Peer Review Assessment Tool
SSH		The Society for Simulation in Healthcare
STA		Society for Technology in Anesthesia
Suxamethonium	Succinylcholine	A short-acting muscle relaxant; often called 'sux'
	TATRC	Telemedicine and Advanced Technology Research Center (US Army)
TCP/IP		Transmission Control Protocol/Internet Protocol (a suite of communications protocols used to connect computers on the internet)
TOE	TEE	Trans (o)esophageal echocardiography
TTV / TTJV		Trans-tracheal ventilation; trans-tracheal jet ventilation
U&E		Urea and electrolytes
	UCLA	University of California at Los Angeles
UPS		Universal Patient Simulator (a Laerdal product)
USB		Universal Serial Bus (an interface standard to allow peripheral devices to be connected to computers)
	USMLE	United States Medical Licensing Examination
	Vital signs	A set of clinical measurements of a patient: temperature, pulse, respirations (rate), blood pressure (and perhaps pain score)
Viva (or *Viva Voce*)		An oral examination
VR		Virtual reality: A computer-simulated environment that gives a sense of being present in the virtual environment and within which a participant can interact in a seemingly real or physical way.
VUCAD		Volatility, uncertainty, complexity, ambiguity and delayed feedback

Index

Pages in bold denote tables

abbreviations 533–40
ACCESS (Anaesthesia Computer Controlled
    Emergency Situation Simulator) 27
adult learning 171–2
    principles **127**
    see also teaching and learning
airline crew training *see* aviation
airway management 468–70
    basic airway manoeuvres 68
    basic life support 67–8
    emergencies, anaesthetic crisis management 493
    endotracheal and tracheostomy tube
        management 469–70
    mask ventilation 68
airway training devices 65–80
    advanced airway interventions 69–72
        airway exchange catheters 73
        endotracheal intubation 70–1
        methods of confirming correct
            intubation **72–3**
        supraglottic airway devices 69
    challenge of airway competence 75–6
    cricothyrotomy 74
    fibreoptic intubation training aids 74
    future 76
    mask ventilation 68
    military medical training 409–10
    nasopharyngeal airway (NPA) 469–70
    part-task trainers 409–11
    settings and materials used **66**
    stages (novice/trainee/competent) 67
    trans-tracheal ventilation 74–5
    useful features of a model **68**
ambulance, vehicle for simulator transport 29–30
amniocentesis/cordocentesis 355
anaesthesia
    behaviour rating systems 311–13
    Comprehensive Anaesthesia Simulation
        Environment (CASE) 281
    nursing simulation 265–7
Anaesthesia Computer Controlled Emergency
    Situation Simulator (ACCESS) 27
Anaesthesia Crisis Resource Management (ACRM)
    281–2, 308–9
anaesthesia performance assessment 501–18
    assessors 507, 510
    competence as marker 504–5
        selection of competencies 504–5
    components of assessment 506–7, **511**
    criteria and grades 510
    hierarchical performance assessment model 503
    key principles of high-stakes global performance
        assessment 505–6
    Miller's model of competence **503**
    numeric scoring sheet 514
    objective structured clinical examination
        (OSCE) 503
    rating methods 507
    reliability and validity 502–4
    reports of assessment 508
    risk reduction strategies 507–8
    scenario design 513–14
    standards against which performance is
        measured 507
    status of simulation-based performance
        assessment 502–3
    Sydney/NSW Medical Board performance
        assessment programme 508–11
    test conditions 507
    understanding of performance 505
anaesthetic crisis management 489–500
    acceptability of simulation 504
        barriers to acceptance 504
    assessment 495
    Effective Management of Anaesthetic Crises
        (EMAC) course 489–90
        accreditation 492
        airway emergencies module 493
        cardiovascular emergencies module 494
        course development and participation 490–2
        EMAC revision and future recommendations 498
        human performance module 493
        instructors 497
        participant evaluations 496–7
        trauma module 494
    ethics of reporting on poor performance in
        EMAC 495
    training for emergencies 490
Anaesthetists' Non-Technical Skills (ANTS)
    structure **312**
    skills taxonomy 308, 311, **312**
animal models, for tendon repair **177**
animals for training 440
Ante Cubital Fossa (ACF) pad 417
apprenticeship model, clinical skills 172
artificial intelligence (AI) 456
assertive communication 322–3
assessment and appraisal
    clinical settings 133–4
    clinical skills 177–9
    competency based 103
    framework for clinical assessment **134**
    self appraisal 135
    SNAPPS acronym 132–3
    see also anaesthesia performance assessment
audiovisual (AV) equipment 85

avatars 253
aviation 37–50, 140, 305–11, 322–3
    acceptance test of simulator 47
    airline crew training, Advanced
        Qualification Program (AQP) 480
    assessment of CRM skills 310–11
    crew/cockpit resource management (CRM) 48,
        279, 304
    flight simulation
        fidelity 44–5
        standards 43–4
    flight training devices, history 38–43
    IATA FSTC 44
    motion sensing system 45–6
    non-technical skills (NTS) training 305–6, 308–11
    origins of CRM 279–80
    simulation 37–50, 322–3
        computer-generated image (CGI) systems 43
        fidelity of simulation 44
        latency or throughput delay 47
        regulation 44
        standards 43
    training programmes 48
    vertigo 46

baby simulators 26
basic life support 67–8
behaviour, *see also* non-technical skills
behaviour rating systems 311–13
    anaesthesia 311–13
    surgery 313
Benner theory, models of nursing 255, 258–9
Best Evidence Medical Education (BEME) 261–2
    Guide-4 141
blocked time concept 19
blood gas interpretation 467
Bristol Medical Simulation Centre (BMSC) 25–34

CAPE (Center for Advanced Pediatric and Perinatal
    Education) 339
cardiopulmonary bypass training 391–406
    current approaches 393
    detection of gas line disconnection (timed events)
        399
    most frequently reported incidents by perfusionists
        302
    no. of cases to proceed to certification **93**
    Orpheus perfusion simulation system 396–400
    role of a high fidelity perfusion simulation system
        393–4
    sample scenario 400–4
cardiopulmonary resuscitation training devices 87–96
    cardiac arrest 150–3
    defibrillation 92–5
    infection control process 89
    repair costs 89
    selection of a mannequin 89–90
cardiovascular emergencies
    anaesthetic crisis management 494
    blood gas interpretation 467
    cardiac arrest, example scenario 150–3
    cardiac tamponade 413
CASE (Comprehensive Anaesthesia Simulation
    Environment) 281

CathSim IV trainer 417–18
Center for Advanced Pediatric and Perinatal Education
    (CAPE) 339
cervical examinations 358–9
chest drain insertion and management 471–2
chest tube placement, military medical training
    411–12
clinical scenarios *see* scenarios
clinical settings 125–37
    assessment and appraisal 133–4
    dialogue and closure 131–3
    educational environment 128–9
    evaluation 135–6
    feedback 134–5, **135**
    learners/learning cycle 127–8, **127, 129**
    orientation/planning 129–30
    SNAPPS, acronym 132–3
clinical skills teaching 171–9
    apprenticeship model 172
        vs structured programme participation **172**
    assessment 177–9
    designing a skills teaching episode 175–7
    evaluation and observation 179
    four-step approach to teaching a skill **174**
    gaining competence 173–4
    instruments and consumables 176, **177**
    learning cycle **173**
    learning environments 175–7
    learning paradigm **174**
    positive critiquing 177
    simulated learning environments 173
closed loop communication 322–3
cognitive aids 287–8
cognitive dissonance 121
cognitive simulation 477–88
    effective medical decision making 480–1
    stimulus–response–feedback loop 481
    technologies 480
cognitive task analysis 141–2
combat casualty care 408–14
communication
    assertive 322–3
    closed loop 322–3
    SBAR 331
    simulation training, crisis management 330–2
competence
    assessment and appraisal 103
    as marker of performance 504–5
    Miller's model 503
    user, virtual reality medical simulations 457–8
Comprehensive Anaesthesia Simulation Environment
    (CASE) 281
computer-generated image (CGI) systems, aviation
    simulation 43
cricoid pressure trainer **69**
cricothyroidotomy simulator, military medical
    training 410
cricothyrotomy 74
crisis resource management (CRM) 277–93, 308–14
    allocate attention 285–6
    anticipation and planning 287
    aviation 308–14
    cognitive aids 287–8
    core concepts 282

course design, and content 309–10
CRM management concepts 282–8, **283**
CRM in medicine 280
effective communication 285, 330–2
effective leadership 284–5
effective use of help 284
fixation errors 286–7
origins of CRM in aviation 279–80
patient crisis simulation and CRM concepts **289–90**
principles 325
simulation systems providing CRM training 288–91
situational awareness 283
skill sets applicable to critical event management **278**
see also Anaesthesia Crisis Resource Management (ACRM)
crisis team training (CTT) 323, 325–8
scoring **328**
critical thinking, models of nursing 257–8
curriculum see medical school curriculum

debriefing 155–79
closure 164–5
crisis resource management **156**
debriefing style 166
educational theory 156–7
foundation
de-roling 160–1
purpose and format 161–2
venting 160
instructor training 166–7
judgement, what to do and avoid 165–6
medical emergency teams (METs) 327–30
participants' discussions 162–3
planning 158
practice
conceptual phases 157
learning environment 158–9
procedure 163
suggested structure 157–65
primary task of debriefing 121
research using simulation 168
room usage, skills training facility 6–7
standardized patients (SPs) as models 187–8
successful debriefing 167–8
using standardized patients (SPs) as models 187–8
video use 164
see also reflection
defibrillators 92–5
resource websites (list of vendors) 94–5
safety 92–3
semi-automatic external defibrillators (SAED) 93–4
diagnostic peritoneal lavage (DPL) 414–15
DISC, personality types, team building training 204–5, **205**
Dreyfuss model, models of nursing 255, 258–9
drugs, clinical scenarios 84

education, airway care 66–7
Effective Management of Anaesthetic Crises (EMAC) course 489–95
electromechanical simulator devices 377
emergency medicine 375–90
anaesthetic crisis management 400

continuing medical education (CME) 382–3
curriculum and practice 376–7
delivery of bad news and disclosure of error 383
management simulations 379
mass casualty situations 386
medical student education 377–8
postgraduate education 379
procedural trainers for medical students 378
real resuscitation equipment in skills training facility 23–4
simulation-based certification of EM practitioners 387
teamwork and communication training 384–6
ultrasound simulator devices 382
see also medical emergency teams (METs)
endoscopy simulators 442
endotracheal intubation 70–1, 469–70
equipment 81–6
acquiring equipment and props 84–5
audiovisual (AV) equipment 85
placement and usability 386
realistic environment 82–3
ethics
reporting on poor performance 495
research using simulation 235–6
European perspective, medical school curriculum 525–8
experimental design, research using simulation 233–4
expert knowledge network, example 459–60
Exsanguinating Limb Hemorrhage simulator 416
eye injuries 418

feedback
and debriefing 327–30, 332–3, **333**
METs 332–3, **333**
multi-source feedback (MSF) 200–1
stimulus–response–feedback loop 481
surgical simulation 439
teaching skills 107–8, 122–3
trainee feedback 300–1
VUCAD 477
fibreoptic bronchoscopy (FOB) 472
fibreoptic intubation training aids 74
Fidelity Implementation Study Group, 1999 report 53
fidelity of simulation 44
First Conference on Simulators in Anesthesiology Education (May 2005) Rochester, NY 530
fixation errors 286–7
Flatland VR environment 455–6
flattening hierarchy 322–3
fluids, medications and body fluids 83–4
Focused Assessment with Sonography for Trauma (FAST) 414

Gaba, David M 280, 530–2
gaming movement, and nursing simulation 249–51
gaming simulation 249–51
glossary 533–40
good medical practice 150, 199–200

haemorrhage
recognition and management 414–16
simulator 416
Harvard Simulation Center 26

health and safety policies 85–6
hierarchical task analysis (HTA), models of nursing 255, 262–3
hierarchy, flattening 322–3
high-quality learning 478
high-quality patient care 478
high-stakes performance assessment 501–18
  key principles 505–6
  see also performance assessment
human patient simulators *see* patient simulators
hybrid simulators
  endoscopy simulators 442
  interventional endovascular simulators 442

induction of labour, problem-based learning (PBL) scenario structure 216–22
industries, non-technical skills (NTS) 305–6
infection control process 89
information and consent, research using simulation 236
integrated procedural performance instrument (IPPI) 210
intern training 295–301
  descriptive data 300–1
  instructors 299–300
  internship programme 296–7
  logistics 299
  trainee feedback 300–1
  training modules 297–9, **298**
  workshop's structure 297
International Airline Flight Simulator Technical Association (IAFSTA) 43
International Meeting on Medical Simulation (IMMS) 531
International Meeting on Simulation in Healthcare (IMSH) 532
interventional endovascular simulators 442
intestinal anastomosis, benchtop testing **178**
intubation
  endotracheal 70–1
  fibreoptic intubation training aids 74
  of newborn **341**
Israel, intern training 295–301

Johns Hopkins Children's Center, simulation training 328–30

Kolb learning styles 338
  models of nursing 255, 260

Laerdal SimMan 27, 82, 410
  acute head injury scenario **31**
  sedation training for non-anaesthesiologists 522
Laerdal-NLN project 256, 259
LapMentor 441
laryngeal mask airway (LMA Classic) 69
learning *see* teaching and learning
Leiden anaesthesia simulator 525
Likert scale 179
Line Oriented Flight Training (LOFT) 48

management simulations 379
managerial skills, team building training 202–3, **202**

mannequin patient simulators 51–64, 81–6
  classifying, integration vs fidelity 54–5
  commercially available simulators 60–2
  design considerations 60–1
  fidelity trap 57–9
  history and development 59–60
  input function and data acquisition 56
  Laerdal SimMan 27, **31**, 82, 410, 522
  Laerdal-NLN project 256, 259
  METI-ECS 27
  METI-HPS 52, 54–5, 60, 82
  models and scripts 56–7
  multi-parameter physiological monitors 55
  outputs generated via monitors 55
  providing a realistic environment 83–4
  standardized patients (SPs) as models 191–2
  terminology 52–4
  VIRGIL chest tube simulator 412
marketing 21
media relations 21
medical decision making 480–1
  respiratory therapy 472
  stimulus–response–feedback loop 481
medical educational simulation 525–8
  curriculum 421–34
medical emergency teams (METs) 321–35
  concepts learned from aviation industry **322**
  crisis resource management principles **325**
  data probes for nine scenarios **327**
  debriefing and feedback 327–30, 332–3, **333**
  examples of simulation training for rapid response systems 325–30
  history (incl. rapid response systems) 324
  lessons learned from high performance teams 323–4
  scoring sheet used in Crisis Team Training (CTT) course **328**
  simulation for aviation team training 322–3
  simulation training to improve team communication in crisis 330–2
medical school curriculum 421–34, 525–8
  European perspective 525–8
  evidence supporting simulation-based learning for medical students 429–32
  simulation orientation checklist **425**
  starting a programme
    essential elements 424
    learning objectives 424
    practical issues 422–3
  UCLA simulation curriculum 424–9
medicine, behaviour rating systems 311–13
METI-ECS 27
METI-HPS 52, 54–5, 60, 82
migration, nurses 244–5
military medical training 407–20
  airway part-task trainers 409–11
  cricothyroidotomy simulator 410
  diagnostic peritoneal lavage (DPL) 414–15
  disabling injuries 418
  future directions 418–19
  simulators for circulatory problems 413–18
  thoracic trauma, chest tube placement 411–12

training for trauma and combat casualty care
  408–14
TraumaMan 408–9, 413, 415
mnemonic exercises 208–9
mobile scenarios 30–2
mobile simulation 25–34
  moving equipment onsite/offsite 28–9
models, *see also* standardized patients (SPs) as models
models of nursing 254–63, **255**
motion sensing systems 45–6
multi-source feedback (MSF) 200–1

nasopharyngeal airway (NPA) 469–70
nephron project, renal simulation 459–60
New South Wales Medical Board performance
  assessment programme 508–11
non-technical skills (NTS) 303–19
  assessment 310–15
    CRM skills in aviation 310–11
    implementation of assessment 313–15
  aviation and other industries 305–14
  background 305–6
  behaviour rating systems
    anaesthesia 311–13
    medicine 311–13
    surgery 313
  data collection techniques 307–8
  definition 303–4
  domain-specific NTS 307–8
  healthcare 306
  identification 306–8
  individual or team skills? 304–5
  safety **304**
  skills taxonomy 308
  training course 308–10
    anaesthesia and surgery 308–9
    content and delivery 309–10
    design/content 309–10
Non-Technical Skills for Surgeons (NOTSS),
  development of rating tool **307, 314**
nuclear industry, non-technical skills (NTS) 305–6
nursing education, USA 242, **243**
nursing shortage
  international nursing shortage 244–6
  USA 243–4
nursing simulation 241–75
  critical care 266–7
  integration of simulation into curricula 246–9,
    247–8, 251–4
    historical perspective, gaming movement 249–51
    vertical and horizontal curricular development
      253–4
  models/frameworks
    Benner theory 258–9
    best practices in education 259–60
    critical thinking 257–8
    Dreyfuss model 258–9
    education and research 254–63, **255**
    hierarchical task analysis 262–3
    Kolb learning styles 260
    nursing process 254–7, **256**
    overlap with Best Evidence Medical Education
      (BEME) 261–2

situated learning 260–1
summary of models **255**
nurse anaesthesia 265–7
  obstetrics 267
  resuscitation 266–7
  sedation training 266, 519–24
  specific clinical problems 263–5
    communication skills 263
    objective structured clinical exams 264–5
    part-task training 263–4
    training in speciality areas 265
  target audience 242–6
  target summary 246

objective structured clinical examination (OSCE) 503
objective structured clinical exams (OSCEs) 264–5
obstetrics 351–74
  amniocentesis/cordocentesis 355
  birthing mannequins 352–6
  clinical scenarios 355–6
  conducting training sessions 356
  counseling for obstetric procedures 360
  didactic handouts 355
  documentation 360
  evaluation/feedback 355
  history and background 351
  instructions for simulations 355
  location of simulation training 357
  nursing simulation 267
  specific procedures 357–63
    artificial rupture of membranes (AROM) 359
    cervical examinations 358–9
    eclamptic seizures 364
    episiotomy and third/fourth-degree lacerations
      354
    fetal scalp electrode (FSE) placement 359
    internal monitor placement and artificial rupture
      of membranes 359–60
    Leopold manoeuvres 359
    operative vaginal delivery 365–6
    postpartum haemorrhage (PPH) 362–4
    shoulder dystocia 360, 369–74
    spontaneous vaginal delivery 359
    vaginal breech delivery 364
  specific task trainers 353–62
    NOELLE and PROMPT birthing trainers 352–4
  teamwork training and evaluation 366
Orpheus perfusion simulation system 396–400
oxygen administration 468

paediatric simulation-based training 337–50
  building a successful programme **340**
  Center for Advanced Pediatric and Perinatal
    Education (CAPE) 339
  extrapolation of adult physiology to paediatric
    patients 344
  future directions 346–8
  identifying the learners 340
  instructors, three groups 345
  sample scenario template **343**
  skills for successful intubation of newborn **341**
  steps in building **340**
part-task training, nursing simulation 263–4

Pathfinder algorithm 452
patient simulators *see* mannequin patient simulators
patient-specific simulation 437
performance assessment *see* assessment and appraisal;,
  see also anaesthesia performance assessment
performance assessment programmes (PAPs) 508–9
pericardiocentesis simulators 413
pigs trotter, model for tendon repair **177**
planning, clinical settings 129–30
portable simulators 25–34
postdoctoral medical training programmes, USA 380
postgraduate education, emergency medicine 379
pressure breathing (IPPB) 470
problem-based learning (PBL) for simulation in
    healthcare 213–25
  background 214–15
  definition 215
  facilitation 223–4
  potential problems 215–16
  scenario development 222–3
  scenario structure examples 216–22
  value 215–16

radio headsets 85
rapid response systems 325–30
  team roles, responsibilities and position 324, **326**
  see also medical emergency teams (METs)
recognizing risks and improving patient safety
    (R2IPS) 210
reflection 121–3
  reflection-on-action 123
  see also debriefing
reliability 234, **235**
  and measurement error 231–2
  sources of evidence **232**
  and validity, test design 504
  see also validity
renal simulation, nephron project 459–60
research using simulation 227–38
  debriefing 168
  ethics, deception and conflicts of interest 235–6
  experimental design 233–4
  flaws in **229**
  information and consent 236
  measurement 229–32
  methods 228–9
  qualitative/quantitative 229–34, **235**
  reliability 234, **235**
    and measurement error 231–2
    sources of evidence **232**
  statistical risk 234
  subject–experimenter effects **233**
  theoretical benefits in healthcare **228**
  validity
    evidence sources **231**
    measurement 230–1
    and reliability 234, **235**
    types **230**
  worthwhile and feasible research 228
respiratory assessment 466–9
  blood gas interpretation 467
  breath sounds 466–7
  percussion of the chest wall 467–8

respiratory therapy 465–76
  bi-level positive airway pressure (BiPAP) 470
  chest drain insertion and management 471–2
  continuous positive airway pressure (CPAP) 470,
    472–3
  CPAP in ICU setting 473
  decision making and team work issues 472
  fibreoptic bronchoscopy (FOB) 472
  future trends 474
  high fidelity simulators 470–1
  intermittent positive
  manual ventilation 470
  oxygen administration 468
  see also airway management; airway training devices
RespiTrainer 471
resuscitation, nursing simulation 266–7

scenarios/scenario design 139–53
  anaesthesia performance assessment 513–14
  cardiac arrest 150–3
  cardiopulmonary bypass training 400–4
  clinical scenario, reflection 121
  cognitive task analysis 141–2
  communication exercises, team building training
    209
  crew resource management 142
  development and programming 16–18
  drugs 84
  evaluation and modification 143
  examples
    Cardiac Arrest and Good Medical
      Practice 150–3
    Foundation Year 2 doctors 143–8
  medical emergency teams (METs) **327**
  mobile scenarios 30–2
  obstetrics 355–6
  one-day simulation course 143–8
  paediatric scenario template **343**
  problem-based learning (PBL)
    induction of labour 216–22
    for simulation in healthcare 222–3
  specification and development of scenario
    event sets 142–3
  stages 142–3
  teaching and learning 118–19
  technical training objectives 142
  template, paediatric simulation-based
    training **343**
  theory 140–1
scoring, standardized patients (SPs) as models 191–2
scripts, teaching 131
sedation training for non-anaesthesiologists 519–24
  airway emergency 523–4
  credentialing guidelines 521
  equipment failure 523
  hemodynamic events 523
  implementation of simulation 521–3
  Laerdal SimMan 522
  nursing 266
  patient evaluation 523
  sedation levels **520**
  trends 524
  unique elements of simulation 521

simulation
  definition and scope 421–2
  enhancing safety and predictability 478
  fidelity 444
  in healthcare, defined 478
  high-stakes performance assessment 501–18
  need for simulations 479
  see also cognitive simulation
simulation centre design *see* skills training facility
simulation gaming movement 249–51
Simulation in Healthcare 530
simulators
  evaluation and validation 444–5
  high fidelity systems 444
  hybrid 442–3
  physical models 441
  virtual reality computing 441–2
situated learning theory, models of
    nursing 255, 260–1
situational awareness 283, 322
skills taxonomy 308
skills training, successful intubation of
    newborn **341**
skills training facility 3–24
  building form 3
    breakout spaces 4, 8
    entrances and exits 5
    external training areas 8
    space planning 4
    technical traffic flow 4–5
  data organization 16
  emergencies, real resuscitation equipment 23–4
  operations and administration 11–24
    back-to-back courses 20
    blocked time concept 19
    calendar and booking system 18–20
    course-specific checklists 12–13
    electronic or web-based scheduling 19–20
    instructor and staff training 20
    performance on the simulation day 13
    post-simulation administration 14–15
    preparations before simulation 12
    reservation process 19
    running multiple rooms simultaneously 20–1
    scheduling: schedule down time 20
    simulator maintenance 15
  publicity 21
  room usage 5
    communication/human factor analysis 7
    control room 6
    debriefing/discussion rooms 6–7
    e-learning pods or carrels 7
    lecture theatre 7
    mock operating theatre 5–6
  scenario development and programming 16–18
  simulation centre website 22–3
  technical aspects 8–9
    acoustics and sound transmission 9
    air handling systems 8
    audiovisual system 9
    broadband connections 9
    lighting 8
    security system 8–9

skin and muscle receptors 46
SNAPPS, acronym 132–3
Society in Europe for Simulation Applied to
    Medicine (SESAM) 525–8
Society for Simulation in Healthcare (SSH) 529–32
Sophus anaesthesia simulator 525
SPRAT (Sheffield Peer Review Assessment Tool)
    factors 200–1
standardized patients (SPs) as models 181–97
  case development 186
  debriefing candidate performance 187–8
  evaluation data/ quality assessment 189–91
  history of assessment 182–3
  mannequin-based simulation 191–2
  performance fidelity 188
  performance measurement 186–7
  programme set-up 183–5
  recruiting and training 187–8
  reliability of evaluation quality 190–1
  scoring 191–2
  simulation centres 183–5
  simulation connectivity systems 185
  simulation content development 185–7
  simulation structure 182
  task specificity 192
  training/ assessment area 184–5
  validation work 192
  validity of evaluation quality 189–90
  virtual patients (VPs) 253
strategic management simulations (SMS) 477
  healthcare applications 485–6
  measurement outputs 483–4
  profile chart 486
  relevance to healthcare and HROs 482–4
  time–event matrix **484**, 485
subject matter experts (SMEs) 454
surgeon's performance *see* Non-Technical Skills for
    Surgeons (NOTSS)
surgery, behaviour rating systems 313
surgical simulation 435–48
  clinician–patient communication 438
  context/climate of learning 439–40
  educational theory 38
  high fidelity systems 444
  hybrid simulators 442–4
  procedure or operation 437
  professional setting 437
  simulator evaluation and validation 444–5
  simulator technology 440–6
  summary of existing commercial systems **443–4**
  technical skills 438–9
  tutor support and feedback 439
  zone of proximal development (ZPD) 439
Sydney Medical Simulation Centre (SMSC),
    performance assessment programme 508

teaching and learning 99–133
  clinical scenarios 118–19
  competency based assessment 103
  confidentiality 120
  development 115–24
  interaction with environment 116
  learners/learning cycle 127–8, **129**

teaching and learning (*cont.*)
  adult learning **127**, 171–2, **173**
  appropriate learning environment 119–20
  facilitating learning 106–8
  needs of learner 117
  objectives 117–18
  outcomes and individual learner 120–1
  planning for learning 99–104
    documenting the planning 103–4
    learning objectives 100
    managing session and students 104–5
    sample teaching plan 112–14
    tasks (summative/formative tasks 100–1
  quality of course and teaching 108–10
  reflection 121–2
    reflection-on-action 123
  teaching skills 127–33
    dialogue and closure 131–3
    flexibility 136
    providing appropriate feedback 107–8, 122–3
    see also clinical skills teaching
  see also problem-based learning (PBL) for
    simulation in healthcare
team, defined 200
team building 199–211
  defined 200
team building training
  background and theories 199–205
  communication exercises 206–9
    interactive team games 207–9
    life raft scenario 209
    mnemonic exercises 208–9
    personal goal setting exercise 207–8
  examples from UK 210–11
  importance and types of teams 201–2
  integrated procedural performance instrument
    (IPPI) 210–11
  managerial skills 202–3, **202**
  outcome measurement 200–1
  personality types and team dynamics, DISC
    acronym 204–5, **205**
  planning and preparation 206, **206**
  recognizing risks and improving patient safety
    (R2IPS) 210
  requirements 203–4
  SBAR for communication 331
  simulator technologies 205
  working with colleagues
    SPRAT (Sheffield Peer Review Assessment Tool)
      factors 201
    UK guidance **200**
teams, *see also* medical emergency teams (METs)
test design
  conditions 507
  psychometrics 504
  rating methods 507
  validity and reliability 504

thoracic trauma, chest tube placement 411–12
time–event matrix, SMS **484**, 485
TOUCH (Telehealth Outreach for Unified Community
  Health) 450–1
tracheostomy tube management 70–1, 469–70
TraumaMan 408–9, 413, 415
  military medical training 408–9, 413

UCLA simulation curriculum 424–9
ultrasound
  Focused Assessment with Sonography for Trauma
    (FAST) 414
  simulator devices, emergency medicine 382
  UltraSim 414
USA
  emergency medicine postgraduate procedural
    requirements 380
  nursing education 242, **243**
    preparation and licensure **243**
  nursing shortage 243–4
  postdoctoral medical training programmes 380

validity
  evidence sources **231**
  measurement 230–1
  and reliability 234, **235**
    test design 504
  sources of evidence **231**
  types **230**, 455
  validation techniques **235**
vehicles, for simulator transport 29–30
vestibular and visual sensory systems 46–7
VIRGIL chest tube simulator 412
virtual patients (VPs) 253
virtual reality computing 441–2, 443
virtual reality medical simulations 449–64
  airway simulators 76
  artificial intelligence (AI) 456
  assessing conceptual understanding 453
  Flatland VR environment 455–6
  future VR simulation developments 460–1
  knowledge representation concepts 451–2
  methods, knowledge-based design
    approach 453–5
  Pathfinder algorithm 452
  preliminary studies of VR simulations 458–9
  TOUCH (Telehealth Outreach for Unified
    Community Health) 450–1, 458
  user competency 457–8
  validation 454–6
Virtual-IV trainer 17–18
visual sensing system 45–6
VUCAD (volatility, uncertainty, complexity,
  ambiguity, and delayed feedback 477

zone of proximal development (ZPD) 439